Nanoparticles in Ocular Drug Delivery Systems

Nanoparticles in Ocular Drug Delivery Systems

Editors

Hugo Almeida
Ana Catarina Silva

MDPI • Basel • Beijing • Wuhan • Barcelona • Belgrade • Manchester • Tokyo • Cluj • Tianjin

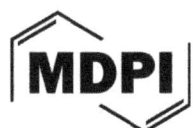

Editors
Hugo Almeida
Pharmaceutical Technology
Laboratory
University of Porto
Porto
Portugal

Ana Catarina Silva
Faculdade de Ciências da Saúde
University Fernando Pessoa
Porto
Portugal

Editorial Office
MDPI
St. Alban-Anlage 66
4052 Basel, Switzerland

This is a reprint of articles from the Special Issue published online in the open access journal *Pharmaceutics* (ISSN 1999-4923) (available at: www.mdpi.com/journal/pharmaceutics/special_issues/ocular_dds).

For citation purposes, cite each article independently as indicated on the article page online and as indicated below:

LastName, A.A.; LastName, B.B.; LastName, C.C. Article Title. *Journal Name* **Year**, *Volume Number*, Page Range.

ISBN 978-3-0365-8003-6 (Hbk)
ISBN 978-3-0365-8002-9 (PDF)

© 2023 by the authors. Articles in this book are Open Access and distributed under the Creative Commons Attribution (CC BY) license, which allows users to download, copy and build upon published articles, as long as the author and publisher are properly credited, which ensures maximum dissemination and a wider impact of our publications.

The book as a whole is distributed by MDPI under the terms and conditions of the Creative Commons license CC BY-NC-ND.

Contents

About the Editors vii

Hugo Almeida and Ana Catarina Silva
Nanoparticles in Ocular Drug Delivery Systems
Reprinted from: *Pharmaceutics* **2023**, *15*, 1675, doi:10.3390/pharmaceutics15061675 1

María Lina Formica, Hamoudi Ghassan Awde Alfonso, Alejandro Javier Paredes, María Elisa Melian, Nahuel Matías Camacho and Ricardo Faccio et al.
Development of Triamcinolone Acetonide Nanocrystals for Ocular Administration
Reprinted from: *Pharmaceutics* **2023**, *15*, 683, doi:10.3390/pharmaceutics15020683 3

Pradeep Singh Rawat, Punna Rao Ravi, Shahid Iqbal Mir, Mohammed Shareef Khan, Himanshu Kathuria and Prasanna Katnapally et al.
Design, Characterization and Pharmacokinetic–Pharmacodynamic Evaluation of Poloxamer and Kappa-Carrageenan-Based Dual-Responsive In Situ Gel of Nebivolol for Treatment of Open-Angle Glaucoma
Reprinted from: *Pharmaceutics* **2023**, *15*, 405, doi:10.3390/pharmaceutics15020405 25

Samir Senapati, Ahmed Adel Ali Youssef, Corinne Sweeney, Chuntian Cai, Narendar Dudhipala and Soumyajit Majumdar
Cannabidiol Loaded Topical Ophthalmic Nanoemulsion Lowers Intraocular Pressure in Normotensive Dutch-Belted Rabbits
Reprinted from: *Pharmaceutics* **2022**, *14*, 2585, doi:10.3390/pharmaceutics14122585 47

Diana Aziz, Sally A. Mohamed, Saadia Tayel and Amal Makhlouf
Enhanced Ocular Anti-Aspergillus Activity of Tolnaftate Employing Novel Cosolvent-Modified Spanlastics: Formulation, Statistical Optimization, Kill Kinetics, Ex Vivo Trans-Corneal Permeation, In Vivo Histopathological and Susceptibility Study
Reprinted from: *Pharmaceutics* **2022**, *14*, 1746, doi:10.3390/pharmaceutics14081746 61

Kaat De Clerck, Geraldine Accou, Félix Sauvage, Kevin Braeckmans, Stefaan C. De Smedt and Katrien Remaut et al.
Photodisruption of the Inner Limiting Membrane: Exploring ICG Loaded Nanoparticles as Photosensitizers
Reprinted from: *Pharmaceutics* **2022**, *14*, 1716, doi:10.3390/pharmaceutics14081716 83

Onyinye Uwaezuoke, Lisa C. Du Toit, Pradeep Kumar, Naseer Ally and Yahya E. Choonara
Linoleic Acid-Based Transferosomes for Topical Ocular Delivery of Cyclosporine A
Reprinted from: *Pharmaceutics* **2022**, *14*, 1695, doi:10.3390/pharmaceutics14081695 101

Telma A. Jacinto, Breno Oliveira, Sónia P. Miguel, Maximiano P. Ribeiro and Paula Coutinho
Ciprofloxacin-Loaded Zein/Hyaluronic Acid Nanoparticles for Ocular Mucosa Delivery
Reprinted from: *Pharmaceutics* **2022**, *14*, 1557, doi:10.3390/pharmaceutics14081557 119

Hay Marn Hnin, Einar Stefánsson, Thorsteinn Loftsson, Rathapon Asasutjarit, Dusadee Charnvanich and Phatsawee Jansook
Physicochemical and Stability Evaluation of Topical Niosomal Encapsulating Fosinopril/γ-Cyclodextrin Complex for Ocular Delivery
Reprinted from: *Pharmaceutics* **2022**, *14*, 1147, doi:10.3390/pharmaceutics14061147 135

Hassan A. Albarqi, Anuj Garg, Mohammad Zaki Ahmad, Abdulsalam A. Alqahtani, Ismail A. Walbi and Javed Ahmad
Recent Progress in Chitosan-Based Nanomedicine for Its Ocular Application in Glaucoma
Reprinted from: *Pharmaceutics* **2023**, *15*, 681, doi:10.3390/pharmaceutics15020681 . . . . **151**

Divyesh H. Shastri, Ana Catarina Silva and Hugo Almeida
Ocular Delivery of Therapeutic Proteins: A Review
Reprinted from: *Pharmaceutics* **2023**, *15*, 205, doi:10.3390/pharmaceutics15010205 . . . . **169**

Amin Orash Mahmoud Salehi, Saeed Heidari-Keshel, Seyed Ali Poursamar, Ali Zarrabi, Farshid Sefat and Narsimha Mamidi et al.
Bioprinted Membranes for Corneal Tissue Engineering: A Review
Reprinted from: *Pharmaceutics* **2022**, *14*, 2797, doi:10.3390/pharmaceutics14122797 . . . . **209**

Elide Zingale, Alessia Romeo, Salvatore Rizzo, Cinzia Cimino, Angela Bonaccorso and Claudia Carbone et al.
Fluorescent Nanosystems for Drug Tracking and Theranostics: Recent Applications in the Ocular Field
Reprinted from: *Pharmaceutics* **2022**, *14*, 955, doi:10.3390/pharmaceutics14050955 . . . . **227**

About the Editors

Hugo Almeida

Hugo Almeida received his degree in Pharmaceutical Sciences from the Faculty of Pharmacy, University of Coimbra (Portugal) in 2006, and a master's degree in Quality Control (branch: Drug Substances and Medicinal Plants) from Faculty of Pharmacy, University of Porto (Portugal) in 2009. In 2016, he received his PhD degree in Pharmaceutical Sciences (branch: Pharmaceutical Technology) from the Faculty of Pharmacy, University of Porto (Portugal).

He has more than 15 years of experience in the medical device industry, as a technical director and head of quality control department, and 1 year in pharmaceutical industry. He has expertise in the execution and supervision of physicochemical and microbiology laboratory test work and in the supervision of the performance of medical devices, ensuring the compliance of the quality and safety standards. He is production manager in a medical device and cosmetic company.

He is researcher at UCIBIO, REQUIMTE, MEDTECH, Department of Drug Sciences, Laboratory of Pharmaceutical Technology, Faculty of Pharmacy, University of Porto, Portugal. He develops his research in the application of stimuli-responsive polymers in controlled and self-regulated drug delivery systems and also on developing lipid-based nanosystems to improve drug delivery. He is author of several scientific articles, editor of one book, author of one book chapter, invited editor of two special issues in the journals *Pharmaceutics* and *Current Pharmaceutical Design*, and invited editor of one topic in MDPI.

Ana Catarina Silva

Associate Professor of Pharmaceutical Technology and Pharmaceutical Biotechnology and Researcher at FP-I3ID, FP-BHS, Faculty of Health Sciences, University Fernando Pessoa, Porto, Portugal.

Senior Researcher at UCIBIO, REQUIMTE, MEDTECH, Laboratory of Pharmaceutical Technology, Faculty of Pharmacy, University of Porto, Portugal.

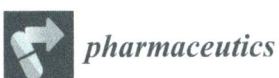

Editorial

Nanoparticles in Ocular Drug Delivery Systems

Hugo Almeida [1,2,3,*] and Ana Catarina Silva [1,2,4,*]

1. UCIBIO (Research Unit on Applied Molecular Biosciences), REQUIMTE (Rede de Química e Tecnologia), MEDTECH (Medicines and Healthcare Products), Laboratory of Pharmaceutical Technology, Department of Drug Sciences, Faculty of Pharmacy, University of Porto, 4050-313 Porto, Portugal
2. Associate Laboratory i4HB-Institute for Health and Bioeconomy, Faculty of Pharmacy, University of Porto, 4050-313 Porto, Portugal
3. Mesosystem Investigação & Investimentos by Spinpark, Barco, 4805-017 Guimarães, Portugal
4. FP-BHS (Biomedical and Health Sciences Research Unit), FP-I3ID (Instituto de Investigação, Inovação e Desenvolvimento), Faculty of Health Sciences, University Fernando Pessoa, 4249-004 Porto, Portugal
* Correspondence: hperas5@hotmail.com (H.A.); anacatsil@gmail.com (A.C.S.)

Conventional ophthalmic formulations lack a prolonged drug release effect and mucoadhesive properties, decreasing their residence time in the precorneal area and, therefore, in drug penetration across ocular tissues, presenting low bioavailability with a consequent reduction in therapeutic efficacy. These limitations are related to the physiological mechanisms of the eye. To increase the residence time in formulations on the surface of ocular tissues and increase their ability to penetrate these tissues, different strategies can be used, namely, the use of viscosifying agents, mucoadhesive polymers, stimuli-responsive polymers, microparticles, and colloidal carriers (e.g., micelles, liposomes, nanosuspensions, nanoemulsions, and polymeric and lipid nanoparticles).

We are delighted to present the latest research and review works reporting on the use of nanoparticles and other nanosystems in ophthalmic formulations to increase the bioavailability of drugs, improving their therapeutic efficacy. The articles selected for this Special Issue are the following:

1. "Development of Triamcinolone Acetonide Nanocrystals for Ocular Administration" [1].
2. "Design, Characterization and Pharmacokinetic–Pharmacodynamic Evaluation of Poloxamer and Kappa-Carrageenan-Based Dual-Responsive In Situ Gel of Nebivolol for Treatment of Open-Angle Glaucoma" [2].
3. "Cannabidiol Loaded Topical Ophthalmic Nanoemulsion Lowers Intraocular Pressure in Normotensive Dutch-Belted Rabbits" [3].
4. "Enhanced Ocular Anti-Aspergillus Activity of Tolnaftate Employing Novel Cosolvent-Modified Spanlastics: Formulation, Statistical Optimization, Kill Kinetics, Ex Vivo Trans-Corneal Permeation, In Vivo Histopathological and Susceptibility Study" [4].
5. "Photodisruption of the Inner Limiting Membrane: Exploring ICG Loaded Nanoparticles as Photosensitizers" [5].
6. "Linoleic Acid-Based Transferosomes for Topical Ocular Delivery of Cyclosporine A" [6].
7. "Ciprofloxacin-Loaded Zein/Hyaluronic Acid Nanoparticles for Ocular Mucosa Delivery" [7].
8. "Physicochemical and Stability Evaluation of Topical Niosomal Encapsulating Fosinopril/γ-Cyclodextrin Complex for Ocular Delivery" [8].
9. "Recent Progress in Chitosan-Based Nanomedicine for Its Ocular Application in Glaucoma" [9].
10. "Ocular Delivery of Therapeutic Proteins: A Review" [10].
11. "Bioprinted Membranes for Corneal Tissue Engineering: A Review" [11].

Citation: Almeida, H.; Silva, A.C. Nanoparticles in Ocular Drug Delivery Systems. *Pharmaceutics* 2023, 15, 1675. https://doi.org/10.3390/pharmaceutics15061675

Received: 2 June 2023
Accepted: 6 June 2023
Published: 8 June 2023

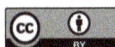

Copyright: © 2023 by the authors. Licensee MDPI, Basel, Switzerland. This article is an open access article distributed under the terms and conditions of the Creative Commons Attribution (CC BY) license (https://creativecommons.org/licenses/by/4.0/).

12. "Fluorescent Nanosystems for Drug Tracking and Theranostics: Recent Applications in the Ocular Field" [12].

The selected articles highlight the use of nanotechnology in ophthalmic formulations to encapsulate molecules with different therapeutic applications, including antibiotics, anti-inflammatory drugs, natural compounds, and proteins. The use of nanosystems in different approaches, such as theranostics and nanobubbles, is also presented, showing their potential for ocular application.

We would like to take this opportunity to thank all the authors and reviewers for their incredible work. Without their contribution, it would not be possible to publish this Special Issue with such high scientific quality. We hope that the readers of this Special Issue enjoy these articles, and that they will serve as a starting point for further research and/or review articles, thus contributing to scientific discovery and progress in this field.

Funding: The Applied Molecular Biosciences Unit—UCIBIO—which is financed by national funds from Fundação para a Ciência e a Tecnologia—FCT—(UIDP/04378/2020 and UIDB/04378/2020), supported this work.

Conflicts of Interest: The authors declare no conflict of interest.

References

1. Formica, M.L.; Awde Alfonso, H.G.; Paredes, A.J.; Melian, M.E.; Camacho, N.M.; Faccio, R.; Tártara, L.I.; Palma, S.D. Development of Triamcinolone Acetonide Nanocrystals for Ocular Administration. *Pharmaceutics* **2023**, *15*, 683. [CrossRef] [PubMed]
2. Rawat, P.S.; Ravi, P.R.; Mir, S.I.; Khan, M.S.; Kathuria, H.; Katnapally, P.; Bhatnagar, U. Design, Characterization and Pharmacokinetic–Pharmacodynamic Evaluation of Poloxamer and Kappa-Carrageenan-Based Dual-Responsive In Situ Gel of Nebivolol for Treatment of Open-Angle Glaucoma. *Pharmaceutics* **2023**, *15*, 405. [CrossRef] [PubMed]
3. Senapati, S.; Youssef, A.A.A.; Sweeney, C.; Cai, C.; Dudhipala, N.; Majumdar, S. Cannabidiol Loaded Topical Ophthalmic Nanoemulsion Lowers Intraocular Pressure in Normotensive Dutch-Belted Rabbits. *Pharmaceutics* **2022**, *14*, 2585. [CrossRef] [PubMed]
4. Aziz, D.; Mohamed, S.A.; Tayel, S.; Makhlouf, A. Enhanced Ocular Anti-Aspergillus Activity of Tolnaftate Employing Novel Cosolvent-Modified Spanlastics: Formulation, Statistical Optimization, Kill Kinetics, Ex Vivo Trans-Corneal Permeation, In Vivo Histopathological and Susceptibility Study. *Pharmaceutics* **2022**, *14*, 1746. [CrossRef] [PubMed]
5. De Clerck, K.; Accou, G.; Sauvage, F.; Braeckmans, K.; De Smedt, S.C.; Remaut, K.; Peynshaert, K. Photodisruption of the Inner Limiting Membrane: Exploring ICG Loaded Nanoparticles as Photosensitizers. *Pharmaceutics* **2022**, *14*, 1716. [CrossRef] [PubMed]
6. Uwaezuoke, O.; Du Toit, L.C.; Kumar, P.; Ally, N.; Choonara, Y.E. Linoleic Acid-Based Transferosomes for Topical Ocular Delivery of Cyclosporine A. *Pharmaceutics* **2022**, *14*, 1695. [CrossRef] [PubMed]
7. Jacinto, T.A.; Oliveira, B.; Miguel, S.P.; Ribeiro, M.P.; Coutinho, P. Ciprofloxacin-Loaded Zein/Hyaluronic Acid Nanoparticles for Ocular Mucosa Delivery. *Pharmaceutics* **2022**, *14*, 1557. [CrossRef] [PubMed]
8. Hnin, H.M.; Stefánsson, E.; Loftsson, T.; Asasutjarit, R.; Charnvanich, D.; Jansook, P. Physicochemical and Stability Evaluation of Topical Niosomal Encapsulating Fosinopril/γ-Cyclodextrin Complex for Ocular Delivery. *Pharmaceutics* **2022**, *14*, 1147. [CrossRef] [PubMed]
9. Albarqi, H.A.; Garg, A.; Ahmad, M.Z.; Alqahtani, A.A.; Walbi, I.A.; Ahmad, J. Recent Progress in Chitosan-Based Nanomedicine for Its Ocular Application in Glaucoma. *Pharmaceutics* **2023**, *15*, 681. [CrossRef] [PubMed]
10. Shastri, D.H.; Silva, A.C.; Almeida, H. Ocular Delivery of Therapeutic Proteins: A Review. *Pharmaceutics* **2023**, *15*, 205. [CrossRef] [PubMed]
11. Orash Mahmoud Salehi, A.; Heidari-Keshel, S.; Poursamar, S.A.; Zarrabi, A.; Sefat, F.; Mamidi, N.; Behrouz, M.J.; Rafienia, M. Bioprinted Membranes for Corneal Tissue Engineering: A Review. *Pharmaceutics* **2022**, *14*, 2797. [CrossRef] [PubMed]
12. Zingale, E.; Romeo, A.; Rizzo, S.; Cimino, C.; Bonaccorso, A.; Carbone, C.; Musumeci, T.; Pignatello, R. Fluorescent Nanosystems for Drug Tracking and Theranostics: Recent Applications in the Ocular Field. *Pharmaceutics* **2022**, *14*, 955. [CrossRef] [PubMed]

Disclaimer/Publisher's Note: The statements, opinions and data contained in all publications are solely those of the individual author(s) and contributor(s) and not of MDPI and/or the editor(s). MDPI and/or the editor(s) disclaim responsibility for any injury to people or property resulting from any ideas, methods, instructions or products referred to in the content.

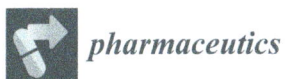

Article

Development of Triamcinolone Acetonide Nanocrystals for Ocular Administration

María Lina Formica [1], Hamoudi Ghassan Awde Alfonso [1], Alejandro Javier Paredes [2], María Elisa Melian [3], Nahuel Matías Camacho [1], Ricardo Faccio [4], Luis Ignacio Tártara [1] and Santiago Daniel Palma [1,*]

[1] Unidad de Investigación y Desarrollo en Tecnología Farmacéutica (UNITEFA), CONICET and Departamento de Ciencias Farmacéuticas, Facultad de Ciencias Químicas, Universidad Nacional de Córdoba, Ciudad Universitaria, Córdoba 5000, Argentina
[2] School of Pharmacy, Queen's University Belfast, 97 Lisburn Road, Belfast BT9 7BL, UK
[3] Área de Farmacología, Departamento de Ciencias Farmacéuticas—CIENFAR, Facultad de Química, Universidad de la República (Udelar), Av. General Flores 2124, Montevideo 11800, Uruguay
[4] Área Física, Departamento de Experimentación y Teoría de la Estructura de la Materia y sus Aplicaciones—DETEMA, Facultad de Química, Universidad de la República (Udelar), Av. General Flores 2124, Montevideo 11800, Uruguay
* Correspondence: sdpalma@unc.edu.ar

Abstract: Triamcinolone acetonide (TA) is a powerful anti-inflammatory drug used in the treatment of inflammatory ocular disorders; however, its poor aqueous solubility and ocular anatomical barriers hinder optimal treatment. The aim of this work was to obtain triamcinolone acetonide nanocrystals (TA-NC) to improve ocular corticosteroid therapy. Self-dispersible TA-NC were prepared by the bead milling technique followed by spray-drying, exhaustively characterized and then evaluated in vivo in an ocular model of endotoxin-induced uveitis (EIU). Self-dispersible TA-NC presented an average particle size of 257 ± 30 nm, a narrow size distribution and a zeta potential of −25 ± 3 mV, which remained unchanged for 120 days under storage conditions at 25 °C. In addition, SEM studies of the TA-NC showed uniform and spherical morphology, and FTIR and XRDP analyses indicated no apparent chemical and crystallinity changes. The subconjunctival administration of TA-NC in albino male white rabbits showed no clinical signs of ocular damage. In vivo studies proved that treatment with self-dispersible TA-NC alleviated the inflammatory response in the anterior chamber and iris in EUI rabbit eyes. Dispersible TA-NC are a promising approach to obtaining a novel nanometric TA formulation for ocular disorders.

Keywords: triamcinolone acetonide; nanocrystals; ocular inflammation; corticosteroids; media milling

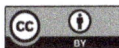

1. Introduction

Corticosteroids are widely used drugs in the treatment of several inflammatory ocular disorders, such as diabetic macular edema (DME), retinal vein occlusion, age-related macular degeneration (AMD) and uveitis [1]. Corticosteroids act by inhibiting inflammation primarily through interaction with glucocorticoid receptors. Although these drugs are considered effective, the duration of their therapeutic effect is conditioned by their pharmaceutical dosage form, the route of administration and their potential side effects. Topical ocular administration is the route of choice for patients; however, less than 5% of the instilled drug is usually absorbed in the ocular tissue, and a minimal amount usually reaches the posterior segment, limiting the treatment of posterior segment pathologies. On the other hand, systemic administration of corticosteroids requires high doses to achieve therapeutic levels of the drug in the eye, which can be accompanied by severe systemic side effects [2].

In this way, the intravitreal administration of corticosteroids as a depot of drug suspensions is usually used to allow effective concentrations in the back of the eye. However, in chronic pathologies, frequent injections are required, which are associated with risks of retinal detachment, endophthalmitis and intravitreal haemorrhage. In addition, chronic treatment with corticosteroids may lead to increased intraocular pressure and predispose to the development of cataracts. A biodegradable intravitreal implant loaded with a corticosteroid has been developed to overcome these drawbacks and allow sustained drug release. Nevertheless, it presented some limitations associated with its administration technique and high cost [3].

Among other corticosteroid therapies, ocular injections of triamcinolone acetonide (TA) are used as an effective and low-cost treatment for different ocular diseases [4,5]. Topical administration of TA to the inner part of the eye is problematic due to ocular barriers and drug properties such as low solubility in body fluids and limited permeability [6]. However, intravitreal or periocular administration of TA increases its delivery to the vitreous cavity, providing prolonged drug action related to a depot effect [7,8]. Thus, the available FDA-approved formulations of TA are applied intravitreally, such as Triescence™-Alcon Research, Ltd. and Trivaris™-Allergan, Inc. Mainly in developing countries, other formulations based on the intravenous suspension of TA are still administered by ocular routes as off-label drugs for the treatment of inflammatory processes of ocular diseases such as DME, uveitis and ADM, among others. Although injectable TA suspension is widely used by clinical ophthalmologists, it presents certain limitations associated with its particle size and preservatives in its formulation, which may hinder its administration and cause ocular discomfort [9]. Therefore, the development of new therapeutic strategies of TA for ocular application is interesting due to its proven efficacy, low cost and the broad range of pathologies for which it is prescribed. Moreover, the limitations related to its route of administration, inclusion in pharmaceutical forms and the need of an effective ocular delivery, must be resolved.

Ocular delivery systems based on nanotechnology have proven to be effective and safe for ocular drug delivery. Different nanotechnological strategies have been developed to obtain TA delivery systems for ocular applications such as liposomes [10], lipid nanocapsules [11], nanostructured lipid carriers [12], microneedles [13] and nanoemulsions [14]. Beyond the fact that these strategies have shown promising results for the ocular delivery of TA, the availability of simpler formulations that allow TA to be maintained as a low-cost therapeutic option is much needed. Hence, the formulation of nanocrystals (NCs) is an interesting strategy to obtain simple nanotechnology-based pharmaceutical formulations that can be prepared by simple and scalable processes.

Drug NCs are solid particles of a drug of nanometric size, typically between 200 and 500 nm [15], surrounded by a stabilizing layer. Usually, stabilizers are amphiphilic surfactants or polymers. NCs can be produced from nanosuspensions (NSs) of drugs, in which nanometric particles of the drug are dispersed in an aqueous medium that can be removed to obtain the NCs as solid nanoparticles.

NCs provide a higher drug dissolution rate, saturation solubility and adhesiveness [16,17]. These physicochemical features allow for improved bioavailability and therapeutic efficacy [18]. Our research group has been working on the development of NC formulations that demonstrate improved biopharmaceutical and pharmacokinetic behaviour of poorly water-soluble drugs via several administration routes [19,20]. Taking into account the above considerations on the need for the development of TA formulations and the advantages of NCs, this work aimed at the development of triamcinolone acetonide nanocrystals (TA-NC) as a novel therapeutic strategy for ocular TA administration. Thus, self-dispersible TA-NC were prepared by media milling followed by spray-drying. Exhaustive physicochemical analyses were performed to characterize the NC, and in vivo studies using albino rabbits were carried out to evaluate the therapeutic efficacy of TA-NC compared to an injectable suspension commonly used off-label for ocular application.

2. Materials and Methods

2.1. Materials and Reagents

The micronized form of triamcinolone acetonide (mTA) with a purity of 99.5% was purchased from Pura Quimica® (Córdoba, Argentina). Poloxamer 188 (P188) was provided by Rupamel S.R.L (Buenos Aires, Argentina), a sales agent of BASF. Ultrapure water was obtained from Water Purification System (HF-Super Easy Series, Heal Force, Shanghai, China). Escherichia coli lipopolysaccharide (LPS) was purchased from Sigma-Aldrich®. Zirmil® Yttrium-stabilized zirconium beads of 0.1 mm size (Saint-Gobain ZirPro, Köln, Germany) were used as a collision agent in the milling process. All other chemicals were extra pure grade and used without further purification.

2.2. Preparation of Triamcinolone Acetonide Nanosuspensions (TA-NS)

Triamcinolone acetonide nanosuspensions (TA-NS) were prepared by the wet bead milling (WBM) technique as described previously [19] using a NanoDisp® laboratory-scale mill (NanoDisp®, Córdoba, Argentina). Briefly, mixtures of mTA and P188 were homogenized in a porcelain mortar for 5 min and ultrapure water was added gradually up to 100 mL to form suspensions. The drug suspensions and 0.1 mm zirconia beads (25% v/v) were then placed in the milling chamber and processed at 1600 rpm for 120 min at a fixed temperature of 15 °C by the circulating cold water with a Thermo Haake® compact refrigerated circulator (Thermo Fisher Scientific, Waltham, MA, USA). The processed samples were evaluated in terms of average particle size (APS) and polydispersity index (PDI) every 30 min. An experimental mixture design was carried out to evaluate the influence of the component ratio of the TA-NS on the colloidal properties. Table 1 shows the ratio of mTA and P188 in the experimental mixture design formulations with a total solids content of 2% w/v (NS1-NS5). In turn, wet milling of a TA-NS with a total solid content of 6% w/v (NS6) composed of TA and P188 with a mass ratio of 1:1 was prepared by WBM with the same process parameters to evaluate the colloidal properties at a higher solids concentration.

2.3. Preparation of Dried Dispersible Triamcinolone Acetonide Nanocrystals

After the WBM process, the water in the TA-NS was immediately removed by spray-drying using a Büchi B-290 mini spray-drier (Büchi Labortechnik AG, Flawil, Switzerland) equipped with a dehumidifier module, using a two-fluid nozzle with a cap orifice diameter of 1.5 mm. The drying process was carried out with the following set conditions: inlet temperature of 45 °C, atomizing air flow rate of 600 L/h, pump speed of 2 mL/min and aspiration at 30 m³/h. In addition, slow magnetic stirring was kept constant during the drying process. The dried powders were weighed to determine the process yield and moisture and stored at 4–8 °C and room temperature (25 °C) under dry conditions.

2.4. Process Yield and Moisture Content

The process yield percentage (PY%) after water removal was calculated by the following equation:

$$PY\,(\%) = \frac{A}{B} \times 100 \quad (1)$$

where A is the solids weighed of TA-NC recovered after drying and B is theoretical initial solids (mTA and P188 weighed), considering the initial dry mixture of powders (drug and P188) as the theoretical 100%.

The moisture of the dried redispersible TA-NC was measured immediately after the removal of water using a halogen heating autoanalyzer (Ohaus M45®, Greifensee, Switzerland) at 90 °C.

2.5. Physical Mixture Preparation

A physical mixture (PM) between broken granules of P188 and mTA was prepared as a control for physicochemical characterization in a mass ratio of 1:1 of both components. Briefly, mTA and P188 were mixed and ground in a porcelain mortar.

2.6. Physicochemical Characterization of NC-TA

Samples from the milling process, TA-NS and dried TA-NC, were analyzed in terms of APS, PDI and zeta potential (ZP) using a Zetasizer NanoSerie DTS 1060 (Malvern Instruments S.A., Worcestershire, UK) at 25 °C in triplicate. Previously, a small fraction (spatula tip) of the dried TA-NC was dispersed in 5 mL of ultrapure water at room temperature. In addition, dried powders were stored at room temperature (~25 °C), while the redispersed TA-NC nanosuspensions were stored at both room temperature (~25 °C) and 4 °C for 30 days. The following parameters were evaluated at different time points: macroscopic aspects (aggregate formation and colour changes), APS, PDI and ZP.

2.7. Scanning Electron Microscopy (SEM)

Images of mTA, PM and dried TA-NC were taken with FE-SEM Σigma (ZEISS, Oberkochen, Germany). Powdered samples were deposited in an aluminum well and sprayed with chromium prior to morphological analysis. Magnification ranges between 500 and 10,000× were used.

2.8. Fourier Transform Infrared Spectroscopy (FTIR)

Powdered samples of mTA, PM, P188 and dried TA-NC were analyzed by FTIR using a Nicolet FTIR 5-SXC® Infrared Spectrophotometer. Four clean-up scans were performed with a threshold of 0.002; 40 background signal scans were made in a spectral range of 650–4000 cm^{-1} and with a deuterated triglycine sulfate detector.

2.9. Differential Scanning Calorimetry (DCS) and Thermogravimetry (TGA)

For DSC analysis, powdered samples of mTA, PM and TA-NC were deposited in aluminum pans and examined at a heating rate of 10 °C/min in the temperature range between 10 and 305 °C using a Discovery DSC 25P instrument (TA Instruments, New Castle, DE, USA) under a dynamic N$_2$ atmosphere (50 mL/min). The DSC cell was calibrated with indium (mp 156.6 °C; ΔHfus = 28.54 J/g). TGA analysis was performed under the same established conditions in the temperature range of 10–350 °C and a dynamic N$_2$ atmosphere (50 mL/min) at a heating rate of 10 °C/min using a TGA instrument (Discovery HP TGA, TA Instruments, New Castle, DE, USA).

2.10. X-ray Powder Diffraction (XRPD)

Powder samples of mTA, P188, PM and TA-NC were examined in terms of crystallinity using a Rigaku Miniflex X-ray powder diffractometer (Rigaku, Tokyo, Japan) with CuKα radiation (λ = 1.5418 Å) operating at 40 kV, 15 mA and utilizing a D/tex Ultra2 1D detector. Measurements were carried out in the scan mode over a 2θ range from 2° to 60° with a step size of 2θ = 0.01° and a speed of 5°/min.

2.11. Confocal Raman Microscopy

Confocal Raman microscopy was performed using WITec Alpha 300-RA confocal Raman microscopy equipment (WITec, Ulm, Germany). The excitation laser wavelength corresponded to λ = 532 nm and the nominal power was adjusted to 45 mW to avoid sample decomposition. Raman spectra of the pure components were obtained by averaging a set of 100 spectra with an integration time of 0.512 s for each spectrum. Two-dimensional confocal Raman microscopy images of the PM and TA-NC samples were collected at random locations of 150 × 150 μm areas with 50 × 50 point grids defining the bitmap image (2500 pixels). Individual Raman spectra were collected for each pixel in the selected areas with an integration time of 0.112 s. The spectrometer operating with 600 lines/mm grating allowed us to obtain spectra with a resolution of ~4 cm^{-1} in the range of 70–4000 cm^{-1}. All images were collected at an optical resolution limit of ~300 nm. True component analysis was used to map the spatial distribution of mTA and P188 in the PM or TA-NC samples using ProjectFive 5.1 Plus software (WITec, Ulm, Germany).

2.12. Drug Saturation Concentration

Excess amounts of mTA, PM and dried dispersible TA-NC were added to tubes containing 1 mL of simulated tear fluid (pH = 7.4) and they were placed in a water bath and shaken at 37 °C. Afterward, they were centrifuged (2990× g, 5 min and 37 °C) and the supernatants were collected and filtered (0.45 μm PVDF membrane). Then, drug concentration was determined by U-Vis. Different time intervals (0.25, 0.5, 0.75, 1, 2, 4, 6, 24, 48 and 72 h) were evaluated in triplicate.

2.13. Animals

Male albino white rabbits (weight, 2.0–2.5 kg) were treated according to the guidelines of the ARVO Statement for the Use of Animals in Ophthalmic and Vision Research. Every effort was made to reduce the number of animals used. All experimental procedures were approved by the Institutional Animal Care and Use Committee (CICUAL) of the Facultad de Medicina, Universidad Nacional de Córdoba (School of Medical Sciences, National University of Cordoba) (No. 44/2017).

2.14. Ocular Tolerance and Irritation Test

Ocular irritation tests were performed using male albino white rabbits (n = 10). Five rabbits were injected subconjunctivally with a dispersible TA-NC suspension (40 mg/mL, 50 μL) in the right eyes, while 50 μL of normal saline solution (NSS) was applied as a control in the left eyes. Fiver other rabbits were subconjunctivally injected with 50 μL of Fortcinolona® 40 suspension (40 mg/mL) in the right eyes, while the left eyes were observed as normal eyes. Clinical signs of damage in the anterior and posterior segments in response to treatments were evaluated using a slit lamp (Huvitz HIS5000, Anyang-si, Gyeonggi-do, Republic of Korea) and indirect ophthalmoscopy by an experienced ophthalmologist. Furthermore, the integrity of the corneal epithelium was checked by fluorescein staining.

2.15. Endotoxin-Induced Uveitis (EIU)

For the preclinical evaluation of TA-NC, we used an EIU rabbit model based on others reported in the literature [21,22], which was previously optimized and adapted in our laboratory [11]. All rabbits were topically anesthetized with 0.5% proparacaine hydrochloride ophthalmic solution and then injected with 60 μL of LPS (Sigma-Aldrich®, Darmstadt, Germany) 1 ng/μL via the intravitreal route using a 30G needle. After 1 h of model induction, the groups of animals were injected subconjunctivally (50 μL) with a single dose as follows: I) a dispersible TA-NC suspension (40 mg/mL) (n = 8), II) Fortcinolona® 40 (40 mg/mL) (n = 8) and III) NSS, the control group of the EUI model (n = 8). The clinical signs of the different groups were compared with IV) normal animals (n = 8) that were neither subjected to the EUI model nor given any treatment. Before determining the clinical signs of different groups, 0.5% topical tropicamide (Alcon Mydril™-Alcon Inc., Fort Worth, TX, USA) and topical anesthesia (0.5% proparacaine hydrochloride ophthalmic solution) were applied to all animals. Two masked experienced ophthalmologists examined the animals by slit-lamp and binocular indirect ophthalmoscopy (Heine small pupil) using a 20D lens (VOLK, Mentor, OH, USA) after 24, 48 and 72 h of the EIU model induction. A clinical inflammation scoring criterion was used to assess the severity of EIU, which took into account the anterior chamber flare, Tyndall effect by anterior chamber cells, fibrine deposits and iris vessel congestion. The anterior chamber flare and Tyndall effect of anterior chamber cells were valued between 0 and 8, while the other parameters were scored between 0 and 4 for each parameter.

Moreover, the aqueous humour fogging in the anterior chamber (flare) was quantified using ImageJ® software (64-bit, Java 8) from ocular photographs taken with Canon EOS Rebel T6 coupled to the slit lamp and calculated as the difference between the mean grey of the corneal light reflection and the anterior camera in each group of animals. An optically cut section of the eye was optically obtained from a very thin parallelepiped slice (3 × 3 mm) of the cornea with a slit lamp microscope (16×) using a 45-degree angle between the illumination and viewing paths. Then, the aqueous humour transparency percentage (AHT%) in the anterior chamber was calculated by the following equation, considering that this difference from mean grey in normal rabbits corresponds to 100%:

$$AHT\% = \frac{D}{E} \times 100 \qquad (2)$$

where D is the aqueous humour fogging of animals after induction of the EIU model and E is the aqueous humour fogging of normal rabbits (baseline response). In addition, the intraocular pressure (IOP) was measured with a calibrated digital ICARe® tonometer.

2.16. Statistical Analysis

For each parameter, ANOVA analysis was performed using Minitab®18 software or Prism-GraphPad, together with the Tukey pairwise comparison, and both ANOVA and Tukey's mean comparison analysis results were expressed as mean values ± standard deviation (SD). $p < 0.05$ was considered to be statistically significant.

3. Results

3.1. Preparation of TA-NS and Dispersible TA-NC

In order to obtain self-dispersible TA-NC, the preparation of TA-NS was first studied. TA-NS were successfully obtained by the WBM technique with the set processing conditions. In order to evaluate the influence of the component ratio of mTA and P188 on the colloidal properties and stability, TA-NS were prepared with different ratios of drug and stabilizer between 0.250 and 1.725%. The results of the experimental mixture design for the preparation of TA-NS (NS1-NS5) with a total solids content of 2% w/v are shown in Table 1.

Table 1. Composition and colloidal parameters of triamcinolone acetonide nanosuspensions (TA-NS) and self-dispersible triamcinolone acetonide nanocrystals (TA-NC) obtained by bead milling and spray-drying, respectively.

	Solid Components of TA-NS			TA-NS after Wet Milling			Dispersed TA-NC after Spray-Drying					
TA-NS	TA (%)	P188 (%)	TSC (%)	Size (nm)	PDI	ZP (mV)	TA-NC	Size (nm)	PDI	ZP (mV)	PY %	MC%
NS1	1.750	0.250	2	250.5 ± 3.2	0.14 ± 0.03	−30.6 ± 0.7	NC1	757.8 ± 13.7	0.52 ± 0.10	−21.0 ± 0.7	51.9	1.28
NS2	1.375	0.625	2	305.3 ± 7.8	0.15 ± 0.03	−25.1 ± 0.5	NC2	326.6 ± 4.2	0.260 ± 0.003	−24.8 ± 0.2	62.2	1.38
NS3	1	1	2	231.8 ± 2.9	0.12 ± 0.02	−25.9 ± 0.3	NC3	260.1 ± 1.6	0.18 ± 0.09	−26.1 ± 0.4	69.2	1.18
NS4	0.625	1.375	2	234.8 ± 2.0	0.12 ± 0.02	−27.2 ± 0.3	NC4	260.1 ± 2.5	0.15 ± 0.02	−25.2 ± 0.9	69.5	1.16
NS5	0.250	1.750	2	312.9 ± 8.3	0.21 ± 0.02	−32.8 ± 0.1	NC5	232.3 ± 1.2	0.14 ± 0.05	−29.9 ± 0.6	68.5	1.57
NS6	3	3	6	274.7 ± 45.8	0.15 ± 0.05	−28.3 ± 3.4	NC6	257.3 ± 30.5	0.15 ± 0.08	−24.9 ± 2.9	60.0	1.26

Abbreviations: APS: Average particle size; MC%: Moisture content percentage; PDI: Polydispersity index; PY%: Process yield percentage; TSC: Total solids content; ZP: Zeta potential.

Despite the composition of the formulation tested, a decreasing trend in particle size and PDI was observed with increasing milling times as shown in Figure 1A. After 2 h of milling at the set parameters, all TA-NS formulations exhibited a particle size below 350 nm and a PDI below 0.2. A decrease in APS was observed in TA-NS with a high proportion of P188 and a low proportion of TA. NS3 and NS4 presented the lowest particle sizes, around 232 nm. Regarding PDI, it seems to decrease with increasing stabilizer concentration up to 1.375% as in NS1 to NS4, while it is the highest in NS5. All PZ values were negative, between −30 and −25 mV, appearing to increase in terms of absolute values with high stabilizer concentration.

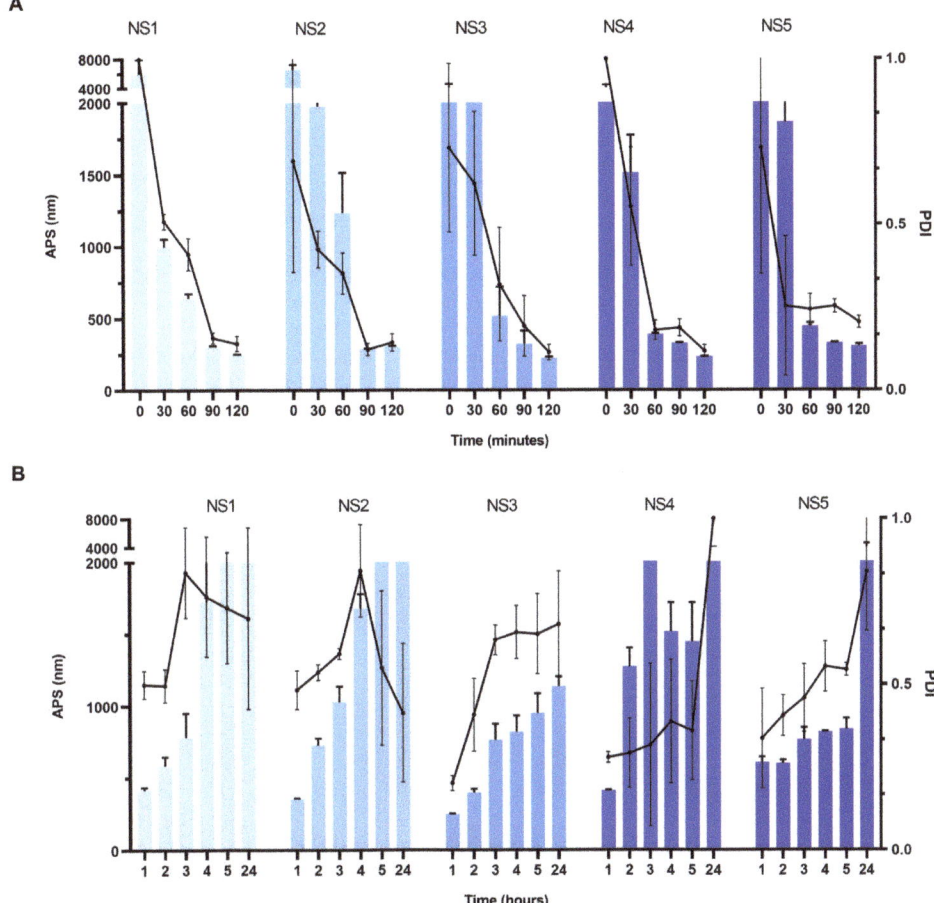

Figure 1. Average particle size (APS) and polydispersity index (PDI) of different drug nanosuspension from mixture design (**A**) during the wet milling process and (**B**) after the wet milling process at room temperature. Results are presented as means ± SD (n = 3) for all tested drug nanosuspensions.

Subsequently, the colloidal stability of different TA-NS under storage conditions at 25 °C was studied. As shown in Figure 1B, there is a progressive increase in the APS and PDI in all nanosuspensions, which doubled their value in the first 2 h and reached micrometric size after 24 h under this storage condition. Based on these results, water removal from TA-NS by the spray-drying process was carried out.

3.2. Dispersible TA-NC

Through the spray-drying process under the established parameters, different dried TA-NC (NC1, NC2, NC3, NC4 and NC5) were efficiently obtained from the respective TA-NS (NS1, NS2, NS3, NS4 and NS5). The spray-drying process yield of different TA-NS was higher than 50%, reaching values of 70% for TA-NC obtained from NS3, NS4 and NS5. Moreover, the moisture content of powder TA-NC was lower than 2%.

Table 1 shows the colloidal parameters of different dried TA-NC in terms of APS, PDI and ZP after dispersion in water. The dried TA-NC prepared with the TA-NS with a high proportion of P188 and a low proportion of TA showed lower APS and PDI and a higher negative ZP in terms of absolute value. Thus, the aqueous dispersed NC1 prepared from the TA-NS with only 0.250% of P188 showed an APS of 758 ± 14 nm and a high polydispersity (PDI = 0.52), presenting a large difference with the parameters of the starting nanosuspension (NS1). On the contrary, the NC5 prepared from the TA-NS with 1.725% of stabilizer exhibited an APS of 232 ± 1 nm and a narrow size distribution (PDI = 0.14), lower than that of the starting nanosuspension (NS5). Regarding the aqueous dispersed NC3 and NC4 prepared from TA-NS with stabilizer concentrations between 1.000 and 1.375% (NS3 and NS4, respectively), both showed an APS of 260 nm, slightly differing (around 30 nm) from the TA-NS (before the spray-drying process). Similarly, water-dispersed NC3 and NC4 exhibited a narrow size distribution, remaining with a PDI below 0.2 after the spray-drying process of NS3 and NS4.

Moreover, all dried TA-NC showed satisfactory aqueous self-dispersion, even those with a high proportion of drug and a low proportion of P188, while faster homogeneous self-dispersion occurs with an increasing amount of stabilizer (Figure 2). As a control, mTA dispersion in ultrapure water was tested under the same experimental conditions, which was not achieved. As illustrated in Figure 2, NC3 containing the same ratio of drug and stabilizer seems to exhibit the most homogeneous powder self-dispersion.

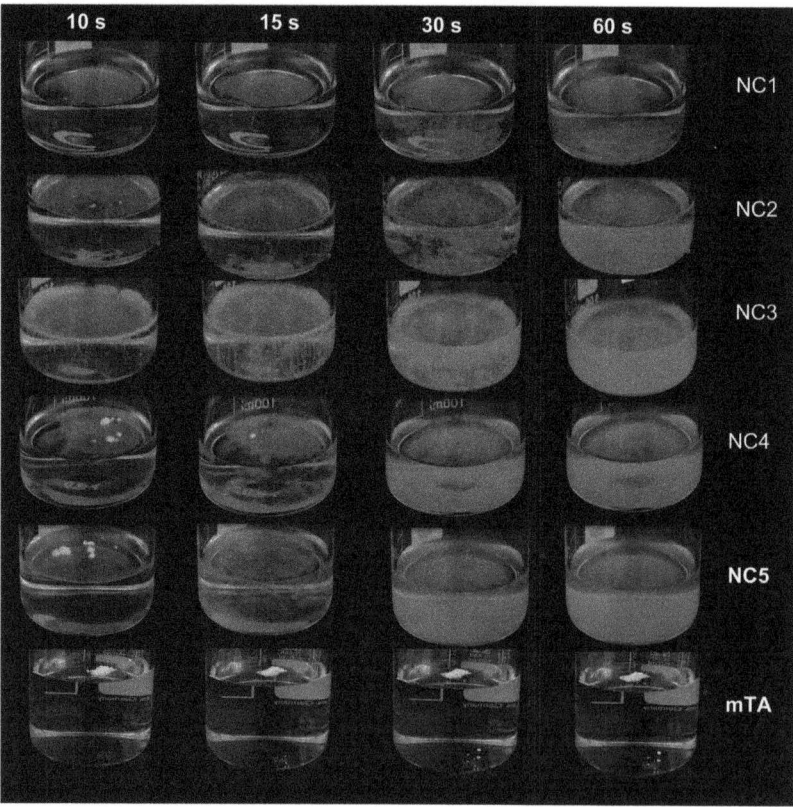

Figure 2. Illustrative images of the aqueous self-dispersion of the powdered TA-NC at 0, 15, 30 and 60 s.

Next, the stability of the different TA-NC stored at room temperature at different times was examined by measuring the particle size after dispersion in water (Figure 3). The TA-NC with the lowest stabilizer concentration exhibited a particle size difference of at least 100 nm between the different studied times after its dispersion in water. In contrast, no significant changes were observed in the APS of the TA-NC with high stabilizer concentration (NC3, NC4 and NC5) after 24 h of its aqueous dispersion. Considering the APS and PDI of TA-NS and dispersible TA-NC, colloidal stability and the use of minimum stabilizer concentration required in ocular pharmaceutical technologies, the TA-NC containing the same ratio of drug and stabilizer (1:1) was selected for further experiments.

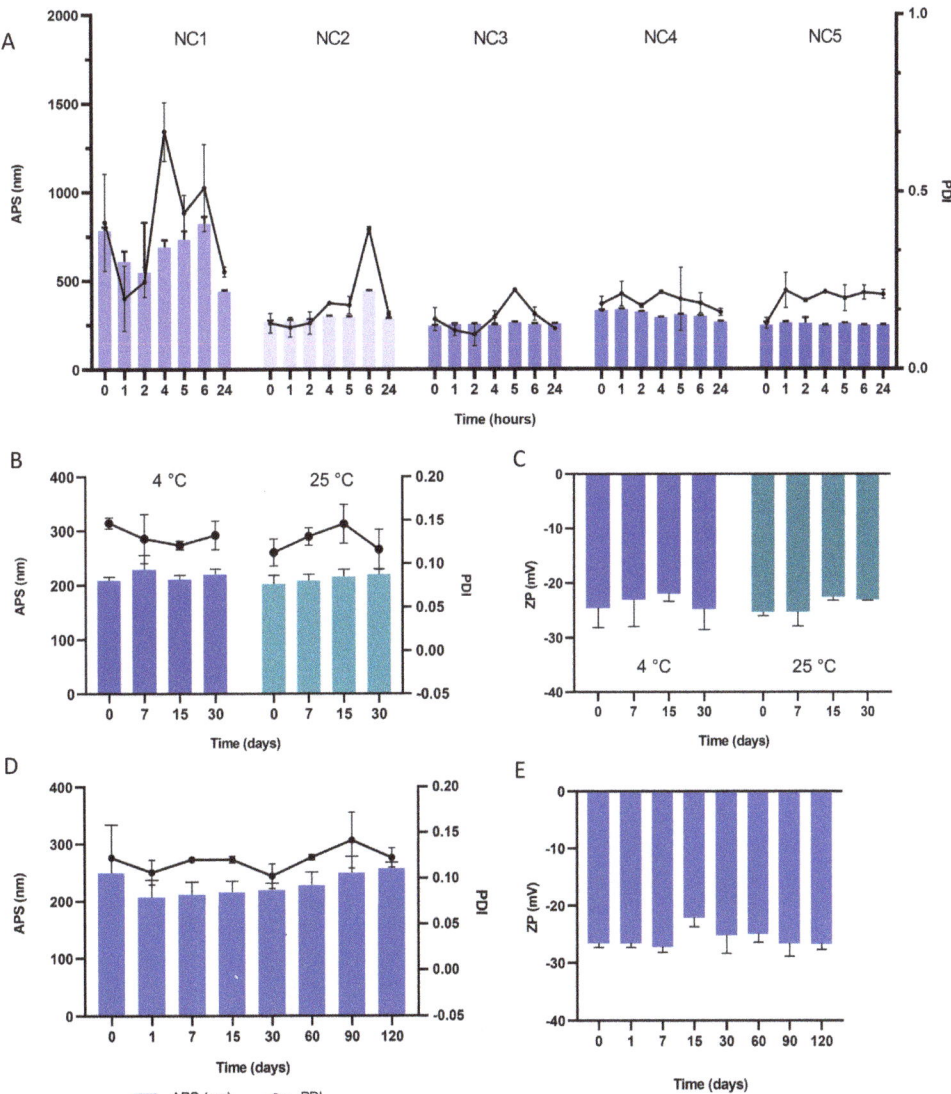

Figure 3. (**A**) Average particle size (APS, bar graph) and polydispersity index (PDI, line graph) of different TA-NC after dispersion in water. (**B**) APS and PDI, and (**C**) zeta potential (ZP) of nanosuspension from TA-NC (NC6) dispersed in water at different times under storage conditions at 4 °C and room temperature (~25 °C). (**D**) APS and (**E**) ZP of TA-NC powder (NC6) at different times under 25 °C storage conditions after water dispersion over time. Results are presented as means ± SD (n = 3) for all TA-NC.

In order to evaluate the preparation of TA-NC from a TA-NS with a higher total solids content (6%) by the described WBM process followed by spray-drying, a drug nanosuspension (NS6) composed of TA and P188 at a mass ratio of 1:1 was prepared. Compared to NC3, which had the same mass ratio with a lower total solids content, NC6 presented slight differences in terms of APS, PDI, ZP and moisture content. Moreover, the previous TA-NS (NS6) presented a comparable size reduction during the milling process resulting in nanoparticles around 275 nm and a PDI lower than 0.2, both slightly higher than those shown by NS3. Therefore, the preparation of TA-NC from the nanosuspension of the drug with a three-fold solids content is feasible at the tested concentrations of TA and P188 with a mass ratio of 1:1.

Subsequently, NC6 dispersed in ultrapure water and stored at 4 °C and 25 °C remained stable for thirty days in terms of APS, PDI and ZP under both storage conditions, showing no significant changes compared to initial values (Figure 3B,C). No macroscopic changes in appearance were observed at the end point of the study. For its part, the dry dispersible NC6 powder retained its APS for at least 120 days under storage at room temperature, as observed in Figure 3D,E.

The formulation corresponding to the dispersible TA-NC obtained from the TA-NS with TA and P188 with a mass ratio of 1:1 was selected to continue with further studies since it showed low APS, a narrow size distribution and low moisture content and was obtained with a high yield from the spray-drying process. In turn, previous TA-NS also exhibited low APS, a narrow size distribution and a lower rate of size increase under room temperature storage conditions after the milling process.

3.3. Scanning Electron Microscopy (SEM)

SEM study performed at 500× and 3000× magnification revealed that TA-NC are homogeneously distributed (Figure 4A) and presented spherical shapes with smooth surfaces (Figure 4B). Under 10,000×, TA-NC were observed to present a rougher surface and were distributed in microclusters of particle sizes around 1 µm (Figure 4C). In contrast to TA-NC, under 500× magnification, no distinct powder particles were observed in the mTA sample (Figure 4D), while at higher magnification (10,000×), particles distributed in heterogeneous macroclusters between 5 and 20 µm were observed (Figure 4B). In addition, PM showed heterogeneous aggregates of mTA and P188 between 5 and 50 µm (Figure 4F).

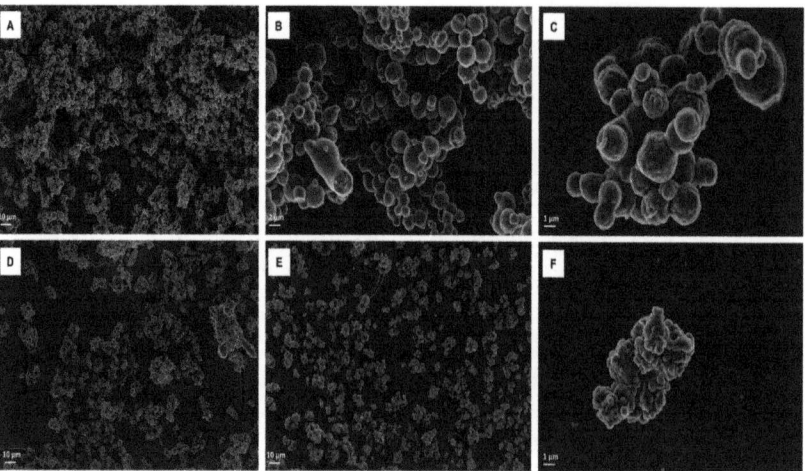

Figure 4. Scanning electron microscope at different magnifications of (**A**)TA-NC at 500×, (**B**) TA-NC at 3000× and (**C**) TA-NC at 10,000×, (**D**) PM at 500×, (**E**) mTA at 1000× and (**F**) mTA at 10,000×.

3.4. Fourier Transform Infrared Spectroscopy (FTIR)

An FTIR spectrometry study was used to analyze the chemical interactions in the chemical structure of the TA-NC and whether there were chemical interactions between the drug and the stabilizer. Figure 5 shows that mTA and TA-NC presented typical infrared absorption bands around 3392 cm^{-1} associated with the O–H stretching vibration and around 1700 cm^{-1} related to the C–O aliphatic ketone present in the TA molecule. In turn, it showed a band at 2950 cm^{-1} that corresponds to the C–H vibrations. Moreover, in the FTIR spectra of mTA and TA-NC, characteristics peaks of TA were observed, such as bands around 1120 cm^{-1} corresponding to the asymmetric axial deformation of C–O–C bond in aliphatic esters and the peak around 1056 cm^{-1} corresponding to C–F stretching of the halogenated ring [13,23].

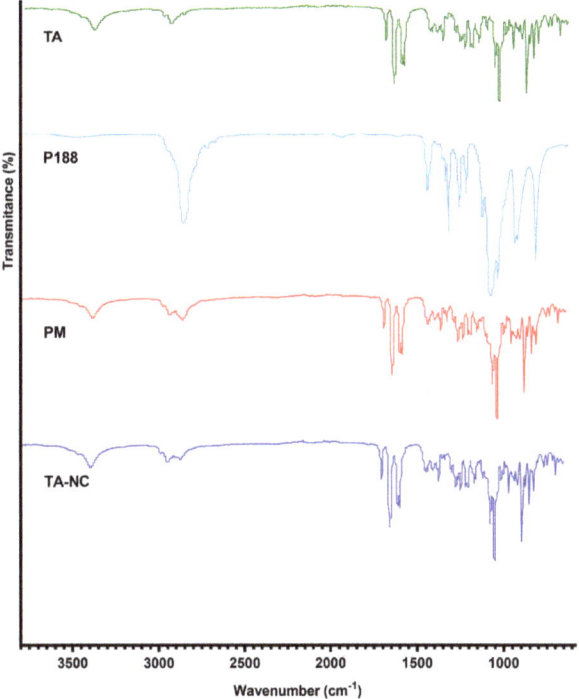

Figure 5. Fourier-transformed infrared (FTIR) spectrometry of mTA, P188, PM and TA-NC.

In addition, P188 showed absorption bands around 2900 cm^{-1}, 1500 cm^{-1} and 1300 cm^{-1} corresponding to the aliphatic chains of the molecule, which were clearly observable in the FTIR spectrum of TA-NC, but with lower intensity. Furthermore, no substantial wavenumbers shifts or additional peaks were observed in the FTIR spectrum of TA-NC. All these results indicate that no detectable chemical interactions between TA and P188 occurred during the preparation process.

3.5. Differential Scanning Calorimetry (DCS) and Thermogravimetry (TGA)

In order to evaluate the thermal properties of TA-NC, DSC and TGA studies were carried out. As shown in Figure 6A, pure mTA presented a characteristic sharp endothermic peak at 293.9 °C associated with the melting point of this drug in the anhydrous crystalline state [23], while pure P188 exhibited a sharp endothermic melting peak at 52.9 °C. Moreover, the TGA study showed that the weight loss of all samples was negligible between 25 and 250 °C, indicating a low moisture content, as also demonstrated above (Table 1). As shown in Figure 6B, mTA exhibited more than a 50% weight loss between 260 and 350 °C, while P188 showed a high weight loss between 300 and 400 °C (80%). Comparing the DSC and TGA thermograms, the results indicate that the melting of TA occurs simultaneously with its decomposition.

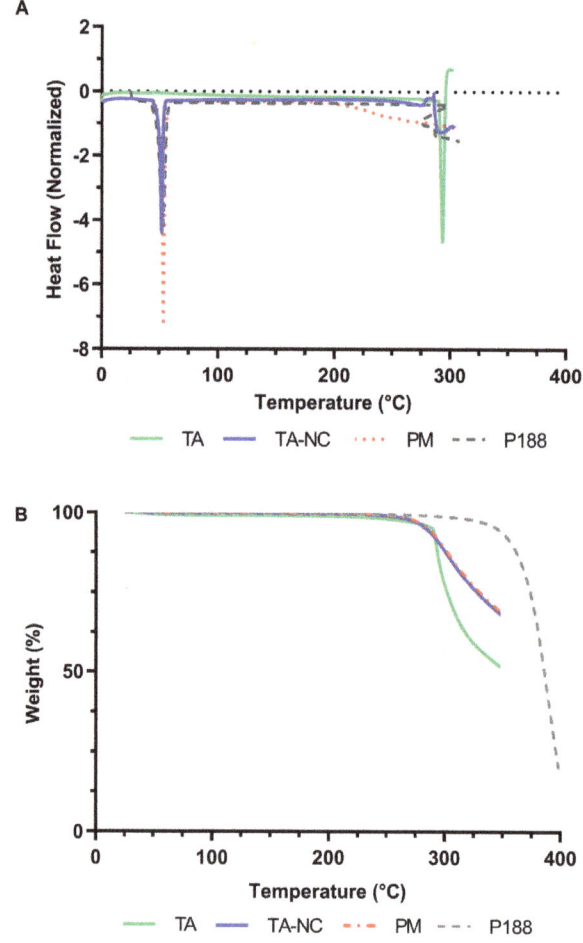

Figure 6. (**A**) Differential scanning calorimetry (DSC) of mTA, P188, PM and TA-NC. (**B**) Thermogravimetric analyses (TGA) of mTA, P188, PM and TA-NC.

In relation to TA-NC, the DSC thermograms exhibited, on the one hand, a well-defined peak at 52.6 °C corresponding to the melting point of P188 and, on the other hand, an endothermic event at 291.9 °C associated with TA, which appears as a poorly defined peak, less intense in terms of endothermic units and slightly shifted in relation to mTA. In the PM sample, endothermic events related to the melting point of the stabilizer and the drug were also observed. Both TA-NC and PM showed a mass loss after the 250 °C range in the TGA study, also evidencing the decomposition of the drug. No significant differences or new peaks associated with glass transition or recrystallization were observed between the DSC thermograms of the TA-NC and the PM.

3.6. X-ray Powder Diffraction (XRPD)

XRPD analysis was carried out to confirm the crystalline state of dried TA-NC. XRPD patterns of mTA, P188, PM and TA-NC are illustrated in Figure 7. Pure mTA exhibited distinctive sharp peaks at 2θ angles of 9–22° and 24–32°, specifically at 9.7°, 14.4°, 17.4°, 19.7°, 24.5° and 30°, indicating the typical crystal structure of the drug [24,25]. On the other hand, P188 presented less crystalline characteristics, with only two main peaks located at 2θ angles of 19.0° and 23.1°. In relation to XRPD patterns of PM and TA-NC, the characteristic peaks of mTA were found in both samples, indicating that the drug remained in crystalline form after the preparation process. Taking into consideration these outcomes with the thermal behaviour observed by DSC, it was concluded that the crystalline structure of TA was largely preserved and neither amorphization nor the formation of polymorphs resulted after bead milling. In reference to the excipient P188, small changes occurred during the PM and TA-NC preparation, evidenced by small changes in the relative intensities of the main two peaks. Nevertheless, the crystallinity of P188 remained almost nonaltered during the preparation of both formulations.

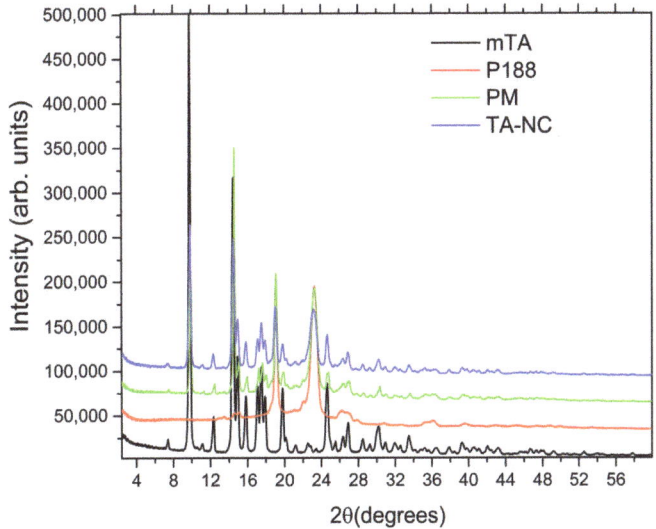

Figure 7. XRPD patterns for mTA, P188, PM and TA-NC.

3.7. Confocal Raman Microscopy

Confocal Raman spectroscopy was very useful to analyze the formulations in the solid state and to evaluate the distribution of components in the TA-NC and PM samples. The Raman analysis of the pure components helped to identify characteristic Raman signals of mTA (most notably ~1670 cm^{-1}) and P188 (~841 cm^{-1}), both signals are important because of their intensity and negligible overlap of signals from both components. The Raman spectra of the pure components are shown in Figure 8B.

The mapping images of the PM and TA-NC samples are shown in Figure 8A,C, respectively. True component analysis (WITec, ProjectFive 5.1 Plus software) of the PM allowed us to identify two different principal components, corresponding to the drug and stabilizer. This reconstructed image (Figure 8A) shows areas where either pure P188 or TA are detected with extensions in the range of ~50 μm and some small areas where the two components are present. On the other hand, the chemical topographic mapping image of the TA-NC sample showed a highly homogeneous distribution of both TA and P188 (Figure 8C), where the spectra collected for each pixel were virtually identical and exclusive areas of the polymer or drug cannot be detected. The mean spectrum of all pixels is shown in Figure 8D. From these results, we can conclude that TA-NC is highly homogeneous, at least at the resolution of the confocal Raman microscope (~300 nm for an excitation laser operating at lambda = 532 nm).

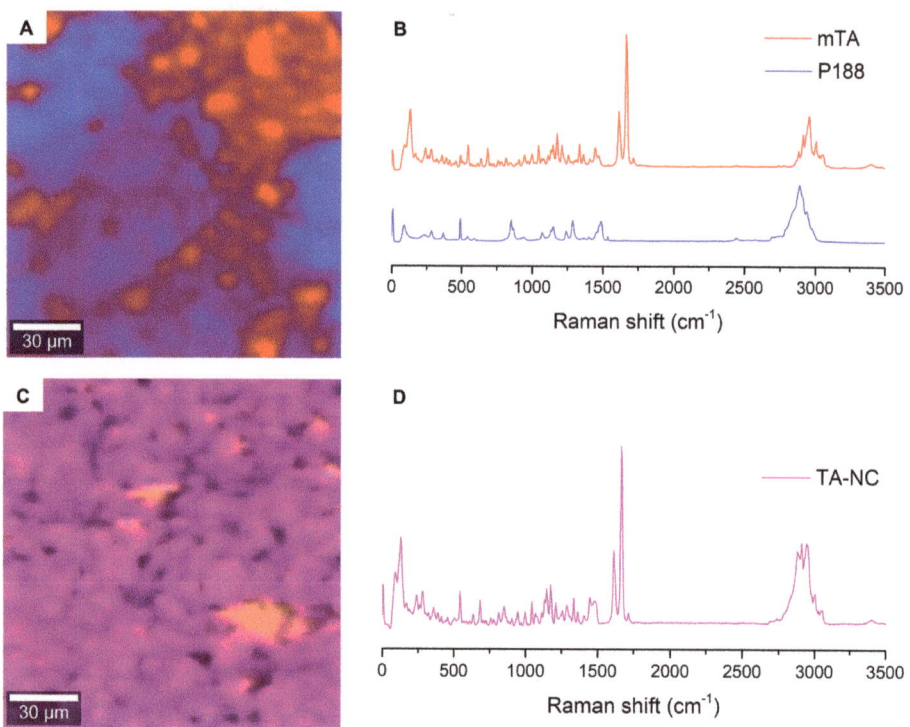

Figure 8. (**A**) Confocal Raman image for PM showing the distribution of the most relevant components (coinciding with mTA and P188) and (**B**) their corresponding averaged spectra according to their selected areas. (**C**) Confocal Raman image for TA-NC, showing a strong homogeneity, as evidenced in (**D**) the average Raman spectra.

3.8. Drug Saturation Concentration

The drug saturation concentration in aqueous media of TA-NC was performed and compared with PM and mTA to evaluate the influence of reducing the particle size on the saturation concentration of TA. The results revealed that TA-NC presented a forty-fold higher drug saturation concentration in a simulated tear fluid than mTA (Figure 9). After incubation at 37 °C, the TA-NC reached a drug saturation concentration of 745 ± 41 µg/mL, while the mTA and PM showed a drug saturation concentration of only 18 ± 1 µg/mL and 11.1 ± 0.3 µg/mL, respectively.

3.9. Ocular Tolerance and Irritation Test

Figure 10 shows rabbit eyes 24 h after the administration of NSS, TA-NC and Fortcinolona® 40. Clinical signs after subconjunctival administration of water-dispersed TA-NC (2 mg) were examined by slit-lamp and binocular indirect ophthalmoscopy. The study revealed the absence of corneal damage, opacity, conjunctival chemosis, conjunctival redness, vitreous haze and retinal damage in all rabbits after 24 h, 48 h, 72 h and 1 week of formulation administration. No conjunctival irritation was observed in any of the groups. Comparable results were observed after subconjunctival administration of NSS and Fortcinolona® 40 at a comparable dose to TA-NC. A group of normal animals was used to compare possible injection-associated alterations. In addition, no apparent lesions were observed in the cornea epithelium by fluorescein staining for either treatment (Figure 10A–C). On the other hand, a delimited deposition of the drug Fortcinolona® 40 could be observed in Figure 10E, while TA-NC seems to be deposited diffusely (Figure 10F).

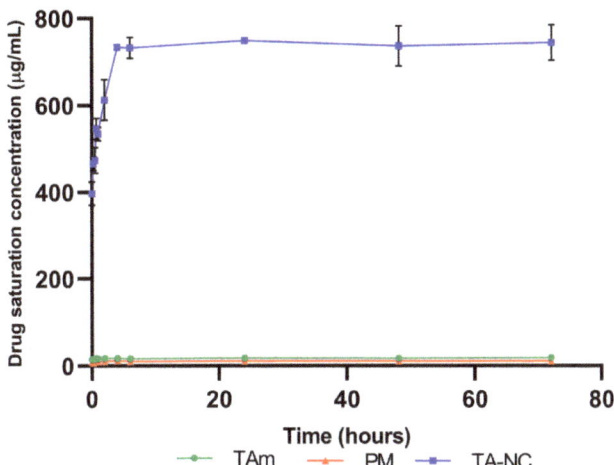

Figure 9. Drug saturation concentration studies of TA-NC, mTA and PM in the simulated tear fluid at 37 °C. Results are presented as means ± SD (n = 3).

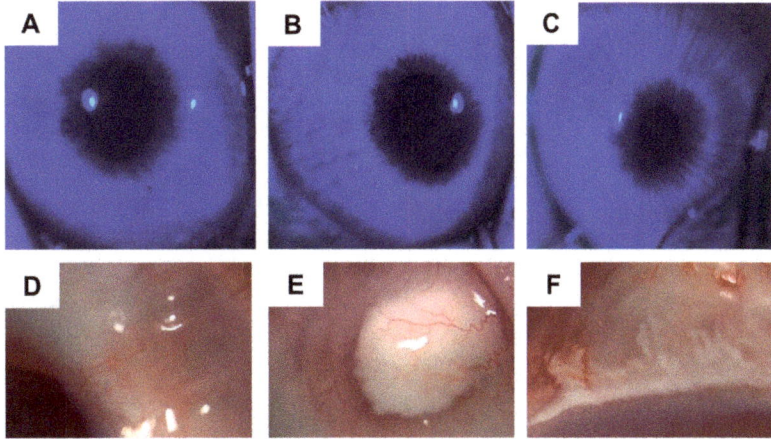

Figure 10. Images of fluorescein staining after 24 h of subconjunctival administration of (**A**) normal saline solution, (**B**) Fortcinolona® 40 and (**C**) aqueous dispersible TA-NC to evaluate corneal damage. Images of conjunctiva rabbit eye after 24 h of subconjunctival administration of (**D**) normal saline solution, (**E**) Fortcinolona® 40 and (**F**) aqueous dispersible TA-NC to evaluate conjunctiva redness.

3.10. In Vivo Therapeutic Efficacy of TA-NC in EIU Model

The in vivo anti-inflammatory efficacy of aqueous dispersible TA-NC was assessed in an EIU rabbit model. As was described above, evaluation of clinical signs revealed maximal intraocular inflammation after 24 h of ocular application of endotoxin. Figure 11A shows the combined mean clinical inflammation score based on clinical signs for the different groups of animals. Rabbits injected with NSS showed clinical inflammatory signs such as conjunctival redness and congestion of iris vessels, protein and fibrin deposits in the cornea and crystalline lens, significant anterior chamber cells (Tyndall effect) and aqueous humour flares. Moreover, IOP decreased after model induction in comparison with baseline IOP in all groups of animals injected with LPS. In contrast, animals injected with an aqueous dispersion of TA-NC significantly alleviated the inflammatory response in the anterior chamber and iris after 24, 48, and 72 h of application compared with animals injected with NSS. Fortcinolona® 40 significantly alleviated clinical inflammatory signs relative to the NSS-injected group after 24 h of model induction; however, no significant differences were observed in clinical scores between these groups after 48 and 72 h. Therefore, TA-NC proved to be the most effective anti-inflammatory treatment under the conditions evaluated.

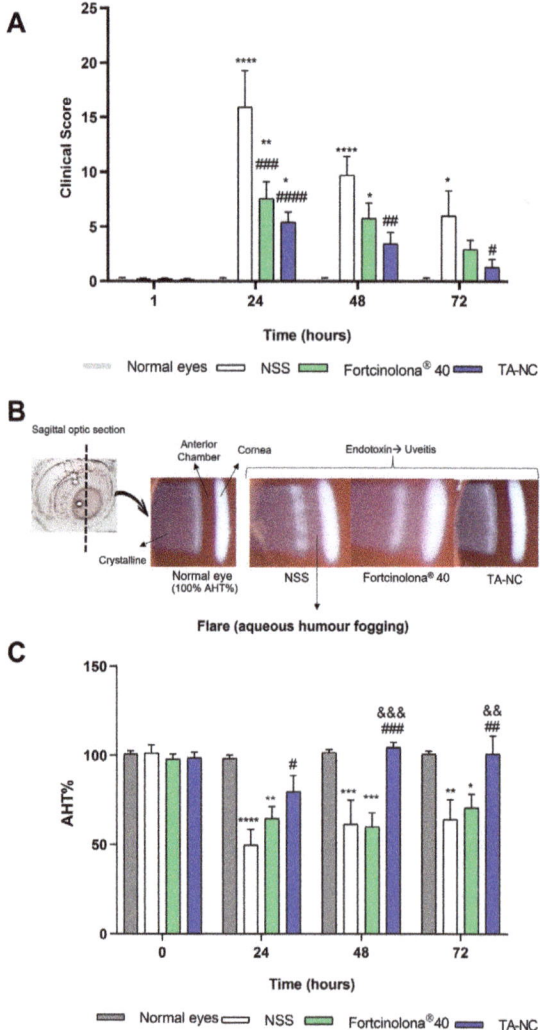

Figure 11. Evaluation of therapeutic efficacy of TA-NC. (**A**) Clinical inflammation score of rabbits treated with normal saline solution (NSS), TA-NC and Fortcinolona® 40 after 24 h, 48 h and 72 h of EUI model in comparison to normal animals. (**B**) Representative photographs taken with slit lamp of the anterior chamber of normal eye and eyes exposed to EIU in vivo model (induced by LPS) after

24 h of subconjunctival treatment with NSS, Fortcinolona® 40 and TA-NC. (**C**) Aqueous humour transparency percentage (AHT%) of the rabbit eye after 24, 48 and 72 h of EIU in vivo model and subconjunctival treatment with NSS (n = 8), Fortcinolona® 40 (n = 8) and TA-NC (n = 8) in comparison with normal eyes (n = 8). AHT% was calculated from the difference in the mean grey between the corneal light reflection and the anterior chamber. Results are presented as means ± SEM for all groups. A two-way ANOVA test was used, and a significant difference was considered to be: * $p < 0.05$; ** $p < 0.005$; *** $p < 0.001$; and **** $p < 0.0001$ in relation to the group of normal eyes. The symbols # $p < 0.05$, ## $p < 0.005$, ### $p < 0.001$, #### $p < 0.0001$ and && $p < 0.005$, &&& $p < 0.001$ are used to refer to significant differences in relation to the NSS group and Fortcinolona® 40 group, respectively.

In uveitis, aqueous humour fogging (flare) in the anterior chamber and the Tyndall effect are the main clinical signs of this ocular disorder, being directly proportional to the observed inflammation. These clinical signs are caused by protein leaking from inflamed blood vessels and cellular infiltration from inflammation of the iris and ciliary body. They can be visualized in the red pupil fondus at maximum slit lamp light intensity. As displayed in Figure 11B, in photographs obtained by a camera attached to the slit lamp, increased fogging was observed in the aqueous humour of the anterior chamber of animals exposed to LPS and injected with NSS. As a brief description of the sagittal optic section of the eye exhibited in the photographs, the cornea is on the right, the anterior chamber is in the centre and the crystalline lens is on the left. In normal eyes, the aqueous humour in the anterior chamber appears transparent, not showing any type of opacity and reflecting the normal red colour of the eye fundus. After 24 h of LPS injection, foggy aqueous humour was observed in the eyes of animals with uveitis and injected with NSS, whereas less fogginess of the aqueous humour was observed when the eyes were treated with TA-NC or Fortcinolona® 40.

The degree of anterior chamber inflammation exhibited in the slit lamp images and aqueous humour fogging of the anterior chamber were analyzed by Image J software and quantified as the mean grey difference between the corneal light reflex and the anterior chamber. The calculated AHT% relative to the basal mean grey difference of the normal eye (which corresponds to 100%) is shown in Figure 11C. The significantly greater AHT% in the TA-NC-treated eye compared with NSS reveals a significant attenuation of the aqueous humour fogging after administration of the nanoparticulate formulation. In contrast, the AHT% in the Fortcinolona® 40-treated eye did not show a significant difference relative to NSS. Thus, TA-NS clearly attenuated ocular inflammation in the animals after the EUI model, with a lower clinical inflammation score and achieving greater aqueous humour transparency. Moreover, TA-NC presented a superior effect relative to Fortcinolona® 40, demonstrating greater therapeutic efficacy in this in vivo model of ocular inflammation.

4. Discussion

TA is a synthetic glucocorticoid widely used as a first-line treatment for several ocular pathologies due to its anti-inflammatory and immunomodulatory effects and low cost. Nevertheless, the TA suspensions commonly used as off-label ophthalmic medicines present certain limitations, mainly associated with their particle sizes, excipients and administration routes. The development of novel therapeutic formulations to improve the ocular efficacy of TA, especially those requiring lower doses and less frequent administration and presenting fewer drug side effects, would be extremely useful. In this regard, the design of an NC-based TA formulation with simple composition obtained by a scalable process is proposed. Thus, a self-dispersible TA-NC was developed as a therapeutic strategy for ocular application produced by WBM followed by the spray-drying process.

The WBM is a top-down method for obtaining NSs that has demonstrated certain advantages associated with the simplicity of the formulation and the ease of scaling up the process and, which is widely accepted by the pharmaceutical industry [26]. In a previous work of our research group, the preparation of NSs of poorly soluble drugs by WBM was studied by exploring different process parameters, showing that the increase in microsphere concentration, high motor speed and low solids content lead to smaller particle sizes and

PDI [19]. In this work, an experimental mixture design for the preparation of TA-NS with a total solids content of 2% w/v was performed to evaluate the ratio of drug and stabilizer using high motor rotation frequencies (1600 rpm) and higher bead content (25%). After 2 h of milling, all TA-NS formulations showed a nanometric particle size of less than 350 nm with a narrow size distribution (PDI less than 0.2). A decrease in APS was observed in TA-NS with a high proportion of P188 and a low proportion of TA, which could be related to the higher availability of P188 to exert steric stabilization between drug particles due to its capacity to bind to their solid surface [27]. TA-NS with P188 concentrations between 1.000 and 1.375% w/v (NS3 and NS4, respectively) showed an APS around 230 nm and PDI = 0.12, while higher APS and PDI were observed with higher stabilizer concentration and lower drug concentration (NS5), which could be related to higher viscosity during the milling process and lower particle breakage efficiency [27]. As described, drug and stabilizer content can influence particle size reduction by media milling.

All TA-NS showed negative surface potentials, which appeared to increase in absolute values with high stabilizer concentration. The decline in zeta potential related to the increasing concentration of P188 could be attributed to the formation of a sterically stabilized polymeric layer. Although TA-NS presented ZP values around −25 mV, an adequate parameter of colloidal stability, APS and PDI were studied after the media milling process. As already described, the formation of nanosized particles creates high-energy surfaces, which can lead to aggregation and Ostwald ripening if stabilization is not at an efficient level. According to the Lifshitz−Slyozov−Wagner theory, in a system where small particles are in equilibrium with larger particles, the overall size and size distribution will increase over time [28]. Thus, a progressive increase in their APS and PDI was observed after 2 h under storage conditions at 25 °C, reaching micrometric sizes after 24 h. Therefore, it was determined that the removal of aqueous media from TA-NS by spray-drying should be performed immediately after bead milling.

Spray-drying is a one-step process that allows the obtainment of a powder from a liquid. The operating parameters were selected considering the process yield achieved for dry NC composed of P188 based on previous research [19], which has been shown to provide a "cryoprotectant effect" for low solids concentrations [29]. Thus, the spray-drying process of different TA-NS showed a process yield of up to 70%, obtaining powders with a moisture content below 2%. In relation to particle size, TA-NC with a low amount of drug and high concentration of stabilizer showed a decrease in APS and PDI after aqueous self-dispersion, remaining without significant changes for at least 24 h and presenting a slight difference (~30 nm) with respect TA-NS before spray-drying. Likewise, TA-NC with equal amounts of drug and stabilizer (1% w/v) exhibited a particle size of 260 nm and a narrow size distribution, resulting in the most useful formulation with which to continue the study since it allowed the obtainment of nanometric sizes without requiring low drug content and high stabilizer content. In this way, it would be possible to minimize the stabilizer concentration as is required in ocular pharmaceutical formulations and, at the same time, ensure complete redispersion of the powders obtained after spray-drying.

In addition, the dispersed TA-NC obtained from TA-NS with a higher total solids content (6%) composed of TA and P188 in a 1:1 ratio (NC6) presented a comparable size and PDI to TA-NC with the same composition and a lower total solids content (2%). As described, stabilization is necessary for the formation of NC as well as for long-term formulation stability during storage. The study of the colloidal stability of NC6 after aqueous self-dispersion revealed that it retains its APS, PDI and ZP at room temperature and 4 °C for at least 30 days, which is the maximum recommended usage time for all ophthalmic formulations once opened; while self-dispersible TA-NC powder remained stable in terms of these assessed parameters at least 120 days.

Concerning the physicochemical characterization of TA-NC, it was revealed that the manufacturing process did not affect the drug properties. TA-NC presented a spherical shape with smooth surfaces, as usually observed for spray-dried powders, and a homogeneous size distribution according to SEM studies, in agreement with results observed for other NCs obtained by WBM and spray-drying processes [19]. Additionally, Raman studies revealed a highly homogeneous distribution of both TA and P188 in TA-NC, which is in line with the analyses of other NCs composed of P188 and obtained by the same process [30]. In addition, no detectable chemical interactions between TA and P188 were observed by FTIR. In turn, XRPD studies revealed that the crystalline structure of TA was largely preserved and that neither amorphization nor polymorph formation occurred after obtaining the TA-NC, while no new peaks associated with glass transition or recrystallization were observed by DSC studies.

Among the main properties of NCs associated with the reduction in the drug particle size to the nanometric range, the increase in surface area is a key factor leading to a faster saturation of the dissolution layer around the particles when they are exposed to the solvent for dissolution and, consequently, to an increase in the dissolution rate, according to the Noyes–Whitney equation [31]. In turn, the increase in drug saturation concentration related to the increase in the curvature and dissolution pressure of the drug from the NC makes a more significant amount of dissolved molecules of the drug compound available [32,33]. Thus, the increased drug saturation concentration of TA-NC was demonstrated, reaching concentration values at least forty times higher in a simulated tear fluid than mTA and PM. Interestingly, TA-NC showed a higher increase in drug saturation concentration than those achieved for lyophilized TA nanosuspensions in other works [13].

Moreover, the satisfactory self-dispersion exhibited by TA-NC could contribute to achieving a drug saturation concentration faster, since particle separation allows exposure of the enlarged surface to aqueous media. In this way, a better spread of particles was observed in the subconjunctival space after subconjunctival injection of dispersed TA-NC compared to Fortcinolona® 40, which forms a defined deposit in the injection site. Adequate particle dispersion could explain this satisfactory spread of particles after ocular administration of TA-NC, which, together with the low particle size, facilitated the injection of the formulation.

Regarding ocular tolerance, the self-dispersible TA-NC did not cause ocular damage after in vivo administration in rabbits, proving to be safe for subconjunctival application. In turn, TA-NC attenuated the clinical signs of the inflammatory response in the in vivo model of EIU, thereby demonstrating its therapeutic efficacy. As the results showed, TA-NC significantly alleviated the inflammatory response in the anterior chamber and iris after 24, 48 and 72 h of subconjunctival injection compared with the group administered with NSS. In turn, it did not show statistically significant differences with the normal eyes after 48 h of injection. Interestingly, the group of animals injected with the commercial TA Fortcinolona® 40 exhibited a significant therapeutic effect on the clinical inflammatory signs relative to the NSS group only after 24 h of its administration and showed statistically significant differences after 24 and 48 h compared with normal eyes. Therefore, TA-NC proved to be the most effective anti-inflammatory treatment under the conditions evaluated.

As described previously, fogging of aqueous humour in the anterior chamber may clinically reflect the degree of inflammation in uveitis. In our study, a single dose of dispersed TA-NC significantly decreased the fogginess, which could be related to the low particle size, easy spread and increased drug saturation concentration. In turn, TA-NC exhibited a superior effect on fogginess attenuation than Fortcinolona® 40 at the same dose, which could be explained by the higher drug saturation concentration that allows a larger amount of available dissolved molecules to exert a pharmacological effect. Similarly, the demonstrated therapeutic efficacy of TA-NC was achieved in this in vivo model by testing half the dose typically used for injection of TA nanosuspensions [34–37] such as off-label Fortcinolona® 40 in the clinical treatment of ocular inflammations such as uveitis. Thus, TA-NC could result in a promising approach to administering lower doses of corticosteroids or decreasing the frequency of administration of the therapeutic scheme. Considering the side effects associated with chronic corticosteroid treatments, such as elevated intraocular pressure and cataract formation as well as those related to frequent intraocular injections, the administration of a lower effective dose of injectable TA is a key achievement. Therefore, TA-NC can be considered a promising alternative in the ocular delivery of TA with demonstrated in vivo efficacy.

5. Conclusions

This work addressed the design of a novel alternative for the treatment of ocular inflammatory disorders. A novel self-dispersible TA-NC was developed by bead milling followed by spray-drying, a method widely used in the pharmaceutical industry that allows the obtainment of self-dispersible powders with a narrow particle size distribution, lower moisture content and a high process yield. In turn, the self-dispersible TA-NC powder remained nanometric-sized for at least 120 days under storage conditions at room temperature, while the aqueous dispersed TA-NC for at least 30 days, the maximum recommended use time for all ophthalmic formulations once opened. Furthermore, a single subconjunctival administration of TA-NC was safe for ocular use and significantly mitigated clinical signs of inflammatory response in the in vivo model at a lower dose of TA than that typically applied in clinical practice. Therefore, self-dispersible TA-NC represents a new approach for ocular use for the treatment of inflammatory processes of various ocular disorders.

Author Contributions: Conceptualization, M.L.F. and S.D.P.; methodology M.L.F., H.G.A.A., A.J.P., L.I.T., M.E.M. and R.F.; validation, M.L.F., H.G.A.A., N.M.C. and L.I.T.; formal analysis, M.L.F., H.G.A.A. and M.E.M.; investigation, M.L.F., A.J.P. and L.I.T.; resources, S.D.P.; data curation, M.L.F.; writing—original draft preparation, M.L.F. and S.D.P.; writing—review and editing, M.L.F., H.G.A.A., A.J.P., L.I.T., M.E.M. and R.F.; visualization, M.L.F.; supervision, S.D.P.; project administration, S.D.P.; funding acquisition, S.D.P. All authors have read and agreed to the published version of the manuscript.

Funding: This research was funded by "Fondo para la Investigación Científica y Tecnológica (FONCyT), funding number PICT 2018. No. 1834", and Consejo Nacional de Investigaciones Científicas y Técnicas (CONICET), funding number PIP 11220200100580CO.

Institutional Review Board Statement: The animal study protocol was approved by the Institutional Animal Care and Use Committee (CICUAL) of the School of Medical Sciences, National University of Cordoba (No. 44/2017) for studies involving animals. In turn, animals were treated according to the guidelines of the ARVO Statement for the Use of Animals in Ophthalmic and Vision Research. All efforts were made to reduce the number of animals used.

Informed Consent Statement: Not applicable.

Data Availability Statement: Not applicable.

Acknowledgments: We thank SeCyT-UNC, FONCyT-ANPCyT and CONICET for financial and technical support. We would also like to acknowledge Egbert Kleinert from Saint-Gobain Ceramics for the advice and the kind donation of zirconia beads. In addition, we thank the technical assistance in the microscopy assays provided by Lamarx-UNC.

Conflicts of Interest: The authors declare no conflict of interest.

References

1. Smithen, L.M.; Ober, M.D.; Maranan, L.; Spaide, R.F. Intravitreal Triamcinolone Acetonide and Intraocular Pressure. *Am. J. Ophthalmol.* **2004**, *138*, 740–743. [CrossRef] [PubMed]
2. Luo, L.; Yang, J.; Oh, Y.; Hartsock, M.J.; Xia, S.; Kim, Y.-C.; Ding, Z.; Meng, T.; Eberhart, C.G.; Ensign, L.M.; et al. Controlled Release of Corticosteroid with Biodegradable Nanoparticles for Treating Experimental Autoimmune Uveitis. *J. Control. Release* **2019**, *296*, 68–80. [CrossRef] [PubMed]
3. Le Merdy, M.; Fan, J.; Bolger, M.B.; Lukacova, V.; Spires, J.; Tsakalozou, E.; Patel, V.; Xu, L.; Stewart, S.; Chockalingam, A.; et al. Application of Mechanistic Ocular Absorption Modeling and Simulation to Understand the Impact of Formulation Properties on Ophthalmic Bioavailability in Rabbits: A Case Study Using Dexamethasone Suspension. *AAPS J.* **2019**, *21*, 65. [CrossRef] [PubMed]
4. Wang, Y.; Friedrichs, U.; Eichler, W.; Hoffmann, S.; Wiedemann, P. Inhibitory Effects of Triamcinolone Acetonide on BFGF-Induced Migration and Tube Formation in Choroidal Microvascular Endothelial Cells. *Graefe's Arch. Clin. Exp. Ophthalmol.* **2002**, *240*, 42–48. [CrossRef] [PubMed]

5. Hirani, A.; Grover, A.; Lee, Y.W.; Pathak, Y.; Sutariya, V. Triamcinolone Acetonide Nanoparticles Incorporated in Thermoreversible Gels for Age-Related Macular Degeneration. *Pharm. Dev. Technol.* **2016**, *21*, 61–67. [CrossRef]
6. Li, J.; Cheng, T.; Tian, Q.; Cheng, Y.; Zhao, L.; Zhang, X.; Qu, Y. A More Efficient Ocular Delivery System of Triamcinolone Acetonide as Eye Drop to the Posterior Segment of the Eye. *Drug Deliv.* **2019**, *26*, 188–198. [CrossRef]
7. Mahran, A.; Ismail, S.; Allam, A.A. Development of Triamcinolone Acetonide-Loaded Microemulsion as a Prospective Ophthalmic Delivery System for Treatment of Uveitis: In Vitro and In Vivo Evaluation. *Pharmaceutics* **2021**, *13*, 444. [CrossRef]
8. Sarao, V.; Veritti, D.; Boscia, F.; Lanzetta, P. Intravitreal Steroids for the Treatment of Retinal Diseases. *Sci. World J.* **2014**, *2014*, 989501. [CrossRef]
9. Yang, Y.; Bailey, C.; Loewenstein, A.; Massin, P. Intravitreal Corticosteroids in Diabetic Macular Edema: Pharmacokinetik Considerations. *Retina* **2015**, *35*, 2440–2449. [CrossRef]
10. Altamirano-Vallejo, J.C.; Navarro-Partida, J.; Gonzalez-De la Rosa, A.; Hsiao, J.H.; Olguín-Gutierrez, J.S.; Gonzalez-Villegas, A.C.; Keller, B.C.; Bouzo-Lopez, L.; Santos, A. Characterization and Pharmacokinetics of Triamcinolone Acetonide-Loaded Liposomes Topical Formulations for Vitreoretinal Drug Delivery. *J. Ocul. Pharmacol. Ther.* **2018**, *34*, 416–425. [CrossRef]
11. Formica, M.L.; Gamboa, G.U.; Tártara, L.I.; Luna, J.D.; Benoit, J.P.; Palma, S.D. Triamcinolone Acetonide-Loaded Lipid Nanocapsules for Ophthalmic Applications. *Int. J. Pharm.* **2020**, *573*, 118795. [CrossRef] [PubMed]
12. Araújo, J.; Garcia, M.L.; Mallandrich, M.; Souto, E.B.; Calpena, A.C. Release Profile and Transscleral Permeation of Triamcinolone Acetonide Loaded Nanostructured Lipid Carriers (TA-NLC): In Vitro and Ex Vivo Studies. *Nanomedicine* **2012**, *8*, 1034–1041. [CrossRef] [PubMed]
13. Wu, Y.; Vora, L.K.; Mishra, D.; Adrianto, M.F.; Gade, S.; Paredes, A.J.; Donnelly, R.F.; Singh, T.R.R. Nanosuspension-Loaded Dissolving Bilayer Microneedles for Hydrophobic Drug Delivery to the Posterior Segment of the Eye. *Biomater. Adv.* **2022**, *137*, 212767. [CrossRef] [PubMed]
14. Fernandes, A.R.; Vidal, L.B.; Sánchez-López, E.; dos Santos, T.; Granja, P.L.; Silva, A.M.; Garcia, M.L.; Souto, E.B. Customized Cationic Nanoemulsions Loading Triamcinolone Acetonide for Corneal Neovascularization Secondary to Inflammatory Processes. *Int. J. Pharm.* **2022**, *623*, 121938. [CrossRef] [PubMed]
15. Müller, R.H.; Keck, C.M. Twenty Years of Drug Nanocrystals: Where Are We, and Where Do We Go? *Eur. J. Pharm. Biopharm.* **2012**, *80*, 1–3. [CrossRef]
16. da, S.; de Jesus, J.I.S.; Lourenço, F.R.; Ishida, K.; Barreto, T.L.; Avino, V.C.; dos, S.; Neto, E.; Bou-Chacra, N.A. Besifloxacin Nanocrystal: Towards an Innovative Ophthalmic Preparation. *Pharmaceutics* **2022**, *14*, 2221. [CrossRef]
17. Chen, M.-L.; John, M.; Lee, S.L.; Tyner, K.M. Development Considerations for Nanocrystal Drug Products. *AAPS J.* **2017**, *19*, 642–651. [CrossRef]
18. Gao, L.; Liu, G.; Ma, J.; Wang, X.; Zhou, L.; Li, X. Drug Nanocrystals: In Vivo Performances. *J. Control. Release* **2012**, *160*, 418–430. [CrossRef]
19. Paredes, A.J.; Camacho, N.M.; Schofs, L.; Dib, A.; del Pilar Zarazaga, M.; Litterio, N.; Allemandi, D.A.; Sánchez Bruni, S.; Lanusse, C.; Palma, S.D. Ricobendazole Nanocrystals Obtained by Media Milling and Spray Drying: Pharmacokinetic Comparison with the Micronized Form of the Drug. *Int. J. Pharm.* **2020**, *585*, 119501. [CrossRef]
20. McGuckin, M.B.; Wang, J.; Ghanma, R.; Qin, N.; Palma, S.D.; Donnelly, R.F.; Paredes, A.J. Nanocrystals as a Master Key to Deliver Hydrophobic Drugs via Multiple Administration Routes. *J. Control. Release* **2022**, *345*, 334–353. [CrossRef]
21. Huang, J.; Yu, X.; Zhou, Y.; Zhang, H.; Song, Q.; Wang, Q.; Li, X. Directing the Nanoparticle Formation by the Combination with Small Molecular Assembly and Polymeric Assembly for Topical Suppression of Ocular Inflammation. *Int. J. Pharm.* **2018**, *551*, 223–231. [CrossRef] [PubMed]
22. Altinsoy, A.; Dilekoz, E.; Kul, O.; Ilhan, S.O.; Tunccan, O.G.; Seven, I.; Bagriacik, E.U.; Sarioglu, Y.; Or, M.; Ercan, Z.S. A Cannabinoid Ligand, Anandamide, Exacerbates Endotoxin-Induced Uveitis in Rabbits. *J. Ocul. Pharm.* **2011**, *27*, 545–552. [CrossRef] [PubMed]
23. García-Millán, E.; Quintáns-Carballo, M.; Otero-Espinar, F.J. Solid-State Characterization of Triamcinolone Acetonide Nanosuspensiones by X-Ray Spectroscopy, ATR Fourier Transforms Infrared Spectroscopy and Differential Scanning Calorimetry Analysis. *Data Brief* **2017**, *15*, 133–137. [CrossRef] [PubMed]
24. García-Millán, E.; Quintáns-Carballo, M.; Otero-Espinar, F.J. Improved Release of Triamcinolone Acetonide from Medicated Soft Contact Lenses Loaded with Drug Nanosuspensions. *Int. J. Pharm.* **2017**, *525*, 226–236. [CrossRef] [PubMed]
25. Sabzevari, A.; Adibkia, K.; Hashemi, H.; Hedayatfar, A.; Mohsenzadeh, N.; Atyabi, F.; Ghahremani, M.H.; Dinarvand, R. Polymeric Triamcinolone Acetonide Nanoparticles as a New Alternative in the Treatment of Uveitis: In Vitro and in Vivo Studies. *Eur. J. Pharm. Biopharm.* **2013**, *84*, 63–71. [CrossRef]
26. Mohammad, I.S.; Hu, H.; Yin, L.; He, W. Drug Nanocrystals: Fabrication Methods and Promising Therapeutic Applications. *Int. J. Pharm.* **2019**, *562*, 187–202. [CrossRef]
27. Tuomela, A.; Hirvonen, J.; Peltonen, L. Stabilizing Agents for Drug Nanocrystals: Effect on Bioavailability. *Pharmaceutics* **2016**, *8*, 16. [CrossRef]
28. Dagtepe, P.; Chikan, V. Quantized Ostwald Ripening of Colloidal Nanoparticles. *J. Phys. Chem. C* **2010**, *114*, 16263–16269. [CrossRef]
29. Paredes, A.J.; Llabot, J.M.; Sánchez Bruni, S.; Allemandi, D.; Palma, S.D. Self-Dispersible Nanocrystals of Albendazole Produced by High Pressure Homogenization and Spray-Drying. *Drug Dev. Ind. Pharm.* **2016**, *42*, 1564–1570. [CrossRef]

30. Melian, M.E.; Paredes, A.; Munguía, B.; Colobbio, M.; Ramos, J.C.; Teixeira, R.; Manta, E.; Palma, S.; Faccio, R.; Domínguez, L. Nanocrystals of Novel Valerolactam-Fenbendazole Hybrid with Improved in Vitro Dissolution Performance. *AAPS PharmSciTech* **2020**, *21*, 237. [CrossRef]
31. Noyes, A.A.; Whitney, W.R. The Rate of Solution of Solid Substances in Their Own Solutions. *J. Am. Chem. Soc.* **1897**, *19*, 930–934. [CrossRef]
32. Real, D.; Formica, M.L.; Picchio, M.; Paredes, A.J. Manufacturing Techniques for Nanoparticles in Drug Delivery. In *Drug Delivery Using Nanomaterials*; Shahzad, Y., Rizvi, S.A.A., Yousaf, A.M., Hussain, T., Eds.; CRC Press: London, UK, 2022; pp. 23–48.
33. Van Eerdenbrugh, B.; Vermant, J.; Martens, J.A.; Froyen, L.; Humbeeck, J.V.; van den Mooter, G.; Augustijns, P. Solubility Increases Associated with Crystalline Drug Nanoparticles: Methodologies and Significance. *Mol. Pharm.* **2010**, *7*, 1858–1870. [CrossRef] [PubMed]
34. Karasu, B.; Kesim, E.; Kaskal, M.; Celebi, A.R.C. Efficacy of Topical Dexamethasone Eye Drops in Preventing Ocular Inflammation and Cystoid Macular Edema Following Uncomplicated Cataract Surgery with or without Injection of a Single Dose Perioperative Subtenon Triamcinolone Acetonide. *Cutan. Ocul. Toxicol.* **2022**, *41*, 310–317. [CrossRef] [PubMed]
35. Hanif, J.; Iqbal, K.; Perveen, F.; Arif, A.; Iqbal, R.N.; Jameel, F.; Hanif, K.; Seemab, A.; Khan, A.Y.; Ahmed, M. Safety and Efficacy of Suprachoroidal Injection of Triamcinolone in Treating Macular Edema Secondary to Noninfectious Uveitis. *Cureus* **2021**, *13*, e20038. [CrossRef] [PubMed]
36. Kim, K.W.; Kusuhara, S.; Tachihara, M.; Mimura, C.; Matsumiya, W.; Nakamura, M. A Case of Panuveitis and Retinal Vasculitis Associated with Pembrolizumab Therapy for Metastatic Lung Cancer. *Am. J. Ophthalmol. Case Rep.* **2021**, *22*, 101072. [CrossRef] [PubMed]
37. Gaballa, S.A.; Kompella, U.B.; Elgarhy, O.; Alqahtani, A.M.; Pierscionek, B.; Alany, R.G.; Abdelkader, H. Corticosteroids in Ophthalmology: Drug Delivery Innovations, Pharmacology, Clinical Applications, and Future Perspectives. *Drug Deliv. Transl. Res.* **2021**, *11*, 866–893. [CrossRef]

Disclaimer/Publisher's Note: The statements, opinions and data contained in all publications are solely those of the individual author(s) and contributor(s) and not of MDPI and/or the editor(s). MDPI and/or the editor(s) disclaim responsibility for any injury to people or property resulting from any ideas, methods, instructions or products referred to in the content.

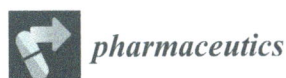

Article

Design, Characterization and Pharmacokinetic–Pharmacodynamic Evaluation of Poloxamer and Kappa-Carrageenan-Based Dual-Responsive In Situ Gel of Nebivolol for Treatment of Open-Angle Glaucoma

Pradeep Singh Rawat [1], Punna Rao Ravi [1,*], Shahid Iqbal Mir [1], Mohammed Shareef Khan [1], Himanshu Kathuria [2], Prasanna Katnapally [3] and Upendra Bhatnagar [3]

[1] Department of Pharmacy, BITS-Pilani Hyderabad Campus, Hyderabad 500078, Telangana, India
[2] Nusmetics Pte Limited, E-Centre@Redhill, 3791 Jalan Bukit Merah, #05-27, Singapore 159471, Singapore
[3] Vimta Labs Limited, 142, Cherlapally Main Rd, IDA Phase II, Hyderabad 500051, Telangana, India
* Correspondence: rpunnarao@hyderabad.bits-pilani.ac.in; Tel.: +91-40-66303539; Fax: +91-40-66303998

Abstract: This study developed a dual-responsive in situ gel of nebivolol (NEB), a selective β-adrenergic antagonist. The gel could achieve sustained concentrations in the aqueous humor to effectively treat glaucoma. The gel was prepared using a combination of poloxamers (Poloxamer-407 (P407) and Poloxamer-188 (P188)) and kappa-carrageenan (κCRG) as thermo-responsive and ion-sensitive polymers, respectively. Box–Behnken design (BBD) was used to optimize the effect of three critical formulation factors (concentration of P407, P188 and κCRG) on two critical response variables (sol-to-gel transition temperature of 33–35 °C and minimum solution state viscosity) of the in situ gel. A desirability function was employed to find the optimal concentrations of P407, P188 and κCRG that yielded a gel with the desired sol-to-gel transition temperature and solution state viscosity. An NEB-loaded gel was prepared using the optimized conditions and evaluated for in vitro drug release properties and ex vivo ocular irritation studies. Furthermore, ocular pharmacokinetic and pharmacodynamics studies were conducted in rabbits for the optimized formulation. The optimized NEB-loaded gel containing P407, P188 and κCRG had a sol-to-gel transition temperature of 34 °C and exhibited minimum viscosity (212 ± 2 cP at 25 °C). The optimized NEB-loaded gel sustained drug release with 86% drug release at the end of 24 h. The optimized formulation was well tolerated in the eye. Ocular pharmacokinetic studies revealed that the optimized in situ gel resulted in higher concentrations of NEB in aqueous humor compared to the NEB suspension. The aqueous humor C_{max} of the optimized in situ gel (35.14 ± 2.25 ng/mL) was 1.2 fold higher than that of the NEB suspension (28.2 ± 3.1 ng/mL), while the $AUC_{0-\infty}$ of the optimized in situ gel (381.8 ± 18.32 ng/mL*h) was 2 fold higher than that of the NEB suspension (194.9 ± 12.17 ng/mL*h). The systemic exposure of NEB was significantly reduced for the optimized in situ gel, with a 2.7-fold reduction in the plasma C_{max} and a 4.1-fold reduction in the plasma $AUC_{0-\infty}$ compared with the NEB suspension. The optimized gel produced a higher and sustained reduction in the intra-ocular pressure compared with the NEB suspension. The optimized gel was more effective in treating glaucoma than the NEB suspension due to its mucoadhesive properties, sustained drug release and reduced drug loss. Lower systemic exposure of the optimized gel indicates that the systemic side effects can be significantly reduced compared to the NEB suspension, particularly in the long-term management of glaucoma.

Keywords: ocular drug delivery; nebivolol; open-angle glaucoma; in situ gel; Box Behnken design; Poloxamer-407; kappa-carrageenan

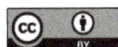

1. Introduction

Glaucoma is a cluster of chronic, progressive optic neuropathies that manifests as an increase in intra-ocular pressure leading to damage of the optic disc and eventually impairing vision [1]. Glaucoma is the second most common cause of blindness globally. The major risk factor for the onset of primary open-angle glaucoma (POAG) is elevated intraocular pressure (IOP) [2]. The main cause of elevated IOP in the anterior chamber of the eye is an ocular drainage system malfunction, which results in blockage and resistance to aqueous humor outflow [3]. Currently, β-blockers account for approximately 70% of all prescriptions for treatment of POAG. This is due to their effectiveness and mechanism of competing with catecholamines for β-2 adrenoreceptors in the ciliary epithelium and decreasing aqueous humor production [4]. However, the non-selective nature of first-generation β-blockers leads to systemic side effects raising concern for long-term management of POAG [5]. Though the second-generation β-1 cardio-selective agents like betaxolol offer a better systemic safety profile as compared to the existing first-generation β-blocking agents, they still suffer from some systemic side effects [6].

Nebivolol (NEB), a third-generation novel selective β-adrenolytic drug, has an unique mechanism of facilitating nitric oxide release that plays a role in the L-Arginine/NO/cGMP pathway, which provides neuroprotective properties while modulating aqueous humor drainage from the trabecular meshwork [7]. These dual mechanisms of lowering IOP as well as providing neuroprotection offer an advantage in the long-term management of POAG [8].

Ophthalmic drops (solutions/suspensions) are the most popular and convenient drug products available for the treatment of ocular diseases. Ophthalmic drops are easy to administer, non-invasive and produce high patient compliance, particularly in ocular diseases which require long-term, multi-dose administration of the drug. Ocular drug delivery is riddled with many challenges due to various physiological, anatomical and enzymatic barriers. These challenges become increasingly difficult as the target site for drug distribution and action moves from superficial layers (layers of cornea/conjunctiva) of the eye to the inner tissue of the eye (iris/ciliary body/vitreous humor). In the management of POAG using conventional ophthalmic drops, the ocular bioavailability for many drugs is very minimal (around 5–10%) while the systemic exposure is very high (50–90%) [9,10].

An in situ gel is an ideal choice for ocular drug delivery because of its ability to undergo rapid sol-to-gel transition via temperature/pH/ion stimuli [11]. Due to its solution state, it is easy to administer while maintaining dose accuracy. Following administration, the in situ gel form a viscous gel which helps in retaining the drug at the surface of the cornea and provides intimate contact with the cornea. In addition, drug dilution by lachrymal fluids and drug loss due to naso-lachrymal drainage is significantly reduced by the viscous gel. This results in higher ocular availability and lower systemic absorption of the drug.

Several synthetic and natural polymers were investigated for their in situ gelling properties based on various stimuli such as temperature, ions and pH [12–14]. In glaucoma, there is dysfunction in aqueous humor circulation leading to variation in the pH and temperature at the precorneal area [15,16]. Therefore, it is crucial to design an ocular in situ gel that can be triggered by more than one stimuli as well as provide mucoadhesive characteristics to sustain drug release for effective management of glaucoma [17].

Poloxamer-407 (P407) is a synthetic thermo-responsive polymer. It is a triblock copolymer, consisting of a central hydrophobic polyoxypropylene (PPO) chain and two lateral hydrophilic polyoxyethylene (PEO) chains. P407 has 70% of PEO and 30% of PPO in its structure [18]. It exhibits thermo-responsive characteristics in the concertation range of 18–22% w/v. The temperature-induced gelation of P407 is due to the hydrophobic interaction of its copolymer chains. As temperature increases, the copolymer chains start aggregating to form a micellar structure, which is the initial step of gelation [19]. However, the gels produced are of low viscosity. Poloxamer-188 (P188) is added to increase the viscosity of the gels formed by P407. P188 has 80% of PEO and 20% of PPO in its structure. P188 produces viscous gels with good mucoadhesive characteristics even at lower concentrations. Therefore, most of the thermo-responsive in situ gels use a combination of P407 and P188 [20].

Carrageenan (CRG) is a long, linear polysaccharide containing D-galactose and D-anhydro-galactose disaccharide repeating units with anionic sulphate groups. Three different grades of CRG are available depending on the number of sulphate groups attached to the disaccharide repeating units. In kappa-carrageenan (κCRG), there is only one sulphate group attached to the disaccharide repeating units. The aqueous solutions of κCRG exhibit ion-sensitive in situ gelling properties in the presence of monovalent ions (such as Na^+ and K^+) [21,22]. κCRG can be combined with P407 + P188 to design dual-responsive ocular in situ gels for effectively delivering drugs towards the inner tissues of the eye. In addition, κCRG, when combined with P407 + P188, forms strong hydrogen bonds with their micellar structure and reinforces the gel structure (Figure 1), resulting in higher gel strength, improved mucoadhesion and slower gel erosion [23,24].

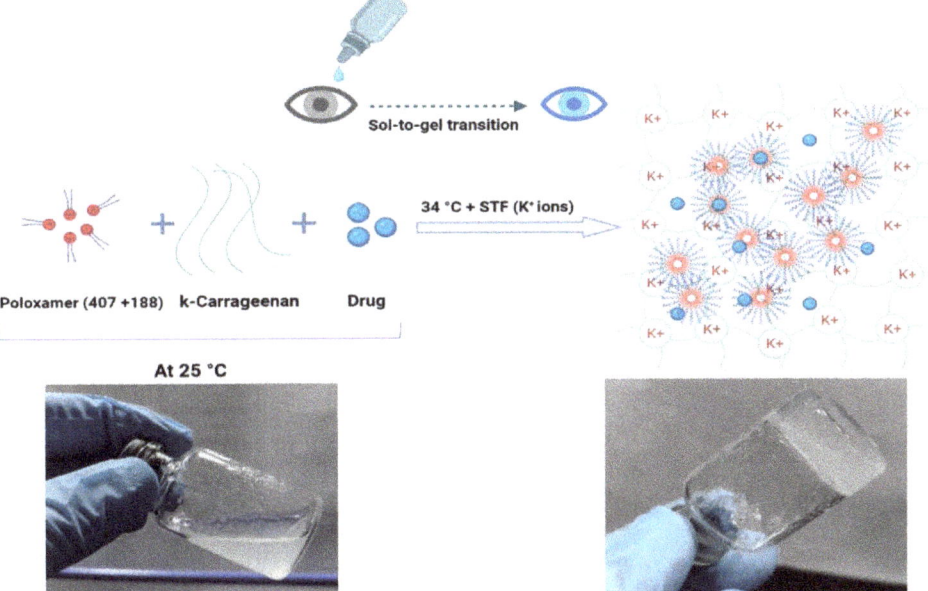

Figure 1. Illustration showing the possible gel matrix formed by the NEB-loaded dual-responsive in situ gel at 34 °C in presence of STF (containing K^+ ions).

In the current research, we designed and optimized an NEB-loaded dual-responsive in situ gel using a mixture of P407 + P188 (as thermo-responsive polymer) and κCRG (as ion-sensitive polymer). The optimized formulation was characterized for mucoadhesion, in vitro drug release and ex vivo ocular toxicity. The ocular pharmacokinetic and pharmacodynamic studies were conducted in New Zealand white rabbits to determine the efficacy of the optimized dual-responsive in situ gel in comparison to the NEB suspension.

2. Materials and Methods
2.1. Materials

Nebivolol (NEB) and nebivolol-d4 (internal standard) were purchased from Vivan life sciences Private limited (Mumbai, India) and BioOrganics Private limited (Bangalore, India), respectively. κCRG, P407, P188 and benzododecinium bromide were procured from Sigma-Aldrich Private Limited (Mumbai, India). Methanol and acetonitrile (LC-MS grade) were purchased from Thermo Fischer Scientific (Mumbai, India). Ammonium acetate, formic acid and disodium EDTA were purchased from SRL Chem Limited (Mumbai, India). Sample analysis was conducted using high-quality HPLC-grade water obtained from the Milli-Q purification system (Millipore®, Burlington, MA, USA). Male New Zealand white rabbits (2–2.5 kg) were procured from Vimta Labs (Hyderabad, India).

2.2. Analytical Method for Analysis of NEB

A validated LC-MS/MS method, reported previously by our group, was used to analyse the concentration of NEB in the aqueous humor and plasma samples obtained in the ocular pharmacokinetic studies [25]. The samples were analysed using an Agilent HPLC (model: 1260 Infinity II, Agilent Technologies Inc., Santa Clara, CA, USA) coupled with a triple quadrupole mass analyser (model: API 4500, AB SCIEX, Redwood City, CA, USA). Chromatographic separation was performed on a reverse phase column (Zorbax SB-C18, 4.6 × 100 mm, 3.5 μm) using a mobile phase consisting of an organic phase (mixture of methanol and acetonitrile in the ratio of 70:30 *v/v*) and an aqueous phase (5 mM ammonium acetate buffer adjusted to pH 3.5 ± 0.05 with formic acid) in the ratio of 75:25 *v/v*. Samples were extracted using a protein precipitation technique. The mass spectrometer was operated in positive electrospray ionization mode with multiple reactions monitoring for NEB at (Q1→Q3) of (406.2→151.1) and for nebivolol-d4 (internal standard) at (Q1→Q3) of (410.2→151.3).

A validated RP-HPLC method was used to determine the concentration of NEB obtained in drug content analysis samples and in vitro drug release study samples. An end-capped C18 column (Luna®, 150 mm × 4.6 mm, 5 μm, Phenomenex, Torrance, CA, USA), maintained at 30 °C inside a column oven, was used in the analysis. The mobile phase consisting of acetonitrile and 0.1% *v/v* orthophosphoric acid in the ratio of 43:57 *v/v* was pumped at a flow rate of 0.8 mL/min to separate the NEB from the interfering peaks. The analyte was detected at a wavelength of 281 nm. The injection volume was fixed at 50 μL. The baseline was stabilized prior to the analysis of the samples.

2.3. Preparation and Optimization of NEB-Loaded Dual-Responsive In Situ Gel

2.3.1. Preparation of NEB-Loaded Dual-Responsive In Situ Gel

The poloxamer solutions were prepared by the cold method [9]. In the first step, the required amounts of P407 (18–20% *w/v*, varied as per the design in BBD) and P188 (1–5% *w/v*, varied as per the design in BBD) were added to pre-cooled (4 °C) deionized water with continuous stirring to ensure proper hydration of the poloxamers. The resultant mixture was kept in the refrigerator for 24 h until the polymers were completely dissolved. The required amount of κCRG (0.3–0.5% *w/v*, varied as per the design in BBD) was added to the above solution and stirred at 500 rpm for 2 h to form a homogenous solution. Finally, NEB (0.3% *w/v*), mannitol (5.2% *w/v*; this was used as an isotonicity-adjusting agent) and benzododecinium bromide (0.01% *w/v*) were added to the resulting solution and stirred for 30 min to form an NEB-loaded dual-responsive in situ gel. The formulation was stored at 4 °C until further use.

2.3.2. Optimization of NEB-Loaded Dual-Responsive In Situ Gel

Box–Behnken design (BBD), a response surface method, was used to analyse and optimize the effect of concentrations of P407, P188 and κCRG on the gelling temperature and solution state viscosity of the dual-responsive in situ gels [26]. BBD was employed at three experimental levels to optimize the three formulation-related factors: X_1—concentration of P407 (18% to 20% *w/v*); X_2—concentration of κCRG (0.3% to 0.5% *w/v*) and X_3—concentration of P188 (1% to 5% *w/v*) as shown in (Table 1). The effect of the three formulation factors was studied on two critical response variables of the in situ gel: Y_1: gelling temperature (°C) and Y_2: solution state viscosity at 25 °C (cP).

Table 1. Experimental design used in BBD for optimization of NEB-loaded dual-responsive in situ gels.

Factors	Levels Used		
Independent Variables	−1	0	+1
X_1 = P407 concentration (% w/v)	18%	19%	20%
X_2 = κCRG concentration (% w/v)	0.3%	0.4%	0.5%
X_3 = P188 concentration (% w/v)	1%	3%	5%
Dependent variables	Constraints		
Y_1 = Gelling temperature	In range of 33–35 °C		
Y_2 = Solution state viscosity at 25 °C	Minimize		

Design Expert software (Version 13, Stat-Ease Inc., Minneapolis, MN, USA) was used to construct the BBD for optimization of the dual-response in situ gel. In the optimization trials, a 17-run BBD (including five centre point runs) was constructed for the three formulation factors (X_1, X_2 and X_3) studied at three levels (−1, 0 and +1) to assess main effects, interaction effects and quadratic effects on response variables (Y_1 and Y_2). In order to evaluate the reproducibility of the method used in the preparation of the in situ gel, five centre point runs were included. Optimization using BBD resulted in a quadratic equation that relates each of the response variables, separately, with the critical factors. The general form of the second-order quadratic equation for a response variable is as follows:

$$Y = \beta_\circ + \beta_1 X_1 + \beta_2 X_2 + \beta_3 X_3 + \beta_{12} X_1 X_2 + \beta_{23} X_2 X_3 + \beta_{13} X_1 X_3 + \beta_{11} X_1^2 + \beta_{22} X_2^2 + \beta_{33} X_3^2 \quad (1)$$

where Y is the response/dependent variable; X_1, X_2 and X_3 are input/independent variables, $\beta_\circ$ is the arithmetic mean response of the seventeen runs. β_i and β_{ij} ($i, j = 1 - 3$) are the coefficients of individual linear and quadratic effects of the factors, respectively.

2.4. Characterization of Blank and NEB-Loaded Dual-Responsive In Situ Gels

2.4.1. Determination of Gelling Temperature and Solution State Viscosity of the In Situ Gels

The 'vial tilting' method, reported in the literature, was used to determine the gelling temperature of the in situ gels [27]. A small tube containing 1 mL of the test formulation was put in a thermostatically controlled water bath. The water bath temperature was raised steadily from 20 °C to 40 °C at a rate of 1 °C/min. The tube was turned 90 degrees at each temperature level. The temperature at which no flow was observed upon tilting the tube was identified as the gelling temperature of the formulation [28].

The solution state viscosity of the in situ gels was measured using a viscometer (Brookfield DV-E, AMETEK, Wilmington, MA, USA) with CP 52 spindle at 10 rpm [29]. The test formulation (in situ gel) was placed in a beaker, and the viscosity was measured at 25 ± 0.5 °C. The experiment was performed in triplicate.

2.4.2. Physical Appearance, pH and Drug Content of Optimized NEB-Loaded Dual-Responsive In Situ Gel

The physical appearance and clarity of the optimized NEB-loaded in situ gel was examined by visual observation. The pH of the formulation (for three replicates) was determined using a calibrated pH meter (Eutech Instruments, Pune, India) [30]. The drug content of the drug-loaded in situ gels was carried out by diluting 100 µL of the formulation in 1 mL of deionized water. The samples were then analysed using HPLC [31]. The drug content was determined for three replicate formulations.

2.5. Rheological Study of Blank and NEB-Loaded Dual-Responsive In Situ Gels

The rheological properties of the blank and NEB-loaded dual-responsive in situ gels were evaluated using a Rheometer (Anton Paar, MCR 302, Graz, Austria) to determine the sol-to-gel transition temperature and the strength of the gel formed by the formulations. The measurements were performed in oscillatory mode using parallel plate geometry with a temperature sweep from 20 °C to 37 °C. The samples were analysed in their linear viscoelastic regions, which were determined by the amplitude and frequency sweep experiments. Three different experimental conditions were used to evaluate the rheological behaviour of the samples: (1) temperature ramp, (2) temperature ramp in the presence of simulated tear fluid (STF) and (3) temperature ramp in the presence of deionized water. The sol–gel transition and gel strength were determined from the data obtained from the plots of 'loss factor (tan δ) vs. temperature' and 'storage modulus (G') vs. temperature' [32–35].

2.6. Mucoadhesion Studies of NEB-Loaded In Situ Gels

The mucoadhesive property of the in situ gels was studied using a Texture analyser (TA-XT plus, Stable Micro Systems, Surrey, UK). A blank P407 + P188 in situ gel and blank κCRG in situ gel were prepared to understand the contribution of the thermo-responsive polymer (mixture of P407 + P188) and ion-responsive polymer (κCRG) towards the overall mucoadhesive properties of the dual-responsive in situ gel. In the study, a filter paper (Whatman filter paper, grade one, Size 110) was cut into a small disc and moistened with mucin dispersion (8% w/w, prepared in STF) to form a mucin disc (which can mimic the mucosal surface of the cornea). The mucin disc was then placed horizontally on the lower end of the texture profile analysis probe using double-sided adhesive tape. Around 100 µL of the test formulation (in situ gel) was poured near the basement probe where the temperature was maintained at 34 °C. The samples were equilibrated and allowed to undergo a sol–gel transition. The probe was lowered at a speed of 1 mm/s until the mucin disc came into contact with the surface of the gel formed by the test formulation. A downward force (0.2 N) was applied for 1 min to ensure proper contact between the mucin disc and the gel. The probe was then moved upwards at a speed of 0.5 mm/s. The force required to detach the mucin disc from the surface of the gel was determined from the force vs. time plot constructed by the instrument software. The study was conducted in triplicate [36,37].

2.7. In Vitro Drug Release Studies of NEB-Loaded In Situ Gels

The dialysis method was used to perform in vitro drug release studies of NEB-loaded in situ gels [30,38]. Drug release studies were conducted for the NEB suspension, NEB-loaded P407 + P188 in situ gel, NEB-loaded κCRG in situ gel and NEB-loaded dual-responsive in situ gel. In the study, 40 µL of the test formulation (equivalent to 3 mg of NEB per mL of formulation) was sealed in a dialysis bag (MWCO: 3.5 kDa). The dialysis bag was incubated in a beaker containing 100 mL of STF (pH 7.4 ± 0.5) with 0.5% w/v Tween 80 as the dissolution media. The dissolution media was stirred at 75 rpm while maintaining the temperature at 34 ± 0.5 °C. Samples of 2 mL were drawn at 0.5, 1, 2, 4, 6, 8, 12, 16, 18 and 24 h during the study. Fresh media (maintained at the same temperature) of equal volume was added each time the sample was drawn from beaker. The samples were centrifuged at 10,000 rpm. The supernatant was collected and analysed, after appropriate dilution, using HPLC to determine the concentration of NEB. The data obtained from the in vitro drug release studies were fit into various kinetic models (i.e., zero-order, first-order, Higuchi and Korsmeyer–Peppas models) to understand the release behaviour of NEB from the different in situ gels [39,40].

2.8. Ex Vivo Ocular Irritation Test (HET-CAM) of the Optimized In Situ Gels

The hen's egg test on chorioallantoic membrane (HET-CAM) method, an inexpensive, rapid and sensitive alternative of the Draize test was performed to study the ocular irritation of optimized in situ gels. Eggs procured from a local hatchery were incubated for nine days for proper growth of the CAM. The eggshells were delicately cracked on each of eggs on the 10th day from the large end to expose the air cell without damaging the inner membrane. The inner membrane was carefully removed with forceps to make the CAM ready for studying the effect of four different treatments. Three eggs (n = 3) were used for each treatment. Group 1 was treated with 0.1 N NaOH (positive control), Group 2 was treated with 0.9% w/v NaCl solution (negative control), Group 3 was treated with the blank dual-responsive in situ gel and Group 4 was treated with the NEB-loaded dual-responsive in situ gel. Blood vessels were examined for 300 s for signs of vascular lysis (disintegration of blood vessels), haemorrhage and coagulation. The irritation score (*IS*) value for each treatment was determined using Equation (2).

$$IS = \left[\frac{(301-H)}{300} \times 5\right] + \left[\frac{(301-L)}{300} \times 7\right] + \left[\frac{(301-C)}{300} \times 9\right] \quad (2)$$

where H is the time (in sec) taken to start haemorrhage reactions, L is the time (in sec) taken to start vessel lysis and C is the time (in sec) taken to start coagulation formation on the CAM [41,42].

The ocular irritation properties of the treatments were identified based on the IS values. A treatment is considered to be 'non-irritating' if the IS value is in the range of 0–0.9, 'slightly irritating' if the IS value is in the range of 1–4.9, 'moderately irritating' if the IS value is in the range of 5–9.9 and 'strongly irritating' if the IS value is in the range of 10–21 [43].

2.9. Hemolysis Study of the Optimized In Situ Gels

The haemolytic study was conducted to evaluate the isotonicity of the optimized in situ gel. Blood (2 mL) was drawn from the marginal ear vein of rabbits using a syringe into centrifuge tubes pre-treated with anticoagulant (4% *w/v* disodium EDTA solution). Red blood cells were separated using centrifugation at 3600 rpm for 15 min. To achieve a haematocrit of 2% (*v/v*), the cells were suspended in a required volume of physiological saline. Then the RBC suspension (1 mL) was mixed with the (1 mL) in situ gel (blank dual-responsive in situ gel or NEB-loaded dual-responsive in situ gel), and the mixture was incubated in water at 37 ± 0.5 °C for 1 h. In positive and negative controls groups, a RBC suspension (1 mL) was mixed with 1 mL of Triton X-100 and 1 mL of 0.9% *w/v* NaCl solution, respectively. For each treatment, the supernatant collected after centrifugation was measured for ultraviolet absorbance at 540 nm, and the absorbance values were substituted in Equation (3) to determine the haemolysis (%). Haemolysis studies of the treatment were carried out in triplicate.

$$\text{Haemolysis (\%)} = \frac{(A_s - A_b)}{(A_c - A_b)} \times 100 \quad (3)$$

where A_c is the absorbance value of the supernatant obtained by treating RBC suspension with Triton X-100, A_s is the absorbance value of the supernatant obtained by treating RBC suspension with in situ gelling formulation and A_b is the absorbance value of the supernatant obtained by treating RBC suspension with a 0.9% *w/v* NaCl solution [44,45].

2.10. Ocular Histopathology Studies of In Situ Gels

Ocular histopathology studies were performed to evaluate the effect of optimized in situ gels on the structural integrity of the corneal epithelium. Fresh goat eyeballs were procured from a local slaughterhouse. The cornea was excised from the goat eyeball. The excised cornea was washed and then incubated with each treatment, separately, for 4 h. The treatments used in the study were: STF (pH 7.4 ± 0.5) (negative control), 75% *v/v* isopropyl alcohol (positive control), blank dual-responsive in situ gel and NEB-loaded dual-responsive in situ gel. After the incubation period, the cornea was again washed and fixed in a 10% formalin solution for 24 h. After fixation, the cornea was subsequently dehydrated for 1.5 h using ethyl alcohol (at each concentration gradient of 30–50–70–90–100%). The cornea was then placed in xylene for 1.5 h and embedded in hot paraffin at 56 °C for 24 h. Paraffin blocks were solidified at room temperature. A rotary microtome (Leica Microsystems SM2400, England) was used to slice paraffin tissue blocks (3–4 μm thick). The sliced tissues were mounted on a glass slide and washed with xylene to remove the paraffin. The tissues were finally stained with haematoxylin and eosin (H-E stain). The stained tissues were observed for histopathological changes under a digital microscope (ZEISS, Axiocam 705 color, Oberkochen, Germany) at 20× magnification [46].

2.11. In Vivo Studies of the Optimized NEB-Loaded Dual-Responsive In Situ Gel

2.11.1. Ocular Pharmacokinetic Studies

Ocular pharmacokinetic studies of the optimized NEB-loaded dual-responsive in situ gel and NEB suspension were performed in male New Zealand white albino rabbits. Animals ($n = 6$ for each treatment group) weighing between 2.5 and 3.0 kg and having clinically normal eyes (free from signs of ocular abnormality) were used in the study. The protocols of conducting the in vivo studies were approved by the Institutional Animal Ethics Committee (IAEC) of Vimta labs, Hyderabad, India (Protocol No.: VLL/1122/NG/1099). All the animals were acclimatized to animal facility conditions ($22 \pm 1\,^\circ$C room temperature, $55 \pm 10\%$ RH, and 12 h light–dark cycle) for one week prior to the study. A calibrated micropipette was used to instil 40 µL of the test formulation (NEB suspension/NEB dual-responsive in situ gel) in the cul-de-sac of each of the eyes in all the rabbits. Immediately following the dosing, the upper and lower eyelids were gently held closed for 10 s to maximize the contact between the cornea and the administered formulation. Aqueous humor samples were collected under mild anaesthesia using isoflurane (2% v/v). Aqueous humor samples (70 µL) were collected from the anterior part of eye by puncturing it with a 30 G sterile hypodermic needle via paracentesis. Blood samples (0.25 mL) were collected from the animals by ear vein puncture and transferred to Eppendorf tubes containing 200 mM K2EDTA (20 µL per mL of blood) as an anticoagulant [47]. Aqueous humor and plasma samples were collected in a sparse sampling manner at 0.5, 1, 2, 4, 8, 12 and 24 h after the formulation instillation. The samples (blood and aqueous humor) obtained from the ocular pharmacokinetic study were analysed using a validated LC-MS method reported by our group [25].

A non-compartmental analysis was used to calculate the pharmacokinetic parameters from the NEB concentration versus time data in each of the matrices [48]. The maximum NEB concentration in the rabbit aqueous humor and plasma (C_{max}, ng/mL), the time to reach C_{max} (T_{max}, h) and the mean residence time ($MRT_{0-\infty}$, h) were determined. The area under the curve from 0 to 24 h ($AUC_{(0-24)}$, ng × h/mL) was calculated using the trapezoidal method.

2.11.2. Pharmacodynamic Studies

In the pharmacodynamic study, the intra-ocular pressure (IOP) in the eye of rabbits was measured using a calibrated tonometer (TONO-PEN XL, Reichert, Germany) [49]. The efficacy of the optimized NEB-loaded dual-responsive in situ gel was compared with the NEB suspension by comparing the time course of percent reduction in IOP [$\Delta IOP(\%)$] of the two formulations. In the study, six rabbits were allocated to the two formulations, with three rabbits for each formulation. The pre-dose IOP values were measured in both the eyes of each rabbit before instilling the formulations. The formulations (NEB-loaded dual-responsive in situ gel and NEB suspension) were instilled at a dosing volume of 40 µL into the lower cul-de-sac of each of the eyes of the rabbits in their group. The IOP was measured at 2, 6 and 12 h after the ocular administration of the formulations. Based on the data obtained in the study, the percentage reduction in *IOP* [$\Delta IOP(\%)$] at different time points was calculated for both the treatments using the following equation:

$$\Delta IOP(\%) = \frac{(IOP_{Pre} - IOP_t)}{IOP_{Pre}} \times 100 \qquad (4)$$

where IOP_{Pre} is the intra-ocular pressure at pre-dose (just before administering the treatment) and IOP_t is the intra-ocular pressure at time t following the administration of the treatment [48].

3. Results

3.1. Optimization of Dual-Responsive In Situ Gels Using BBD

A total of 17 independent runs (including 5 centre point runs) were constructed using BBD to examine three critical formulation factors on the two response variables. NEB-loaded dual-responsive in situ gels were prepared, in triplicate, for each run separately based on the composition of the run given by the BBD. The prepared in situ gels were evaluated to determine their gelling temperature (Y_1) and solution state viscosity at 25 °C (Y_2). The data obtained for each of the runs are presented in Table 2.

Table 2. Design matrix of the 17 experimental runs generated by BBD and responses obtained from characterization of NEB-loaded dual-responsive in situ gels in terms of gelling temperature and solution state viscosity.

Run	Critical Factors			Response	
	P407 Concentration (X_1, %w/v)	κCRG Concentration (X_2, %w/v)	P188 Concentration (X_3, %w/v)	Gelling Temperature (Y_1, °C)	Sol State Viscosity (Y_2, cP)
1	19	0.4	3	41	212
2	19	0.4	3	41	205
3	19	0.5	1	34	217
4	18	0.3	3	42	183
5	19	0.5	5	46	209
6	19	0.3	5	45	199
7	20	0.4	5	45	227
8	18	0.4	1	35	195
9	19	0.4	3	41	204
10	19	0.3	1	34	211
11	20	0.4	1	33	233
12	18	0.4	5	47	179
13	20	0.5	3	40	227
14	19	0.4	3	40	210
15	19	0.4	3	41	205
16	18	0.5	3	42	187
17	20	0.3	3	40	224

3.1.1. Effect of Critical Formulation Factors on the Gelling Temperature (Y_1) of In Situ Gels

Regression analysis was used to model the gelling temperature (Y_1) as a function of the three critical formulation factors (X_1, X_2 and X_3) for the NEB-loaded dual-responsive in situ gels obtained from the 17 runs generated by BBD. The quadratic equation, with statistically significant terms, relating the gelation temperature of the in situ gels and the three critical factors, in the coded form, is given below:

$$Gelling\ temperature\ (Y_1) = 40.80 - 1.00 X_1 + 0.125 X_2 + 5.88 X_3 + 0.25 X_2 X_3 + 0.225 X_1^2 - 1.02 X_3^2 \quad (5)$$

The statistical significance of the regression model and the various model terms was evaluated using analysis of variance (ANOVA). The ANOVA results of the regression model for gelling temperature are presented in Table 3. The F_{cal} value (214.12) of the model was statistically significant, with $P_{cal} < 0.0001$. The regression coefficients, R^2_{adj} (adjusted R^2) and R^2_{press} (predicted error sum of square R^2) of the model were 0.9917 and 0.9819, respectively. High R^2_{adj} and R^2_{press} indicate that the regression equation obtained in the optimization can predict the gelling temperature (Y_1) values within a less than 2% deviation from the experimental/observed values. The lack of fit of the model was insignificant (F_{cal} value = 0.417 and $P_{cal} = 0.751$). The lowest and highest gelling temperatures were

33 ± 0.5 °C and 47 ± 0.5 °C for the in situ gels prepared using the conditions given in the 11th and 12th experimental runs, respectively (Table 2).

Table 3. Results obtained from ANOVA of BBD for optimization of gelling temperature and solution state viscosity of NEB-loaded dual-responsive in situ gels.

Source	Gelling Temperature (Y_1, °C)				Sol State Viscosity at 25 °C (Y_2, cP)			
	Sum of Squares	DF	F-Value	p-Value	Sum of Squares	DF	F-Value	p-Value
Model	289.07	9	214.12	<0.0001	3835.69	91	46.22	<0.0001
X_1	8.00	1	53.33	0.0002	3486.13	1	378.05	<0.0001
X_2	0.125	1	0.833	0.3917	66.13	1	7017	0.0316
X_3	276.13	1	1840.83	<0.0001	220.50	1	23.91	0.0018
$X_1 X_2$	0.000	1	0.000	1.000	0.25	1	0.0271	0.8739
$X_1 X_3$	0.000	1	0.000	1.000	25	1	2.71	0.1436
$X_2 X_3$	0.250	1	1.67	0.2377	4.16	1	0.433	0.5312
X_1^2	0.213	1	1.42	0.2721	6.32	1	0.6852	0.4351
X_2^2	0.0026	1	0.0175	0.8984	2.21	1	0.240	0.6392
X_3^2	4.42	1	29.49	0.0010	26.84	1	2.91	0.1317
Residual	1.05	7			64.45	7		
Lack of fit	0.2500	3	0.4167	0.751	13.75	3	0.3609	0.7856
Pure error	0.800	4			50.80	4		
Total	290.12	16			3900.24	16		

3.1.2. Effect of Critical Formulation Factors on the Solution State Viscosity (Y_2) of In Situ Gels

The quadratic equation relating the effect of the three critical formulation factors (X_1, X_2 and X_3) on the solution state viscosity (Y_2) of the NEB-loaded dual-responsive in situ gels obtained from the 17 runs generated by BBD, in the coded form, is presented in Equation (6) given below:

$$\text{Solution state vicosity } (Y_2) = 207.2 + 0.88X_1 + 2.88X_2 - 5.25X_3 + X_2X_3 - 1.23X_1^2 + 2.53X_3^2 \quad (6)$$

The results obtained from the ANOVA of the regression equation for solution state viscosity (Y_2) suggest that the model was statistically significant (F_{cal} value = 46.22 and P_{cal} < 0.0001) while the lack of fit was insignificant (F_{cal} value = 0.361 and P_{cal} = 0.786) (Table 3). The regression equation for solution state viscosity (Y_2) appeared to have very high predictability as suggested by R^2_{adj} (0.963) and R^2_{press} (0.923) values, which are closer to 1.

In the optimization design, the in situ gels prepared using the experimental conditions given in the 12th run exhibited minimum viscosity (179 ± 2.3 cP at 25 °C), while the formulation prepared using the 11th experimental run conditions had maximum viscosity (233 ± 4.1 cP at 25 °C) (Table 2).

The effect of concentration of P407 and concentration of P188, at a fixed concentration of κCRG, on gelling temperature of the in situ gels is presented as a response surface graph in Figure 2a. The gelling temperature decreased slightly with an increase in concentration of P407 (from 18 to 20% w/v) at higher concentrations of P188 (3 to 5% w/v). Increasing the concentration of P188 (from 1 to 5% w/v) had a positive impact on the gelling temperature of the in situ gels at any given concentration of P407 studied in the design. As depicted in Figure 2b, at a fixed concentration of P407, increase in the concentration of κCRG (from 0.3 to 0.5% w/v) did not have any significant effect on the gelling temperature of the in situ gels at any given concentration of P188 (1 to 5% w/v). It was expected κCRG, being an ion-sensitive polymer, should not have much impact on the gelling temperature of the in situ gels. Though P407 is a thermo-sensitive polymer, the concentration ranges in which it was studied had a smaller impact on gelling temperature. However, the gelling temperature increased with an increase in concentration of P188. This could be due to the increase in the polyethylene oxide content in the poloxamer polymers mixture (P407 + P188) in the vehicle, which then prevents the water molecules from moving away from PPO chains and thereby reduces the chances of micelle formation followed by gelling [50].

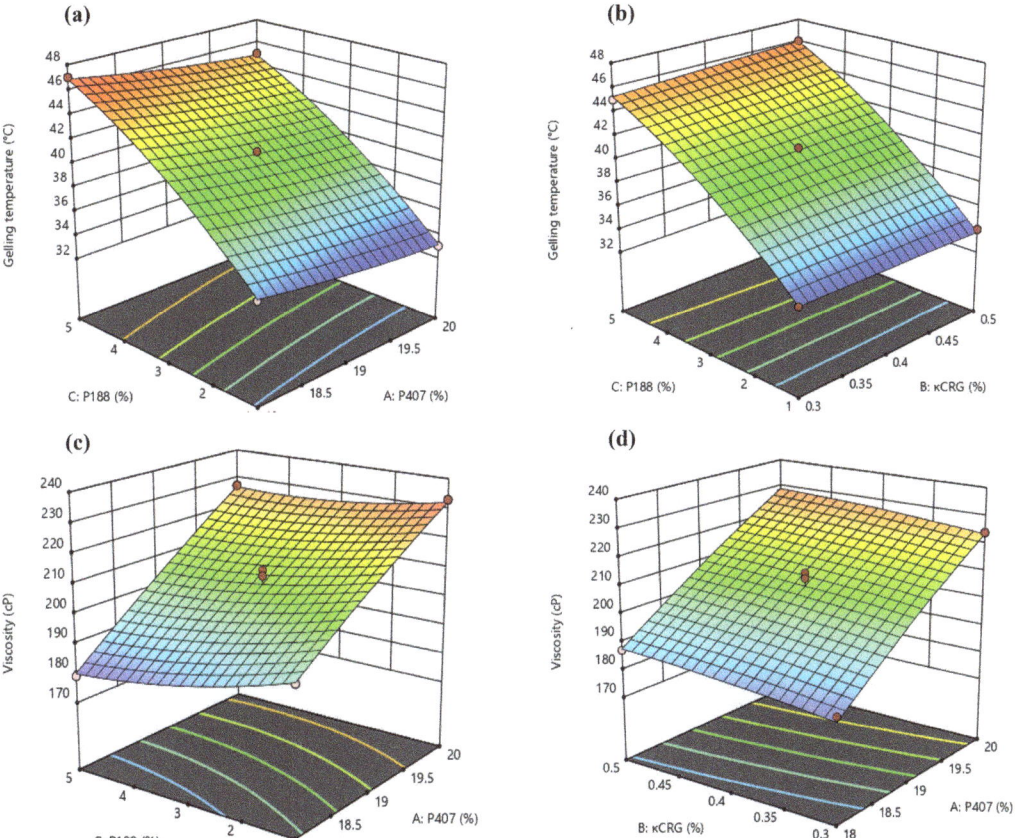

Figure 2. Response surface 3D plots showing the effect of (**a**) concentration of P407 and P188 on gelling temperature; (**b**) concentration of P188 and κCRG on gelling temperature; (**c**) concentration of P188 and P407 on solution state viscosity and (**d**) concentration of P407 and κCRG on solution state viscosity of NEB-loaded dual-responsive in situ gels.

Figure 2c presents the response surface of solution state viscosity (at 25 °C) of the in situ gels as a function of the concentration of P188 and concentration of P407 (at a fixed concentration of κCRG). As depicted in the graph, the solution state viscosity decreased significantly with an increase in the concentration of P407 (from 18 to 20% *w/v*) at any given concentration of P188 (1 to 5% *w/v*). Increasing the concentration of P188 (from 1 to 5% *w/v*) marginally decreased the solution state viscosity of the in situ gels at any given concentration of P407 (18 to 20% *w/v*). At a fixed concentration of P188, an increase in the concentration of κCRG (from 0.3 to 0.5% *w/v*) resulted in a slight increase in the solution state viscosity of the in situ gels at any given concentration of P407 (18 to 20% *w/v*) (Figure 2d). The solution state viscosity of the in situ gels (at 25 °C) was more affected by the concentration of P407 than the concentration of P188 or κCRG. This could be due to the higher concentration of P407 relative to the other polymers used in the in situ gels. As the concentration of P407 increased, the solution state viscosity of the in situ gels (at 25 °C) increased. The results obtained in our study are consistent with the observations made by Hirun et al. in their work [26].

3.1.3. Identification of Optimized Conditions Using Desirability Function

A simultaneous optimization technique involving a desirability function was employed to determine the optimal conditions for the preparation of NEB-loaded dual-responsive in situ gels. The objective for gelling temperature (Y_1) was set as a range between 33 and 35 °C, and for solution state viscosity, the goal was set to minimize while applying the desirability function. At the highest overall desirability value, the optimized conditions for the preparation of the NEB-loaded dual-responsive in situ gel were as follows: concentration of P407 = 19% w/v, concentration of κCRG = 0.3% w/v and concentration of P188 = 1% w/v.

3.2. Characterization of Optimized NEB-Loaded Dual-Responsive In Situ Gel

3.2.1. Gelling Temperature and Solution State Viscosity

The gelling temperature and the solution state viscosity (25 °C) of the optimized NEB-loaded dual-responsive in situ gel were 34 ± 0.5 °C and 212 ± 2 cP, respectively. These results were close to the predicted values determined from the regression equations of gelling temperature (Y_1) and the solution state viscosity (Y_2), affirming the validity of the optimization model. The optimized NEB-loaded dual-responsive in situ gel exhibited desirable flow properties in the solution state (at 25 °C) while undergoing rapid sol-to-gel transition and forming a firm gel in the presence of STF at 34 ± 0.5 °C (Figure 3).

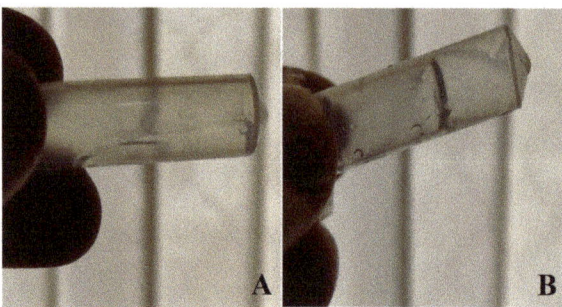

Figure 3. Image showing the flow properties of an optimized NEB-loaded dual-responsive in situ gel. (**A**) Free flowing properties at 25 °C suitable for easy and accurate dosing and (**B**) forming a firm gel at 34 ± 0.5 °C in presence of STF.

3.2.2. Physical Appearance, pH, Osmolarity and Drug Content of the Optimized Dual-Responsive In Situ Gels

The blank dual-responsive in situ gel was transparent, while the optimized NEB-loaded dual-responsive in situ gel was translucent due to suspended NEB particles. The pH of both formulations was 7.2 ± 0.5, which is compatible with the pH of lachrymal fluids. The osmolarity of the optimized formulation was calculated based on the molarity equation and was found to be 285.44 mOsm/L. The osmolarity of the optimized in situ gel lies in the range reported for lachrymal fluids [51]. The drug content of the optimized NEB-loaded dual-responsive in situ gel was found to be 96.5 ± 1% for three independent batches of the formulation. This suggests that the method of preparation of the in situ gels was reliable and reproducible.

3.3. Rheological Studies of Blank and NEB-Loaded Dual-Responsive In Situ Gels

Figure 4a,b depict the rheological behaviour of the optimized blank and NEB-loaded dual-responsive in situ gels, respectively, as a function of temperature in the presence of STF and deionized water. Figure 4a presents the loss factor (tan δ) vs. temperature behaviour of the formulations, while Figure 4b shows the storage modulus (G') of the formulations as a function of temperature. The tan δ values of optimized blank and NEB-loaded dual-responsive in situ gels, without the addition of STF/deionised water, were more than one in the temperature range of 20 to 30 °C, indicating the free-flowing nature of the formulations. The tan δ values dropped below one between 32 and 34 °C for the optimized blank and NEB-loaded dual-responsive in situ gels in the presence of deionised water. This suggests a clear sol-to-gel transition due to the thermo-responsive component (P407 + P188) of dual-responsive in situ gels. In the presence of STF, tan δ values of the optimized blank and NEB-loaded dual-responsive in situ gels were more than one in the temperature range of 20 to 37 °C, with a drop in the range of 32 to 34 °C. Due to the presence of the cations (K^+ and Na^+) in STF, the ion-responsive component (κCRG) of the dual-responsive in situ gels caused the in situ gels to undergo sol-to-gel transition even at 20 °C. In the temperature range of 32 to 34 °C, the thermo-responsive component added to the increase in viscosity of the gel that was formed. These results indicate that both thermo-responsive and ion-responsive polymers were able to cause a sol-to-gel transition of the in situ gels independently and synergistically (Table 4).

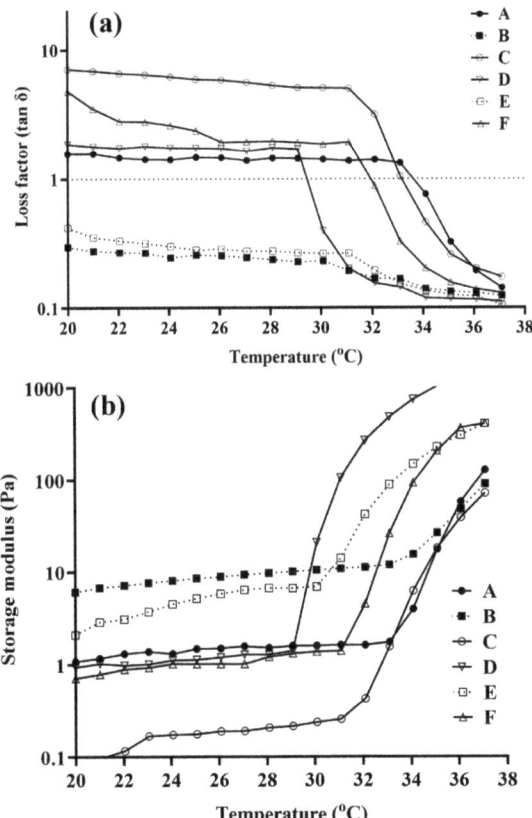

Figure 4. Semi-logarithmic plots of (a) loss tangent (tan δ) and (b) storage modulus (G') of an optimized blank dual-responsive in situ gel and an NEB-loaded dual-responsive in situ gel as a function of temperature in presence of STF and deionized (DI) water. Rheological studies of optimized blank and NEB-loaded in situ gels. Note: A—blank dual-responsive in situ gel; B—blank dual-responsive in situ gel in the presence of STF; C—blank dual-responsive in situ gel in the presence of DI water; D—NEB-loaded dual-responsive in situ gel; E—NEB-loaded dual-responsive in situ gel in the presence of STF and F—NEB-loaded dual-responsive in situ gel in the presence of DI water.

Table 4. Loss tangent (tan δ) of optimized blank dual-responsive in situ gel and NEB-loaded dual-responsive in situ gel as a function of temperature (20 to 37 °C) in presence of STF and deionized (DI) water.

Formulation	Experimental Condition Used in Rheological Study		
	Only Temp Ramp	Temp Ramp in Presence of DI Water	Temp Ramp in Presence of STF
Blank dual-responsive in situ gel	tan δ > 1 in the range of 20–33 °C and tan δ = 1 at 34 °C	tan δ >> 1 in the range of 20–33 °C and tan δ = 1 at 34 °C	tan δ < 1 in the range of 20–30 °C and tan δ << 1 in the range of 30–37 °C
NEB-loaded dual-responsive in situ gel	20–30 tan δ > 1 At 32 °C tan δ = 1	tan δ >> 1 in the range of 20–32 °C and tan δ = 1 at 33 °C	tan δ < 1 in the range of 20–31 °C and tan δ << 1 in the range of 31–37 °C

Note—tan δ >> 1 indicates low storage modulus with no gelation (liquid state); tan δ > 1 indicates increased storage modulus with no gelation; tan δ = 1 indicates gelling point; tan δ < 1 indicates gelling with high storage modulus (gel with low viscosity) and tan δ << 1 indicates gelling with very high storage modulus (gel with high viscosity).

The data obtained from the storage modulus (G′) of the in situ gels further supported the inferences made from the loss factor values. The G′ values of NEB-loaded dual-responsive in situ gels, in the presence of deionised water, were low in the temperature range of 20–31 °C. However, the G′ values increased steeply in the temperature range of 31 to 34 °C, suggesting a significant increase in the viscosity of the formulation due to the sol-to-gel transition caused by the thermo-responsive polymer. In the presence of STF, NEB-loaded dual-responsive in situ gels exhibited higher G′ values even in the temperature range of 20 to 30 °C, which further increased in temperature range of 30 to 34 °C. Higher G′ values even in the temperature range of 20 to 30 °C were due to the gelation of the ion-responsive polymer (κCRG) caused by the cations present in STF. The spike in G′ values in the temperature range of 30 to 34 °C was due to the increase in viscosity caused by the thermo-responsive polymer mixture (P407 + P188).

3.4. Mucoadhesion Study of the Blank In Situ Gels

In situ gels with good mucoadhesive characteristics can improve the overall permeation of the drug through the corneal membrane by providing intimate contact with the corneal membrane and also increasing the residence time. A texture analyser was used to evaluate the mucoadhesive properties of blank in situ gels. The blank P407 + P188 in situ gel (0.145 N) exhibited relatively low mucoadhesive properties compared to the bank κCRG in situ gel (0.253 N). This can be attributed to the large molecular weight and secondary interactions (hydrogen bonding) of κCRG with the mucin [52]. The blank dual-responsive in situ gel showed slightly more mucoadhesion compared to the blank κCRG in situ gel (0.289 N), possibly due to the additive effect of the individual polymers in the dual-responsive in situ gel (Figure 5).

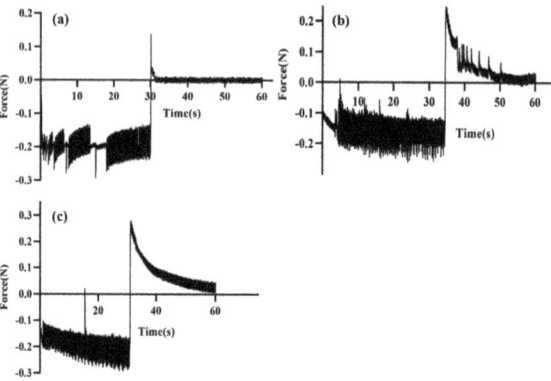

Figure 5. Mucoadhesive behaviour of (**a**) blank (P407 + P188) in situ gel, (**b**) blank κCRG in situ gel and (**c**) blank dual-responsive in situ gel, expressed in terms of mucoadhesion force (N).

3.5. In Vitro Drug Release Studies of NEB-Loaded In Situ Gels

In vitro drug release studies were performed in STF (pH 7.4 ± 0.5) containing Tween 80 (0.5% *w/v*). The solubility of the NEB in STF was 28.62 µg/mL. Therefore, to maintain the sink condition, 100 mL of STF containing 0.5% *w/v* of Tween 80 was used in the study. The mean cumulative percentage of drug released vs. time was plotted from the in vitro dissolution data (Figure 6). The NEB suspension was dissolved completely within 30 min. The NEB-loaded P407 + P188 in situ gel and NEB-loaded κCRG in situ gel showed 90% drug release within 8 h and 12 h, respectively. The optimized NEB-loaded dual-responsive in situ gel slowed and prolonged the drug release, with 86% drug release at the end of 24 h. This can be attributed to the interaction of κCRG with the micelles of (P407 + P188) through secondary bonds, such as hydrogen bonds, resulting in increased viscosity of the gel formed, which is in line with the observations made from the rheological evaluation of the in situ gels. Increase in gel viscosity reduced the diffusivity of the drug through the gel matrix [23]. The drug release from the NEB-loaded dual-responsive in situ gel as well as the NEB-loaded P407 + P188 in situ gel and NEB-loaded κCRG in situ gel followed Higuchi kinetics. The value of n in the Korsmeyer–Peppas equation for the NEB-loaded dual-responsive in situ gel was found to be 0.77, suggesting the release of NEB was due to the combined effect of Fickian diffusion and matrix erosion.

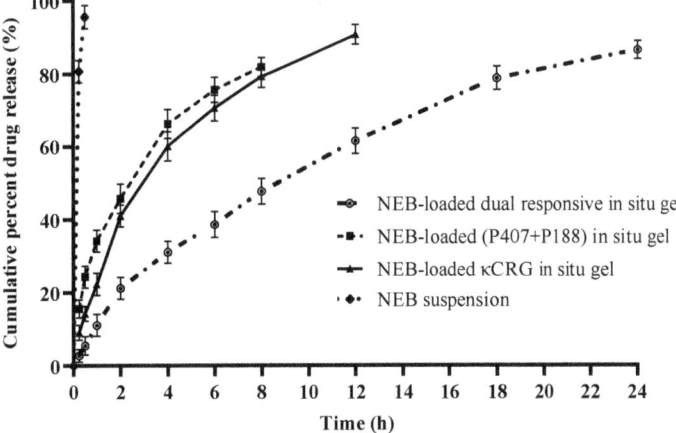

Figure 6. In vitro drug release profiles of an NEB suspension, NEB-loaded (P407 + P188) in situ gel, NEB-loaded κCRG in situ gel and NEB-loaded dual-responsive in situ gel. Each data point is the mean cumulative percent of NEB released (± SD) of three independent formulations (*n* = 3).

3.6. Ex Vivo Ocular Irritation Test (HET-CAM) of the Optimized In Situ Gels

The images obtained from the HET-CAM test of the various treatments are presented in Figure 7. The positive control caused significant damage to the CAM within 30 s, resulting in coagulation and haemorrhages followed by the lysis of blood vessels in the CAM (Figure 5B). The irritation severity score of the positive control was found to be 18. The negative control (0.9% *w/v* NaCl solution), blank and NEB-loaded dual-responsive in situ gels did not cause any inflammatory changes in the CAM. No visible changes were observed in terms coagulation/haemorrhage/lysis of the blood vessels in the CAM upon treatment with the negative control or in situ gels. The irritation severity score of the negative control, blank and NEB-loaded dual-responsive in situ gels were 0. Based on the results obtained from the HET-CAM test, it can be inferred that the optimized NEB-loaded dual-responsive in situ gel is safe and well tolerated by ocular tissues.

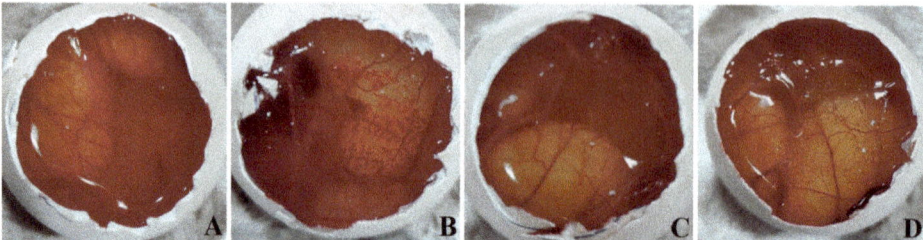

Figure 7. Images obtained from the HET-CAM test following the exposure of the CAM membrane to (**A**) negative control (0.9% *w/v* NaCl); (**B**) positive control (0.1 N NaOH); (**C**) blank dual-responsive in situ gel and (**D**) NEB-loaded dual-responsive in situ gel.

3.7. Hemolysis Study of the Optimized In Situ Gels

The RBCs treated with the optimized in situ gels (blank and NEB-loaded dual-responsive in situ gel) were checked for their shape and size (40× magnification). The morphology of the RBCs was found to be intact when treated with the negative control sample (STF pH 7.4), blank and NEB-loaded in situ gels. However, the RBCs incubated with Triton X-100 were completely lysed, as shown in Figure 8. The haemolysis (%) values of the RBCs incubated with the blank and NEB-loaded dual-responsive in situ gels were found to be 1.1% and 1.16%, respectively. These results suggest that optimized the NEB-loaded dual-responsive in situ gel is isotonic and biocompatible with no/minimal detectable disruption of RBCs.

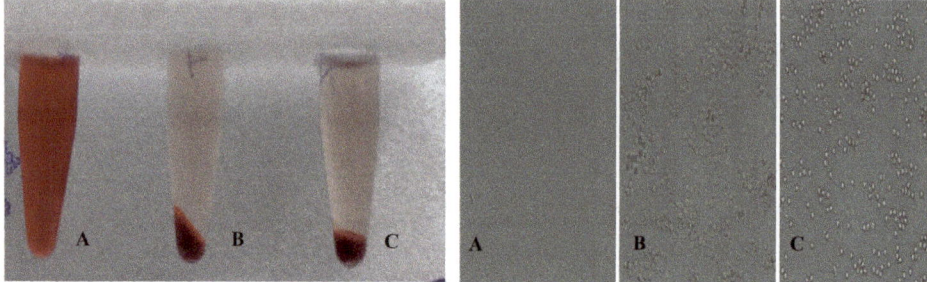

Figure 8. Results obtained from haemolysis studies of RBCs treated with (**A**) positive control (Triton X-100); (**B**) negative control (0.9% *w/v* NaCl) and (**C**) NEB-loaded dual-responsive in situ gel.

3.8. Ocular Histopathology Studies of the Optimized In Situ Gels

Microscopic examinations of the corneal structure incubated with STF (negative control) showed intact epithelium and stroma without any sign of tissue damage (Figure 9). There was visible disruption of the epithelium and stroma with tissue necrosis in the presence of 75% *v/v* isopropyl alcohol (positive control). The cornea treated with the optimized in situ gels (blank and NEB-loaded dual-responsive in situ gel) did not show any significant difference as compared to the STF-treated cornea. We can infer that the optimized formulations are safe and do not alter the structural integrity of the cornea.

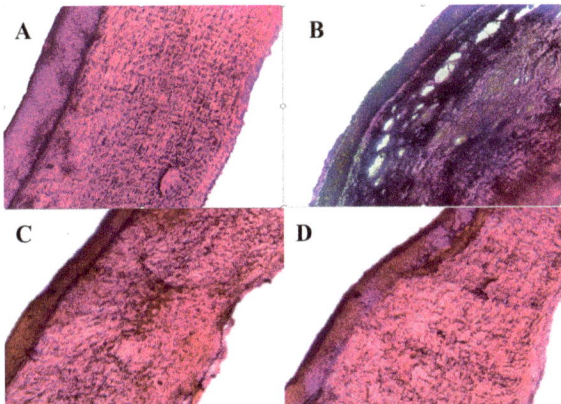

Figure 9. Microscopic images of the cornea exposed to (**A**) negative control (STF, pH 7.4); (**B**) positive control (IPA, 75% *v/v*); (**C**) blank dual-responsive in situ gel and (**D**) NEB-loaded dual-responsive in situ gel.

3.9. In Vivo Studies of the Optimized NEB-Loaded Dual-Responsive In Situ Gel

3.9.1. Pharmacokinetic Study

The time course profiles of NEB in aqueous humor and plasma following the ocular administration of the NEB suspension and the optimized NEB-loaded dual-responsive in situ gel (at drug dose of 0.05 mg/kg) are shown in Figure 10a,b, respectively. The ocular and plasma pharmacokinetic data obtained in the study were subjected to non-compartmental analysis using Pheonix WinNonLin software (version 8.3.3.33, Pharsight Corporation, Raleigh, NC, USA) to determine pharmacokinetic parameters such as maximum concentration of NEB (C_{max}), time to reach maximum concentration of NEB (T_{max}), area under the course curve between zero to time 't' (AUC_{0-t}), area under the curve between 't = 0' and 't = ∞' ($AUC_{0-\infty}$) and mean residence time between 't = 0' and 't = ∞' ($MRT_{0-\infty}$). The pharmacokinetic parameters are presented in Table 5.

Table 5. Pharmacokinetic parameters of NEB in aqueous humor and plasma following ocular administration of an NEB suspension and optimized NEB-loaded dual-responsive in situ gel in male New Zealand white rabbits.

Biological Matrix	Parameters	Units	Treatments	
			NEB Suspension	NEB In Situ Gel
Aqueous humor	C_{max}	ng/mL	28.2 ± 3.1	35.14 ± 2.25 *
	T_{max}	h	2	4
	AUC_{0-24}	ng/mL * h	189.0 ± 13.14	364.1 ± 16.76 ***
	$AUC_{0-\infty}$	ng/mL * h	194.9 ± 12.17	381.8 ± 18.32 ***
	$MRT_{0-\infty}$	h	6.12 ± 0.178	8.11 ± 0.12 ***
Plasma	C_{max}	ng/mL	1.8 ± 0.01	0.6 ± 0.01 ***
	T_{max}	h	0.5	1
	AUC_{0-24}	ng/mL * h	20.2 ± 2.7	4.1 ± 0.2 ***
	$AUC_{0-\infty}$	ng/mL * h	33.2 ± 2.1	8.0 ± 0.43 ***
	$MRT_{0-\infty}$	h	25.8 ± 1.5	11.01 ± 0.6 ***

Each value represents the mean ± SD of four independent determinations ($n = 4$). * Statistically significant difference ($P_{cal} < 0.05$) was observed when compared against the NEB suspension. *** Statistically significant difference ($P_{cal} < 0.0001$) was observed when compared against the NEB suspension.

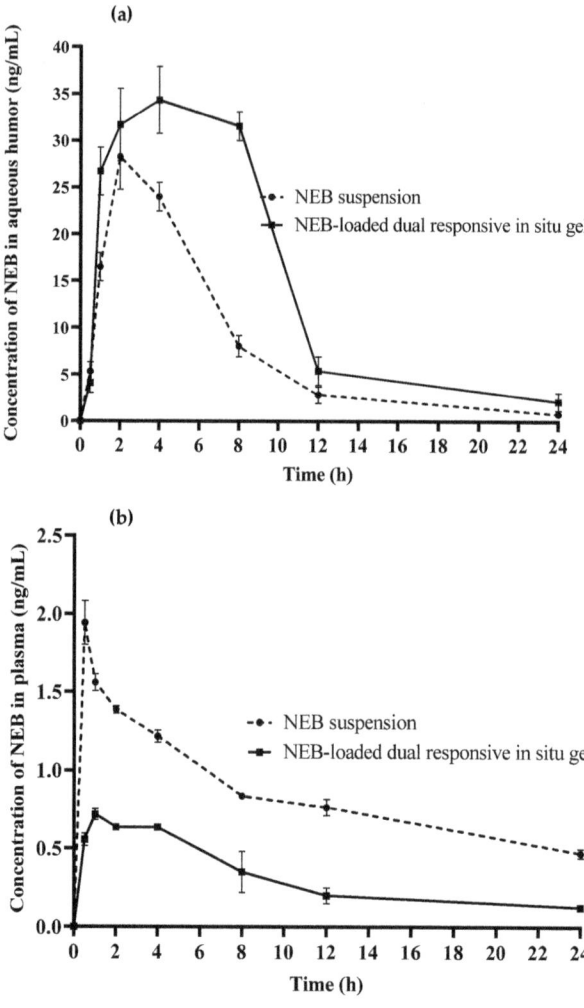

Figure 10. Mean concentration versus time profiles obtained following ocular administration of NEB suspension and optimized NEB in-situ gel in male New Zealand white rabbits (**a**) in aqueous humor and (**b**) in plasma. Each data point represents the mean of four independent determinations ($n = 4$).

The aqueous humor C_{max} (35.14 ± 2.25 ng/mL) and $AUC_{0-\infty}$ (381.8 ± 18.32 ng/mL*h) of the NEB-loaded dual-responsive in situ gel were 1.2 fold ($P_{cal} < 0.05$) and 2 fold ($P_{cal} < 0.0001$) higher as compared with the C_{max} (28.2 ± 3.1 ng/mL) and $AUC_{0-\infty}$ (194.9 ± 12.17 ng/mL*h) of the NEB suspension, respectively. Higher C_{max} and $AUC_{0-\infty}$ suggests that a greater amount of NEB could permeate across the cornea and reach the aqueous humor in the case of the NEB-loaded dual-responsive in situ gel compared with the NEB suspension. This could be due to the lesser drug loss, lesser drug dilution and intimate contact between the gel and cornea for efficient permeation of the drug offered by the in situ gel compared to the suspension. Furthermore, the $MRT_{0-\infty}$ values of the in situ gel (8.11 ± 0.12 h) were significantly higher ($P_{cal} < 0.0001$) than those of the NEB suspension (6.12 ± 0.18 h). This indicates that the in situ gel sustained the concentrations of NEB in the aqueous humor for a longer duration compared with the NEB suspension. This could be due to the ability of the in situ gel to resist nasolacrimal drainage for a longer duration compared to the suspension by forming a viscous gel at the precorneal area. Since the in situ gel remained in the precorneal area for a longer duration, the drug permeation into the aqueous humor was more sustained.

In ocular drug delivery, systemic side effects resulting from unwanted absorption of the drug into systemic circulation is a major cause of concern. Ocular drug products of β-adrenergic antagonists (like timolol, betaxolol etc.) used in the long-term treatment of glaucoma suffer from systemic side effects like bradycardia, reduced blood pressure and an irregular pulse [53]. An ocular drug product which results in lesser systemic exposure of the drug will have a relatively low side effect profile.

The C_{max} (0.69 ± 0.01 ng/mL) and $AUC_{0-\infty}$ (8.05 ± 0.43 ng/mL*h) in plasma of the NEB-loaded dual-responsive in situ gel were 2.7 fold (P_{cal} < 0.0001) and 4.1 fold (P_{cal} < 0.0001) lower as compared with the C_{max} (1.86 ± 0.01 ng/mL) and $AUC_{0-\infty}$ (33.21 ± 2.1 ng/mL*h) in plasma of the NEB suspension, respectively. Based on the data obtained, we can infer that the in situ gel resulted in significantly lower systemic exposure compared to the NEB suspension. Following ocular administration, the in situ gel forms a viscous gel layer with mucoadhesive properties on the surface of cornea through which the drug permeates into the aqueous humor. This pathway of drug permeation is considered more productive in reaching the target sites of the iris/ciliary body for the treatment of glaucoma. In the case of suspension, the drug present in a dissolved state in the lachrymal fluids could spread on the cornea and conjunctiva. Since the conjunctival membranes are highly vascularized, drugs that are in contact with conjunctiva permeate through it and reach systemic circulation. In addition, the naso-lachrimal drainage system can draw drugs present in the dissolved state into the lachrymal fluids and into the nasal cavity, from which the drug can get absorbed into systemic circulation. The plasma $MRT_{0-\infty}$ of the in situ gel (11.0 ± 0.6 h) was significantly (P_{cal} < 0.0001) lower than that of the NEB suspension (25.8 ± 1.5 h). The concentrations of NEB in systemic circulation were sustained for more time in the case of the NEB suspension compared to the in situ gel. This suggests that the in situ gel significantly decreases the duration for which the systemic side effects would be experienced by the patients compared to the NEB suspension. Overall, the pharmacokinetic studies indicate that NEB-loaded dual-responsive in situ gels produce higher and sustained concentrations of NEB at the aqueous humor as well as reduce the intensity and duration of systemic side effects of the drug.

3.9.2. Pharmacodynamic Study

The percentage reduction in IOP [$\Delta IOP(\%)$] versus time profiles of the NEB-loaded dual-responsive in situ gel and NEB suspension are presented in Figure 11. The pharmacodynamic data [$\Delta IOP(\%)$ versus time] of the two formulations was analysed using NCA to determine parameters such as area under the curve between 't = 0' and 't = 12 h' (AUC_{0-12h}) and mean response time between 't = 0' and 't = 12 h' (MRT_{0-12h}). The AUC_{0-12h} of the NEB-loaded dual-responsive in situ gel (137.04) was 1.85 fold higher (P_{cal} < 0.0001) compared with that of the NEB suspension (74.21). A higher pharmacodynamic response was observed for the in situ gel compared to the NEB suspension. In addition, the MRT_{0-12h} of the in situ gel (6.1 h) was higher compared to the that of the NEB suspension (4.06 h). The NEB-loaded dual-responsive in situ gel could provide a sustained pharmacodynamic effect compared to the NEB suspension. These results are in line with the data obtained in the pharmacokinetic studies, which clearly indicated a higher and sustained concentration of NEB in the aqueous humor for NEB-loaded dual-responsive in situ gel compared to NEB suspension.

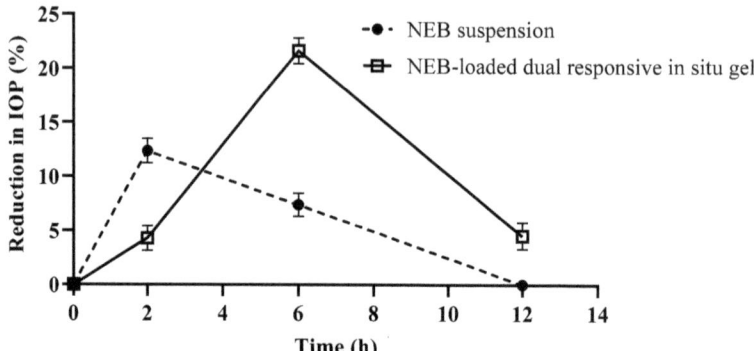

Figure 11. Percentage reduction in intra-ocular pressure [ΔIOP (%)] versus time profiles obtained following ocular administration of an NEB suspension and optimized NEB-loaded dual-responsive in situ gel at a drug dose of 0.05 mg/kg in male New Zealand white rabbits ($n = 6$).

4. Conclusions

In the present study, NEB-loaded dual-responsive in situ gels containing a mixture of P407 + P188 as a thermo-responsive polymer and κCRG as an ion-responsive polymer was successfully developed and optimized using BBD. The optimized dual-responsive in situ gel exhibited the desired flow properties at room temperature while undergoing rapid sol-to-gel transition at physiological temperature in the presence of STF. The dual-responsive in situ gel was well tolerated with no signs of irritation/inflammation of the eye. The formulation showed good mucoadhesive characteristics. Ocular pharmacokinetic studies revealed that the optimized NEB-loaded dual-responsive in situ gel could enhance the ocular bioavailability with minimum systemic exposure compared to NEB suspensions. The pharmacodynamic studies established the efficacy of the NEB-loaded dual-responsive in situ gel in reducing the IOP compared to the NEB suspension. The results obtained in the current research showed that optimized NEB-loaded dual-responsive in situ gels can be a promising drug delivery system for the effective treatment of glaucoma.

Author Contributions: Conceptualization, P.S.R. and P.R.R.; methodology, S.I.M., P.S.R. and P.R.R.; software, S.I.M., P.S.R. and P.R.R.; validation, S.I.M., P.S.R. and P.R.R.; formal analysis, S.I.M., P.S.R., M.S.K., P.K. and U.B.; investigation, S.I.M., P.S.R., M.S.K., P.K. and U.B.; resources, P.S.R. and P.R.R.; data curation, P.R.R. and H.K.; writing—original draft preparation, S.I.M. and P.S.R.; writing—review and editing, P.R.R. and H.K.; visualization, P.R.R. and H.K.; supervision, P.R.R.; project administration, P.R.R.; funding acquisition, P.S.R. and P.R.R. All authors have read and agreed to the published version of the manuscript.

Funding: This research received no external funding. All the resources were provided by BITS Pilani Hyderabad Campus.

Institutional Review Board Statement: The animal study protocol was approved by the Institutional Animal Ethics Committee of VIMTA Labs, Hyderabad, India (Protocol No.: VLL/1122/NG/1099 dated 22 November 2022) for studies involving animals.

Informed Consent Statement: Not applicable.

Data Availability Statement: Not applicable.

Conflicts of Interest: The authors declare no conflict of interest.

References

1. Weinreb, R.N.; Aung, T.; Medeiros, F.A. The Pathophysiology and Treatment of Glaucoma: A Review. *Jama* **2014**, *311*, 1901–1911. [CrossRef] [PubMed]
2. Gazzard, G.; Foster, P.J.; Devereux, J.G.; Oen, F.; Chew, P.; Khaw, P.T.; Seah, S. Intraocular Pressure and Visual Field Loss in Primary Angle Closure and Primary Open Angle Glaucomas. *Br. J. Ophthalmol.* **2003**, *87*, 720–725. [CrossRef] [PubMed]

3. Toris, C.B.; Gagrani, M.; Ghate, D. Current Methods and New Approaches to Assess Aqueous Humor Dynamics. *Expert Rev. Ophthalmol.* **2021**, *16*, 139–160. [CrossRef]
4. Anne, M.V.; Gillies, W.E. Ocular β-Blockers in Glaucoma Management. *Drugs Aging* **1992**, *2*, 208–221.
5. Taniguchi, T.; Kitazawa, Y. The Potential Systemic Effect of Topically Applied Beta-Blockers in Glaucoma Therapy. *Curr. Opin. Ophthalmol.* **1997**, *8*, 55–58. [CrossRef]
6. Buckley, M.M.-T.; Goa, K.L.; Clissold, S.P. Ocular Betaxolol. *Drugs* **1990**, *40*, 75–90. [CrossRef]
7. Szumny, D.; Szelag, A. The Influence of New Beta-Adrenolytics Nebivolol and Carvedilol on Intraocular Pressure and Iris Blood Flow in Rabbits. *Graefe's Arch. Clin. Exp. Ophthalmol.* **2014**, *252*, 917–923. [CrossRef]
8. Wareham, L.K.; Buys, E.S.; Sappington, R.M. The Nitric Oxide-Guanylate Cyclase Pathway and Glaucoma. *Nitric Oxide* **2018**, *77*, 75–87. [CrossRef]
9. Qi, H.; Chen, W.; Huang, C.; Li, L.; Chen, C.; Li, W.; Wu, C. Development of a Poloxamer Analogs/Carbopol-Based in Situ Gelling and Mucoadhesive Ophthalmic Delivery System for Puerarin. *Int. J. Pharm.* **2007**, *337*, 178–187. [CrossRef]
10. Gupta, H.; Jain, S.; Mathur, R.; Mishra, P.; Mishra, A.K.; Velpandian, T. Sustained Ocular Drug Delivery from a Temperature and PH Triggered Novel in Situ Gel System. *Drug Deliv.* **2007**, *14*, 507–515. [CrossRef]
11. Nagarwal, R.C.; Kant, S.; Singh, P.N.; Maiti, P.; Pandit, J.K. Polymeric Nanoparticulate System: A Potential Approach for Ocular Drug Delivery. *J. Control. Release* **2009**, *136*, 2–13. [CrossRef] [PubMed]
12. Chowhan, A.; Giri, T.K. Polysaccharide as Renewable Responsive Biopolymer for in Situ Gel in the Delivery of Drug through Ocular Route. *Int. J. Biol. Macromol.* **2020**, *150*, 559–572. [CrossRef] [PubMed]
13. Yoshida, M.; Langer, R.; Lendlein, A.; Lahann, J. From Advanced Biomedical Coatings to Multi-functionalized Biomaterials. *J. Macromol. Sci. Part C Polym. Rev.* **2006**, *46*, 347–375. [CrossRef]
14. Nastyshyn, S.; Stetsyshyn, Y.; Raczkowska, J.; Nastishin, Y.; Melnyk, Y.; Panchenko, Y.; Budkowski, A. Temperature-Responsive Polymer Brush Coatings for Advanced Biomedical Applications. *Polymers* **2022**, *14*, 4245. [CrossRef]
15. Goel, M.; Picciani, R.G.; Lee, R.K.; Bhattacharya, S.K. Aqueous Humor Dynamics: A Review. *Open Ophthalmol. J.* **2010**, *4*, 52. [CrossRef]
16. Fabiani, C.; Li Voti, R.; Rusciano, D.; Mutolo, M.G.; Pescosolido, N. Relationship between Corneal Temperature and Intraocular Pressure in Healthy Individuals: A Clinical Thermographic Analysis. *J. Ophthalmol.* **2016**, *2016*, 3076031. [CrossRef] [PubMed]
17. Chassenieux, C.; Tsitsilianis, C. Recent Trends in PH/Thermo-Responsive Self-Assembling Hydrogels: From Polyions to Peptide-Based Polymeric Gelators. *Soft Matter* **2016**, *12*, 1344–1359. [CrossRef]
18. Carlfors, K.E.J.; Petersson, R. Rheological Evaluation of Poloxamer as an in Situ Gel for Ophthalmic Use. *Eur. J. Pharm. Sci.* **1998**, *6*, 105–112. [CrossRef]
19. Dumortier, G.; Grossiord, J.L.; Agnely, F.; Chaumeil, J.C. A Review of Poloxamer 407 Pharmaceutical and Pharmacological Characteristics. *Pharm. Res.* **2006**, *23*, 2709–2728. [CrossRef]
20. Swain, G.P.; Patel, S.; Gandhi, J.; Shah, P. Development of Moxifloxacin Hydrochloride Loaded In-Situ Gel for the Treatment of Periodontitis: In-Vitro Drug Release Study and Antibacterial Activity. *J. Oral Biol. Craniofacial Res.* **2019**, *9*, 190–200. [CrossRef]
21. Zia, K.M.; Tabasum, S.; Nasif, M.; Sultan, N.; Aslam, N.; Noreen, A.; Zuber, M. A Review on Synthesis, Properties and Applications of Natural Polymer Based Carrageenan Blends and Composites. *Int. J. Biol. Macromol.* **2017**, *96*, 282–301. [CrossRef]
22. Bhowmick, B.; Sarkar, G.; Rana, D.; Roy, I.; Saha, N.R.; Ghosh, S.; Bhowmik, M.; Chattopadhyay, D. Effect of Carrageenan and Potassium Chloride on an in Situ Gelling Ophthalmic Drug Delivery System Based on Methylcellulose. *RSC Adv.* **2015**, *5*, 60386–60391. [CrossRef]
23. Liu, Y.; Zhu, Y.; Wei, G.; Lu, W.-Y. Effect of Carrageenan on Poloxamer-Based in Situ Gel for Vaginal Use: Improved in Vitro and in Vivo Sustained-Release Properties. *Eur. J. Pharm. Sci.* **2009**, *37*, 306–312. [CrossRef] [PubMed]
24. Li, C.; Li, C.; Liu, Z.; Li, Q.; Yan, X.; Liu, Y.; Lu, W. Enhancement in Bioavailability of Ketorolac Tromethamine via Intranasal in Situ Hydrogel Based on Poloxamer 407 and Carrageenan. *Int. J. Pharm.* **2014**, *474*, 123–133. [CrossRef] [PubMed]
25. Rawat, P.S.; Ravi, P.R.; Kaswan, L.; Raghuvanshi, R.S. Development and Validation of a Bio-Analytical Method for Simultaneous Quantification of Nebivolol and Labetalol in Aqueous Humor and Plasma Using LC-MS/MS and Its Application to Ocular Pharmacokinetic Studies. *J. Chromatogr. B* **2020**, *1136*, 121908. [CrossRef]
26. Hirun, N.; Kraisit, P.; Tantishaiyakul, V. Thermosensitive Polymer Blend Composed of Poloxamer 407, Poloxamer 188 and Polycarbophil for the Use as Mucoadhesive In Situ Gel. *Polymers* **2022**, *14*, 1836. [CrossRef]
27. Vijaya, C.; Goud, K.S. Ion-Activated in Situ Gelling Ophthalmic Delivery Systems of Azithromycin. *Indian J. Pharm. Sci.* **2011**, *73*, 615. [CrossRef]
28. Xiong, W.; Gao, X.; Zhao, Y.; Xu, H.; Yang, X. The Dual Temperature/PH-Sensitive Multiphase Behavior of Poly (N-Isopropylacrylamide-Co-Acrylic Acid) Microgels for Potential Application in in Situ Gelling System. *Colloids Surf. B Biointerfaces* **2011**, *84*, 103–110. [CrossRef]
29. Mandal, S.; Thimmasetty, M.K.M.J.; Prabhushankar, G.L.; Geetha, M.S. Formulation and Evaluation of an in Situ Gel-Forming Ophthalmic Formulation of Moxifloxacin Hydrochloride. *Int. J. Pharm. Investig.* **2012**, *2*, 78. [CrossRef]
30. Okur, N.Ü.; Yozgatli, V.; Okur, M.E. In Vitro–in Vivo Evaluation of Tetrahydrozoline-loaded Ocular in Situ Gels on Rabbits for Allergic Conjunctivitis Management. *Drug Dev. Res.* **2020**, *81*, 716–727. [CrossRef]
31. Kaur, H.; Ioyee, S.; Garg, R. Formulation and Evaluation of In-Situ Ocular Gel of Gatifloxacin. *Int. J. Pharm. Res. Heal. Sci.* **2016**, *4*, 1365–1370. [CrossRef]

32. Ceulemans, J.; Ludwig, A. Optimisation of Carbomer Viscous Eye Drops: An in Vitro Experimental Design Approach Using Rheological Techniques. *Eur. J. Pharm. Biopharm.* **2002**, *54*, 41–50. [CrossRef] [PubMed]
33. Gratieri, T.; Gelfuso, G.M.; Rocha, E.M.; Sarmento, V.H.; de Freitas, O.; Lopez, R.F.V. A Poloxamer/Chitosan in Situ Forming Gel with Prolonged Retention Time for Ocular Delivery. *Eur. J. Pharm. Biopharm.* **2010**, *75*, 186–193. [CrossRef]
34. Destruel, P.-L.; Zeng, N.; Maury, M.; Mignet, N.; Boudy, V. In Vitro and in Vivo Evaluation of in Situ Gelling Systems for Sustained Topical Ophthalmic Delivery: State of the Art and Beyond. *Drug Discov. Today* **2017**, *22*, 638–651. [CrossRef]
35. Weng, L.; Chen, X.; Chen, W. Rheological Characterization of in Situ Crosslinkable Hydrogels Formulated from Oxidized Dextran and N-Carboxyethyl Chitosan. *Biomacromolecules* **2007**, *8*, 1109–1115. [CrossRef] [PubMed]
36. Woertz, C.; Preis, M.; Breitkreutz, J.; Kleinebudde, P. Assessment of Test Methods Evaluating Mucoadhesive Polymers and Dosage Forms: An Overview. *Eur. J. Pharm. Biopharm.* **2013**, *85*, 843–853. [CrossRef]
37. Kiss, E.L.; Berkó, S.; Gácsi, A.; Kovács, A.; Katona, G.; Soós, J.; Csányi, E.; Gróf, I.; Harazin, A.; Deli, M.A. Development and Characterization of Potential Ocular Mucoadhesive Nano Lipid Carriers Using Full Factorial Design. *Pharmaceutics* **2020**, *12*, 682. [CrossRef]
38. Lin, H.-R.; Sung, K.C. Carbopol/Pluronic Phase Change Solutions for Ophthalmic Drug Delivery. *J. Control. Release* **2000**, *69*, 379–388. [CrossRef]
39. Abrego, G.; Alvarado, H.; Souto, E.B.; Guevara, B.; Bellowa, L.H.; Parra, A.; Calpena, A.; Garcia, M.L. Biopharmaceutical Profile of Pranoprofen-Loaded PLGA Nanoparticles Containing Hydrogels for Ocular Administration. *Eur. J. Pharm. Biopharm.* **2015**, *95*, 261–270. [CrossRef]
40. Peppas, N.A.; Sahlin, J.J. A Simple Equation for the Description of Solute Release. III. Coupling of Diffusion and Relaxation. *Int. J. Pharm.* **1989**, *57*, 169–172. [CrossRef]
41. Moosa, R.M.; Choonara, Y.E.; du Toit, L.C.; Tomar, L.K.; Tyagi, C.; Kumar, P.; Carmichael, T.R.; Pillay, V. In Vivo Evaluation and In-Depth Pharmaceutical Characterization of a Rapidly Dissolving Solid Ocular Matrix for the Topical Delivery of Timolol Maleate in the Rabbit Eye Model. *Int. J. Pharm.* **2014**, *466*, 296–306. [CrossRef] [PubMed]
42. Batista-Duharte, A.; Jorge Murillo, G.; Pérez, U.M.; Tur, E.N.; Portuondo, D.F.; Martínez, B.T.; Téllez-Martínez, D.; Betancourt, J.E.; Pérez, O. The Hen's Egg Test on Chorioallantoic Membrane: An Alternative Assay for the Assessment of the Irritating Effect of Vaccine Adjuvants. *Int. J. Toxicol.* **2016**, *35*, 627–633. [CrossRef]
43. Terreni, E.; Chetoni, P.; Burgalassi, S.; Tampucci, S.; Zucchetti, E.; Chipala, E.; Alany, R.G.; Al-Kinani, A.A.; Monti, D. A Hybrid Ocular Delivery System of Cyclosporine-A Comprising Nanomicelle-Laden Polymeric Inserts with Improved Efficacy and Tolerability. *Biomater. Sci.* **2021**, *9*, 8235–8248. [CrossRef] [PubMed]
44. Arruda, I.R.S.; Albuquerque, P.B.S.; Santos, G.R.C.; Silva, A.G.; Mourão, P.A.S.; Correia, M.T.S.; Vicente, A.A.; Carneiro-da-Cunha, M.G. Structure and Rheological Properties of a Xyloglucan Extracted from Hymenaea Courbaril Var. Courbaril Seeds. *Int. J. Biol. Macromol.* **2015**, *73*, 31–38. [CrossRef]
45. Kaur, G.; Singh, D.; Brar, V. Bioadhesive Okra Polymer Based Buccal Patches as Platform for Controlled Drug Delivery. *Int. J. Biol. Macromol.* **2014**, *70*, 408–419. [CrossRef] [PubMed]
46. Kimna, C.; Winkeljann, B.; Hoffmeister, J.; Lieleg, O. Biopolymer-Based Nanoparticles with Tunable Mucoadhesivity Efficiently Deliver Therapeutics across the Corneal Barrier. *Mater. Sci. Eng. C* **2021**, *121*, 111890. [CrossRef] [PubMed]
47. Li, J.; Liu, H.; Liu, L.; Cai, C.; Xin, H.; Liu, W. Design and Evaluation of a Brinzolamide Drug-Resin in Situ Thermosensitive Gelling System for Sustained Ophthalmic Drug Delivery. *Chem. Pharm. Bull.* **2014**, c14-00451. [CrossRef] [PubMed]
48. Diwan, R.; Ravi, P.R.; Agarwal, S.I.; Aggarwal, V. Cilnidipine Loaded Poly (ε-Caprolactone) Nanoparticles for Enhanced Oral Delivery: Optimization Using DoE, Physical Characterization, Pharmacokinetic, and Pharmacodynamic Evaluation. *Pharm. Dev. Technol.* **2021**, *26*, 278–290. [CrossRef]
49. Reddy, I.K.; Vaithiyalingam, S.R.; Khan, M.A.; Bodor, N.S. Intraocular Pressure-Lowering Activity and in Vivo Disposition of Dipivalyl Terbutalone in Rabbits. *Drug Dev. Ind. Pharm.* **2001**, *27*, 137–141. [CrossRef]
50. Huang, W.; Zhang, N.; Hua, H.; Liu, T.; Tang, Y.; Fu, L.; Yang, Y.; Ma, X.; Zhao, Y. Preparation, Pharmacokinetics and Pharmacodynamics of Ophthalmic Thermosensitive in Situ Hydrogel of Betaxolol Hydrochloride. *Biomed. Pharmacother.* **2016**, *83*, 107–113. [CrossRef]
51. Bron, A.J.; Willshire, C. Tear Osmolarity in the Diagnosis of Systemic Dehydration and Dry Eye Disease. *Diagnostics* **2021**, *11*, 387. [CrossRef] [PubMed]
52. Yermak, I.M.; Davydova, V.N.; Kravchenko, A.O.; Chistyulin, D.A.; Pimenova, E.A.; Glazunov, V.P. Mucoadhesive Properties of Sulphated Polysaccharides Carrageenans from Red Seaweed Families Gigartinaceae and Tichocarpaceae. *Int. J. Biol. Macromol.* **2020**, *142*, 634–642. [CrossRef] [PubMed]
53. Inoue, K. Managing Adverse Effects of Glaucoma Medications. *Clin. Ophthalmol.* **2014**, *8*, 903. [CrossRef] [PubMed]

Disclaimer/Publisher's Note: The statements, opinions and data contained in all publications are solely those of the individual author(s) and contributor(s) and not of MDPI and/or the editor(s). MDPI and/or the editor(s) disclaim responsibility for any injury to people or property resulting from any ideas, methods, instructions or products referred to in the content.

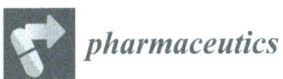 *pharmaceutics*

Article

Cannabidiol Loaded Topical Ophthalmic Nanoemulsion Lowers Intraocular Pressure in Normotensive Dutch-Belted Rabbits

Samir Senapati [1,†], Ahmed Adel Ali Youssef [1,2,†], Corinne Sweeney [1], Chuntian Cai [1], Narendar Dudhipala [1] and Soumyajit Majumdar [1,3,*]

1. Department of Pharmaceutics and Drug Delivery, School of Pharmacy, University of Mississippi, Oxford, MS 38677, USA
2. Department of Pharmaceutical Technology, Faculty of Pharmacy, Kafrelsheikh University, Kafrelsheikh 33516, Egypt
3. Research Institute of Pharmaceutical Sciences, University of Mississippi, Oxford, MS 38677, USA
* Correspondence: majumso@olemiss.edu; Tel.: +1-662-9153793
† These authors contributed equally to this work.

Citation: Senapati, S.; Youssef, A.A.A.; Sweeney, C.; Cai, C.; Dudhipala, N.; Majumdar, S. Cannabidiol Loaded Topical Ophthalmic Nanoemulsion Lowers Intraocular Pressure in Normotensive Dutch-Belted Rabbits. *Pharmaceutics* **2022**, *14*, 2585. https://doi.org/10.3390/pharmaceutics14122585

Academic Editors: Ana Catarina Silva and Hugo Almeida

Received: 30 October 2022
Accepted: 21 November 2022
Published: 24 November 2022

Publisher's Note: MDPI stays neutral with regard to jurisdictional claims in published maps and institutional affiliations.

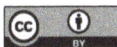

Copyright: © 2022 by the authors. Licensee MDPI, Basel, Switzerland. This article is an open access article distributed under the terms and conditions of the Creative Commons Attribution (CC BY) license (https://creativecommons.org/licenses/by/4.0/).

Abstract: Cannabidiol (CBD) is the major non-psychoactive and most widely studied of the cannabinoid constituents and has great therapeutic potential in a variety of diseases. However, contradictory reports in the literature with respect to CBD's effect on intraocular pressure (IOP) have raised concerns and halted research exploring its use in ocular therapeutics. Therefore, the current investigation aimed to further evaluate CBD's impact on the IOP in the rabbit model. CBD nanoemulsions, containing Carbopol® 940 NF as a mucoadhesive agent (CBD-NEC), were prepared using hot-homogenization followed by probe sonication. The stability of the formulations post-moist-heat sterilization, in terms of physical and chemical characteristics, was studied for three different storage conditions. The effect of the formulation on the intraocular pressure (IOP) profile in normotensive Dutch Belted male rabbits was then examined. The lead CBD-NEC formulation (1% w/v CBD) exhibited a globule size of 259 ± 2.0 nm, 0.27 ± 0.01 PDI, and 23.2 ± 0.4 cP viscosity, and was physically and chemically stable for one month (last time point tested) at 4 °C, 25 °C, and 40 °C. CBD-NEC significantly lowered the IOP in the treated eyes for up to 360 min, with a peak drop in IOP of 4.5 mmHg observed at the 150 min time point, post-topical application. The IOP of the contralateral eye (untreated) was also observed to be lowered significantly, but the effect lasted up to the 180 min time point only. Overall, topically administered CBD, formulated in a mucoadhesive nanoemulsion formulation, reduced the IOP in the animal model studied. The results support further exploration of CBD as a therapeutic option for various inflammation-based ocular diseases.

Keywords: cannabidiol; nanoemulsion; carbopol® 940 NF; autoclave; IOP; rabbits

1. Introduction

Cannabis contains more than 100 cannabinoids [1]. Δ^9-tetrahydrocannabinol (THC) is the major psychoactive component while cannabidiol (CBD) is the major non-psychoactive and most widely studied of the other cannabinoid constituents. CBD is known to act on various receptor targets such as peroxisome proliferator-activated receptor gamma (PPARγ) and 5-hydroxytryptamine 1A receptor (5-HT1A), and shows anti-inflammatory (by interacting with the CB_2 receptor and inhibiting immune cell migration), neuroprotective, and antioxidant properties (by scavenging reactive oxygen species (ROS) and blocking NADPH oxidase) [2–4]. CBD, thus, holds tremendous potential as a therapeutic candidate in multiple ocular diseases.

In recent years, however, contradictory reports in the literature and the lack of rigor in most prior studies make it difficult to conclude the impact of CBD on intraocular pressure (IOP). Concerns about CBD increasing IOP on topical application have generated questions about the safety of CBD for ocular use. A review of the literature reveals that, prior to 2022, a total of nine studies investigated the effect of CBD on the IOP. These investigations were conducted in rabbits, cats, monkeys, and humans, and were administered via topical ocular, oral, sublingual, or intravenous routes of administration. Intravenous CBD administration in rabbits [5–7] and oral administration in monkeys [6] did not demonstrate any effect on the IOP. On the other hand, topical application of CBD in rabbits, using mineral-oil-based formulations [8], continuous topical application in cats using a mini pump [9], and intravenous CBD application in human subjects [10] all led to transient drop in IOP.

Two studies, however, have reported an increase in IOP after CBD application [11,12]. Tomida et al. investigated sublingual administration of CBD in humans through oromucosal spray and observed a transient rise in the IOP with a CBD dose of 40 mg but not with 20 mg [11]. In 2018, a report by Miller et al. raised serious concerns about the safety of topical ocular CBD application [12]. The authors studied the effect of THC (5 mM; 0.16% w/v) and CBD (5 mM; 0.16% w/v), alone and in combination, on the IOP in C57BL/6J (C57) mice and CB1 knockout (CB1 KO) mice on CD1 strain background. THC lowered the IOP in C57 male mice for 8 h whereas CBD increased the IOP in C57 male mice. However, when CBD was administered to CB1 KO mice, this resulted in a decrease in IOP 1 h after administration, but there was no effect observed 4 h post-administration. When CBD/THC mixture was administration to C57 mice, CBD blocked the effect of THC and there was no effect on IOP observed in the treated and contralateral eyes (no statistically significant difference). Based on the above observations, Miller et al. concluded that, unlike THC, CBD increases the IOP upon topical application and on co-administration with THC, CBD counteracts the IOP lowering effect of THC.

Contrary to the observation by Miller et. al. [12], Rebibo et al., in 2022, reported that a CBD nanoemulsion (NE) decreased IOP when administered three times a day for two weeks. At 0.4% CBD concentration, IOP decreased significantly in female C57BL/6 mice after 7 and 14 days compared to the baseline values within the group [13]. A reduction in IOP was also observed with 1.6% CBD after 3 and 14 days of topical application. Additionally, 0.4% CBD significantly lowered the IOP at 7, 10, and 14 treatment days compared to the blank NE group, whereas the 1.6% NE reduced the IOP after 3, 10, and 14 days compared to the blank NE group. However, a reduction in IOP was not seen in the 0.8% CBD treated groups. Thus, although there are some questions in this report as to why the middle dose did not show any effect on the IOP, the data suggests that topically administered CBD did not increase the IOP in mice.

Thus, except for the two studies conducted by Miller et al. and Tomida et al. [11,12], all other studies indicate that CBD does not increase IOP but rather has an IOP lowering effect. However, based on the report by Miller et al. [12], the development of CBD as a therapeutic candidate for ocular diseases has almost come to a halt because of IOP related safety concerns.

CBD's site of action is at the trabecular meshwork or the iris-ciliary (IC) bodies, or both, depending upon the molecular mechanisms involved based on the current understanding [14,15]. Thus, for CBD to mediate local activity following topical application, it has to penetrate across the corneal epithelium and reach the anterior segment ocular tissues, especially the aqueous humor (AH) and IC bodies to achieve a therapeutic effect. Our earlier investigations explored the penetration of CBD into the ocular tissues through the topical route [16]. In that investigation, Tocrisolve-based CBD formulations (0.47% w/v) were prepared and tested in New Zealand White (NZW) rabbits and the study revealed that the CBD levels in the ocular tissues, 90 min post-administration, were very low [16]. Unfortunately, in that study, the effect of the Tocrisolve–based CBD formulations on the IOP was not monitored. However, to better understand the effect of CBD on the IOP in rabbits, a formulation allowing better delivery of CBD into the intraocular tissues would be needed.

Previously, we encountered similar transcorneal delivery challenges with THC from mineral oil or Tocrisolve-based THC NE formulations and resultant lack of an IOP lowering effect through the topical administration route [17–19]. This ultimately led to the development of a Carbopol® 940 NF containing THC NE formulation (THC-NEC) with low oil (5% instead of the 20% in Tocrisolve) and different surfactant concentrations [20]. With this THC-NEC formulation we were able to demonstrate consistent IOP lowering activity of THC in New Zealand White (NZW) rabbits [20,21].

Thus, the first aim of this study was to formulate CBD into the THC-NEC formulation vehicle, to enhance drug retention on the ocular surface and allow better permeation through the corneal membrane [20]. The second aim was to understand the effect of CBD on the IOP of pigmented Dutch Belted (DB) rabbits. The DB rabbits show a higher IOP than the NZW rabbits and thus serve as a better model to study the effect on IOP. Additionally, the role of pigmentation, if any, on the duration of activity would be evident in this model.

2. Materials and Methods

2.1. Materials

2.1.1. Chemicals and Glassware

Cannabidiol (CBD) derived from hemp was used in this study and was a gift from ElSohly Laboratories, Inc. (Oxford, MS, USA). Optical rotation, melting point test, mass spectroscopy, and nuclear magnetic resonance spectroscopy studies were performed to ensure that this investigation was carried out with the (-) normal CBD isomer. Poloxamer 407 NF grade, sesame oil NF grade, Carbopol® 940 NF grade, glycerin NF grade, and Tween® 80 (Polysorbate 80) NF grade were purchased from Spectrum Chemicals (New Brunswick, NJ, USA). All other chemicals, including Vitamin E-d-alpha-tocopherol polyethylene glycol 1000 succinate (TPGS), were purchased from Fisher Scientific (St. Louis, MO, USA). Solvents used for the instrumental analysis were of high-performance liquid chromatography (HPLC) grade and were purchased from Fischer Scientific (St. Louis, MO, USA). Centrifuge tubes, scintillation glass vials, and Slide-A-Lyzer™ MINI Dialysis Devices (10 K molecular weight cutoff) were purchased from Fischer Scientific (Hampton, NH, USA). Screw top clear class A (Type I) borosilicate glass HPLC vials (12 × 32 mm, 2.0 mL) with pre-slit silicone septa were purchased from Waters (Waters, Milford, CA, USA).

2.1.2. Animals

Dutch Belted (DB) male rabbits (weight; 4.75–5.75 lbs and age; 8–12 weeks) were purchased from ENVIGO (Denver, PA, USA). All animal experiments conformed to the tenets of the Association for Research in Vision and Ophthalmology statement on the Use of Animals in Ophthalmic and Vision Research and followed the University of Mississippi Institutional Animal Care and Use Committee approved protocols (18-029).

2.2. Methods

2.2.1. HPLC Method

CBD was quantified using an HPLC-UV system comprising of a Waters® Alliance e2695 separations module and a Waters® 2489 UV/Vis dual absorbance detector. Stock solutions of CBD were prepared in acetonitrile. A detection wavelength (λ_{max}) of 210 nm was set. The mobile phase, consisting of a mixture of solution A and B (75:25 v/v), was pumped isocratically at a flow rate of 1.2 mL/min. Solution A consisted of a mixture of acetonitrile and methanol (75:25 v/v) containing 0.05% v/v formic acid, while solution B was Milli-Q water containing 0.05% v/v trifluoroacetic acid. Chromatographic separation was achieved within 10 min on a Waters Symmetry® C18 column (150 × 4.6 mm, 5 µm) as a stationary phase with a retention time of 7.5 min. The injection volume was set to 20 µL and the detector sensitivity was set to 2.0 AUFS (absorbance units full scale). The column temperature was kept at 40 °C while the sample holder temperature was kept at 25 °C. The HPLC method was linear over a CBD concentration range of 1–20 µg/mL.

2.2.2. Preparation of CBD-NE Formulations

The composition of the CBD-NE formulation is presented in Table 1. Oil in water (O/W) NE was prepared using hot homogenization followed by the probe sonication method [22,23]. The oil phase was prepared by dissolving an accurately weighed amount of CBD in sesame oil, with heating at 70 ± 2 °C, to obtain a clear oily solution. The aqueous phase comprising glycerin (tonicity adjusting agent), Poloxamer 407 and Tween® 80 (surfactants), TPGS (antioxidant), and water was placed in another glass vial and simultaneously heated at 70 °C under continuous stirring in a water bath. The hot aqueous phase was then added to the heated oil phase dropwise under continuous magnetic stirring at 2000 rpm for 5 min to form pre-emulsion. This pre-emulsion was then homogenized using a T25 digital Ultra-Turrax (IKA Works, Inc., Wilmington, NC, USA) at 11,000 rpm for 5 min at 65.0 ± 2.0 °C to form a coarse emulsion. The coarse emulsion was allowed to cool at room temperature before being subjected to probe sonication in an ice bath for 10 min with a 3 mm stepped microtip at 500 watts power supply and 115 volts (40% amplitude, pulse on: 10 s and pulse off: 15 s) using a Sonics Vibra-Cell™ Sonicator (Newtown, CT, USA) to form NE.

Table 1. Composition of cannabidiol-loaded nanoemulsion formulations.

Ingredients (% w/v)	Formulations	
	CBD-NE	CBD-NEC
CBD	1.0	1.0
Sesame oil NF	5.0	5.0
Tween® 80 NF	2.0	2.0
Poloxamer 407 NF	0.2	0.2
Glycerin NF	2.25	2.25
Carbopol® 940 NF	-	0.4
TPGS	0.002	0.002
Milli-Q water q.s (mL)	10	10

2.2.3. Preparation of the Mucoadhesive CBD-NE (CBD-NEC)

The NE preparation method, as described above, was followed for the preparation of the NEC formulations (Table 1). However, the volume of Milli-Q water used to prepare NE was split into two equal parts: one part was used to prepare the aqueous solution of the mucoadhesive agent (Carbopol® 940 NF) and the other half was used to prepare the aqueous phase as described above. They were both heated to 70 °C and added into the oily phase containing the drug in a drop-by-drop fashion, using two different pipettes, under constant magnetic stirring at 2000 rpm for 5 min to form a pre-emulsion. This pre-emulsion was then homogenized using a T25 digital Ultra-Turrax (IKA Works, Inc., Wilmington, NC, USA) at 11,000 rpm for 5 min at 65.0 ± 2.0 °C to form a coarse emulsion. The coarse emulsion was allowed to cool at room temperature before being subjected to probe sonication in an ice bath for 10 min with a 3 mm stepped microtip at 500 watts power supply and 115 volts (40% amplitude, pulse on: 10 s and pulse off: 15 s) using Sonics Vibra-Cell™ Sonicator (Newtown, CT, USA) to form NE [21,24].

2.2.4. Measurement of Globule Size, Polydispersity Index (PDI), and Zeta Potential (ZP)

The NE and NEC formulations were evaluated for their globule size, PDI, and ZP using Zetasizer (Nano ZS Zen3600, Malvern Panalytical Inc., Westborough, MA, USA) at 25 °C in disposable, folded, clear, and solvent-resistant micro-cuvettes (ZEN0040). The NE and NEC formulations were diluted (100-fold) with Milli-Q water [25]. The same diluted formulations were transferred to Zetasizer disposable folded capillary DTS1070 cells for performing zeta potential measurement after globule size and PDI measurement [26,27]. All globule size, PDI, and zeta potential measurements were conducted in triplicate.

2.2.5. Assay (CBD Content)

Fifty microliters (50 µL) of the CBD-NE and CBD-NEC formulations were transferred into a volumetric flask (5 mL) and the volume was adjusted with acetonitrile (extracting solvent, 100-fold dilution). The extract was vortexed (5 min, 2000 rpm, Vortex-Genie® 2, Scientific Industries, Inc., Bohemia, NY, USA) and sonicated (Bransonic® ultrasonic cleaner, Branson Ultrasonics corporation, Brookfield, CT, USA) for 10 min. The extract was then centrifuged (AccuSpin 17R centrifuge, Fisher Scientific, Hanover, IL, USA) for 20 min at 13,000 rpm. Then, the supernatant was diluted (10-fold) with acetonitrile before being analyzed for CBD content using the HPLC method mentioned above.

2.2.6. pH Measurement

The pH was measured with a Mettler Toledo pH meter (FiveEasy™, Columbus, OH, USA) equipped with an Inlab® Micro Pro-ISM probe. Before measurement, the pH meter was calibrated using different buffers with known pH values of 4.01, 7.00, and 10.01 (Orion™ Standard All-in-One™ pH Buffer Kit, Thermo Fisher Scientific, Chelmsford, MA, USA). The pH measurements were carried out in triplicate.

2.2.7. Viscosity Measurement

A Brookfield cone and plate viscometer (LV-DV-II+ Pro Viscometer, Middleborough, MA, USA) was used to measure the viscosity of the prepared NE and NEC formulations in the presence and absence of simulated tear fluid (STF). STF was prepared by dissolving 0.0084% calcium chloride, 0.138% potassium chloride, 0.678% sodium chloride, and 0.218% sodium bicarbonate in Milli-Q water and the pH was adjusted to 7.0 ± 0.2 with 0.1 N hydrochloric acid. STF was mixed with the formulation in a ratio of 7:50 prior to viscosity measurement. The STF to formulation ratio was selected based on the expectation that a standard eyedropper dispenses 0.05 mL (50 µL) while the precorneal tear fluid volume is about 7 to 10 µL [25]. The cup was thermally equilibrated at 25 ± 0.5 °C for 15 min with the aid of a circulating water bath before the test. The sample (0.5 mL) was placed in the viscometer cup plate and rotated at a constant speed of 5.0 rpm using a CPE 52 spindle. The torque required to maintain this speed was measured and translated to viscosity values (centipoise, cP). Rheology analysis was performed using Rheocalc® software (Version 3.3 Build 49-1, USA). The viscosity measurements of all samples were carried out in triplicate.

2.2.8. Sterilization Process and Stability Assessment

CBD-NE and CBD-NEC formulations were subjected to terminal moist heat sterilization (121 °C under 15 psi for 15 min, 3850ELP-B/L-D Tuttnauer autoclave, Heidolph, Germany) process in glass vials. The sterilization cycle was confirmed by the color change of the indicator tapes attached to the glass vials.

2.2.9. Stability Studies

The physicochemical stability of NE and NEC formulations was evaluated at refrigerated (4 ± 2 °C), room temperature (25 ± 2 °C), and accelerated (40 °C ± 2 °C) storage conditions pre- and post-moist heat sterilization process. The formulations were evaluated for any change in globule size, PDI, ZP, pH, and CBD content over the one month of storage.

2.2.10. Scanning Transmission Electron Microscopy (STEM)

The analysis was carried out using a JSM-7200FLV Scanning Electron Microscope (JOEL, Peabody, MA, USA) attached to a STEM detector with an accelerating voltage of 30 kV. STEM samples were examined following a negative staining protocol with a solution of UranyLess. A carbon-plated copper grid was placed on top of one drop (20 µL) of the formulation for 60 s and the excess sample was blotted off with a filter paper after grid removal from the formulation surface to remove any excess sample. The grid was then washed by dipping it in distilled water and the grid was blotted with filter paper to remove excess water. Next, the grid was placed sample down on top of one drop (20 µL) of the staining solution for 60 s and then was blotted with a filter paper to remove any excess stain. The grid was allowed to dry for a few minutes by air. The grid was examined under the scanning transmission electron microscope at 30 K times magnification power.

2.2.11. In Vivo Single Dose Efficacy Studies—IOP Measurement

IOP was measured following our earlier published protocols [20,21]. Pigmented DB rabbits were acclimatized to the environment, personnel, and measurement procedure for 14 days to establish the IOP baseline. The CBD-NEC and NEC placebo formulations were individually instilled (50 µL) into the lower cul-de-sac of the left eye (treated eye) of the DB rabbits, while the right eye (contralateral) was kept untreated. Following topical instillation, the eyelids were kept closed (5–10 s) to decrease spillage of the NE formulations. The IOP was measured before instillation (to establish a baseline IOP) and every 30 min up to 180 min, and then every 60 min up to 480 min post-instillation. The IOP value displayed on the TONOVET Plus tonometer (Icare® Finland Oy, Finland) was an average of six readings and at each time point was measured in triplicate. The IOP measurements at each time point are reported as percent change in IOP (Equation (1)).

$$\Delta IOP = \frac{\text{Baseline IOP} - \text{Measured IOP}}{\text{Baseline IOP}} \times 100 \qquad (1)$$

Ocular irritation was qualitatively evaluated through visual monitoring of redness and changes in tearing or blinking rate.

2.2.12. Statistical Analysis

Statistical comparisons of the means were performed using one-way analysis of variance (ANOVA). The difference was considered significant when the p-value was <0.05. SPSS 28 software (IBM®, Armonk, NY, USA) was used for the statistical evaluations.

3. Results and Discussion

NE formulations are nanosized (20–200 nm), thermodynamically stable, isotropic systems [22]. NEs have a high solubilizing capacity for therapeutic moieties, excellent physicochemical stability, and are biocompatible [28,29]. NEs can improve ocular permeation, extend drug release, and enable drug distribution to the deeper ocular tissues [22,28]. The low surface tension of these nanocarriers facilitate excellent spreading on the ocular surface and excellent mixing with the tear film, thus prolonging the residence time of the drug on the ocular surface and improving ocular permeation [30]. All these factors led to considering these nanocarriers as the vehicle of choice for this investigation.

Mucoadhesive agents prolong the ocular surface residence time of topically applied therapeutics by adhering to the mucin layer of the tear film, thus enabling uniform distribution of the applied eyedrops above the cornea [20,31]. Therefore, the addition of a mucoadhesive agent to the developed NE could result in prolonging the activity and improving the therapeutic outcomes of CBD. Many mucoadhesive agents that have been reported and used in many Food and Drug Administration (FDA) approved ophthalmic dosage forms such as chitosan, Carbopol®, hydroxyl propyl methyl cellulose, sodium carboxy methyl cellulose, hyaluronan, and xanthan gum.

Carbomer copolymer type A (Pemulen TR-2 NF Carbopol® 71G NF, Carbopol® 971P NF, and Carbopol® 981 NF) and B (Pemulen TR-1 NF) and Carbomer homopolymer type B (Carbopol® 974P NF, Carbopol® 5984 EP, and Carbopol® 934 NF) and C (Carbopol® 940 NF, and Carbopol® 980 NF) have been used in many FDA approved ophthalmic formulations [20]. Carbomer homopolymer type C (Carbopol® 940 NF) gives the highest viscosity at pH 7.5 and has been used up to 4.0% w/w in FDA approved ophthalmic formulations according to the FDA inactive ingredients database. Besides its mucoadhesive properties, Carbopol® 940 NF undergoes a pH-dependent *sol-to-gel* transition to form a viscoelastic gel above a pH of 5.5. The normal pH range of human tear fluid is 6.5 to 7.6 with an average value of 7.0 [23,32]. In the alkaline environment of human tears, the carboxyl groups ionize and generate many negative charges along the Carbopol® polymer backbone. The electrostatic repulsion of the similar negative charges of the anionic carboxyl group triggers the uncoiling and expansion of the polymeric chains, thus resulting in polymer swelling and gel formation [33].

Our earlier investigation studied the effect of inclusion of Carbopol® 940 NF on the intensity and duration of IOP lowering activity of Δ^9-tetrahydrocannabinol-valine-hemisuccinate (THC-VHS) loaded in a nanoemulsion formulation [20]. The THC-VHS-NEC formulation demonstrated a significant ($p < 0.05$) improvement in the duration of IOP lowering activity, compared to THC-VHS-NE. Moreover, THC-VHS-NEC was more effective than the marketed latanoprost ophthalmic eyedrops in terms of both duration and intensity of IOP lowering. Thus, with the main objective of increased ocular surface residence of the topically applied eye drops, Carbopol® 940 NF was the best choice for this study with its dual mechanism for serving the objective.

3.1. Formulation Development

CBD-NE and CBD-NE formulations were prepared according to our previously established protocols [20]. The composition of the prepared NE formulations is presented in Table 1. The NE formulations were prepared using sesame oil as the oily phase as CBD possesses adequate solubility in this oil. Moreover, Epidiolex®, the only FDA approved commercial product (oral) for CBD, is provided as a solution in sesame oil. The selected Carbopol® 940 NF concentration (0.4% w/w) increases the viscosity of the prepared NE while facilitating easy topical ocular application ($\leq$50 cP) based on our earlier investigations [20].

3.2. Physicochemical Characteristics of CBD-NE and CBD-NEC Formulations

The globule size, PDI, ZP, and drug content of CBD-NE and CBD-NEC formulations are illustrated in Table 2. The globule size is an important factor for adhesion and interaction with ocular epithelial cells. The reduction in globule size provides a larger surface area for contact with the ocular surface, which can significantly enhance bioavailability [34]. Smaller globules (<200 nm) are transported by receptor-mediated endocytosis uptake whereas larger particles are transported by phagocytosis [23]. PDI values show the width of globule size distribution and PDI values < 0.3 demonstrate that the NE formulations were uniform dispersions with narrow globule size distribution [35]. ZP values of more than ±30 mV indicate good physical stability for the prepared NEs [23,36].

Table 2. Globule size, PDI, zeta potential, drug content, pH, and viscosity of the CBD-NE and CBD-NEC formulations (mean ± SD, n = 3).

Parameter	Formulation	
	CBD-NE	CBD-NEC
Globule size (d. nm)	167.2 ± 4.2	259.5 ± 2.0
Polydispersity index	0.20 ± 0.01	0.27 ± 0.01
Zeta potential (mV)	−19.8 ± 1.1	−37.9 ± 0.8
Drug content (%)	100.0 ± 0.3	101.9 ± 0.1
pH	5.6 ± 0.02	3.6 ± 0.02
Viscosity (cP) without STF	11.6 ± 0.5	23.2 ± 0.4
Viscosity (cP) with STF	12.3 ± 1.0	31.2 ± 1.2

Carbopol® 940 NF addition changed ZP significantly from −19.8 ± 1.1 for CBD-NE to −37.9 ± 0.8 for CBD-NEC, probably due to the negatively charged carboxylic acid groups along the polymer backbone. The change in ZP suggests that Carbopol® 940 NF is adsorbed on the surface of the oil droplets [20]. The significant increase ($p < 0.05$) in globule size from

167.2 ± 4.2 for CBD-NE to 259.5 ± 2.0 for CBD-NEC also supports surface adsorption of Carbopol® 940 NF [20]. Both NE formulations demonstrated CBD content, 100.0 ± 0.3 for CBD-NE and 101.9 ± 0.1 for CBD-NEC, within the acceptance limits of the label's content (90–110%).

3.3. pH and Viscosity

Although physiological pH ranges are always preferred, the eye can tolerate topical formulations with low buffering capacity over a pH range of 3.0–8.6. In this study, incorporation of the mucoadhesive agent, Carbopol® 940 NF, significantly ($p < 0.05$) affected the pH of the formulation (Table 2). The decrease in pH from 5.6 ± 0.02 (CBD-NE) to 3.6 ± 0.02 (CBD-NEC) would be due to the acidic carboxylic groups of Carbopol® 940 NF. The pH values of both formulations were within the acceptable range. Moreover, in our earlier studies with THC-VHS using the same vehicle, there were no signs of discomfort, ocular irritation, or redness in the treated eye during the in vivo single-dose efficacy study period (8 h study) based on visual examination [20]. This suggests the lower pH of the CBD-NEC formulation would not cause any ocular irritation or redness in the treated eye.

Viscosity is a critical parameter of topical ophthalmic dosage forms because it can affect the performance of the applied product as well as patient comfort. Generally, viscosity values up to 50 cP have been established to be most favorable in terms of patient compliance, ease of topical ocular application, and prolonging retention at the ocular surface, thus leading to improved ocular bioavailability [37]. The viscosity of both NE formulations was measured using a Brookfield cone and plate viscometer (Table 2). It was observed that the viscosity of the CBD-NE formulation (11.6 ± 0.5 cP) was significantly ($p < 0.05$) increased, expectedly, after the incorporation of Carbopol® 940 NF (CBD-NEC; 23.2 ± 0.4 cP) within the formulation. Moreover, the addition of STF increased the viscosity (31.2 ± 1.2) of CBD-NEC significantly ($p < 0.05$) because the alkaline environment (7.0 ± 0.2) resulted in Carbopol® 940 NF swelling and gel formation. All measured viscosity values were favorable for ocular application.

3.4. STEM

The surface morphology of CBD-NEC was studied using STEM and the result is shown in Figure 1. The globules were spherical in shape with a globule size around 250 d.nm, which is consistent with the results obtained from dynamic light scattering studies.

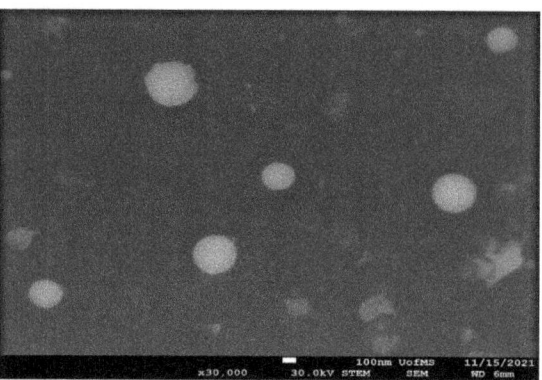

Figure 1. STEM micrograph of CBD-NEC formulation.

3.5. Stability Studies

The physicochemical stability of both NE formulations was evaluated at 4, 25, and 40 °C storage conditions over 30 days (last time point tested). Both formulations did not show any change in color, precipitation, creaming, or cracking during the testing period upon visual examination.

Addition of Carbopol® 940 NF makes filtration of the NEC formulation very challenging, necessitating aseptic manufacturing if not autoclavable. Terminal sterilization of the final dosage form is always more preferred than aseptic manufacturing. Thus, moist-heat sterilization was also investigated for the NE and NEC formulations. The pre- and post-moist-heat sterilization physicochemical characteristics are provided in Table 3. The autoclaved formulations remained stable under the test conditions employed; globule size, PDI, ZP, pH, and drug content did not show a significant ($p < 0.05$) change in comparison to the pre-autoclaved formulation for one month.

Table 3. Stability data for CBD-NE and CBD-NEC nanoemulsion formulations pre- and post- sterilization over one month of storage at 4, 25, and 40 °C (mean ± SD, $n = 3$).

Formulation	Day	Storage at 4 ± 2 °C									
		DS (d, nm)		PDI		ZP (mV)		pH		Drug Content (%)	
		Sterilization Stage									
		Pre	Post	Pre	Post	Pre	Post	Pre	Post	Pre	Post
CBD-NE	0	167.2 ± 4.2	167.9 ± 2.0	0.20 ± 0.01	0.21 ± 0.02	−19.8 ± 1.1	−21.6 ± 0.2	5.60 ± 0.02	5.62 ± 0.01	100.0 ± 0.3	97.0 ± 0.2
	30	166.0 ± 3.7	163.6 ± 2.6	0.20 ± 0.02	0.23 ± 0.01	−21.7 ± 0.5	−20.6 ± 0.4	5.60 ± 0.02	5.64 ± 0.02	99.5 ± 2.1	99.0 ± 0.5
CBD-NEC	0	259.5 ± 2.0	258.5 ± 0.4	0.26 ± 0.01	0.25 ± 0.02	−33.9 ± 0.8	−34.7 ± 0.3	3.60 ± 0.01	3.59 ± 0.03	101.9 ± 0.1	98.2 ± 0.3
	30	252.9 ± 2.8	251.7 ± 3.7	0.25 ± 0.01	0.26 ± 0.01	−35.2 ± 0.2	−33.6 ± 0.4	3.60 ± 0.01	3.65 ± 0.01	101.9 ± 1.4	102.6 ± 1.5
		Storage at 25 ± 2 °C									
CBD-NE	0	165.7 ± 1.8	166.4 ± 2.0	0.21 ± 0.01	0.22 ± 0.01	−19.8 ± 0.9	−21.6 ± 0.8	5.62 ± 0.02	5.63 ± 0.01	99.8 ± 0.1	97.0 ± 0.1
	30	164.9 ± 1.0	161.9 ± 3.0	0.22 ± 0.01	0.22 ± 0.02	−21.2 ± 0.3	−20 ± 0.6	5.64 ± 0.02	5.62 ± 0.01	98.2 ± 1.7	97.6 ± 0.6
CBD-NEC	0	262.9 ± 1.3	259.4 ± 0.8	0.25 ± 0.02	0.24 ± 0.02	−34.3 ± 2.1	−35.7 ± 0.8	3.61 ± 0.01	3.60 ± 0.02	100.8 ± 0.1	101.0 ± 0.1
	30	256.8 ± 4.7	256.1 ± 0.8	0.26 ± 0.01	0.26 ± 0.01	−35.8 ± 0.6	−34.3 ± 0.8	3.64 ± 0.01	3.65 ± 0.02	100.2 ± 2.0	99.6 ± 2.1
		Storage at 40 ± 2 °C									
CBD-NE	0	166.8 ± 2.2	170.2 ± 2.4	0.19 ± 0.01	0.21 ± 0.01	−21.2 ± 0.5	−19.6 ± 0.3	5.55 ± 0.01	5.64 ± 0.02	99.6 ± 0.1	98.0 ± 0.3
	30	160.9 ± 2.0	162.2 ± 2.6	0.21 ± 0.01	0.21 ± 0.00	−20.8 ± 0.6	−20.6 ± 0.5	5.58 ± 0.01	5.62 ± 0.01	100.3 ± 3.1	99.8 ± 0.2
CBD-NEC	0	263.1 ± 1.8	256.9 ± 2.9	0.24 ± 0.03	0.25 ± 0.01	−34.4 ± 2.1	−35.4 ± 0.3	3.60 ± 0.03	3.62 ± 0.01	99.9 ± 0.2	101.6 ± 0.5
	30	254.9 ± 4.0	254.7 ± 1.8	0.25 ± 0.01	0.26 ± 0.01	−34.6 ± 1.6	−36.2 ± 0.8	3.64 ± 0.01	3.65 ± 0.03	102.9 ± 0.3	102.4 ± 1.2

Surfactant composition, globule size, and surface charge are directly related to the physical stability of NEs. The combined effect of these three parameters determines the formulation stability. A suitable surfactant combination provides an elastic interface between the two immiscible liquids, allowing the dispersed phase to be suspended in the form of small globules in the dispersion medium [38]. The oil globules become elastic and can survive a high degree of tension during deformation. In addition, smaller dispersed oil globules are not affected by gravitational force and become suspended continuously in the dispersion medium [39]. Moreover, numerous surface charges over the smaller oil globules keep them separate due to the presence of strong interglobular repulsive forces [40].

The continuous motion of oil globules within the dispersion medium makes oil globules approach each other, and the globules become subjected to strong repulsive force and finally move apart after the elastic collision [40]. This phenomenon improves kinetic stability by Brownian motion [38]. Although high-molecular-weight surfactants such as Tween® 80 and Poloxamer 407 provide a lower magnitude of ZP, these surfactants keep the NE stable by the additive effects of steric hindrance and the repulsive force between similarly charged globules [38]. Based on the HLB theory reported by Griffin, a mixture of surfactants with a final HLB value between 9 and 12 is sufficient to prepare stable O/W Nes [41,42]. Hence, it seems that the 1:10 ratio of Poloxamer 407: Tween® 80 (HLB: ~15.6) could provide excellent physical stability. It is worth mentioning that the same formulation composition loaded with THC-VHS provided excellent stability with respect to globule size, PDI, ZP, pH, and drug content pre- and post-sterilization in our earlier investigation [20].

3.6. In Vivo Single-Dose Efficacy Studies—IOP Measurement

In earlier studies, Miller et al. reported there was an increase in IOP in mice after administering CBD [12], whereas Rebibo et al. [13] reported a decrease in IOP when mice were dosed with a CBD emulsion. Both groups administered a blank vehicle to the contralateral eye and a drug loaded formulation to the treated eye; however, they report contrasting results. This could be attributed to how the change in IOP was determined. Miller et al. compared the IOP of the treated eye to that of the contralateral eye, whereas Rebibo et al. [13] compared the IOP of the treated eye to the baseline values. As the literature indicates, IOP lowering agents applied to one eye can significantly reduce IOP in the contralateral eye also [17,20,43–48]. This has also been observed in the mouse model [49,50]. CBD, like THC, is seen to lower the IOP in the contralateral eye. Thus, concluding the effect of CBD on the IOP, or a change in IOP, based on a comparison between the contralateral and treated eye IOPs could be erroneous.

Miller et al. and Rebibo et al. both used a mouse model to demonstrate the impact of CBD on IOP. The mouse model is particularly attractive due to the ease of husbandry, the extensive genomic resources available, and the potential for genetic manipulation [51]. However, the mouse model for glaucoma also presents challenges with obtaining an accurate determination of IOP due to the small size of the mouse eye. Both research groups have used anesthesia to measure the IOP. Anesthesia has been reported to influence the IOP in rodents. The type and quantity of the anesthesia used determines how much the IOP is influenced [52]. Kim et al. reported that the mean IOP decreases rapidly during the first 10 min after the loss of the lid reflex and remains unchanged thereafter. Both groups have reported measurements taken after the successful induction of anesthesia, which could impact the IOP reading [12,13].

Figure 2 illustrates the IOP vs. time profile following topical administration of CBD-NEC (treated eye and contralateral eye), NEC placebo (treated eye), and baseline of left eye in Dutch Belted male rabbits. The IOP versus time profile of the baseline of the left eye (test eye) was established prior to application of NEC formulations. There were no significant ($p > 0.05$) differences found in the baseline of the test eye over the 8 h and an average IOP of 23.1 ± 0.2 mmHg was maintained. The NEC-placebo formulation exhibited a similar IOP vs. time profile as the baseline and maintained an average IOP of 23.5 ± 0.3 mmHg. The CBD-NEC formulation demonstrated a significant IOP-lowering effect in the DB rabbits following a topical application ($p < 0.05$). A drop of more than 10% was observed for both the contralateral and test eye 30 min after the application of CBD-NEC formulation in the test eye as well as the contralateral eye. The maximum drops in IOP (% drop from time 0) for the test eye and contralateral eye after the instillation of CBD-NEC were 19.9% and 17.4%, respectively, at 150 min post-application. The durations of action (considered only if the drop in IOP was more than 10% from baseline) for the test eye and contralateral eye were 240 min and 150 min, respectively. The IOP began returning to baseline after 180 min post-application. The IOP of the treated eye after application of CBD-NEC was significantly lower than the established left eye baseline from the 30 min time point ($p < 0.005$) and this effect lasted until 300 min ($p < 0.001$). The statistical difference between the treatments can be found in Table 4. Based on previous data that suggest the addition of the mucoadhesive agent to a nanoemulsion prolongs the duration of action compared to the nanoemulsion alone, CBD-NE was not tested [20].

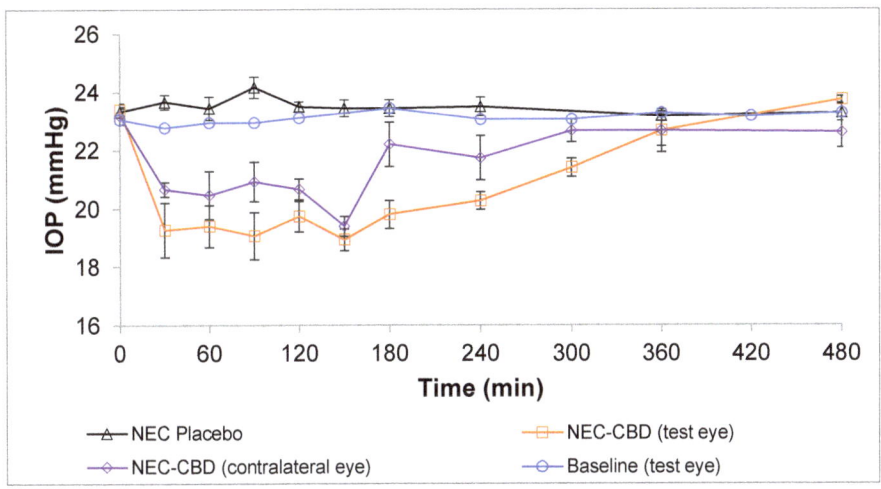

Figure 2. IOP vs. time profile following topical administration of CBD-NEC (treated eye and contralateral eye), NEC placebo (treated eye), and baseline of left eye in Dutch Belted male rabbits (mean ± SEM, $n = 6$).

Table 4. p-values associated with the difference in the IOP values of treated and contralateral eyes from the baseline value post-instillation of CBD-NEC or placebo formulations in the Dutch Belted male rabbits ($n = 6$).

Time Point (min)	CBD-NEC Treated Eye vs. NEC-Placebo p-Value	CBD-NEC Treated Eye vs. CBD-NEC Contralateral Eye p-Value	CBD-NEC Treated Eye vs. Baseline Treated Eye p-Value	CBD-NEC Contralateral Eye vs. Baseline Treated Eye p-Value
0	0.211	0.625	1.000	1.000
30	0.003	0.235	0.005	<0.001
60	0.003	0.397	0.001	0.024
90	<0.001	0.155	0.001	0.024
120	<0.001	0.226	<0.001	0.001
150	<0.001	0.431	<0.001	<0.001
180	<0.001	0.045	<0.001	0.309
240	<0.001	0.144	<0.001	0.149
300	–	0.051	<0.001	0.356
360	0.566	1.000	0.271	0.564
480	0.323	0.088	0.045	0.396

4. Conclusions

This study is the first to report—to the author's knowledge—that CBD lowers the IOP in normotensive Dutch Belted rabbits following topical application. The CBD-NEC formulation exhibited a max drop of 19.9% with a duration of 300 min. The CBD-NE and CBD-NEC formulations were successfully prepared using Carbopol® 940 NF as a mucoadhesive agent and were evaluated for stability at 4, 25, and 40 °C. Both formulations were sterilized via moist heat and the pre- and post-autoclaved formulations were stable for at least one month (last time point tested) after the sterilization process. The ocular tissue biodistribution profile, dose–effect relationship, effect of sex on the pharmacodynamic activity, and investigations into the IOP lowering mechanism are the topics of additional studies that are underway. In summary, the prepared NE formulations could provide a promising CBD delivery platform for the treatment of glaucoma or other ocular indications.

Author Contributions: Conceptualization, S.S., A.A.A.Y., N.D., C.S. and S.M.; methodology, experimentation, and interpretation, A.A.A.Y., C.S., S.S., C.C. and N.D.; writing—original draft, A.A.A.Y., S.S. and C.S.; writing—review and editing, A.A.A.Y., N.D., C.C., S.S. and S.M.; supervision, S.M. All authors have read and agreed to the published version of the manuscript.

Funding: This work was supported in part by grant #P30GM122733 from the National Institute of General Medical Sciences, National Institutes of Health. The content is solely the responsibility of the authors and does not necessarily represent the official views of the National Institutes of Health.

Institutional Review Board Statement: All animal experiments conformed to the tenets of the Association for Research in Vision and Ophthalmology statement on the Use of Animals in Ophthalmic and Vision Research and followed the University of Mississippi Institutional Animal Care and Use Committee approved protocols (18-029).

Informed Consent Statement: Not applicable.

Data Availability Statement: The data presented in this study are available upon request from the corresponding author.

Acknowledgments: The authors thank Vijayasankar Raman for his assistance with the scanning transmission electron microscopy images presented in this work that were generated using the instruments and services at the Microscopy and Imaging Center, University of Mississippi. This facility is supported in part by grant 1726880, National Science Foundation.

Conflicts of Interest: The authors declare that they have no conflict of interest to disclose.

References

1. Radwan, M.M.; ElSohly, M.A.; Slade, D.; Ahmed, S.A.; Khan, I.A.; Ross, S.A. Biologically Active Cannabinoids from High-Potency Cannabis Sativa. *J. Nat. Prod.* **2009**, *72*, 906–911. [CrossRef]
2. De Almeida, D.L.; Devi, L.A. Diversity of Molecular Targets and Signaling Pathways for CBD. *Pharmacol. Res. Perspect.* **2020**, *8*, e00682. [CrossRef]
3. El-Remessy, A.B.; Al-Shabrawey, M.; Khalifa, Y.; Tsai, N.-T.; Caldwell, R.B.; Liou, G.I. Neuroprotective and Blood-Retinal Barrier-Preserving Effects of Cannabidiol in Experimental Diabetes. *Am. J. Pathol.* **2006**, *168*, 235–244. [CrossRef]
4. Liou, G.I.; Auchampach, J.A.; Hillard, C.J.; Zhu, G.; Yousufzai, B.; Mian, S.; Khan, S.; Khalifa, Y. Mediation of Cannabidiol Anti-Inflammation in the Retina by Equilibrative Nucleoside Transporter and A2A Adenosine Receptor. *Investig. Ophthalmol. Vis. Sci.* **2008**, *49*, 5526–5531. [CrossRef]
5. Green, K.; Symonds, C.M.; Oliver, N.W.; Elijah, R.D. Intraocular Pressure Following Systemic Administration of Cannabinoids. *Curr. Eye Res.* **1982**, *2*, 247–253. [CrossRef]
6. Elsohly, M.A.; Harland, E.C.; Benigni, D.A.; Waller, C.W. Cannabinoids in Glaucoma II: The Effect of Different Cannabinoids on Intraocular Pressure of the Rabbit. *Curr. Eye Res.* **1984**, *3*, 841–850. [CrossRef]
7. Liu, J.H.; Dacus, A.C. Central Nervous System and Peripheral Mechanisms in Ocular Hypotensive Effect of Cannabinoids. *Arch. Ophthalmol.* **1987**, *105*, 245–248. [CrossRef]
8. Green, K.; Wynn, H.; Bowman, K.A. A Comparison of Topical Cannabinoids on Intraocular Pressure. *Exp. Eye Res.* **1978**, *27*, 239–246. [CrossRef]
9. Colasanti, B.K.; Powell, S.R.; Craig, C.R. Intraocular Pressure, Ocular Toxicity and Neurotoxicity after Administration of Δ9-Tetrahydrocannabinol or Cannabichromene. *Exp. Eye Res.* **1984**, *38*, 63–71. [CrossRef]
10. Grotenhermen, F. Clinical Pharmacokinetics of Cannabinoids. *J. Cannabis Ther.* **2003**, *3*, 3–51. [CrossRef]
11. Tomida, I.; Azuara-Blanco, A.; House, H.; Flint, M.; Pertwee, R.G.; Robson, P.J. Effect of Sublingual Application of Cannabinoids on Intraocular Pressure: A Pilot Study. *J. Glaucoma* **2006**, *15*, 349–353. [CrossRef]
12. Miller, S.; Daily, L.; Leishman, E.; Bradshaw, H.; Straiker, A. Δ9-Tetrahydrocannabinol and Cannabidiol Differentially Regulate Intraocular Pressure. *Investig. Ophthalmol. Vis. Sci.* **2018**, *59*, 5904–5911. [CrossRef]
13. Rebibo, L.; Frušić-Zlotkin, M.; Ofri, R.; Nassar, T.; Benita, S. The Dose-Dependent Effect of a Stabilized Cannabidiol Nanoemulsion on Ocular Surface Inflammation and Intraocular Pressure. *Int. J. Pharm.* **2022**, *617*, 121627. [CrossRef]
14. Vallée, A.; Lecarpentier, Y.; Vallée, J.-N. Cannabidiol and the Canonical WNT/β-Catenin Pathway in Glaucoma. *Int. J. Mol. Sci.* **2021**, *22*, 3798. [CrossRef]
15. Straiker, A.; Miller, S. Δ9-THC and CBD Differentially Regulate Intraocular Pressure. *Investig. Ophthalmol. Vis. Sci.* **2018**, *59*, 6040.

16. Taskar, P.; Adelli, G.; Patil, A.; Lakhani, P.; Ashour, E.; Gul, W.; ElSohly, M.; Majumdar, S. Analog Derivatization of Cannabidiol for Improved Ocular Permeation. *J. Ocul. Pharmacol. Ther.* **2019**, *35*, 301–310. [CrossRef] [PubMed]
17. Taskar, P.S.; Patil, A.; Lakhani, P.; Ashour, E.; Gul, W.; ElSohly, M.A.; Murphy, B.; Majumdar, S. ∆9-Tetrahydrocannabinol Derivative-Loaded Nanoformulation Lowers Intraocular Pressure in Normotensive Rabbits. *Trans. Vis. Sci. Tech.* **2019**, *8*, 15. [CrossRef]
18. Adelli, G.R.; Bhagav, P.; Taskar, P.; Hingorani, T.; Pettaway, S.; Gul, W.; ElSohly, M.A.; Repka, M.A.; Majumdar, S. Development of a ∆9-Tetrahydrocannabinol Amino Acid-Dicarboxylate Prodrug with Improved Ocular Bioavailability. *Investig. Ophthalmol. Vis. Sci* **2017**, *58*, 2167–2179. [CrossRef]
19. Hingorani, T.; Adelli, G.R.; Punyamurthula, N.; Gul, W.; ElSohly, M.A.; Repka, M.A.; Majumdar, S. Ocular Disposition of the Hemiglutarate Ester Prodrug of ∆9-Tetrahydrocannabinol from Various Ophthalmic Formulations. *Pharm. Res.* **2013**, *30*, 2146–2156. [CrossRef] [PubMed]
20. Sweeney, C.; Dudhipala, N.; Thakkar, R.; Mehraj, T.; Marathe, S.; Gul, W.; ElSohly, M.A.; Murphy, B.; Majumdar, S. Impact of Mucoadhesive Agent Inclusion on the Intraocular Pressure Lowering Profile of ∆9-Tetrahydrocannabinol-Valine-Hemisuccinate Loaded Nanoemulsions in New Zealand White Rabbits. *Int. J. Pharm.* **2022**, *616*, 121564. [CrossRef]
21. Sweeney, C.; Dudhipala, N.; Thakkar, R.; Mehraj, T.; Marathe, S.; Gul, W.; ElSohly, M.A.; Murphy, B.; Majumdar, S. Effect of Surfactant Concentration and Sterilization Process on Intraocular Pressure–Lowering Activity of ∆9-Tetrahydrocannabinol-Valine-Hemisuccinate (NB1111) Nanoemulsions. *Drug Deliv. Transl. Res.* **2021**, *11*, 2096–2107. [CrossRef]
22. Youssef, A.A.A.; Cai, C.; Dudhipala, N.; Majumdar, S. Design of Topical Ocular Ciprofloxacin Nanoemulsion for the Management of Bacterial Keratitis. *Pharmaceuticals* **2021**, *14*, 210. [CrossRef] [PubMed]
23. Youssef, A.A.A.; Thakkar, R.; Senapati, S.; Joshi, P.H.; Dudhipala, N.; Majumdar, S. Design of Topical Moxifloxacin Mucoadhesive Nanoemulsion for the Management of Ocular Bacterial Infections. *Pharmaceutics* **2022**, *14*, 1246. [CrossRef] [PubMed]
24. Tatke, A.; Dudhipala, N.; Janga, K.Y.; Balguri, S.P.; Avula, B.; Jablonski, M.M.; Majumdar, S. In Situ Gel of Triamcinolone Acetonide-Loaded Solid Lipid Nanoparticles for Improved Topical Ocular Delivery: Tear Kinetics and Ocular Disposition Studies. *Nanomaterials* **2019**, *9*, 33. [CrossRef]
25. Youssef, A.A.A.; Dudhipala, N.; Majumdar, S. Dual Drug Loaded Lipid Nanocarrier Formulations for Topical Ocular Applications. *IJN* **2022**, *17*, 2283–2299. [CrossRef] [PubMed]
26. Youssef, A.; Dudhipala, N.; Majumdar, S. Ciprofloxacin Loaded Nanostructured Lipid Carriers Incorporated into In-Situ Gels to Improve Management of Bacterial Endophthalmitis. *Pharmaceutics* **2020**, *12*, 572. [CrossRef]
27. Marathe, S.; Shadambikar, G.; Mehraj, T.; Sulochana, S.P.; Dudhipala, N.; Majumdar, S. Development of α-Tocopherol Succinate-Based Nanostructured Lipid Carriers for Delivery of Paclitaxel. *Pharmaceutics* **2022**, *14*, 1034. [CrossRef] [PubMed]
28. Lallemand, F.; Daull, P.; Benita, S.; Buggage, R.; Garrigue, J.-S. Successfully Improving Ocular Drug Delivery Using the Cationic Nanoemulsion, Novasorb. *J. Drug Deliv.* **2012**, *2012*, 604204. [CrossRef]
29. Singh, M.; Bharadwaj, S.; Lee, K.E.; Kang, S.G. Therapeutic Nanoemulsions in Ophthalmic Drug Administration: Concept in Formulations and Characterization Techniques for Ocular Drug Delivery. *J. Control. Release* **2020**, *328*, 895–916. [CrossRef] [PubMed]
30. Ammar, H.O.; Salama, H.A.; Ghorab, M.; Mahmoud, A.A. Nanoemulsion as a Potential Ophthalmic Delivery System for Dorzolamide Hydrochloride. *AAPS PharmSciTech* **2009**, *10*, 808–819. [CrossRef] [PubMed]
31. Naik, J.B.; Pardeshi, S.R.; Patil, R.P.; Patil, P.B.; Mujumdar, A. Mucoadhesive Micro-/Nano Carriers in Ophthalmic Drug Delivery: An Overview. *BioNanoScience* **2020**, *10*, 564–582. [CrossRef]
32. Abelson, M.B.; Udell, I.J.; Weston, J.H. Normal Human Tear PH by Direct Measurement. *Arch. Ophthalmol.* **1981**, *99*, 301. [CrossRef]
33. Ban, M.M.; Chakote, V.R.; Dhembre, G.N.; Rajguru, J.R.; Joshi, D.A. In-Situ Gel for Nasal Drug Delivery. *Int. J. Dev. Res.* **2018**, *8*, 18763–18769.
34. Dhahir, R.K.; Al-Nima, A.M.; Yassir Al-bazzaz, F. Nanoemulsions as Ophthalmic Drug Delivery Systems. *Turk. J. Pharm. Sci.* **2021**, *18*, 652–664. [CrossRef]
35. Lin, L.; Gu, Y.; Cui, H. Moringa Oil/Chitosan Nanoparticles Embedded Gelatin Nanofibers for Food Packaging against Listeria Monocytogenes and Staphylococcus Aureus on Cheese. *Food Packag. Shelf Life* **2019**, *19*, 86–93. [CrossRef]
36. Mitri, K.; Shegokar, R.; Gohla, S.; Anselmi, C.; Müller, R.H. Lipid Nanocarriers for Dermal Delivery of Lutein: Preparation, Characterization, Stability and Performance. *Int. J. Pharm.* **2011**, *414*, 267–275. [CrossRef]
37. Uddin, M.S.; Mamun, A.A.; Kabir, M.T.; Setu, J.R.; Zaman, S.; Begum, Y.; Amran, M.S. Quality Control Tests for Ophthalmic Pharmaceuticals: Pharmacopoeial Standards and Specifications. *J. Adv. Med. Pharm. Sci.* **2017**, *14*, 1–17. [CrossRef]
38. Rai, V.K.; Mishra, N.; Yadav, K.S.; Yadav, N.P. Nanoemulsion as Pharmaceutical Carrier for Dermal and Transdermal Drug Delivery: Formulation Development, Stability Issues, Basic Considerations and Applications. *J. Control. Release* **2018**, *270*, 203–225. [CrossRef] [PubMed]
39. Komaiko, J.S.; McClements, D.J. Formation of Food-Grade Nanoemulsions Using Low-Energy Preparation Methods: A Review of Available Methods. *Compr. Rev. Food Sci. Food Saf.* **2016**, *15*, 331–352. [CrossRef]
40. Mishra, N.; Yadav, K.S.; Rai, V.K.; Yadav, N.P. Polysaccharide Encrusted Multilayered Nano-Colloidal System of Andrographolide for Improved Hepatoprotection. *AAPS PharmSciTech* **2017**, *18*, 381–392. [CrossRef]

41. Santos, J.; Calero, N.; Trujillo-Cayado, L.A.; Martín-Piñero, M.J.; Muñoz, J. Processing and Formulation Optimization of Mandarin Essential Oil-Loaded Emulsions Developed by Microfluidization. *Materials* **2020**, *13*, 3486. [CrossRef]
42. Griffin, W.C. Calculation of HLB Values of Non-Ionic Surfactants. *J. Soc. Cosmet. Chem.* **1954**, *5*, 249–256.
43. Kiel, J.W.; Kopczynski, C.C. Effect of AR-13324 on episcleral venous pressure in Dutch belted rabbits. *J. Ocul. Pharmacol. Ther.* **2015**, *31*, 146–151. [CrossRef] [PubMed]
44. Dong, Y.-R.; Huang, S.-W.; Cui, J.-Z.; Yoshitomi, T. Effects of Brinzolamide on Rabbit Ocular Blood Flow in Vivo and Ex Vivo. *Int. J. Ophthalmol.* **2018**, *11*, 719.
45. Rao, H.L.; Senthil, S.; Garudadri, C.S. Contralateral Intraocular Pressure Lowering Effect of Prostaglandin Analogues. *Indian J. Ophthalmol.* **2014**, *62*, 575–579. [CrossRef]
46. Piltz, J.; Gross, R.; Shin, D.H.; Beiser, J.A.; Dorr, D.A.; Kass, M.A.; Gordon, M.O. Contralateral Effect of Topical β-Adrenergic Antagonists in Initial One-Eyed Trials in the Ocular Hypertension Treatment Study. *Am. J. Ophthalmol.* **2000**, *130*, 441–453. [CrossRef] [PubMed]
47. Dunham, C.N.; Spaide, R.F.; Dunham, G. The Contralateral Reduction of Intraocular Pressure by Timolol. *Br. J. Ophthalmol.* **1994**, *78*, 38–40. [CrossRef] [PubMed]
48. Arfaee, F.; Armin, A. A Comparison between the Effect of Topical Tafluprost and Latanoprost on Intraocular Pressure in Healthy Male Guinea Pigs. *J. Exot. Pet Med.* **2021**, *39*, 91–95. [CrossRef]
49. Aihara, M.; Lindsey, J.D.; Weinreb, R.N. Reduction of Intraocular Pressure in Mouse Eyes Treated with Latanoprost. *Investig. Ophthalmol. Vis. Sci.* **2002**, *43*, 146–150.
50. Ota, T.; Murata, H.; Sugimoto, E.; Aihara, M.; Araie, M. Prostaglandin Analogues and Mouse Intraocular Pressure: Effects of Tafluprost, Latanoprost, Travoprost, and Unoprostone, Considering 24-Hour Variation. *Investig. Ophthalmol. Vis. Sci.* **2005**, *46*, 2006–2011. [CrossRef] [PubMed]
51. Weinreb, R.N.; Lindsey, J.D. The Importance of Models in Glaucoma Research. *J. Glaucoma* **2005**, *14*, 302–304. [CrossRef]
52. Kim, C.Y.; Kuehn, M.H.; Anderson, M.G.; Kwon, Y.H. Intraocular Pressure Measurement in Mice: A Comparison between Goldmann and Rebound Tonometry. *Eye* **2007**, *21*, 1202–1209. [CrossRef]

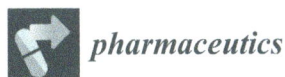

Article

Enhanced Ocular Anti-Aspergillus Activity of Tolnaftate Employing Novel Cosolvent-Modified Spanlastics: Formulation, Statistical Optimization, Kill Kinetics, Ex Vivo Trans-Corneal Permeation, In Vivo Histopathological and Susceptibility Study

Diana Aziz [1], Sally A. Mohamed [2], Saadia Tayel [1] and Amal Makhlouf [1,*]

[1] Department of Pharmaceutics and Industrial Pharmacy, Faculty of Pharmacy, Cairo University, Cairo 11562, Egypt
[2] Department of Microbiology and Immunology, Faculty of Pharmacy, Cairo University, Cairo 12613, Egypt
* Correspondence: amal.makhlouf@pharma.cu.edu.eg

Abstract: Tolnaftate (TOL) is a thiocarbamate fungicidal drug used topically in the form of creams and ointments. No ocular formulations of TOL are available for fungal keratitis (FK) treatment due to its poor water solubility and unique ocular barriers. Therefore, this study aimed at developing novel modified spanlastics by modulating spanlastics composition using different glycols for enhancing TOL ocular delivery. To achieve this goal, TOL basic spanlastics were prepared by ethanol injection method using a full 3^2 factorial design. By applying the desirability function, the optimal formula (BS6) was selected and used as a nucleus for preparing and optimizing TOL-cosolvent spanlastics according to the full $3^1.2^1$ factorial design. The optimal formula (MS6) was prepared using 30% propylene glycol and showed entrapment efficiency percent (EE%) of 66.10 ± 0.57%, particle size (PS) of 231.20 ± 0.141 nm, and zeta potential (ZP) of −32.15 ± 0.07 mV. MS6 was compared to BS6 and both nanovesicles significantly increased the corneal permeation potential of TOL than drug suspension. Additionally, in vivo histopathological experiment was accomplished and confirmed the tolerability of MS6 for ocular use. The fungal susceptibility testing using *Aspergillus niger* confirmed that MS6 displayed more durable growth inhibition than drug suspension. Therefore, MS6 can be a promising option for enhanced TOL ocular delivery.

Keywords: tolnaftate; spanlastics; cosolvent; fungal keratitis; kill kinetics; susceptibility

Citation: Aziz, D.; Mohamed, S.A.; Tayel, S.; Makhlouf, A. Enhanced Ocular Anti-Aspergillus Activity of Tolnaftate Employing Novel Cosolvent-Modified Spanlastics: Formulation, Statistical Optimization, Kill Kinetics, Ex Vivo Trans-Corneal Permeation, In Vivo Histopathological and Susceptibility Study. *Pharmaceutics* 2022, 14, 1746. https://doi.org/10.3390/pharmaceutics14081746

Academic Editors: Ana Catarina Silva and Hugo Almeida

Received: 29 June 2022
Accepted: 16 August 2022
Published: 22 August 2022

Publisher's Note: MDPI stays neutral with regard to jurisdictional claims in published maps and institutional affiliations.

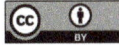

Copyright: © 2022 by the authors. Licensee MDPI, Basel, Switzerland. This article is an open access article distributed under the terms and conditions of the Creative Commons Attribution (CC BY) license (https://creativecommons.org/licenses/by/4.0/).

1. Introduction

Fungal keratitis (FK) is one of the serious corneal infections that can cause eye damage and blindness if not treated effectively. Ocular trauma is considered the most common cause of FK as it can introduce fungi directly into the cornea [1]. It is evident that the most common causative organisms of FK are *Candida* and filamentous fungi (like *Fusarium species* and *Aspergillus species*) [2]. *Aspergillus* spp., if not diagnosed early, can result in macular involvement, damage of the choroid, and necrosis in the retina with subsequent reduction in visual capacity [3]. The spectrum of *Aspergillus* spp. is causing FK to become broader than previously believed [4]. Furthermore, *Aspergillus* is resistant to hot and dry conditions [5]. Hence, FK caused by *Aspergillus* spp. significantly increased over the last few years.

Tolnaftate (TOL) is a synthetic thiocarbamate antifungal agent that acts selectively against filamentous fungi, e.g., *Aspergillus* spp. Its fungicidal activity is mediated by inhibiting squalene epoxidase, which is an important enzyme in the biosynthesis of ergosterol (an important constituent of the fungal membrane). Therefore, squalene accumulates in the fungal plasma membrane and ergosterol is diminished resulting in negative effects on the membrane permeability and fungus growth resulting in cell death [6]. However, the conventionally available topical dosage forms of TOL, e.g., creams, gels, and ointments are of limited efficacy due to their poor penetration potential which requires long-term therapy and consequently decreases patient compliance [7]. Hence, several researchers have put forward their efforts in designing novel topical particulate carriers for enhancing the penetration of TOL for better therapeutic efficacy and increased patient compliance. These carriers include solid lipid nanoparticles [8], nanostructured lipid carriers [8], proniosomes [9,10], niosomal gels [11], and liposomal gels [7]. TOL is predictable to be a favorable therapeutic agent for the treatment of FK due to its selective fungicidal activity, lipophilic character (log P 5.5), and intermediate molecular weight (307.4). These physico-chemical properties enhance TOL permeability through the lipid-rich fungal cell membrane [12]. However, there is no satisfactory data in earlier literature about the use of TOL in an appropriate ocular delivery system for FK treatment due to its poor water solubility (0.00054 mg/mL) and the unique ocular barriers which consequently limit its ocular efficacy [13]. Our research team formulated TOL in novel polymeric pseudorotaxans and confirmed its superiority over TOL suspension in enhancing its ocular permeation and retention [14]. The challenge in this article is to formulate TOL in another novel delivery system for enhancing its water solubility with resultant enhancing its ocular permeation and retention.

The blinking reflex of the eye and its tear film turnover reduce the amount of the applied dose available to be absorbed. The remaining drug must then penetrate through the corneal epithelial constricted junction to be therapeutically effective [15]. Hence, to achieve satisfactory antifungal activity, an ideal topical drug delivery system should possess high corneal penetration, prolonged retention time with the eye, simplicity of installation, decreased frequency of administration with minimal side effects, and better patient compliance [16]. Accordingly, several novel drug delivery systems have been adopted for enhancing the ocular delivery of antifungal agents and improving their ocular bioavailability such as nanovesicles (niosomes, liposomes), elastic vesicles (transferosomes, spanlastics), microemulsions, solid lipid nanoparticles, and polymeric mixed micelles.

Spanlastics, span-based elastic vesicles, are referred to as modified niosomes. Like niosomes, spanlastics are uni/multilamellar spherical structures composed mainly of lipophilic non-ionic surfactant (span) with an additional edge activator that imparts flexibility to their walls [17]. Edge activators (single chain surfactants) can destabilize the vesicles and improve their vesicular bilayer deformability by lowering their surface tension [18]. Hence, the high elasticity of spanlastics helped them to enhance drug permeation through different mucosal bio-membranes (skin, cornea, gastrointestinal mucosa, etc.), by squeezing themselves through membrane pores with minimal risk of vesicular rupture [19]. Spanlastics had been investigated previously for their capability to augment the ocular, trans-duodenal, and transdermal drug absorption [17,20,21].

In the last two decades, great progress has been made in the field of formulating vesicular nano-carriers. For example, water was partially replaced with a cosolvent, e.g., ethanol, glycerol, and propylene glycol in order to induce a degree of elasticity to the vesicular bilayer [22]. In addition to enhancing the vesicular bilayer fluidity, these additives can enhance TOL water solubility due to their high solubilizing power [23]. It had been reported that the transdermal delivery of diclofenac and baicalin was enhanced via the incorporation of cosolvents in the vesicular constructs [22,24]. Up to date, the use of cosolvent-tailored nanovesicles for enhancing ocular delivery has not been yet investigated. Therefore, this research was conducted for accomplishing two main goals; the first one was to formulate TOL spanlastics according to 3^2 factorial designs using Design-Expert® software in order to study the effect of various formulation variables on the prepared spanlastics properties and to select the optimal formulation using desirability function. Secondly, to confirm the hypothesized capacity of cosolvents in enhancing the vesicular deformability, the optimal basic spanlastics were utilized as the nucleus for fashioning novel tailored spanlastics by modifying their composition using various cosolvents. Tailored spanlastics were prepared using a full $2^1 3^1$ factorial design for studying the effect of the type and proportion of the used cosolvent on the vesicular properties and selecting the optimal one based on the desirability function.

2. Materials and Methods

2.1. Materials

Tolnaftate (TOL) was supplied by Hikma pharmaceuticals (Cairo, Egypt). Span 60 (sorbitan monostearate) and Tween 80 (polyoxyethylene sorbitan monooleate) were acquired from Sigma Chemical Co. (St. Louis, MO, USA). Absolute methanol, absolute ethanol, glycerol, and propylene glycol were acquired from El-Nasr Pharmaceutical Chemicals Co. (Abu-Zaabal, Cairo, Egypt).

2.2. Preparation of TOL Basic Spanlastics

TOL basic spanlastics (prepared without the incorporation of cosolvents) were formulated using ethanol injection method [25]. Precisely, Span 60 and TOL (10 mg) were dissolved in 5 mL of absolute ethanol which was sonicated for 5 min at 80 °C to obtain a clear solution. The resultant alcoholic solution was then rapidly injected into the pre-heated aqueous solution (Tween 80, as edge activator, dissolved in 10 mL ultra-pure distilled water and heated to the temperature of 80 °C at 600 rpm using a 30 gauze syringe). The ratio of Span 60 to Tween 80 was optimized using Design-Expert® software (Version 7, Stat-Ease, Inc., Minneapolis, MN, USA) according to full 3^2 factorial design (Table 1). Post hoc analysis was performed using Tukey's honest significant difference (HSD) test using SPSS software 17.0 (SPSS Inc., Chicago, IL, USA). Stirring was continued at 80 °C for 30 min. Spanlastics were formed spontaneously turning the solution slightly turbid. Then, the resultant turbid solution was left for another 30 min on a magnetic stirrer at room temperature for ethanol removal by evaporation. For reduction of PS, the prepared formulae were sonicated in a bath sonicator at 25 °C for 10 min. TOL basic spanlastics formulations were then left overnight to equilibrate at 4 °C.

Table 1. Full 3^2 factorial design for TOL basic spanlastics optimization.

Factors	Levels		
X_1: Span 60 amount (mg)	200	300	400
X_2: Tween 80 amount (mg)	50	100	150
Responses (dependent variables)	Desirability Constraints		
Y_1: EE%	Maximize		
Y_2: PS (nm)	Minimize		
Y_3: ZP (mV)	Maximize (as absolute value)		

Abbreviations: EE%, entrapment efficiency; PS, particle size; ZP, zeta potential.

2.3. In Vitro TOL Basic Spanlastics Characterization

2.3.1. Entrapment Efficiency (EE%)

TOL basic spanlastics formulae were filtered using Whatman filter paper (grade No. 1, 11 µm) to separate the unentrapped drug due to the extremely low solubility of TOL in water [17,26,27] whereas vesicles loaded with TOL passed through the filter paper to the filtrate. Then, 0.3 mL of the filtrate were then sonicated with methanol, and the entrapped TOL concentration was measured spectrophotometrically at 257 nm. Each result was expressed as the mean of three measurements ± SD. TOL EE% was calculated by the following formula:

$$EE\% = \frac{\text{Incorporated amount of TOL}}{\text{Totlal amount of TOL}} \times 100$$

2.3.2. Particle Size (PS), Polydispersity Index (PDI), and Zeta Potential (ZP)

Zetasizer Nano ZS (Malvern Instrument Ltd., Worcestershire, UK) was used in the determination of PS, PDI, and ZP of the prepared TOL basic spanlastics applying dynamic light scattering technique. The formulations were diluted with deionized water prior to measurement to produce proper scattering intensity. Each measurement was carried out in triplicates.

2.4. TOL Basic Spanlastics Formulation Optimization

Desirability function was applied to select the optimum TOL basic spanlastics. The optimization process targeted to achieve a formula with the highest EE% and ZP (as absolute value) and the least PS as presented in Table 1. The formula with the highest desirability value (near to one) was chosen. To check whether the responses predicted by the software are valid or not, the optimized TOL basic spanlastics formula was prepared and characterized and its responses were compared to the predicted ones [28].

2.5. Modification of the Optimal TOL Basic Spanlastics Using Cosolvents

Cosolvent-modified spanlastics (TOL-cosolvent spanlastics) were prepared using the same components of the optimal basic spanlastics together with different cosolvents (glycerol and propylene glycol in different concentrations). Formulations were prepared using the same ethanol injection technique employed for the preparation of the basic spanlastics, and the cosolvent was added to the pre-heated aqueous medium.

2.6. Statistical Design for the Preparation of TOL-Cosolvent Spanlastics

A full factorial design ($3^1.2^1$) was utilized using Design-Expert® software to prepare TOL-cosolvent spanlastics. Changing the utilized cosolvent (X_1) and its percentage (%v/v) (X_2) were considered as the independent variables X_1 and X_2, respectively. On the other hand, EE% (Y_1), PS (Y_2), and ZP (Y_3) were the selected dependent variables as shown in Table 2. For the percentage of the used cosolvent (X_2), post hoc analysis was performed by Tukey's HSD test utilizing SPSS software 17.0.

Table 2. Full ($3^1.2^1$) factorial design for optimization of TOL-cosolvent spanlastics.

Factors	Levels		
X_1: Type of cosolvent	Glycerol		Propylene glycol
X_2: Percentage of cosolvent	10	20	30
Responses (dependent variables)	**Desirability Constraints**		
Y_1: EE%	Maximize		
Y_2: PS (nm)	Minimize		
Y_3: ZP (mV)	Maximize (as absolute value)		

Abbreviations: EE%, entrapment efficiency percent; PS, particle size; ZP, zeta potential.

2.7. In Vitro TOL-Cosolvent Spanlastics Characterization

2.7.1. Entrapment Efficiency (EE%)

EE% of TOL-cosolvent spanlastics was determined using the same procedures followed for determination of EE% of TOL spanlastics.

2.7.2. Particle Size (PS), Polydispersity Index (PDI), and Zeta Potential (ZP)

As previously mentioned, PS, ZP, and PDI were determined using Zetasizer at 25 °C.

2.8. TOL-Cosolvent Spanlastics Optimization

The optimum TOL-cosolvent spanlastics composition was predicted by applying the desirability function method using Design-Expert® software (Version 7, Stat-Ease, Inc., Minneapolis, MN, USA). The optimization criteria were the smallest PS, the highest EE%, and absolute value of ZP (Table 2). The formulation with the highest desirability value was chosen for further characterizations. After selection, the optimal formulation was prepared, characterized, and compared with the predicted responses to confirm the model efficacy. Thereafter, to explore the effect of the added cosolvent on the vesicular physico-chemical properties, the characteristics of the optimal cosolvent tailored spanlastics (PS, ZP, and

EE%) were compared to those of the optimal basic spanlastics. Student's *t*-test was used to statistically analyze the results.

2.9. Transmission Electron Microscopy (TEM)

The morphological features of the selected optimal TOL-cosolvent spanlastics were assessed using TEM (Joel JEM 1230, Tokyo, Japan). One drop of the undiluted sample was placed on a carbon-coated copper grid and allowed to dry for about 10 min at room temperature and subsequently investigated.

2.10. Differential Scanning Calorimetry (DSC)

Thermal analysis of TOL, Span 60, the optimum TOL-cosolvent spanlastics formula, and the physical mixture of TOL with spanlastics ingredients was accomplished by a previously calibrated differential scanning calorimeter (DSC-60, Shimadzu, Kyoto, Japan). Each sample ($\approx$5 mg) was placed in a standard aluminum pan and heated in a temperature range of 10–300 °C at a heating rate of 10 °C/min with continuous purging of nitrogen (25 mL/min).

2.11. Ex Vivo Studies

2.11.1. Corneas Preparation

The Research Ethics Committee of the Faculty of Pharmacy, Cairo University, Egypt approved the study (PI 2982). Adult male New Zealand albino rabbits (2.5–3.0 kg) were used to extract the corneas. The rabbits were decapitated following anesthesia with an intramuscular injection of ketamine 35 mg/kg, and a relaxing agent: xylazine 5 mg/kg [29]. The eyes were enucleated immediately, and the corneas were excised and cautiously cleaned with saline and checked for being free from any pores before using in the test. The permeation experiment was conducted within half an hour of corneas extraction [25].

2.11.2. Corneal Permeation Study

A modified static Franz diffusion cell (area = 0.64) was used in TOL corneal permeation studies. The excised corneas were sandwiched between the donor and receptor chamber. The receptor medium was 100 mL of methanol: water (3:2), and it was kept under continuous stirring (100 rpm) at 37 °C [30]. Accurate volume of each of the optimal TOL-cosolvent spanlastics, TOL basic spanlastics, and TOL aqueous suspension (equivalent to 300 µg TOL) was loaded under non-occlusive conditions on the corneal surface (donor compartment). At different time intervals (0.5, 1, 2, 4, 6, and 8 h), 3 mL volumes were withdrawn from the receptor compartment and fresh medium was added to replace the withdrawn samples. The study was performed three times and the results were presented as mean ± SD. TOL amount in the samples was determined by a validated HPLC system (Shimadzu, Kyoto, Japan) equipped with L-7110 pump unit and an X Terra™ column (Reversed C18:4.6 mm × 250 mm) having 5 µm size adsorbent as stationary phase (Milford, CT, USA). We used methanol 80% (v/v) as a mobile phase which flowed with a rate of 1.2 mL/min, and the drug was detected at 258 nm [31]. The assay procedures were validated for linearity, accuracy, and precision.

The cumulative amount of TOL permeated per unit area (µg/cm^2) was plotted against time (h). The flux (J$_{max}$) at 8 h and the enhancement ratio (ER) were calculated using the following equations [32].

$$J_{max} = \frac{\text{Amount of drug permeated}}{\text{Time} \times \text{Area of membrane}}$$

$$ER = \frac{J_{max} \text{of the optimal nanoformulation}}{J_{max} \text{of the drug suspension}}$$

The differences in J$_{max}$ and total TOL permeated were statistically analyzed using SPSS software 17.0. Post hoc analysis was performed using Tukey's HSD test. The difference was considered significant when $p \leq 0.05$.

2.12. In Vitro Antifungal Activity

2.12.1. Fungal Strain and Inoculum Preparation

In this study, *Aspergillus niger* standard strain (ATCC32656) was tested. Sabouraud Dextrose Agar (SDA) (Oxoid, Hampshire, UK) was used as the growth medium and the plates were incubated for 48–96 h at 28 ± 2 °C. The germinating spores were harvested in sterile normal saline solution, and the inoculum size was adjusted to 10^5–10^6 CFU/mL count.

2.12.2. Tested Samples

For the in vitro antifungal activity, the tested treatments were (i) the optimum TOL-cosolvent spanlastics (MS6) (treatment A), (ii) TOL aqueous suspension (1 mg/mL) (treatment B), and (iii) placebo solution (TOL-free optimum cosolvent-spanlastics formula).

2.12.3. Minimum Inhibitory Concentration (MIC)

The determination of MIC was performed utilizing microbroth dilution technique according to Sayed et al. [30,33]. Two-fold serially diluted treatments A and B were set in double strength Sabouraud Dextrose Broth (SDB) (500–0.24 µg/mL), dispensed into U-shaped bottom 96-well plates, then 10 µL of the spore suspension (inoculum size of 10^5–10^6 CFU/mL) was added to each well. Negative control (double strength SDB only) and positive control (double strength SDB and two-fold serial dilution of placebo solution with 10 µL of the inoculum) were adopted. The microplates were incubated at 28 ± 2 °C for 48 h. The MIC was determined as the lowest concentration having no observable fungal growth. Triplicates of the experiment were conducted.

2.12.4. Minimum Fungicidal Concentration (MFC)

For treatment A and treatment B, the determination of MFC was performed using broth microdilution method according the Clinical and Laboratory Standards Institute guidelines [33]. Briefly, 2-fold serially diluted treatment A or B till the MIC together with the 10 µL spore suspension at 28 ± 2 °C were incubated in 96-well plates for 24 h. Then, 10 µL of mixture was spotted on SDA plates. The plates were then incubated at 28 ± 2 °C for 48 h then the fungal colony count (as CFU/mL) was determined. The MFC was expressed as the lowest treatment concentration that shows no fungal growth.

2.12.5. Kill Kinetics Assay

Time–kill kinetics of treatment A and treatment B against *Aspergillus niger* (ATCC32656) were conducted according to the method described by Ismail et al., with some modifications [34]. Briefly, the killing kinetics of treatment A and treatment B were assayed at the fungicidal concentrations. In a 96-well microtiter plate, 100 µL of the double strength SDB and 100 µL of treatment A or treatment B in its MFC concentration together with 10 µL of the spore suspension (inoculum size of 10^5–10^6 CFU/mL). Ten microliters of this mixture were added to 90 µL of saline solution, 10-fold serially diluted, and subjected to viable colony count on SDA medium (0 time sample). The 96-well microtiter plate containing the mixture of treatment and fungal spores was incubated at 28 ± 2 °C for up to 24 h. Then, samples of each test were withdrawn at time intervals of 4, 6, 10, 16, and 24 h, diluted, and subjected to viable colony count on SDA medium. The test was performed in triplicates.

2.13. In Vivo Studies

2.13.1. Animals

The Research Ethics Committee at Faculty of Pharmacy, Cairo University, Egypt (PI 2982) approved the study. Twelve male albino rabbits (2–3 kg) were used in the study. The rabbits were individually caged under proper conditions of humidity, temperature (25 ± 2 °C), and 12 h light/dark cycles. The animals were on a standard dry food and water ad libitum. Examination of the rabbits by a slit lamp was performed to exclude animals with ocular inflammation or disorder before the study.

2.13.2. Draize Test

In order to assess the irritation potential of the optimal formula, a scoring system was applied using three male albino New Zealand rabbits [29]. An aliquot of 100 µL of the optimal TOL-cosolvent spanlastics was added to the right eye (in the conjunctival sac) and the left eye was treated with normal saline to serve as control. We examined the right eye visually at 1, 2, 5, 8, and 24 h after installation for any irritation, and the eye was scored according to Draize scale [19,29]. The Draize scale was given as follows: 0, no reaction; 1, very slight erythema; 2, well-defined erythema; 3, moderate to severe erythema [19].

2.13.3. Histopathology

Male albino New Zealand rabbits (3 animals) were utilized to assess the safety of the prepared spanlastics. The optimum TOL-cosolvent spanlastics (one drop) were dropped into the rabbit's right eye and normal saline was installed into the left eye as control. The treatments were repeated at one-hour intervals for a total of six hours [35]. Then, the rabbits were anesthetized and euthanized and their eyeballs were extracted, washed with normal saline solution, and fixed in 10% formalin in saline for 24 h. Then, the samples were washed with tap water followed by serial dilutions of alcohols to dehydrate the samples. Then, specimens were cleared in xylene and fixed in paraffin for 24 h at 56 degrees in hot air oven. A sledge microtome (Leica Microsystems SM2400, Cambridge, UK) was used to prepare paraffin beeswax tissue blocks by sectioning at 4 microns thickness. Then tissue sections were presented on glass slides, deparaffinized, stained by hematoxylin and eosin stain to be examined under light electric microscope [36].

2.13.4. Susceptibility Test

The tested microorganism was *Aspergillus niger* (ATCC32656). A parallel design of two groups each composed of three rabbits was applied. The study was performed according to Albash et al. [37]. Group I was administered the optimal TOL-cosolvent spanlastics (treatment A) and group II was administered TOL suspension (treatment B). Equal volumes (50 µL containing 50 µg TOL) of treatment A and treatment B were applied in the lower conjunctival sac of the rabbit's right eye using micropipette. No treatment was applied in the left eye of all rabbits to serve as the control. At predetermined intervals (2–24 h), four sterile filter paper discs (Whatman no. 5, 6 mm in diameter) were wetted by placing the discs under the eyelid of each eye. For each eye (right and left), two discs were placed in a 1.5 mL Eppendorf tube containing 500 µL SDB inoculated with 10% v/v fungal spore suspension (10^5–10^6 CFU/mL). The other two discs were placed in a 1.5 mL Eppendorf tube containing 500 µL uninoculated SDB as a blank for measuring the optical densities. All tubes were then incubated at $28 \pm 2\ °C$ for 48 h under aerobic conditions. At the end of the incubation period, 200 µL of each tube was transferred to a sterile 96-well plate and the optical densities ($OD_{600\ nm}$) were read on an automated spectrophotometric plate reader (Biotek, Synergy 2, Winooski, VT, USA). The results were presented as growth inhibition % calculated according to the following equation:

$$\text{Growth inhibition \%} = \frac{\text{Control (left eye) OD600 nm} - \text{Test (right eye) OD600 nm}}{\text{Control (left eye) OD600 nm}} \times 100$$

3. Results and Discussion

3.1. Preparation of TOL Basic Spanlastics

Based on the preliminary studies, the ethanol injection method was the most appropriate method for preparing TOL spanlastics. Span 60, a lipophilic non-ionic surfactant (HLB = 4.7), was selected due to the lipophilicity of its saturated alkyl chain which cards the formation of multi-lamellar vesicles [21]. Furthermore, the surface-active nature of Span 60 would boost the action of the edge activator in reducing the interfacial tension with the subsequent production of fine spanlastics dispersion. In contrast, it was shown that Span 40 and Span 80 formed vesicles with a high degree of instability and aggregation [38]. The incorporation of edge activators would enhance the vesicular elastic nature and increase their deformability. Different edge

60 (film-forming material), multiple layers would have accumulated over each other and consequently, PS increased. These results can also be correlated with the noticeable increase in EE% by increasing the amount of Span 60. As previously mentioned, increasing Span 60 amount increased the amount of TOL incorporated in vesicles' hydrophobic region and consequently increased the distance between the vesicular lipid bilayer with the resultant increase in PS [43]. Oppositely, the PS of TOL basic spanlastics was not significantly affected by the amount of Tween 80 (X_2) (p = 0.1270).

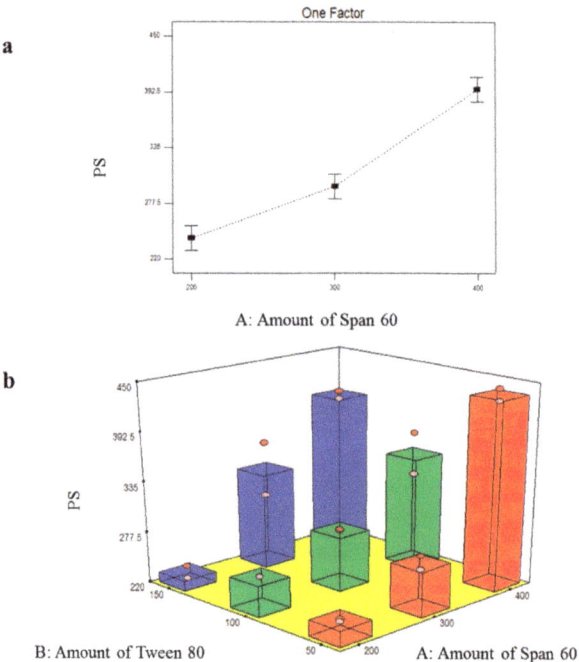

Figure 2. Line plot of the significant effect of Span 60 amount (X_1) (**a**) and response 3D plot for the combined effect of Span 60 amount (X_1) and Tween 80 amount (X_2) (**b**) on PS of TOL basic spanlastics.

3.2.3. Formulation Variables Effect on ZP of TOL Basic Spanlastics

The nanosystem stability is related directly to the magnitude of the electric charge adsorbed on its surface. It was observed that TOL basic spanlastics were with negative ZP values which fluctuated from -23.25 ± 0.78 to -39.45 ± 0.92 mV (Table 3). This negative charge will prevent aggregation and give more stable dispersion. The influence of the amount of Span 60 (X_1) and the amount of Tween 80 (X_2) on the ZP of TOL basic spanlastics is illustrated in Figure 3. Statistical analysis showed that both X_1: the amount of Span 60 and X_2: the amount of Tween 80 had a significant effect on ZP of TOL basic spanlastics ($p < 0.0001$ and = 0.0047, respectively) (Table 4). With respect to the effect of the amount of Span 60 (X_1) on ZP, post hoc analysis revealed that spanlastics prepared using 400 mg Span 60 had the highest ZP and that ZP increased by increasing the amount of Span 60 in a concentration-dependent manner. This might be attributed to the ionizable carboxylate group present within the polar head of Span 60, which is normally directed towards the aqueous external phase creating net negative ZP [46]. Hence, by increasing Span 60 amount, more negative carboxylate groups would reside on the vesicular surface, and consequently, ZP increases. With respect to the effect of the amount of Tween 80 (X_2) on ZP of TOL basic spanlastics, the post hoc test showed that spanlastics containing 100 mg Tween 80 possessed the highest ZP compared to spanlastics prepared using 50 and 150 mg. The higher ZP values of spanlastics containing 100 mg compared to those of 50 mg are referred to as the EE% which increased when the Tween

80 amount increased as previously stated. TOL, containing an ionizable thiocarbamate group, could ionize and obtain a negative charge in alkaline and neutral pH. Hence, by increasing the amount of Tween 80 from 50 to 100 mg, more TOL would be entrapped within the vesicles with further ionization of the thiocarbamate group and consequently increased negative charge acquired by the formed spanlastics [47]. As previously mentioned, there was no significant difference in EE% of spanlastics containing 100 mg and those of 150 mg Tween 80. However, the latter showed significantly lower ZP values. Tween 80, being a non-ionic surfactant, can reside on the surface of the vesicles' bilayer due to its hydrophilicity and consequently shield the acquired negative surface charge [48]. Hence, by increasing the amount of Tween 80, the negative ZP values gradually decreased due to the accumulation of the hydrophilic non-ionic surfactant (Tween 80) on the vesicular bilayer surface with consequent shielding of the surface negative charge [20,21].

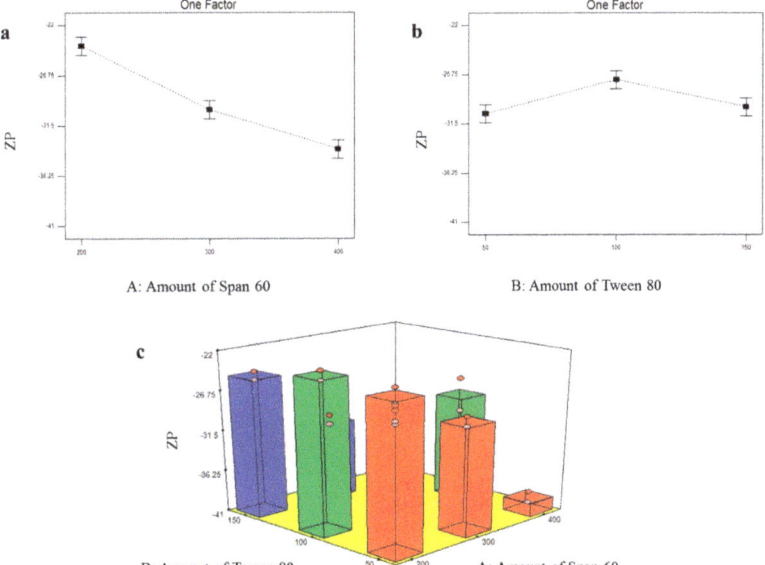

Figure 3. Line plots of the significant effect of Span 60 amount (X_1) (**a**), Tween 80 amount (X_2) (**b**), response 3D plot for the combined effect of Span 60 amount (X_1) and Tween 80 amount (X_2) (**c**), on ZP of TOL basic spanlastics.

3.3. Selection of the Optimal TOL Basic Spanlastics

In order to select the optimal formula from the nine prepared spanlastics formulations, a response surface analysis of the factorial design was performed using Design-Expert® software. The predetermined constraints for optimization (minimizing PS and maximizing EE% and ZP, as absolute value), were achieved in BS6 with total desirability of 0.633. BS6 was composed of 400 mg Span 60 and 100 mg Tween 80 and showed EE% of 76.80 ± 7.07%, PS of 349.55 ± 34.44 nm, and ZP of −28.75 ± 2.76 mV. Therefore, BS6 was selected as a nucleus formula for preparing and optimizing novel cosolvent-modified spanlastics.

3.4. Factorial Design Analysis of TOL-Cosolvent Spanlastics

To assess the effect of using different cosolvents on the physicochemical properties of spanlastics and to evaluate the effect of cosolvent amount on these properties, a full $3^1.2^1$ factorial design was utilized and statistically analyzed through Design-Expert® software. The model selected was 2FI. The measured responses of the six experimental runs are presented in Table 5. As shown in Table 6, adequate precision is greater than 4 (the desirable value) in all responses except ZP which was a non-significant model term. It was also noted that the predicted R^2 values came in reasonable agreement with the adjusted R^2 in all responses except ZP (Table 6). The negative predicted R^2 value of ZP indicates that the overall mean is a better predictor of the response [49]. This might be due to the fact that the ZP of the prepared tailored spanlastics was not significantly influenced by any of the tested factors.

Table 5. Experimental runs, independent variables, and measured responses of $3^1.2^1$ full factorial experimental design of TOL-cosolvent spanlastics.

Runs	X_1	X_2	Y_1	Y_2	Y_3
	Cosolvent Type	Cosolvent Percentage	EE% [a]	PS (nm) [a]	ZP (mV) [a]
MS1	Glycerol	10	71 ± 5.66	416.5 ± 33.23	−30.9 ± 1.13
MS2	Glycerol	20	37.8 ± 1.56	285.5 ± 11.17	−29.75 ± 2.90
MS3	Glycerol	30	72.5 ± 2.83	581.5 ± 2.55	−31.9 ± 1.13
MS4	Propylene glycol	10	56.73 ± 15.09	328.55 ± 14.21	−31.8 ± 0.71
MS5	Propylene glycol	20	57.45 ± 2.76	374.85 ± 32.74	−28.7 ± 2.12
MS6	Propylene glycol	30	66.1 ± 0.57	231.2 ± 0.141	−32.15 ± 0.07

Abbreviations: EE%, entrapment efficiency percent; PS, particle size ZP, zeta potential; MS, modified spanlastics.
[a] Data represented as mean ± SD (n = 3).

Table 6. Output data of the full factorial analysis of TOL-cosolvent spanlastics.

Responses	R^2	Adjusted R^2	Predicted R^2	Adequate Precision	Significant Factors
EE%	0.8557	0.7354	0.4226	7.209	X_2 (=0.0089)
PS (nm)	0.9836	0.9699	0.9342	24.226	X_1 (<0.0001), X_2 (=0.0009)
ZP (mV)	0.5441	0.1641	−0.8238	2.991	—

Abbreviations: EE%, entrapment efficiency percent; PS, particle size; ZP, zeta potential.

3.4.1. Effect of Formulation Variables on EE% of TOL-Cosolvent Spanlastics

EE% of all TOL-cosolvent spanlastics ranged from 37.80 ± 1.56 to 72.50 ± 2.83% as demonstrated in Table 5. The influence of type of cosolvent (X_1) and percentage of cosolvent (X_2) is graphically illustrated in Figure 4. Results of the ANOVA test revealed that type of cosolvent (X_1) did not significantly affected EE% of TOL-modified spanlastics ($p = 0.9339$). On the other side, the percentage of the cosolvent (X_2) possessed significant effect on EE% ($p = 0.0089$). By increasing the percentage of cosolvent (glycerol or propylene glycol), EE% significantly increased. This could be attributed to the cosolvent positive effect on TOL solubility in the lipid phase [50]. Furthermore, the higher concentration of cosolvent allowed a superior lipid packing and more efficient drug loading [51].

3.4.2. Formulation Variables Effect on PS of TOL-Cosolvent Spanlastics

As shown in Table 5, the PS of the prepared TOL-cosolvent spanlastics fluctuated from 231.20 ± 0.141 to 581.50 ± 2.55 nm. Figure 5 illustrates the effect of type of cosolvent (X_1) and percentage of cosolvent (X_2) on PS of the prepared tailored spanlastics. Statistical analysis showed that type of cosolvent (X_1) had a significant effect on PS ($p < 0.0001$). Due to the higher viscosity of glycerol, it was shown that it formed significantly larger vesicles compared to propylene glycol-modified spanlastics [52]. Additionally, Manconi et al. reported the reduction in PS by incorporation of glycols [51]. It was also shown that the percentage of cosolvent (X_2) significantly affected the PS of the prepared spanlastics ($p = 0.0009$). With respect to glycerol-based vesicles, the ANOVA test revealed that increasing concentration of glycerol caused the formation of bigger vesicles due to the glycerol viscous nature [52]. In contrast, 30% propylene glycol-based vesicles showed the smallest PS. This could be related to that the incorporation of propylene glycol caused reduction in vesicular size due to its interaction with vesicular bilayer causing more bilayer flexibility and small vesicle size. Hence, increasing propylene glycol percentage showed significant negative effect on vesicular size [50]. These results also came in agreement with Manconi et al. who reported that diclofenac-loaded vesicles showed significant decrease in PS by increasing the percentage of propylene glycol to 40 and 50% [51].

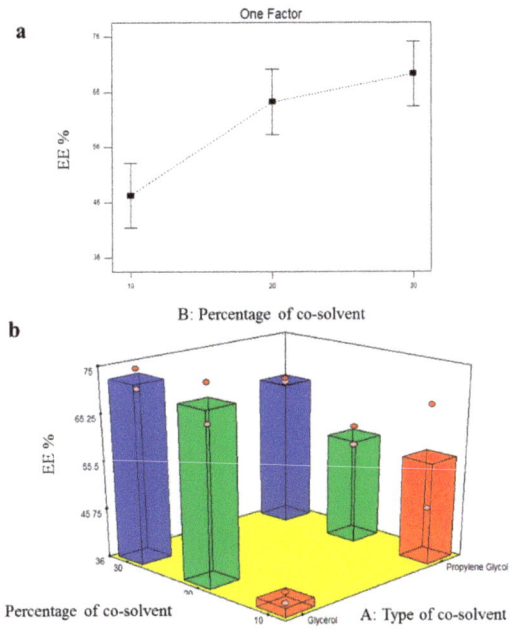

Figure 4. Line plots of the significant effect of cosolvent percentage (X_2) (**a**) and response 3D plot for the combined effect of cosolvent type (X_1) and cosolvent percentage (X_2) (**b**), on EE% of TOL-cosolvent spanlastics.

3.4.3. Formulation Variables Effect on ZP of TOL-Cosolvent Spanlastics

The ZP of TOL-cosolvent spanlastics fluctuated between -28.70 ± 2.12 and -32.15 ± 0.07 mV as shown in Table 5. The ZP of the prepared spanlastics was not affected significantly by the studied factors ($p > 0.05$).

3.5. Selection of the Optimal TOL-Cosolvent Spanlastics

Desirability was determined by identifying the optimal formula that has the highest EE% and ZP, as the absolute value, and the lowest PS. These desirability constraints were established in MS6 with overall desirability of 0.895. MS6 was prepared using 30% propylene glycol and showed EE% of 66.10 ± 0.57%, PS of 231.20 ± 0.141 nm, and -32.15 ± 0.07 mV. By comparing the measured responses for both BS6 and MS6, MS6 showed significantly smaller PS compared to BS6 ($p = 0.04$) due to the influence of the incorporated cosolvent (propylene glycol) on enhancing the vesicular bilayer flexibility and consequently producing vesicles with smaller PS [50]. Hence, MS6 was selected for further characterization. Oppositely both vesicles showed was no significant difference in EE% and ZP ($p = 0.167$ and 0.223, respectively).

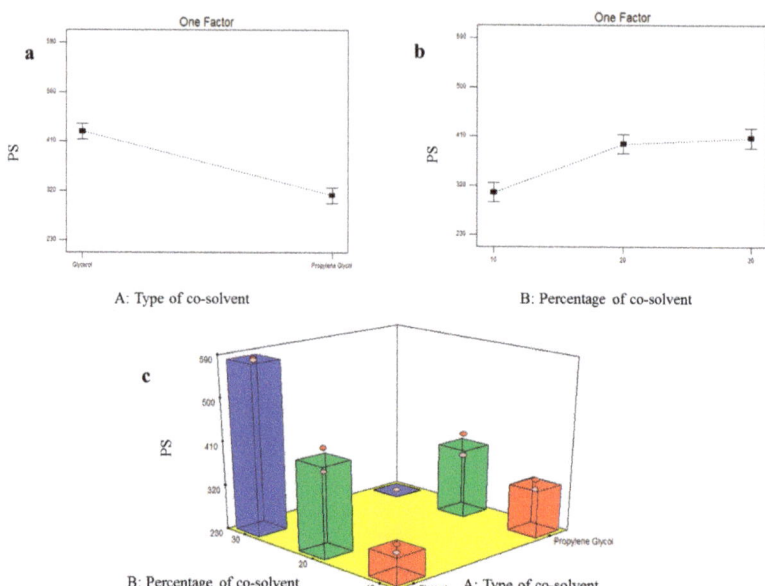

Figure 5. Line plots of the significant effect of type of cosolvent (X_1) (**a**), percentage of cosolvent (X_2) (**b**), response 3D plot for the combined effect of type of cosolvent (X_1), and percentage of cosolvent (X_2) (**c**) on PS of TOL-cosolvent spanlastics.

3.6. Transmission Electron Microscopy (TEM)

TEM imaging is valuable for describing the morphological features of the prepared system [41]. Illustrative photomicrographs of MS6 are exemplified in Figure 6. The developed modified spanlastics were well scattered without any aggregations. Furthermore, the vesicular diameter observed by TEM was in line with that previously measured using a Zetasizer and ranged from 200–300 nm.

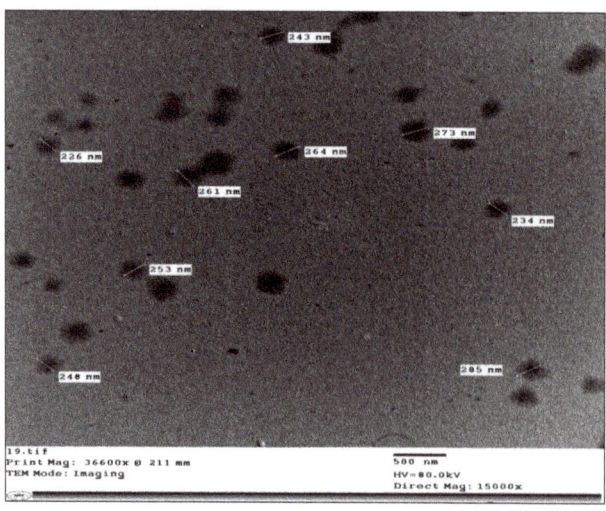

Figure 6. Transmission electron micrograph of MS6.

3.7. Differential Scanning Calorimetry (DSC)

The DSC thermograms of TOL, Span 60, TOL-Span 60-Tween 80-propylene glycol physical mixture, and MS6 are shown in Figure 7. Since the measuring temperature of DSC equipment ranged from 25 to 725 °C, the thermotropic properties of Tween 80 and propylene glycol, being liquids at room temperature, could not be assessed in this work [17]. The DSC thermogram of pure TOL showed a single endothermic peak at 112.31 °C corresponding to its melting point due to the TOL crystallinity [53]. The endothermic peak at 55.05 °C was for Span 60 and corresponded to its melting point [54]. Regarding the DSC thermogram of the physical mixture of TOL with cosolvent-modified spanlastics components, it showed the endothermic transition of TOL but with lower intensity compared to the pure drug. This might be attributed to the dilution of the drug with the used excipients [55]. Oppositely, the TOL endothermic peak was completely absent in the thermogram of MS6 confirming that TOL was entrapped in cosolvent-modified spanlastics and perfectly interacted with the vesicular bilayer. Furthermore, the development of a less-ordered lattice arrangement in the case of MS6 compared to pure excipients was evidenced by the changes in the positions of the melting peak (lowering of the melting enthalpies) of both TOL and Span 60 together with the appearance of a broad endothermic peak at 91.38 °C [20]. It could also be related to the effect of Tween 80 as an edge activator in perturbing the packing characteristics of Span 60 and consequently fluidizing the vesicular bilayer [56]. Hence, the aforementioned results confirmed that TOL dispersed homogenously within spanlastics in an amorphous form.

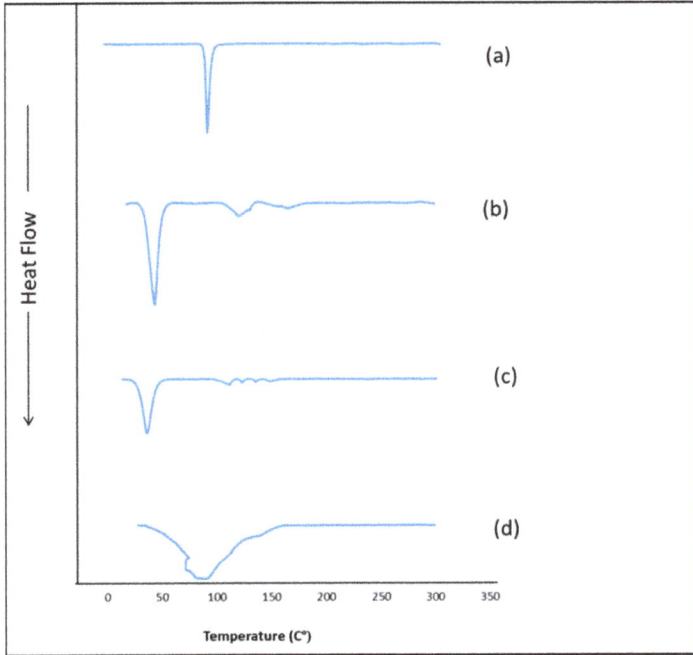

Figure 7. DSC thermograms of (**a**) TOL, (**b**) Span 60, (**c**) physical mixture of TOL-cosolvent spanlastics components, and (**d**) formula MS6.

3.8. Ex Vivo Corneal Permeation

TOL permeability from MS6 was examined using excised rabbits' corneas and its corneal permeation profile was constructed and compared to that of BS6 and drug suspension (Figure 8). By comparing the corneal permeability parameters, it was shown that both MS6 and BS6 significantly enhanced the drug flux and resulted in a higher amount of TOL permeated in 8 h compared to TOL suspension ($p < 0.05$) (Table 7). This significantly enhanced TOL ocular delivery through cosolvent-modified spanlastics as well as basic spanlastics could be related to the hydrophilic ingredients of these elastic vesicles (edge activators and propylene glycol) which are attracted preferentially to the area of high water content such as the aqueous humor and the vitreous of the eye which constitutes a majority of water (≈90%). Hence, edge activators enhance the vesicular deep migration in the water-rich environment, carrying drug molecules to secure and acceptable hydration conditions [25,57]. In addition, the nanometric size of these elastic vesicles eased their passage through the narrow hydrated corneal stromal network as a fine dispersion compared to coarse PS of drug suspension [58].

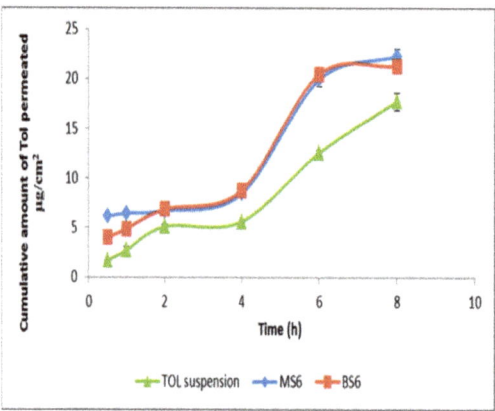

Figure 8. Ex vivo corneal permeation profile of TOL-cosolvent spanlastics (MS6) and basic spanlastics (BS6) compared to TOL suspension.

Table 7. Ex vivo corneal permeability parameters of TOL-cosolvent spanlastics (MS6) and basic spanlastics (BS6) compared to a drug suspension.

Formulation	Total Amount of TOL Permeated per Unit Area in 8 h (µg/cm^2) [a]	J_{max} (µg/cm^2/h) [a]	ER
MS6	22.33 ± 0.67	4.36 ± 0.13	1.26
BS6	21.30 ± 0.07	4.16 ± 0.01	1.20
Drug suspension	17.74 ± 0.89	3.46 ± 0.17	1

Abbreviations: J_{max}, flux; ER, enhancement ratio; MS, modified spanlastics; BS, basic spanlastics. [a] Data presented as mean ± SD (n = 3).

3.9. In Vitro Antifungal Activity

3.9.1. Minimum Inhibitory Concentration (MIC)

The microbroth dilution technique was applied in the antifungal assays in order to investigate whether the optimal TOL-cosolvent spanlastics (MS6) impacts the antifungal activity of TOL. The MIC of MS6 (treatment A) was 0.49 µg/mL, while TOL suspension (treatment B) had a higher MIC (1.95 µg/mL) and that for the placebo solution was 125 µg/mL. Hence, the antifungal activity of MS6 was improved in comparison to that of TOL suspension. This might be related to the ability of MS6 to enhance TOL solubility, which consequently enhanced TOL penetration through the fungal cell wall and inhibited ergosterol biosynthesis which is responsible for its activity [16,30].

3.9.2. Minimum Fungicidal Concentration (MFC)

The broth microdilution technique was used to determine MFC for treatment A and B. Both MS6 and TOL suspension exhibited fungicidal effect after 48 h of incubation at 28 °C ± 2 for. MS6 (treatment A) showed a more powerful fungicidal effect at 3.9 µg/mL

(8× MIC), whereases MFC of TOL suspension (treatment B) was higher with a value of 125 µg/mL (64× MIC). Therefore, TOL suspension had inferior fungicidal activity compared to that of MS6.

3.9.3. Kill Kinetics Assay

The killing kinetics of *Aspergillus niger* (ATCC32656) by treatment A and treatment B were investigated. Treatment A (MS6) killed *Aspergillus niger* (ATCC32656) after 16 h incubation at its MFC concentration (3.9 µg/mL) (9× MIC), while longer time (24 h) was needed for treatment B (TOL suspension) to kill *Aspergillus niger* (ATCC32656) at its MFC concentration (125 µg/mL) (64× MIC) (Figure 9). This confirmed the superior anti-aspergillus activity of TOL-cosolvent spanlastics compared to the drug suspension.

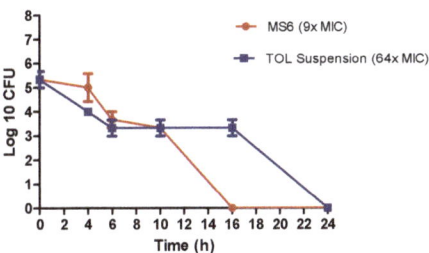

Figure 9. The killing kinetics of treatment A (MS6) and treatment B (TOL suspension) tested against *Aspergillus niger* (ATCC32656). Treatment A tested at concentration of (3.9 µg/mL) (9× MIC), treatment B (TOL suspension) tested at concentration of (125 µg/mL) (64× MIC). Data are represented by means of the number of recovered colonies counted at each time point ± SD, n = 3. The chart was generated using GraphPad Prism (v5) (GraphPad, California, CA, USA).

3.10. In Vivo Studies

3.10.1. Draize Test

The obtained results of the Draize test showed that corneas treated with MS6 did not show irritation, lacrimation, or any sign of inflation compared to the control eye at all tested time points. Hence, they scored zero on the Draize scale. These results suggested the ocular tolerance of the optimally modified spanlastics.

3.10.2. Histopathology

The obtained photomicrographs exhibited the absence of any histopathological changes in the cornea (the lining corneal epithelium, the underlying stroma, and endothelium) (Figure 10(a2)). The same results were observed in the iris (Figure 10(b2)), retina, choroid, and sclera (Figure 10(c2)) compared to control (Figure 10(a1–c1)). The absence of any histopathological abnormalities in ocular tissues after treatment with TOL-cosolvent spanlastics confirmed its tolerability and safety for ocular application.

3.10.3. Susceptibility Test

The retention time of the drug on the surface of eye following ocular administration strongly affects the percentage growth inhibition of *Aspergillus niger* (Figure 11). The percentage inhibition of MS6 was maximum (45.7 ± 33.66%) after 6 h of administration. Similarly, after 6 h, the TOL suspension reached its maximum inhibition (50.75 ± 20.15%) but then it decreased to 0% inhibition after 8 h and 27 ± 38.18% after 24 h. The percentage growth inhibition of MS6 was significantly greater than that of TOL suspension after 8 h ($p = 0.005$) of administration (one-way ANOVA, $p < 0.05$).

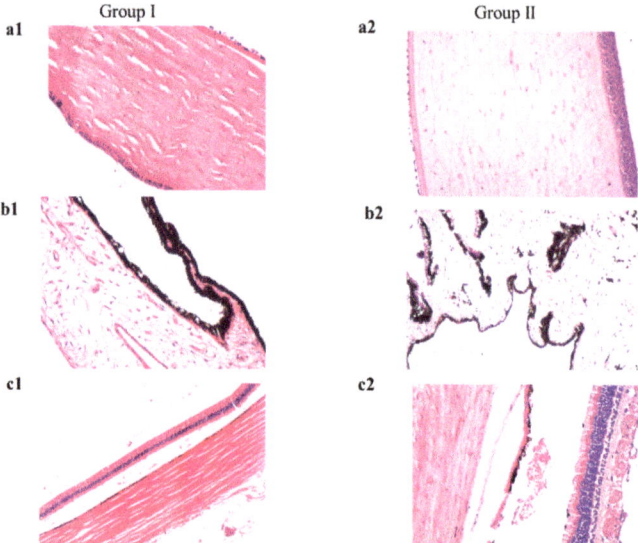

Figure 10. Histopathological photomicrographs (stained with hematoxylin and eosin) showing control rabbit eye (group I) and MS6-treated eye (group II); (**a1,a2**) show the cornea, (**b1,b2**) show the iris, (**c1,c2**) demonstrate the retina, choroid and sclera with normal histological structure (×40 magnification power). Photomicrographs of Group I ((**a1,b1,c1**)) were adopted from Aziz et al. [14].

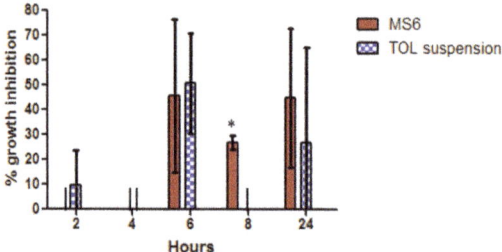

Figure 11. In vivo percentage growth inhibition of MS6 (treatment A) compared to TOL suspension (treatment B) on *Aspergillus niger* (ATCC32656). * Indicates statistically significant difference between the columns applying one-way ANOVA test ($p < 0.05$, n = 3).

TOL-cosolvent spanlastics had prolonged antifungal activity in the eye compared to TOL suspension. The area under the curve for MS6 was 1.5 folds greater than that of TOL suspension ($AUC_{2\,h-24\,h}$ = 458.6 and 300.3, respectively). This might be related to the PS of MS6 which was smaller than that of drug suspension which consequently increased the residence of TOL on the cornea [15,20]. In addition, the components of the modified spanlastics formula such as the cosolvent and edge activators enhanced the corneal penetration of TOL. Therefore, MS6 is an encouraging substitute for eye drops due to its prolonged antifungal effect.

4. Conclusions

In this work, TOL basic spanlastics were formulated using the ethanol injection method according to a full 3^2 factorial design to analyze the formulation variable's effect on the characteristics of TOL spanlastics characteristics and to select the optimal formulation for further modification. BS6 was selected as the nucleus for developing novel TOL-modified spanlastics by incorporating different cosolvent in different concentrations in their constructs. TOL-modified spanlastics were prepared using the same procedures of preparing basic spanlastics according to $3^1 2^1$ full factorial designs. MS6, prepared using 30% propylene glycol, was the optimized TOL-cosolvent spanlastics with a desirability value of 0.895. MS6 was compared to BS6 and both of them presented superior corneal permeation potential compared to a drug suspension. The safety and tolerability of MS6 were confirmed by the in vivo histopathological studies. The fungal susceptibility of *Aspergillus niger* (ATCC32656) to TOL using confirmed the superior residence of MS6 in the cornea compared to a drug suspension. Concisely, it can be concluded that modified spanlastics can be an effective ocular treatment for *Aspergillus niger*-induced fungal keratitis.

Author Contributions: Conceptualization, D.A. and A.M.; methodology, D.A., A.M. and S.A.M.; software, D.A., S.A.M. and A.M.; validation, D.A., S.A.M. and A.M.; formal analysis, D.A., S.A.M. and A.M.; investigation, D.A., S.A.M. and A.M.; resources, D.A., S.A.M. and A.M.; data curation, D.A., S.A.M. and A.M.; writing—original draft preparation, D.A. and S.A.M.; writing—review and editing, A.M.; visualization, D.A., A.M. and S.A.M.; supervision, S.T.; project administration, A.M. and S.T.; funding acquisition, D.A., S.A.M. and A.M. All authors have read and agreed to the published version of the manuscript.

Funding: This research received no external funding.

Institutional Review Board Statement: The animal study protocol was approved by The Research Ethics Committee-Faculty of Pharmacy, Cairo University, Egypt (PI 2982-25/04/2022).

Informed Consent Statement: Not applicable.

Data Availability Statement: Not applicable.

Conflicts of Interest: The authors declare no conflict of interest.

References

1. Acharya, Y.; Acharya, B.; Karki, P. Fungal keratitis: Study of increasing trend and common determinants. *Nepal J. Epidemiol.* **2017**, *7*, 685–693. [CrossRef] [PubMed]
2. Younes, N.F.; Abdel-Halim, S.A.; Elassasy, A.I. Corneal targeted Sertaconazole nitrate loaded cubosomes: Preparation, statistical optimization, in vitro characterization, ex vivo permeation and in vivo studies. *Int. J. Pharm.* **2018**, *553*, 386–397. [CrossRef] [PubMed]
3. Spadea, L.; Giannico, M.I. Diagnostic and management strategies of Aspergillus endophthalmitis: Current insights. *Clin. Ophthalmol.* **2019**, *13*, 2573. [CrossRef]
4. Öz, Y.; Özdemir, H.G.; Gökbolat, E.; Kiraz, N.; Ilkit, M.; Seyedmousavi, S. Time-kill kinetics and in vitro antifungal susceptibility of non-fumigatus Aspergillus species isolated from patients with ocular mycoses. *Mycopathologia* **2016**, *181*, 225–233. [CrossRef] [PubMed]
5. Sherwal, B.; Verma, A. Epidemiology of ocular infection due to bacteria and fungus-a prospective study. *JK Sci.* **2008**, *10*, 127–131.
6. Abdelbary, A.A.; Abd-Elsalam, W.H.; Al-Mahallawi, A.M. Fabrication of novel ultradeformable bilosomes for enhanced ocular delivery of terconazole: In vitro characterization, ex vivo permeation and in vivo safety assessment. *Int. J. Pharm.* **2016**, *513*, 688–696. [CrossRef]
7. Gunda, S.R.C.; Ganesh, G. Formulation and evaluation of tolnaftate loaded topical liposomal gel for effective skin drug delivery to treat fungal diseases. *J. Chem. Pharm. Res.* **2014**, *6*, 856–866.
8. Abousamra, M.M.; Mohsen, A.M. Solid lipid nanoparticles and nanostructured lipid carriers of tolnaftate: Design, optimization and in-vitro evaluation. *Int. J. Pharm. Pharm. Sci.* **2016**, *8*, 380–385.
9. Viswanath, V.; Reddy, R.; Surekha, M.; Bhuvaneswari, S. Effect of edge actuators on the formulation and characterization of tolnaftate proniosomes. *Int. J. Res. Pharm. Sci.* **2015**, *6*, 344–357.
10. AbouSamra, M.M.; Salama, A.H. Enhancement of the topical tolnaftate delivery for the treatment of tinea pedis via provesicular gel systems. *J. Liposome Res.* **2017**, *27*, 324–334. [CrossRef]
11. Ramya, M.G.; Akki, R.; Kumar, P.D. Formulation and evaluation of tolnaftate loaded topical niosomal gel. *Pharma Innov. J.* **2017**, *6*, 29–34.
12. Kaur, I.P.; Rana, C.; Singh, H. Development of effective ocular preparations of antifungal agents. *J. Ocul. Pharmacol. Ther.* **2008**, *24*, 481–493. [CrossRef] [PubMed]
13. Akhtar, N.; Sahu, S.; Pathak, K. Antifungal potential of tolnaftate against Candida albicans in the treatment of onychomycosis: Development of nail lacquer and ex vivo characterization. *Pharm. Biomed. Res.* **2016**, *2*, 1–12. [CrossRef]

14. Aziz, D.; Mohamed, S.; Tayel, S.; Makhlouf, A. Implementing polymeric pseudorotaxanes for boosting corneal permeability and antiaspergillus activity of tolnaftate: Formulation development, statistical optimization, ex vivo permeation and in vivo assessment. *Drug Deliv.* **2022**, *29*, 2162–2176. [CrossRef]
15. Fahmy, A.M.; Hassan, M.; El-Setouhy, D.A.; Tayel, S.A.; Al-Mahallawi, A.M. Statistical optimization of hyaluronic acid enriched ultradeformable elastosomes for ocular delivery of voriconazole via Box-Behnken design: In vitro characterization and in vivo evaluation. *Drug Deliv.* **2021**, *28*, 77–86. [CrossRef]
16. Li, J.; Li, Z.; Liang, Z.; Han, L.; Feng, H.; He, S.; Zhang, J. Fabrication of a drug delivery system that enhances antifungal drug corneal penetration. *Drug Deliv.* **2018**, *25*, 938–949. [CrossRef]
17. Fahmy, A.M.; El-Setouhy, D.A.; Habib, B.A.; Tayel, S.A. Enhancement of Transdermal Delivery of Haloperidol via Spanlastic Dispersions: Entrapment Efficiency vs. Particle Size. *AAPS PharmSciTech* **2019**, *20*, 95. [CrossRef]
18. Duangjit, S.; Opanasopit, P.; Rojanarata, T.; Ngawhirunpat, T. Evaluation of meloxicam-loaded cationic transfersomes as transdermal drug delivery carriers. *AAPS PharmSciTech* **2013**, *14*, 133–140. [CrossRef]
19. ElMeshad, A.N.; Mohsen, A.M. Enhanced corneal permeation and antimycotic activity of itraconazole against Candida albicans via a novel nanosystem vesicle. *Drug Deliv.* **2016**, *23*, 2115–2123. [CrossRef]
20. Basha, M.; Abd El-Alim, S.H.; Shamma, R.N.; Awad, G.E. Design and optimization of surfactant-based nanovesicles for ocular delivery of Clotrimazole. *J. Liposome Res.* **2013**, *23*, 203–210. [CrossRef]
21. Tayel, S.A.; El-Nabarawi, M.A.; Tadros, M.I.; Abd-Elsalam, W.H. Duodenum-triggered delivery of pravastatin sodium via enteric surface-coated nanovesicular spanlastic dispersions: Development, characterization and pharmacokinetic assessments. *Int. J. Pharm.* **2015**, *483*, 77–88. [CrossRef] [PubMed]
22. Manconi, M.; Caddeo, C.; Nacher, A.; Diez-Sales, O.; Peris, J.E.; Ferrer, E.E.; Fadda, A.M.; Manca, M.L. Eco-scalable baicalin loaded vesicles developed by combining phospholipid with ethanol, glycerol, and propylene glycol to enhance skin permeation and protection. *Colloids Surf. B Biointerfaces* **2019**, *184*, 110504. [CrossRef]
23. Chessa, M.; Caddeo, C.; Valenti, D.; Manconi, M.; Sinico, C.; Fadda, A.M. Effect of Penetration Enhancer Containing Vesicles on the Percutaneous Delivery of Quercetin through New Born Pig Skin. *Pharmaceutics* **2011**, *3*, 497–509. [CrossRef] [PubMed]
24. Manca, M.L.; Zaru, M.; Manconi, M.; Lai, F.; Valenti, D.; Sinico, C.; Fadda, A.M. Glycerosomes: A new tool for effective dermal and transdermal drug delivery. *Int. J. Pharm.* **2013**, *455*, 66–74. [CrossRef] [PubMed]
25. Kakkar, S.; Kaur, I.P. Spanlastics—A novel nanovesicular carrier system for ocular delivery. *Int. J. Pharm.* **2011**, *413*, 202–210. [CrossRef] [PubMed]
26. Fahmy, A.M.; El-Setouhy, D.A.; Ibrahim, A.B.; Habib, B.A.; Tayel, S.A.; Bayoumi, N.A. Penetration enhancer-containing spanlastics (PECSs) for transdermal delivery of haloperidol: In vitro characterization, ex vivo permeation and in vivo biodistribution studies. *Drug Deliv.* **2018**, *25*, 12–22. [CrossRef]
27. Aburahma, M.H.; Abdelbary, G.A. Novel diphenyl dimethyl bicarboxylate provesicular powders with enhanced hepatocurative activity: Preparation, optimization, in vitro/in vivo evaluation. *Int. J. Pharm.* **2012**, *422*, 139–150. [CrossRef]
28. Fares, A.R.; ElMeshad, A.N.; Kassem, M.A.A. Enhancement of dissolution and oral bioavailability of lacidipine via pluronic P123/F127 mixed polymeric micelles: Formulation, optimization using central composite design and in vivo bioavailability study. *Drug Deliv.* **2018**, *25*, 132–142. [CrossRef]
29. Eldeeb, A.E.; Salah, S.; Ghorab, M. Formulation and evaluation of cubosomes drug delivery system for treatment of glaucoma: Ex-vivo permeation and in-vivo pharmacodynamic study. *J. Drug Deliv. Sci. Technol.* **2019**, *52*, 236–247. [CrossRef]
30. Sayed, S.; Elsayed, I.; Ismail, M.M. Optimization of β-cyclodextrin consolidated micellar dispersion for promoting the transcorneal permeation of a practically insoluble drug. *Int. J. Pharm.* **2018**, *549*, 249–260. [CrossRef]
31. Kezutyte, T.; Kornysova, O.; Maruska, A.; Briedis, V. Assay of tolnaftate in human skin samples after in vitro penetration studies using high performance liquid chromatography. *Acta Pol. Pharm.* **2010**, *67*, 327–334. [PubMed]
32. El Zaafarany, G.M.; Awad, G.A.; Holayel, S.M.; Mortada, N.D. Role of edge activators and surface charge in developing ultradeformable vesicles with enhanced skin delivery. *Int. J. Pharm.* **2010**, *397*, 164–172. [CrossRef]
33. Humphries, R.M.; Ambler, J.; Mitchell, S.L.; Castanheira, M.; Dingle, T.; Hindler, J.A.; Koeth, L.; Sei, K. CLSI methods development and standardization working group best practices for evaluation of antimicrobial susceptibility tests. *J. Clin. Microbiol.* **2018**, *56*, e01934-17. [CrossRef] [PubMed]
34. Ismail, M.M.; Samir, R.; Saber, F.R.; Ahmed, S.R.; Farag, M.A. Pimenta oil as a potential treatment for Acinetobacter baumannii wound infection: In vitro and in vivo bioassays in relation to its chemical composition. *Antibiotics* **2020**, *9*, 679. [CrossRef] [PubMed]
35. Yousry, C.; Zikry, P.M.; Salem, H.M.; Basalious, E.B.; El-Gazayerly, O.N. Integrated nanovesicular/self-nanoemulsifying system (INV/SNES) for enhanced dual ocular drug delivery: Statistical optimization, in vitro and in vivo evaluation. *Drug Deliv. Transl. Res.* **2020**, *10*, 801–814. [CrossRef]
36. Bancroft, J.; Stevens, A.; Turner, D. *Theory and Practice of Histopathological Techniques*, 4th ed.; Churchill Livingstone: New York, NY, USA; London, UK; Madrid, Spain, 1996.
37. Albash, R.; Al-Mahallawi, A.M.; Hassan, M.; Alaa-Eldin, A.A. Development and optimization of terpene-enriched vesicles (Terpesomes) for effective ocular delivery of fenticonazole nitrate: In vitro characterization and in vivo assessment. *Int. J. Nanomed.* **2021**, *16*, 609. [CrossRef]

38. Kaur, I.P.; Rana, C.; Singh, M.; Bhushan, S.; Singh, H.; Kakkar, S. Development and evaluation of novel surfactant-based elastic vesicular system for ocular delivery of fluconazole. *J. Ocul. Pharmacol. Ther. Off. J. Assoc. Ocul. Pharmacol. Ther.* **2012**, *28*, 484–496. [CrossRef]
39. Rao, Y.; Zheng, F.; Zhang, X.; Gao, J.; Liang, W. In vitro percutaneous permeation and skin accumulation of finasteride using vesicular ethosomal carriers. *AAPS PharmSciTech* **2008**, *9*, 860–865. [CrossRef]
40. Lieberman, H. *Pharmaceutical Dosage Forms: Disperse Systems*; CRC Press: Boca Raton, FL, USA, 1998.
41. Abd-Elsalam, W.H.; El-Zahaby, S.A.; Al-Mahallawi, A.M. Formulation and in vivo assessment of terconazole-loaded polymeric mixed micelles enriched with Cremophor EL as dual functioning mediator for augmenting physical stability and skin delivery. *Drug Deliv.* **2018**, *25*, 484–492. [CrossRef]
42. De Lima, L.S.; Araujo, M.D.M.; Quináia, S.P.; Migliorine, D.W.; Garcia, J.R. Adsorption modeling of Cr, Cd and Cu on activated carbon of different origins by using fractional factorial design. *Chem. Eng. J.* **2011**, *166*, 881–889. [CrossRef]
43. Aziz, D.E.; Abdelbary, A.A.; Elassasy, A.I. Implementing Central Composite Design for Developing Transdermal Diacerein-Loaded Niosomes: Ex vivo Permeation and In vivo Deposition. *Curr. Drug Deliv.* **2018**, *15*, 1330–1342. [CrossRef] [PubMed]
44. El Menshawe, S.F.; Nafady, M.M.; Aboud, H.M.; Kharshoum, R.M.; Elkelawy, A.; Hamad, D.S. Transdermal delivery of fluvastatin sodium via tailored spanlastic nanovesicles: Mitigated Freund's adjuvant-induced rheumatoid arthritis in rats through suppressing p38 MAPK signaling pathway. *Drug Deliv.* **2019**, *26*, 1140–1154. [CrossRef] [PubMed]
45. Aboud, H.M.; Hassan, A.H.; Ali, A.A.; Abdel-Razik, A.H. Novel in situ gelling vaginal sponges of sildenafil citrate-based cubosomes for uterine targeting. *Drug Deliv.* **2018**, *25*, 1328–1339. [CrossRef] [PubMed]
46. Abdelrahman, F.E.; Elsayed, I.; Gad, M.K.; Elshafeey, A.H.; Mohamed, M.I. Response surface optimization, Ex vivo and In vivo investigation of nasal spanlastics for bioavailability enhancement and brain targeting of risperidone. *Int. J. Pharm.* **2017**, *530*, 1–11. [CrossRef]
47. Younes, N.F.; Abdel-Halim, S.A.; Elassasy, A.I. Solutol HS15 based binary mixed micelles with penetration enhancers for augmented corneal delivery of sertaconazole nitrate: Optimization, in vitro, ex vivo and in vivo characterization. *Drug Deliv.* **2018**, *25*, 1706–1717. [CrossRef]
48. Wilson, B.; Samanta, M.K.; Santhi, K.; Kumar, K.P.S.; Paramakrishnan, N.; Suresh, B. Poly (n-butylcyanoacrylate) nanoparticles coated with polysorbate 80 for the targeted delivery of rivastigmine into the brain to treat Alzheimer's disease. *Brain Res.* **2008**, *1200*, 159–168. [CrossRef]
49. Alexander, D.L.; Tropsha, A.; Winkler, D.A. Beware of R(2): Simple, Unambiguous Assessment of the Prediction Accuracy of QSAR and QSPR Models. *J. Chem. Inf. Modeling* **2015**, *55*, 1316–1322. [CrossRef]
50. Elmoslemany, R.M.; Abdallah, O.Y.; El-Khordagui, L.K.; Khalafallah, N.M. Propylene glycol liposomes as a topical delivery system for miconazole nitrate: Comparison with conventional liposomes. *AAPS PharmSciTech* **2012**, *13*, 723–731. [CrossRef]
51. Manconi, M.; Mura, S.; Sinico, C.; Fadda, A.; Vila, A.; Molina, F. Development and characterization of liposomes containing glycols as carriers for diclofenac. *Colloids Surf. A Physicochem. Eng. Asp.* **2009**, *342*, 53–58. [CrossRef]
52. Salem, H.F.; Kharshoum, R.M.; Sayed, O.M.; Abdel Hakim, L.F. Formulation design and optimization of novel soft glycerosomes for enhanced topical delivery of celecoxib and cupferron by Box-Behnken statistical design. *Drug Dev. Ind. Pharm.* **2018**, *44*, 1871–1884. [CrossRef]
53. Kumari, P.; Misra, S.; Pandey, S. Formulation and Evaluation of Tolnaftate Microsponges Loaded Gels for Treatment of Dermatophytosis. *Eur. J. Pharm. Med. Res.* **2017**, *4*, 326–335.
54. Al-Mahallawi, A.M.; Abdelbary, A.A.; Aburahma, M.H. Investigating the potential of employing bilosomes as a novel vesicular carrier for transdermal delivery of tenoxicam. *Int. J. Pharm.* **2015**, *485*, 329–340. [CrossRef] [PubMed]
55. Elsayed, I.; Abdelbary, A.A.; Elshafeey, A.H. Nanosizing of a poorly soluble drug: Technique optimization, factorial analysis, and pharmacokinetic study in healthy human volunteers. *Int. J. Nanomed.* **2014**, *9*, 2943–2953. [CrossRef]
56. Kakkar, S.; Kaur, I.P. A novel nanovesicular carrier system to deliver drug topically. *Pharm. Dev. Technol.* **2013**, *18*, 673–685. [CrossRef]
57. Aziz, D.E.; Abdelbary, A.A.; Elassasy, A.I. Fabrication of novel elastosomes for boosting the transdermal delivery of diacerein: Statistical optimization, ex-vivo permeation, in-vivo skin deposition and pharmacokinetic assessment compared to oral formulation. *Drug Deliv.* **2018**, *25*, 815–826. [CrossRef]
58. Zhou, T.; Zhu, L.; Xia, H.; He, J.; Liu, S.; He, S.; Wang, L.; Zhang, J. Micelle carriers based on macrogol 15 hydroxystearate for ocular delivery of terbinafine hydrochloride: In vitro characterization and in vivo permeation. *Eur. J. Pharm. Sci. Off. J. Eur. Fed. Pharm. Sci.* **2017**, *109*, 288–296. [CrossRef]

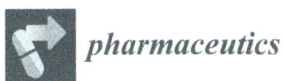

Article

Photodisruption of the Inner Limiting Membrane: Exploring ICG Loaded Nanoparticles as Photosensitizers

Kaat De Clerck [1,2], Geraldine Accou [3], Félix Sauvage [1,2], Kevin Braeckmans [1,2], Stefaan C. De Smedt [1,2], Katrien Remaut [1,2,*] and Karen Peynshaert [1,2]

[1] Lab of General Biochemistry and Physical Pharmacy, Faculty of Pharmaceutical Sciences, Ghent University, Ottergemsesteenweg 460, 9000 Ghent, Belgium
[2] Ghent Research Group on Nanomedicines, Ghent University, Ottergemsesteenweg 460, 9000 Ghent, Belgium
[3] Department of Ophthalmology, Ghent University Hospital, 9000 Ghent, Belgium
* Correspondence: katrien.remaut@ugent.be; Tel.: +32-9-264-8046; Fax: +32-9-2648189

Abstract: The inner limiting membrane (ILM) represents a major bottleneck hampering efficient drug delivery to the retina after intravitreal injection. To overcome this barrier, we intend to perforate the ILM by use of a light-based approach which relies on the creation of vapor nanobubbles (VNBs) when irradiating photosensitizers with high intensity laser pulses. Upon collapse of these VNBs, mechanical effects can disrupt biological structures. As a photosensitizer, we explore indocyanine green (ICG) loaded nanoparticles (NPs) specifically designed for our application. In light of this, ICG liposomes and PLGA ICG NPs were characterized in terms of physicochemical properties, ICG incorporation and VNB formation. ICG liposomes were found to encapsulate significantly higher amounts of ICG compared to PLGA ICG NPs which is reflected in their VNB creating capacity. Since only ICG liposomes were able to induce VNB generation, this class of NPs was further investigated on retinal explants. Here, application of ICG liposomes followed by laser treatment resulted in subtle disruption effects at the ILM where zones of fully ablated ILM were alternated by intact regions. As the interaction between the ICG liposomes and ILM might be insufficient, active targeting strategies or other NP designs might improve the concept to a further extent.

Keywords: retinal drug delivery; inner limiting membrane; photodisruption; vapor nanobubbles; indocyanine green; nanotechnology; pulsed laser

1. Introduction

The global burden of vision impairment and blindness is estimated to afflict the increasingly elderly population on a continuous basis in the coming years with the most prominent pathologies being glaucoma, age-related macular degeneration, diabetic retinopathy along with several inherited disorders [1,2]. All these diseases share the origin of their underlying mechanism at the level of the retina, a key player in visual processing. Although, while worldwide scientific effort continuously uncovers potential therapies such as gene- and stem cell therapy products to treat retinal diseases [3,4], efficient delivery to the posterior segment of the eye is essential for their clinical translation. Following the footsteps of the first FDA approved retinal gene therapy product Luxturna, clinical trials are currently to a large extent monopolized by gene augmentation strategies targeting the outer retina via subretinal injection. However, while highly effective to target photoreceptor cells (PRs) and the retinal pigment epithelium (RPE), new pioneering therapeutic strategies such as neuroprotection [5], optogenetics [6] and reprogramming [7] demand delivery to target cells located in the inner retina. In this regard, intravitreal (IVT) injection is increasing in interest given its low-invasive and easy-to-perform character which is exemplified by its routinely clinical use to deliver antibodies [8]. Despite these attractive features, large therapeutics in the nanosized-range and beyond struggle to reach their target cells after

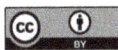

injection into the vitreous. The major culprit challenging retinal delivery after IVT injection is the inner limiting membrane (ILM), a thin membrane located in front of the retina [9–11]. While several inventive approaches to overcome this barrier such as subILM injection [12], ILM peeling [13] and enzymatic digestion [10] indeed elicit enhanced drug delivery, the lack of tunability and/or highly invasive nature of these approaches block the road to clinical translation.

Conscious of the need for new perspectives, our group recently explored an innovative light-based approach to disrupt the ILM in a controlled manner. In general, this physical technique is based on pulsed laser irradiation combined with photothermal molecules or nanoparticles (NPs) and is mainly investigated as a tool to enhance intracellular drug delivery, termed photoporation for this purpose [14–16]. The procedure is usually initiated by incubation of cells with a photosensitizer followed by application of extremely short laser pulses (<10 ns). Thereby, an ultrafast increase in temperature is induced resulting in evaporation of the surrounding water. Consequently, nanoscopic bubbles, known as vapor nanobubbles (VNBs), are created which expand by consuming their thermal energy. Finally, upon their collapse, high-pressure shock waves are released which can create transient pores in the cell membrane. Seeing that the concept recently broadened its applications to destruct larger biological structures such as biofilms [17] and collagen aggregates in the vitreous ('eye floaters') [18–20], laser-induced VNB formation also offers an interesting alternative to locally disrupt the main delivery bottleneck after IVT injection, i.e., the ILM.

Based on their intrinsic capacity to efficiently convert absorbed laser light into photothermal phenomena, plasmonic materials—e.g., gold nanoparticles (AuNPs)—are well suited to expertly mediate VNB formation due to their localized surface plasmon resonance (LSPR). However, as toxicity-concerns [21] as well as lack of biodegradability interfere clinical translation, a shift toward the design of photosensitizing materials with biodegradable and biocompatible characteristics is on the rise [22]. For ILM disruption specifically, the FDA approved organic dye indocyanine green (ICG) concerns an interesting candidate given its history in the ophthalmologic field as a dye to stain the ILM during ILM peeling. Moreover, it is favored with photothermal properties operating in the near-infrared (NIR) range which is beneficial in an in vivo setting [23–26]. Triggered by this potential match, we recently revealed the strength of the photosensitizing capacity of free ICG as proof of principle was established to disrupt the ILM via ICG-mediated photoporation resulting in enhanced retinal drug delivery [27]. Although these results highlight the potential of this photodisruption concept, several aspects must be considered in view of clinical translation. Firstly, after IVT injection, ICG might be captured into the network of the vitreous cavity due to its affinity for collagen resulting in loss of a fraction of ICG that is able to reach the ILM. Thus, laser application can potentially affect the collagen network of the vitreous. Secondly, due to its molecular weight of 775 Da, ICG is able to cross the ILM and enter the retina implying that the VNB effects might not remain restricted to the ILM [28]. The current design of the treatment could, consequently, induce collateral damage at the level of retinal cells and/or vitreous. Therefore, to boost this promising concept to a further extent, we intended to load ICG into nanoparticles unable of crossing the ILM to strive for a more localized treatment and smoothen the migration through the vitreous.

Interestingly, owing to ICG's profitable spectral properties, incorporation of ICG into NPs is a highly investigated topic; It is researched in context of light triggered drug release, imaging purposes, photodynamic and photothermal therapy for cancer treatment. As a result, an expanded set of NP designs are discussed in literature as ICG is compatible with different materials attributable to its amphiphilic nature—e.g., mesoporous silica [29], polymeric [30], lipid [31]- as well as protein-based [32] nanoparticles. As IVT injection of ICG NPs would be preferred, optimal mobility in the vitreous should be guaranteed which is dictated by the size and surface charge of NPs. In this regard, a size below 550 nm is required to be able to traverse through the collagen network while a negative to neutral charge should prevent binding to vitreous components [33,34]. On top of that, a second criterium implies that ILM penetration of ICG NPs must be excluded requiring a size above

100 nm [35,36]. Accordingly, to design the ideal NP for our approach the following criteria must be met: (1) a negative to neutral charge and a size below 550 nm to allow mobility through the vitreous, (2) a size above 100 nm to prevent ILM penetration as well as (3) a high ICG loading for efficient VNB generation.

In this study, we explore two types of ICG NPs with biodegradable and biocompatible characteristics for photodisruption of the ILM (Figure 1). We incorporated ICG in different types of poly (lactic-co-glycolic acid) (PLGA) NPs and liposomes which were screened in terms of physicochemical and ICG incorporating characteristics. The VNB creating capacity was furthermore investigated by use of dark field microscopy in two different settings: in buffer and accumulated onto patient-derived human ILM. Since ICG liposomes emerged as the most encouraging photothermal NP, their VNB effects were finally evaluated in an ex vivo setting on bovine retinal explants.

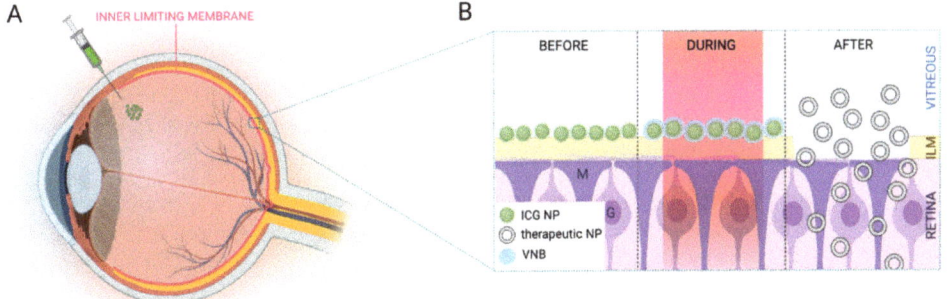

Figure 1. (**A**) Schematic overview of IVT injection of ICG NPs. (**B**) After migration through the vitreous, ICG NPs accumulate at the level of the ILM. Application of high intensity laser pulses results in VNB formation. Upon collapse of these VNBs, mechanical effects can disrupt the ILM paving the way for therapeutics to enter the retina. Image created with BioRender.

2. Experimental Section

2.1. Materials

1,2-dipalmitoyl-sn-glycero-3-phosphocholine (DPPC), 1,2-distearoyl-sn-glycero-3-phosphocholine (DSPC), 1-stearoyl-2-hydroxy-sn-glycero-3-phosphocholine (Lyso PC), 1,2-distearoyl-sn-glycero-3 phosphoethanolamine (DSPE), 1,2-distearoyl-sn-glycero-3-phosphoethanolamine-N-[methoxy (polyethylene glycol)-2000] (DSPE-PEG), 1,2-dioleoyl-3-trimethylammonium-propane (DOTAP) and cholesterol were purchased from Avanti Polar Lipids, Inc. (Alabaster, AL, USA). Poly (vinyl alcohol) (PVA, M_w 13,000–23,000) 88–89% hydrolyzed, poly (D,L-lactide-co-glycolide) (PLGA, M_w 7000–17,000) 50:50, dimethylsulfoxide (DMSO) and acetonitrile were obtained from Sigma-Aldrich (St. Louis, MO, USA). Dichloromethane was purchased from Carl Roth (Karlsruhe, Germany). Paraformaldehyde (PFA) and methanol were purchased from Honeywell Research Chemicals (Charlotte, NC, USA).

2.2. Synthesis of ICG NPs

2.2.1. ICG Liposomes

Three types of ICG liposomes composed of varying lipid components were synthesized via the thin-film hydration method based on previous reports in literature [36,37]. Lipids were dissolved in chloroform and mixed in different ratios (Table 1). The lipid mixture was placed in a rotary evaporation system to exclude the organic solvent by gradually reducing the pressure below 100 mbar at 40 °C. Next, the lipid film was hydrated with 500 µL of a water phase composed of ICG dissolved in HEPES (N-2-hydroxyethylpiperazine-N-2-ethane sulfonic acid) buffer (20 mM, pH 7.4). To solubilize the lipid film, this hydration step was performed in a water bath at 60 °C for 1 h under continuous rotation. Subsequently, the liposomes were downsized by applying a tip sonication cycle (3× 10 s, 10% amplitude (A), Branson digital sonifier, Danbury, CT, USA). After removal of free components by dialysis for 24 h at 4 °C (20 kDa, Float-A-Lyzer® G2, Spectrum laboratories), the ICG liposomes were stored at 4 °C.

Table 1. Composition, molar ratios and starting concentrations of ICG liposomes.

ICG LIPOSOMES				
Type	Composition	Molar Ratio	ICG Concentration (mg/mL)	Total Lipid Concentration (mg/mL)
DPPC	DPPC/DSPC/Lyso PC/DSPE	75/15/10/4	0.22	7.2
DPPC-PEG	DPPC/DSPC/Lyso PC/DSPE-PEG	75/15/10/4	0.37	7.2
DOTAP-PEG	CHOL/DOTAP/DSPE-PEG	10/9/1	0.53	25

2.2.2. PLGA ICG NPs

Based on the spontaneous emulsification solvent evaporation method, three types of PLGA ICG NPs were investigated according to previous described protocols with slight modifications [38–40]. A detailed overview of the solvents, volume ratios as well as ICG, PLGA and PVA concentrations for each type is displayed in Table 2. Briefly, varying amounts of PLGA and ICG were independently dissolved in an appropriate organic solvent and gently pooled together to obtain the organic phase. Next, the ICG/PLGA mixture was added dropwise to the aqueous phase composed of MilliQ water with varying concentrations of PVA as a stabilizer. For type 2 specifically, a proper emulsion was obtained by an extra tip sonication step (10 s, 10% A). Next, the organic phase was allowed to evaporate by continuous stirring for 4 h at room temperature. In order to collect the PLGA ICG NPs and eliminate free components, 3 washing steps with MilliQ water were performed by use of centrifugation (type 1:3 min at 4000× g; type 2:5 min at 7000× g; type 3:5 min at 10,000× g).

Table 2. Solvents, starting concentrations and volume ratios of PLGA ICG NPs. (I: organic solvent ICG, P: organic solvent PLGA, O: total organic phase, W: total aqueous phase).

PLGA ICG NPs							
Type	Concentration ICG (mg/mL)	ICG Solvent	Concentration PLGA (mg/mL)	Solvent PLGA	PVA	Volume Ratio I/P	Volume Ratio O/W
1	10	Methanol	50	Acetonitrile	4%	1:1	1:4
2	1	Methanol/DCM	30	Methanol/DCM	0.25%	3:7	1:10
3	10	DMSO	10	Acetonitrile	-	1:10	1:5

2.3. Characterization of ICG NPs

2.3.1. Size and Zeta Potential

Dynamic light scattering (DLS, Zetasizer Nano ZS, Malvern instruments Co., Worcestershire, UK) was used in order to screen the hydrodynamic diameter as well as the zeta potential of ICG NPs. Prior to analysis, ICG NPs were diluted 1/100 in HEPES buffer for ICG liposomes or MilliQ water for PLGA ICG NPs. The size distribution was reported as the Z-average value.

2.3.2. ICG Concentration and Encapsulation Efficiency

The ICG concentration was determined based on fluorescence measurements by use of a microplate reader (Victor^3, PerkinElmer, Waltham, MA, USA). In order to measure the encapsulated amount of ICG, ICG NPs were dissolved in DMSO to release the ICG. Based on a standard curve (0.08–5 µg/mL) of free ICG in DMSO, we were able to measure the ICG concentration of the individual ICG NPs. The encapsulation efficiency (EE%) was furthermore calculated based on Equation (1).

$$EE\% = \frac{\text{Initial mass ICG}}{\text{mass ICG in formulation}} \times 100 \qquad (1)$$

2.4. VNB Generation ICG NPs in Buffer and on Isolated Patient-Derived Human ILM

To determine whether ICG NPs are suitable photothermal entities to induce ILM photodisruption, VNB generation was evaluated in two different settings: ICG NPs in buffer as well as ICG NPs accumulated onto the ILM. Depending on the type of particle, a proper dilution in MilliQ or HEPES buffer was made to be able to visualize potential VNBs. In case of studying the effects on the ILM, patient-derived human ILM isolated during ILM peeling was obtained from Ghent University Hospital. Protocols were approved by the Ethical Committee of Ghent University Hospital (dossier number: BC-10642). After an incubation period of 15 min for the NPs to sediment and/or attach to the ILM, VNBs were detected via dark field microscopy. Since the home built 800 nm picosecond set-up is not connected to a dark field microscope, another laser set-up was used to detect VNB formation. With this set-up, laser pulses of 7 ns were applied tuned to a wavelength of 561 or 647 nm (Opolette HE 355 LD, OPOTEK Inc., Carlsbad, CA, USA). The laser pulse energy was monitored by an energymeter (J-25MB-HE&LE, Energy Max-USB/RS sensors, Coherent, Santa Clara, CA, USA) synchronized with the pulsed laser. Images and/or movies were recorded via MicroManager and Free Cam software, respectively.

2.5. Isolation of Bovine Retinal Explants

The entire procedure of explant isolation, laser treatment, cryopreservation, sectioning and immunostaining was performed as described earlier [27]. Bovine eyes were obtained from a local slaughterhouse and transported in cold CO_2 independent medium (Gibco®, Paisly, UK). The excess muscle and glandular tissue were removed in order to allow for a smooth dissection. After submerging the eye in 20% ethanol, the sclera was punctured 10 mm below the limbus with a 21G needle to create an entrypoint to bisect the eye with curved scissors followed by separation of the anterior segment. After gently removing the vitreous, the posterior eyecup was filled with CO_2 independent medium. Three relaxing cuts were made to flatten the entire structure to be able to isolate retinal explants by use of an 11 mm trephine blade (Beaver-Visitec International, Waltham, MA, USA). After carefully removing the surrounding retina, the explants were isolated by pipetting CO_2 independent medium below the explants.

2.6. Laser Treatment of Bovine Retinal Explants

Bovine retinal explants were transferred to a 35 mm glass bottom dish (Nunc™, Thermo Fisher Scientific, Waltham, MA, USA) making sure the ILM was positioned upwards. The dish was placed in the laser set-up and 20 µL of ICG NPs was added on top of the explants. Next, the entire explant was scanned with 2 picosecond laser pulses of 800 nm at a frequency of 1 kHz. For this purpose, a home built set-up was used powered by a Ti:Sapphire regenerative amplifier (Spitfire-Ace PM1K, Spectra-Physics, Milpitas, CA, USA) seeded by a Ti:Sapphire solid state laser (Mai Tai HP, Spectra-Physics, Milpitas, CA, USA) and pumped by a diode Nd:YLF laser (Ascend 40, Spectra-Physics, Milpitas, CA, USA). The total scanning time of one retinal explant was approximately 6 min. After laser treatment, the fixation and cryopreservation process was immediately initiated.

2.7. Cryopreservation, Sectioning and Immunostaining

After completing the laser treatment, bovine retinal explants were fixed with 4% PFA for 2 h at 4 °C. After removal of the PFA, cryopreservation was performed which includes three steps. Sequentially, retinal explants were incubated with 30% sucrose overnight (4 °C), 1:1 30% sucrose/O.C.T (Tissue Tek®, Sakura Finetek, Antwerp, Belgium) for 3 h (4 °C) and O.C.T for 3 h (25 °C). Next, the explants were transferred to cryomolds embedded in fresh O.C.T followed by snap freezing in cooled isopentane and stored at −20 °C. Using a cryostat (Leica), 10 µm cryosections were cut followed by mounting onto SuperFrost® Plus microscopy slides (Thermo Fisher Scientific, Waltham, MA, USA). In order to obtain an overview of the entire retina, 6 different locations at a distance of 1 mm from each other were investigated per sample.

The ILM was visualized by use of an indirect immunostaining method with collagen IV antibodies, a main constituent of the ILM. As a first step, the sections were washed 10 min with phosphate buffered saline (PBS) at room temperature. Next, the tissue was permeabilized by submerging the sections in 0.1% Triton for 5 min followed by another washing step with PBS for 10 min. After a blocking step with 5% goat serum for 1 h at room temperature, the sections were incubated overnight with a 1:200 dilution of rabbit anti-collagen IV antibody (Ab6586, Abcam, Cambridge, UK) at 4 °C. The primary antibody was removed by a washing step with PBS for 10 min. Subsequently, the sections were incubated with a 1:500 dilution of Hoechst as well as secondary anti-rabbit AlexaFluor 568 antibody (Invitrogen). A last washing step in PBS was executed to finally mount the slides with 1:1 PBS/glycerol solution. Retinal cryosections were imaged via confocal microscopy (Nikon A1R) using a 60x water objective (SR plan apo IR 60X WI). Further processing of the images was achieved with Fiji software.

3. Results

3.1. Synthesis of ICG Nanoparticles with Suitable Physicochemical Characteristics

In the search for a suitable nanosized-photosensitizer for localized ILM photodisruption, two main classes of ICG NPs with biodegradable and biocompatible features were evaluated: ICG liposomes and PLGA ICG NPs. By varying several parameters during synthesis, three individual sub-types were investigated for each class (Tables 1 and 2).

As proper physicochemical characteristics are of utmost significance to reach the ILM after IVT injection, the different ICG NP formulations were screened in terms of size and charge by measuring the hydrodynamic diameter and zeta potential, respectively. Based on Figure 2A, it can be noted that all the ICG NPs exceed the lower size limit criterium of 100 nm to be able to accumulate at the level of the ILM. While the sizes of all ICG liposomes are consistently leaning towards the lower limit independent of the lipid composition, with values ranging between 113 ± 8 nm and 124 ± 9 nm, PLGA ICG NPs are clearly found in a higher size-order. In the latter class, amending the organic solvents, PLGA and PVA concentration during synthesis gave rise to relevant differences. Type 1 and 2 resulted in the largest particles with values of 467 ± 24 nm and 428 ± 32 nm, respectively, in vicinity of the upper size limit of 550 nm. On the contrary, type 3 is characterized by a significantly lower size of 233 ± 48 nm.

In addition to size, surface charge is considered as another key parameter dictating the fate of NPs after IVT injection. According to literature, it is known that a negative to neutral charge is favorable to permit sufficient mobility in the vitreous [41]. When analyzing the zeta potential, Figure 2C indicates that all ICG NPs meet this requirement–except for the DOTAP-PEG liposomes. All PLGA ICG NPs were found to be highly negatively charged (<−20 mV) independent of changed parameters during synthesis, while the charge of ICG liposomes is lipid dependent. Evidently, incorporating neutral lipids such as DPPC and DSPC should result in neutral liposomes. However, due to incorporation of negatively charged ICG in the lipid layer this value shifted to slightly negative values (>−20 mV). When changing to a positively charged lipid system, the overall surface charge of the DOTAP-PEG liposomes was found to be slightly positive.

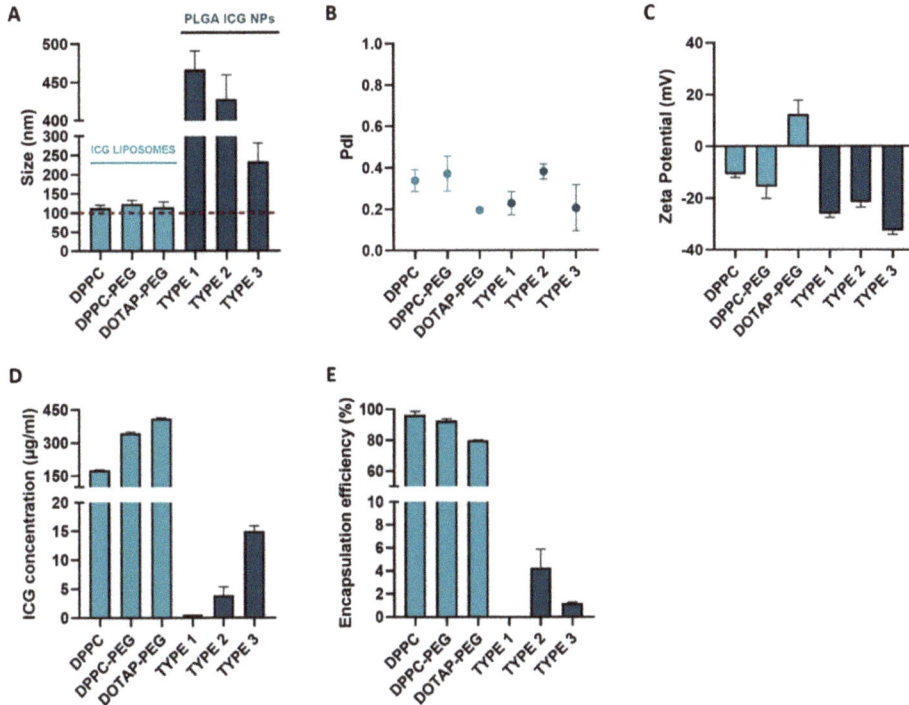

Figure 2. Physicochemical and ICG incorporating characterization of ICG liposomes (DPPC, DPPC-PEG and DOTAP-PEG) and PLGA ICG NPs (types 1–3). (**A**) Hydrodynamic diameter. (**B**) PdI. (**C**) Zeta Potential. (**D**) Total ICG concentration. (**E**) Encapsulation efficiency of ICG.

As sufficient ICG encapsulation could possibly be a prelude to identify the most successful particle in terms of VNB creating capacity, the ICG concentration as well as the encapsulation efficiency (EE%) of ICG NPs were evaluated (Figure 2D,E). Remarkably, ICG liposomes indistinctly outclass PLGA ICG NPs in terms of both parameters. Type 1 PLGA ICG NPs embodies the least impressive candidate as both values of ICG concentration and EE% are almost negligible. Although types 1 and 2 perform slightly better, the highest ICG concentration in this class of NPs does not exceed 15 µg/mL and encapsulation efficiencies remain below 10% indicating that a large fraction of ICG is lost during synthesis. Interestingly, ICG liposomes were able to ascend ICG concentrations to 180 µg/mL for DPPC liposomes and even 343 µg/mL for DPPC-PEG liposomes combined with efficient encapsulation with values above 90%. Although for DOTAP-PEG liposomes higher concentrations up to 411 µg/mL were obtained, it is of note that this is probably due to the increase of the lipid concentration. Hence, the number of liposomes is probably higher compared to the DPPC-(PEG) liposomes. Moreover, the encapsulation for this type of liposome was the lowest within this class with a value of 79.8%.

3.2. ICG Liposomes Are Manifested as the Most Promising Photosensitizer

To reveal whether ICG NPs display intrinsic VNB creating capacities, dark field microscopy was performed before and during application of a 7 ns laser pulse to detect the presence of VNBs for all formulations in buffer solution (Figure 3). In this regard, the suspected trends founded by the ICG incorporating characteristics are largely confirmed. Indeed, PLGA ICG NPs are not able to generate VNBs despite application of powerful 3.6 J/cm^2 pulses of 561 nm indicating ICG concentrations lower than 15 µg/mL do not suffice for the rapid temperature increase to generate VNBs. On the contrary, the three types of liposomes emerge as efficient mediators of photodisruption since bubble formation was observed (Figure 3, white arrowheads). In order to acquire an impression of differences in efficiency between the individual types of ICG liposomes, the lowest laser fluences able to induce apparent VNB formation were determined. Therefore, the wavelength was tuned to 647 nm to approximate ICG's absorption maximum of 800 nm as close as possible. However, no appreciable difference is observed as the values remain between 1.04 and 1.46 J/cm^2 for all liposomes. Lastly, another important remark to make is that, given the size of the liposomes, the observed generated bubbles are possibly not originating from individual liposomes but rather provoked by aggregation of NPs.

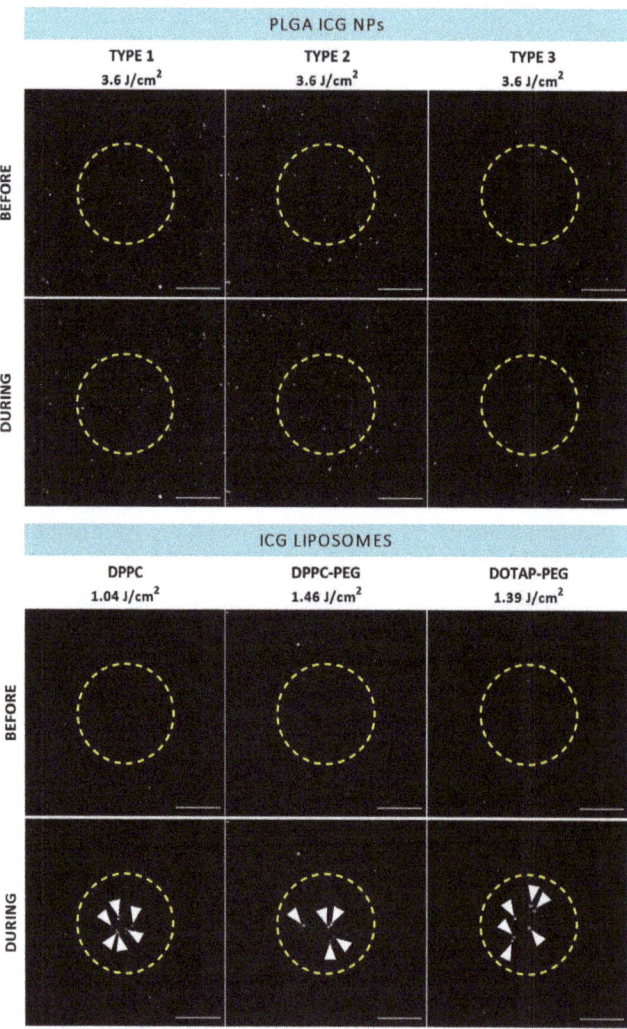

Figure 3. Dark field microscopy images of ICG NPs in buffer before and during application of a 7 ns laser pulse (ICG liposomes: 647 nm, ~1.3 J/cm^2, PLGA ICG NPs: 561 nm, ~3.6 J/cm^2). White arrowheads indicate the presence of VNBs. Yellow dotted line represents the size of the laser beam. Scale bar = 75 µm.

Since the actual target of ICG NP-mediated photodisruption is in a biological environment, the interaction between ICG NPs and the ILM could possibly change the observed effects. Therefore, the same process was repeated after incubation with patient-derived isolated human ILM as displayed in Figure 4. Although accumulation of PLGA ICG NPs onto the ILM could possibly boost VNB generation, there was still a lack of VNBs for each type. On the other hand, the three different types of ICG liposomes were still able to form VNBs at the human ILM. However, when revolving around effects on the ILM itself after VNB formation, no persuasive impact such as pore formation is observed for any type of ICG liposome as the human ILM seems to remain intact.

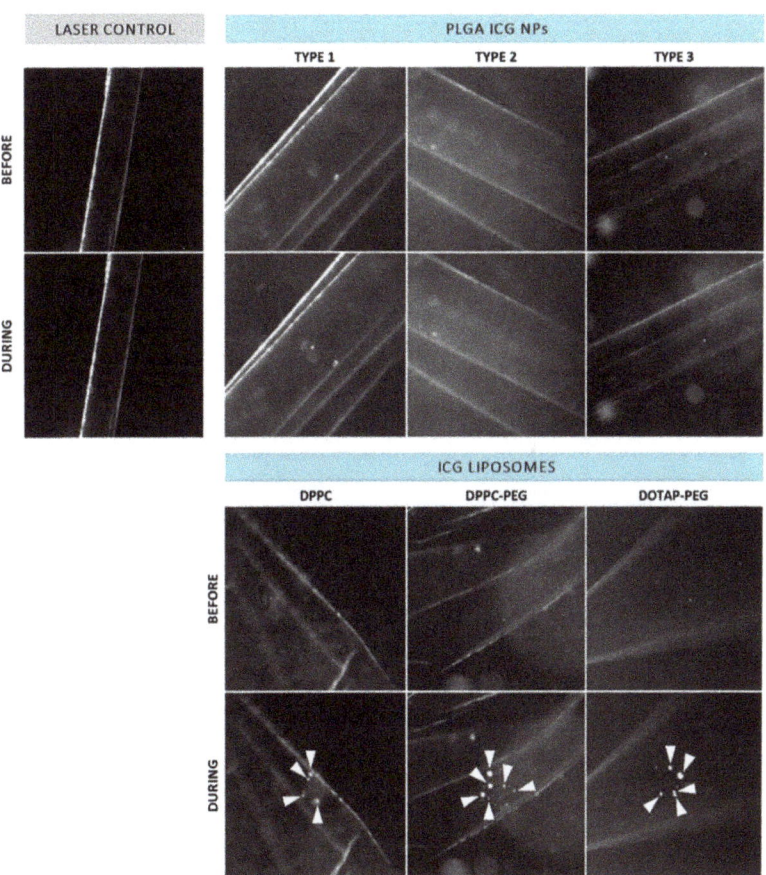

Figure 4. Dark field microscopy images of patient-derived isolated human ILM incubated with ICG NPs before and during application of a laser pulse (561 nm, ~3.6 J/cm^2). White arrowheads indicate presence of VNBs.

Although application of a single pulse resulted in creation of VNBs but did not elicit noticeable effects at the level of the ILM, we investigated whether this could be improved by use of repeated pulses. Remarkably, we did observe some effects when multiple pulses were applied as highlighted in Figure 5. Application of three individual pulses resulted in some structural changes as indicated by the green dotted circle. However, this feature was only obtained for DPPC-PEG liposomes probably due to the fact that the ICG incorporation per individual liposome is the highest compared to the other liposomes based on the ICG:lipid ratio.

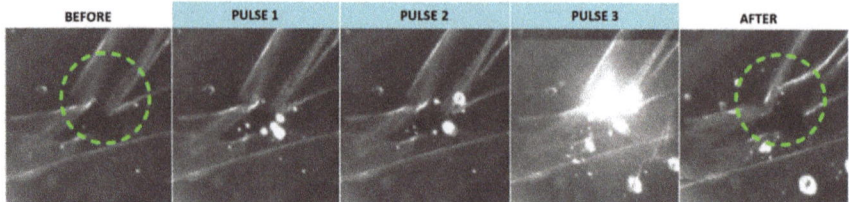

Figure 5. Dark field microscopy images of patient-derived ILM incubated with DPPC-PEG liposomes before, during and after application of three individual laser pulses (561 nm, ~3.6 J/cm^2). Green dotted circle indicates structural changes of the ILM.

3.3. ILM Integrity Is Slightly Affected after Laser Treatment with ICG Liposomes

To further investigate the possible impact of our treatment on ILM integrity from a different perspective, the approach was tested on bovine retinal explants. To this end, a picosecond setup was used tunable to a wavelength of 800 nm matching the absorption maximum of ICG. As based on the preceding experiments ICG liposomes surfaced as the most promising photothermal agent, the next set of experiments was continued with this class of NPs. After laser treatment, bovine explants were further processed into retinal cryosections stained with collagen IV antibodies, a main constituent of the ILM. As depicted in Figure 6A, an intact ILM is observed in untreated samples. Similar observations are made when explants underwent laser treatment without the presence of a photosensitizer implying that laser only is insufficient to affect the ILM. Interestingly, we did observe subtle effects when laser treatment was mediated with ICG liposomes as clarified in Figure 6B (two representative images). For all ICG liposomes, regions can be found where a large portion of the ILM is fully ablated (top row, white dotted lines). However, locations where the ILM remains mainly intact (bottom row, few dotted lines) are also present. It is of note that in the latter case it appears that the ILM occurs less bright compared to control samples. Interestingly, this observation can denote that an "ILM thinning" effect, where part of the ILM is removed without fully ablating it, might be provoked by our treatment. For each tested NP, both ILM ablation and thinning are occurring in approximately equal proportion concluding that no specific ICG liposome is surpassing its competitors. In general, the structural organization of the retina is retained in all cases.

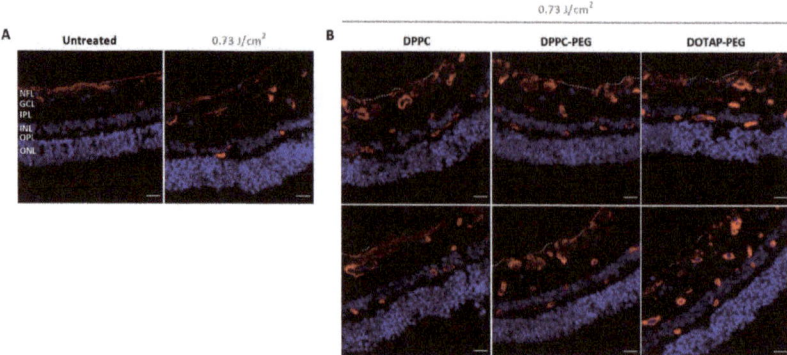

Figure 6. Visualization of retinal cryosections via confocal microscopy. (**A**) Control samples: untreated and laser treated. (**B**) Treated samples: application of ICG liposomes on top of bovine retinal explants followed by laser treatment with 800 nm pulsed laser light. Blue: Hoechst staining to visualize nuclei. Red: immunostaining for Collagen IV to show the ILM and blood vessels. White dotted line indicates complete absence of the ILM. Scale bar = 20 µm.

4. Discussion

Visual perception is enabled by an intricate process which involves entry of light in the eye and its translation into an image at the level of the brain. To bring this to a successful conclusion, the neurosensory retina vouches for the key task to translate light into an electric message. Unfortunately, several acquired and inherited disorders find their origin at the level of the retina. Yet, the evolving expertise in the field of nucleic acid based- and stem cell therapy opens increasing perspectives to develop promising therapeutics to combat retinal diseases. While PRs and RPE cells located in the outer retina have a well-known history as target cells for gene augmentation strategies, other interesting modes of action such as neuroprotection, optogenetics and reprogramming require inner retinal targeting. To reach these cells, IVT injection is the most attractive delivery route from a targeting as well as a safety perspective [8]. Large therapeutics are, unfortunately, in many cases blocked at the level of the ILM while heading for the retina. Excitingly, our research group recently revealed the power of ICG-mediated photodisruption to bypass this barrier in a controlled and tunable manner [27]. Although this concept has proven its worth to enhance retinal drug delivery, opportunities to further boost or fine-tune the technique more in depth are still in place. A potential hurdle in view of clinical translation is that, due to affinity of ICG for collagen in the vitreous and its ability to diffuse into the retina, ICG might not efficiently reach or remain strictly localized at the ILM which may lower the potency of the technique or induce collateral damage, respectively. To eliminate these potential concerns, we explore loading of ICG into NPs unable of crossing the ILM to efficiently guide ICG in the direction of the ILM aiming for a localized treatment.

In order to pursuit localized disruption effects at the level of the ILM, optimization of a suitable ICG-nanocarrier is the first pivotal step. To be able to traverse through the mesh network of the vitreous after IVT injection a size below 550 nm and negative to neutral charge are a must. On top of that, ILM passage should be avoided by targeting a size above 100 nm. Two main classes of biodegradable and biocompatible NPs eligible to meet these requirements were scrutinized: ICG liposomes and PLGA ICG NPs. For each individual class, three independent sub-types were evaluated to find the ideal match for our approach. Interestingly, all screened formulations were characterized by a size within our effective window of 100–550 nm. ICG liposomes were all featured by a size narrowly exceeding the lower limit of 100 nm, independent of the lipid composition, ICG and lipid concentration. On the other hand, PLGA ICG NPs clearly yielded larger particles yet remaining below the 550 nm upper limit. Since the PLGA ICG NPs were all synthesized based on emulsification, the NP size is mainly dependent on the stability of the emulsion droplets governed by several formulation parameters such as the type of solvents, polymer and stabilizer concentration [42–44]. By varying several of these parameters, the size could be tuned to large sizes for type 1 and 2 (>400 nm) while type 3 resulted in significantly smaller NPs (~233 nm) which is in accordance with the differences observed when comparing the respective sizes obtained by other research groups [38–40]. In terms of kinetic mobility, it is evident that given their larger size PLGA ICG NPs type 1 and 2 will migrate at a slower pace through the vitreous which potentially lowers the odds to effectively reach the ILM compared to the other ICG NPs. While diffusion might be retarded to some extent in consequence of size, different reports in literature state the importance of surface charge of NPs as the main decisive factor for diffusion behavior [33,45,46]. Indeed, as the vitreous is a negatively charged network, positively charged nanoparticles might be immobilized to a large extent due to electrostatic interaction while negative and neutral NPs are in general not restricted. Interestingly, all formulations were marked by a slightly negative to negative charge, except for the DOTAP-PEG liposomes which are slightly positively charged. Yet, in the latter case, an extra coating step with negatively charged components, e.g., hyaluronic acid, might facilitate vitreal migration [47]. Since, as evidenced by Martens et al., PEGylation of NPs might improve the diffusion rate even more, DPPC-PEG liposomes might be most preferred in terms of mobility in the vitreous.

Although ICG NPs might be equipped with the desired physicochemical characteristics, sufficient incorporation of ICG into the NP is possibly a critical factor to ensure ILM destructing capacities. Therefore, ICG concentration and encapsulation efficiency were evaluated as indicator to predict whether ICG NPs can operate in the VNB mode. ICG liposomes were found to be discernibly more skilled to incorporate higher ICG amounts, ranging between 180 and 411 µg/mL, compared to PLGA ICG NPs which are not able to exceed values of 15 µg/mL. For the latter class attempts to increase ICG incorporation by varying synthesis parameters were unsuccessful. As the synthesis of PLGA ICG NPs was performed based on emulsification, it is likely that ICG does not remain confined to the organic phase based on its amphiphilic nature resulting in loss of a large fraction of ICG. Additionally, as both PLGA and ICG are negatively charged, electrostatic repulsion might hamper proper incorporation. For ICG liposomes, on the contrary, ICG's amphiphilic properties are profitable as it is reported that ICG is able to interact with phospholipids as well as liposomes [25]. While it is estimated that ICG is inserted in the lipid bilayer [48], Lajunen et al. revealed via molecular dynamics simulation that ICG is able to interact with hydrophilic PEG chains present on the surface of PEGylated liposomes [31]. The fact that we were able to incorporate a higher ICG concentration into PEGylated DPPC liposomes compared to their PEG-lacking counterparts accompanied by a more negative zeta potential is underpinned by this hypothesis. In an attempt to increase ICG concentration, positively DOTAP-PEG liposomes were investigated to explore the contribution of electrostatic interaction. Although the group of Miranda et al. claimed almost full complexation of ICG, we observed a significantly lower EE value of 79.8%. Considering the difference between the loading method, it is plausible that our passive loading could be less efficient. It should be taken into account that although the absolute ICG concentration of this type is the highest, the lipid concentration of this type of liposome was elevated whereby the ICG loading per individual particle is potentially lower. In this regard, the highest value is probably achieved with the DPPC-PEG formulation.

When turning to photothermal effects, two "modes" can be distinguished: direct heating mode and VNB mode [15,16]. While the direct heating mode is generally observed with continuous wave (CW) irradiation or low intensity pulsed laser light inducing thermal effects, high intensity laser pulses can provoke the creation of nanoscopic bubbles resulting in mechanical phenomena. Although the state-of-the art photothermal agents are often plasmonic NPs such as AuNPs favored with substantial absorbing capacities based on their localized surface plasmon resonance (LSPR) [14–16], these characteristics do not apply for ICG NPs. However, owing to ICG's absorbing capacities in the NIR range, ICG NPs are widely investigated as photothermal NPs in the field of photothermal therapy to induce hyperthermia after CW irradiation to destroy tumor cells. These findings have spurred to investigate how ICG NPs behave after irradiation with high intensity laser pulses. In buffer solution, PLGA ICG NPs were not found to trigger VNB generation probably due to the low concentrations of ICG encapsulated into this type of NP (between 0.5 and 15 µg/mL). As a result, this class of particles is possibly only able to operate in the direct heating mode. In this regard, Della Pelle et al. observed a modest temperature rise of 7.5 °C when irradiating a 5 µg/mL ICG solution for 5 min with a CW laser (3 W/cm^2, 808 nm) while further ascending to 50 µg/mL was accompanied by an elevated temperature rise of 50.7 °C [49]. This indicates that, although the actual temperature increase might be higher due to the use of high intensity laser pulses in our case, this is not sufficient to induce the rapid temperature increase needed for VNB generation. Although we believe that operating in the heating mode might be able to permeabilize the ILM to some extent as thermal denaturation of ILM proteins might be provoked, reaching the VNB mode is an advantage both in terms of efficacy and safety. Sauvage et al. demonstrated that less laser pulses are required to fully destroy vitreous floaters when the bubble mode is achieved. Most importantly, since Haritoglou et al. observed severe disorganization of the human inner retina after application of ICG followed by halogen illumination, the close proximity of the retinal cells makes us strive to reach the VNB mode to tune the approach as safe as possible [50].

Due to the insulating nature of gas combined with the very short bubble lifetime of VNBs, dissipation of heat to the surrounding tissue is negligible which should temper retinal toxicity. Intriguingly, this objective was achieved when irradiating ICG liposomes in buffer with 7 ns laser pulses. Based on the feature of ICG liposomes to incorporate higher amounts of ICG, higher increases in temperature are possibly obtained able to exceed the critical temperature of the buffer to induce evaporation. Interestingly, these values are in agreement with the ICG concentrations found to be effective in inducing VNB formation after accumulation of free ICG onto the ILM (0.1 mg/mL) and vitreous floaters (0.5 mg/mL) [19,27]. Given the size of the liposomes and number of bubbles, however, it is possible that we are not able to detect individual VNBs as it is more difficult to form VNBs with smaller NPs [22], but observing VNBs resulting from aggregated liposomes.

In a next step, to investigate possible changes in VNB-behavior in a biological setting and to detect structural damage at the level of the ILM, the same set of experiments was performed in presence of patient-derived human ILM. However, the same trends were sustained. While PLGA ICG NPs were still lacking the capacity to induce VNB formation, ICG liposomes preserved their assets to do so. Despite VNB generation for all ICG liposomes, no discernible effects at the level of the ILM were elicited such as the creation of holes as earlier observed for free ICG [27]. Since free ICG molecules, renowned for their high affinity for the human ILM, are able to cluster in the ILM-network, ICG NPs are rather "in touch" with the membrane implying that larger VNB formation should be obtained to provoke more pronounced effects. Yet, it is probable that more subtle effects, e.g., permeabilization or structural disorganization of the protein network of the membrane, are not retraceable via dark field microscopy. Remarkably, DPPC-PEG liposomes were able to disrupt the ILM to some extent after repetition of 3 individual laser pulses which was not the case for the other types of liposomes likely attributable to the highest ICG:lipid ratio of this liposome. While the efficacy of the approach might be upgraded by use of multiple pulses, a downgrade in terms of toxicity cannot be excluded.

Since ICG liposomes outperformed their polymeric PLGA NP counterparts at each stage, only ICG liposomes were included to evaluate ICG NP-mediated photodisruption on bovine retinal explants. While zones with absent parts of ILM were observed, areas with intact ILM were retrieved in almost equal amounts. Based on empirical evaluation, we suggest that the intact ILM might be thinned to some extent. Since the same trend was observed for all liposomes, none of them emerges as the most efficient photosensitizer which is expected based on the insignificant difference in the lowest laser fluence able to elicit VNBs. The fact that we were only able to observe mild effects, lacking a clear trend, might be explained by several hypotheses. Firstly, since leakage of ICG from the liposomes was not determined, we can not exclude the contribution of free ICG to the observed results. Secondly, as previously mentioned, we suggest that VNBs are rather generated due to aggregation of individual NPs. The difficult to control nature of this process might explain the irregularity of the observed effects. Lastly, another important parameter determining the probability of success is the affinity of the ICG NPs for the ILM. Since the ILM itself is considered to be negatively charged, electric repulsion might limit the affinity of the NPs for the ILM. However, since the ILM is a complex matrix composed of different extracellular proteins [9] where other mechanisms such as hydrophobic interactions may come into play, it is difficult to predict which physicochemical properties are most suitable for optimal interaction with the ILM. Moreover, steric hindrance due to PEGylation might further interfere with the affinity. Seeing that mild effects were observed on bovine retinal explants while almost no damage is provoked on isolated human ILM, we expect that the mild effects are not powerful enough to permeabilize the significantly thicker human ILM. In conclusion, the current approach with ICG liposomes is not able to disrupt the ILM in a consistent and reproducible manner. However, since it is probable that we still miss out subtle effects undetectable via dark field microscopy or imaging of cryosections, no clear statements can be made whether or not the observed effects are adequate to boost retinal drug delivery which should be investigated more into depth with advanced microscopy techniques or evaluation of entrance of model drugs.

An important point to consider is that only one type of synthesis was evaluated for both ICG liposomes and PLGA ICG NPs as the goal was to screen different types of NPs. Nevertheless, we are aware that other types of synthesis are attractive in terms of upscaling, avoiding the use of organic solvents and surfactants, controlling the size or might improve the ICG encapsulation. Although increase of ICG concentration might boost VNB generation even more, our observations suggest that the major obstacle is the interaction between the ILM and the NPs. Active targeting strategies might solve this issue, however, attachment of antibodies to the liposomes is possibly challenging and this extra step can complicate market translation. On top of that, switching to other types of ICG NPs can be another perspective to intrinsically improve the affinity of ICG NPs for the ILM. While mesoporous silica NPs are also widely investigated to incorporate ICG, other types of NPs matching the biological environment of the ILM, e.g., albumin- or hyaluronic acid based NPs, or more neutrally charged ones could be promising. Hence, the possible influence of the nature and charge of ICG NPs on the interaction with the complex protein matrix of the ILM is an interesting topic which should be investigated more into depth.

5. Conclusions

The main objective of this study was to screen the potential of different types of ICG NPs as photothermal entities to boost the ILM photodisruption concept, previously established by our research group, in terms of restricting the treatment to the ILM only. In this way, collateral damage to other structures could be bypassed and toxicity concerns tempered. We were able to successfully synthesize a set of PLGA ICG NPs and ICG liposomes characterized by suitable physicochemical properties that qualify for our approach. ICG liposomes towered above PLGA ICG NPs in terms of ICG incorporating features which was shown to determine their potential to induce VNBs. Generation of VNBs was only observed for ICG liposomes both in buffer and after accumulation onto the human ILM. Nevertheless, laser treatment on bovine retinal explants mediated by ICG liposomes merely resulted in limited effects including small areas of ablated ILM alternated by zones of mainly intact but possibly thinned ILM. Whether or not these effects are satisfactory to enhance retinal drug delivery is the next question that should be answered. However, based on our results we hypothesize that the major obstacle involves the interaction between the ICG NPs and the complex ILM matrix, an important subject which demands further investigation. In addition to active targeting strategies of ICG liposomes to enhance this interaction, exploring other NP types with different building blocks and/or more neutral charges might gain more insight into NP-ILM interaction and hence improve the concept to a further extent.

Author Contributions: Conceptualization, K.D.C., K.B., S.C.D.S., K.R. and K.P.; methodology, K.D.C. and K.P.; validation, K.D.C. and K.P.; formal analysis, K.D.C.; investigation, K.D.C.; resources, G.A.; writing—original draft preparation, K.D.C.; writing—review and editing, F.S., K.R. and K.P.; visualization, K.D.C.; supervision, K.R. and K.P.; funding acquisition, K.R. All authors have read and agreed to the published version of the manuscript.

Funding: Karen Peynshaert is a postdoctoral fellow of the Research Foundation Flanders, Belgium (FWO-Vlaanderen, grant 12Y2719N) and received a 'Krediet aan Navorsers' grant (1508120N). Félix Sauvage is a postdoctoral fellow of the Research Foundation Flanders (FWO, grant 12X3222N). The authors would like to acknowledge funding from IOF (grant F2021/IOF-Advanced/112).

Institutional Review Board Statement: The study was conducted in accordance with the Declaration of Helsinki, and approved by the Ethical Committee of Ghent University Hospital (dossier number: BC-10642).

Informed Consent Statement: Informed consent was obtained from all subjects involved in the study.

Data Availability Statement: The data presented in this study are available in this article: Photodisruption of the Inner Limiting Membrane: Exploring ICG Loaded Nanoparticles as Photosensitizers.

Conflicts of Interest: The authors declare no conflict of interest.

References

1. Burton, M.J.; Ramke, J.; Marques, A.P.; Bourne, R.R.A.; Congdon, N.; Jones, I.; Tong, B.A.M.A.; Arunga, S.; Bachani, D.; Bascaran, C.; et al. The Lancet Global Health Commission on Global Eye Health: Vision beyond 2020. *Lancet Glob. Health* **2021**, *9*, e489–e551. [CrossRef]
2. Steinmetz, J.D.; Bourne, R.R.; Briant, P.S.; Flaxman, S.R.; Taylor, H.R.; Jonas, J.B.; Abdoli, A.A.; Abrha, W.A.; Abualhasan, A.; Abu-Gharbieh, E.G.; et al. Causes of blindness and vision impairment in 2020 and trends over 30 years, and prevalence of avoidable blindness in relation to VISION 2020: The Right to Sight: An analysis for the Global Burden of Disease Study. *Lancet Glob. Health* **2021**, *9*, e144–e160. [CrossRef]
3. Askou, A.L.; Jakobsen, T.S.; Corydon, T.J. Retinal gene therapy: An eye-opener of the 21st century. *Gene Ther.* **2020**, *28*, 209–216. [CrossRef]
4. Zhang, K.; Aguzzi, E.; Johnson, T. Retinal Ganglion Cell Transplantation: Approaches for Overcoming Challenges to Functional Integration. *Cells* **2021**, *10*, 1426. [CrossRef]
5. Devoldere, J.; Peynshaert, K.; De Smedt, S.; Remaut, K. Müller cells as a target for retinal therapy. *Drug Discov. Today* **2019**, *24*, 1483–1498. [CrossRef]
6. Sahel, J.-A.; Boulanger-Scemama, E.; Pagot, C.; Arleo, A.; Galluppi, F.; Martel, J.N.; Degli Esposti, S.; Delaux, A.; de Saint Aubert, J.-B.; de Montleau, C.; et al. Partial recovery of visual function in a blind patient after optogenetic therapy. *Nat. Med.* **2021**, *27*, 1223–1229. [CrossRef]
7. Lu, Y.; Brommer, B.; Tian, X.; Krishnan, A.; Meer, M.; Wang, C.; Vera, D.L.; Zeng, Q.; Yu, D.; Bonkowski, M.S.; et al. Reprogramming to recover youthful epigenetic information and restore vision. *Nature* **2020**, *588*, 124–129. [CrossRef]
8. Ofri, R.; Ross, M. The future of retinal gene therapy: Evolving from subretinal to intravitreal vector delivery. *Neural Regen. Res.* **2021**, *16*, 1751–1759. [CrossRef]
9. Peynshaert, K.; Devoldere, J.; Minnaert, A.-K.; De Smedt, S.C.; Remaut, K. Morphology and Composition of the Inner Limiting Membrane: Species-Specific Variations and Relevance toward Drug Delivery Research. *Curr. Eye Res.* **2019**, *44*, 465–475. [CrossRef]
10. Dalkara, D.; Kolstad, K.D.; Caporale, N.; Visel, M.; Klimczak, R.R.; Schaffer, D.V.; Flannery, J.G. Inner Limiting Membrane Barriers to AAV-mediated Retinal Transduction from the Vitreous. *Mol. Ther.* **2009**, *17*, 2096–2102. [CrossRef]
11. Zhang, K.Y.; Johnson, T.V. The internal limiting membrane: Roles in retinal development and implications for emerging ocular therapies. *Exp. Eye Res.* **2021**, *206*, 108545. [CrossRef] [PubMed]
12. Gamlin, P.D.; Alexander, J.J.; Boye, S.L.; Witherspoon, C.D.; Boye, S.E. SubILM Injection of AAV for Gene Delivery to the Retina. *Methods Mol. Biol.* **2019**, *1950*, 249–262. [PubMed]
13. Takahashi, K.; Igarashi, T.; Miyake, K.; Kobayashi, M.; Yaguchi, C.; Iijima, O.; Yamazaki, Y.; Katakai, Y.; Miyake, N.; Kameya, S.; et al. Improved Intravitreal AAV-Mediated Inner Retinal Gene Transduction after Surgical Internal Limiting Membrane Peeling in Cynomolgus Monkeys. *Mol. Ther.* **2016**, *25*, 296–302. [CrossRef] [PubMed]
14. Ramon, J.; Xiong, R.; De Smedt, S.C.; Raemdonck, K.; Braeckmans, K. Vapor nanobubble-mediated photoporation constitutes a versatile intracellular delivery technology. *Curr. Opin. Colloid Interface Sci.* **2021**, *54*, 10145. [CrossRef]
15. Xiong, R.; Samal, S.K.; Demeester, J.; Skirtach, A.G.; De Smedt, S.C.; Braeckmans, K. Laser-assisted photoporation: Fundamentals, technological advances and applications. *Adv. Phys. X* **2016**, *1*, 596–620. [CrossRef]
16. Xiong, R.; Raemdonck, K.; Peynshaert, K.; Lentacker, I.; De Cock, I.; Demeester, J.; De Smedt, S.C.; Skirtach, A.G.; Braeckmans, K. Comparison of Gold Nanoparticle Mediated Photoporation: Vapor Nanobubbles Outperform Direct Heating for Delivering Macromolecules in Live Cells. *ACS Nano* **2014**, *8*, 6288–6296. [CrossRef]
17. Teirlinck, E.; Xiong, R.; Brans, T.; Forier, K.; Fraire, J.; Van Acker, H.; Matthijs, N.; De Rycke, R.; De Smedt, S.C.; Coenye, T.; et al. Laser-induced vapour nanobubbles improve drug diffusion and efficiency in bacterial biofilms. *Nat. Commun.* **2018**, *9*, 1–12. [CrossRef]
18. Sauvage, F.; Fraire, J.C.; Remaut, K.; Sebag, J.; Peynshaert, K.; Harrington, M.; Van de Velde, F.J.; Xiong, R.; Tassignon, M.-J.; Brans, T.; et al. Photoablation of Human Vitreous Opacities by Light-Induced Vapor Nanobubbles. *ACS Nano* **2019**, *13*, 8401–8416. [CrossRef]
19. Sauvage, F.; Nguyen, V.P.; Li, Y.; Harizaj, A.; Sebag, J.; Roels, D.; Van Havere, V.; Peynshaert, K.; Xiong, R.; Fraire, J.C.; et al. Laser-induced nanobubbles safely ablate vitreous opacities in vivo. *Nat. Nanotechnol.* **2022**, *17*, 552–559. [CrossRef]
20. Barras, A.; Sauvage, F.; de Hoon, I.; Braeckmans, K.; Hua, D.; Buvat, G.; Fraire, J.C.; Lethien, C.; Sebag, J.; Harrington, M.; et al. Carbon quantum dots as a dual platform for the inhibition and light-based destruction of collagen fibers: Implications for the treatment of eye floaters. *Nanoscale Horiz.* **2021**, *6*, 449–461. [CrossRef]
21. Pan, Y.; Neuss, S.; Leifert, A.; Fischler, M.; Wen, F.; Simon, U.; Schmid, G.; Brandau, W.; Jahnen-Dechent, W. Size-Dependent Cytotoxicity of Gold Nanoparticles. *Small* **2007**, *3*, 1941–1949. [CrossRef] [PubMed]

22. Harizaj, A.; Wels, M.; Raes, L.; Stremersch, S.; Goetgeluk, G.; Brans, T.; Vandekerckhove, B.; Sauvage, F.; De Smedt, S.C.; Lentacker, I.; et al. Photoporation with Biodegradable Polydopamine Nanosensitizers Enables Safe and Efficient Delivery of mRNA in Human T Cells. *Adv. Funct. Mater.* **2021**, *31*, 2102472. [CrossRef]
23. Burk, S.E.; Da Mata, A.P.; Snyder, M.E.; Rosa, R.H.; Foster, R.E. Indocyanine green–assisted peeling of the retinal internal limiting membrane. *Ophthalmology* **2000**, *107*, 2010–2014. [CrossRef]
24. Farah, M.E.; Maia, M.; Penha, F.M.; Rodrigues, E.B. The Use of Vital Dyes during Vitreoretinal Surgery—Chromovitrectomy. *Dev. Ophthalmol.* **2015**, *55*, 365–375. [PubMed]
25. Desmettre, T.; Devoisselle, J.; Mordon, S. Fluorescence Properties and Metabolic Features of Indocyanine Green (ICG) as Related to Angiography. *Surv. Ophthalmol.* **2000**, *45*, 15–27. [CrossRef]
26. Reinhart, M.B.; Huntington, C.R.; Blair, L.J.; Heniford, B.T.; Augenstein, V.A. Indocyanine Green: Historical Context, Current Applications, and Future Considerations. *Surg. Innov.* **2016**, *23*, 166–175. [CrossRef] [PubMed]
27. Peynshaert, K.; Vanluchene, H.; De Clerck, K.; Minnaert, A.-K.; Verhoeven, M.; Gouspillou, N.; Bostan, N.; Hisatomi, T.; Accou, G.; Sauvage, F.; et al. ICG-mediated photodisruption of the inner limiting membrane enhances retinal drug delivery. *J. Control. Release* **2022**, *349*, 315–326. [CrossRef] [PubMed]
28. Jackson, T.; Antcliff, R.J.; Hillenkamp, J.; Marshall, J. Human Retinal Molecular Weight Exclusion Limit and Estimate of Species Variation. *Investig. Opthalmology Vis. Sci.* **2003**, *44*, 2141–2146. [CrossRef]
29. Lee, C.-H.; Cheng, S.-H.; Wang, Y.-J.; Chen, Y.-C.; Chen, N.-T.; Souris, J.; Chen, C.-T.; Mou, C.-Y.; Yang, C.-S.; Lo, L.-W. Near-Infrared Mesoporous Silica Nanoparticles for Optical Imaging: Characterization and In Vivo Biodistribution. *Adv. Funct. Mater.* **2009**, *19*, 215–222. [CrossRef]
30. Saxena, V.; Sadoqi, M.; Shao, J. Enhanced photo-stability, thermal-stability and aqueous-stability of indocyanine green in polymeric nanoparticulate systems. *J. Photochem. Photobiol. B Biol.* **2004**, *74*, 29–38. [CrossRef]
31. Lajunen, T.; Kontturi, L.-S.; Viitala, L.; Manna, M.; Cramariuc, O.; Róg, T.; Bunker, A.; Laaksonen, T.; Viitala, T.; Murtomäki, L.; et al. Indocyanine Green-Loaded Liposomes for Light-Triggered Drug Release. *Mol. Pharm.* **2016**, *13*, 2095–2107. [CrossRef] [PubMed]
32. Sheng, Z.; Hu, D.; Zheng, M.; Zhao, P.; Liu, H.; Gao, D.; Gong, P.; Gao, G.; Zhang, P.; Ma, Y.; et al. Smart Human Serum Albumin-Indocyanine Green Nanoparticles Generated by Programmed Assembly for Dual-Modal Imaging-Guided Cancer Synergistic Phototherapy. *ACS Nano* **2014**, *8*, 12310–12322. [CrossRef]
33. del Amo, E.M.; Rimpelä, A.K.; Heikkinen, H.E.; Kari, O.K.; Ramsay, E.; Lajunen, T.; Schmitt, M.; Pelkonen, L.; Bhattacharya, M.; Richardson, D.; et al. Pharmacokinetic aspects of retinal drug delivery. *Prog. Retin. Eye Res.* **2017**, *57*, 134–185. [CrossRef] [PubMed]
34. Xu, Q.; Boylan, N.J.; Suk, J.S.; Wang, Y.-Y.; Nance, E.A.; Yang, J.-C.; McDonnell, P.J.; Cone, R.A.; Duh, E.J.; Hanes, J. Nanoparticle diffusion in, and microrheology of, the bovine vitreous ex vivo. *J. Control. Release* **2013**, *167*, 76–84. [CrossRef]
35. Peynshaert, K.; Devoldere, J.; Forster, V.; Picaud, S.; Vanhove, C.; De Smedt, S.C.; Remaut, K. Toward smart design of retinal drug carriers: A novel bovine retinal explant model to study the barrier role of the vitreoretinal interface. *Drug Deliv.* **2017**, *24*, 1384–1394. [CrossRef]
36. Tavakoli, S.; Peynshaert, K.; Lajunen, T.; Devoldere, J.; del Amo, E.M.; Ruponen, M.; De Smedt, S.C.; Remaut, K.; Urtti, A. Ocular barriers to retinal delivery of intravitreal liposomes: Impact of vitreoretinal interface. *J. Control. Release* **2020**, *328*, 952–961. [CrossRef] [PubMed]
37. Miranda, D.; Wan, C.; Kilian, H.I.; Mabrouk, M.T.; Zhou, Y.; Jin, H.; Lovell, J.F. Indocyanine Green Binds to DOTAP Liposomes for Enhanced Optical Properties and Tumor Photoablation simple mixing of ICG with DOTAP liposomes results in full dye binding to the liposomes and enhanced ICG optical properties. *Biomater. Sci.* **2019**, *7*, 3158–3164. [CrossRef]
38. Saxena, V.; Sadoqi, M.; Shaoa, J. Indocyanine green-loaded biodegradable nanoparticles: Preparation, physicochemical characterization and in vitro release. *Int. J. Pharm.* **2004**, *278*, 293–301. [CrossRef]
39. Chen, Q.; Xu, L.; Liang, C.; Wang, C.; Peng, R.; Liu, Z. Photothermal therapy with immune-adjuvant nanoparticles together with checkpoint blockade for effective cancer immunotherapy. *Nat. Commun.* **2016**, *7*, 13193. [CrossRef]
40. Lee, Y.-H.; Lai, Y.-H. Synthesis, Characterization, and Biological Evaluation of Anti-HER2 Indocyanine Green-Encapsulated PEG-Coated PLGA Nanoparticles for Targeted Photothearpy of Breast Cancer Cells. *PLoS ONE* **2016**, *11*, e0168192.
41. Peynshaert, K.; Devoldere, J.; De Smedt, S.C.; Remaut, K. In vitro and ex vivo models to study drug delivery barriers in the posterior segment of the eye. *Adv. Drug Deliv. Rev.* **2018**, *126*, 44–57. [CrossRef] [PubMed]
42. Song, X.; Zhao, Y.; Hou, S.; Xu, F.; Zhao, R.; He, J.; Cai, Z.; Li, Y.; Chen, Q. Dual agents loaded PLGA nanoparticles: Systematic study of particle size and drug entrapment efficiency. *Eur. J. Pharm. Biopharm.* **2008**, *69*, 445–453. [CrossRef]
43. Song, K.C.; Lee, H.S.; Choung, I.Y.; Cho, K.I.; Ahn, Y.; Choi, E.J. The effect of type of organic phase solvents on the particle size of poly(d,l-lactide-co-glycolide) nanoparticles. *Colloids Surf. A Physicochem. Eng. Asp.* **2006**, *276*, 162–167. [CrossRef]
44. Yesenia, K.; Rodríguez-Córdova, R.J.; Gutiérrez-Valenzuela, C.A.; Peñuñuri-Miranda, O.; Zavala-Rivera, P.; Guerrero-Germán, P.; Lucero-Acuña, A. PLGA nanoparticle preparations by emulsification and nanoprecipitation techniques: Effects of formulation parameters. *RSC Adv.* **2020**, *10*, 4218–4231.
45. Tavakoli, S.; Kari, O.K.; Turunen, T.; Lajunen, T.; Schmitt, M.; Lehtinen, J.; Tasaka, F.; Parkkila, P.; Ndika, J.; Viitala, T.; et al. Diffusion and Protein Corona Formation of Lipid-Based Nanoparticles in the Vitreous Humor: Profiling and Pharmacokinetic Considerations. *Mol. Pharm.* **2020**, *18*, 699–713. [CrossRef] [PubMed]

46. Martens, T.F.; Vercauteren, D.; Forier, K.; Deschout, H.; Remaut, K.; Paesen, R.; Ameloot, M.; Engbersen, J.F.; Demeester, J.; De Smedt, S.C.; et al. Measuring the intravitreal mobility of nanomedicines with single-particle tracking microscopy. *Nanomedicine* **2013**, *8*, 1955–1968. [CrossRef] [PubMed]
47. Martens, T.F.; Remaut, K.; Deschout, H.; Engbersen, J.F.; Hennink, W.E.; van Steenbergen, M.J.; Demeester, J.; De Smedt, S.C.; Braeckmans, K. Coating nanocarriers with hyaluronic acid facilitates intravitreal drug delivery for retinal gene therapy. *J. Control. Release* **2015**, *202*, 83–92. [CrossRef]
48. Kraft, J.C.; Ho, R.J.Y. Interactions of Indocyanine Green and Lipid in Enhancing Near-Infrared Fluorescence Properties: The Basis for Near-Infrared Imaging in Vivo. *Biochemistry* **2014**, *53*, 1275–1283. [CrossRef]
49. Della Pelle, G.; López, A.D.; Fiol, M.S.; Kostevšek, N. Cyanine Dyes for Photo-Thermal Therapy: A Comparison of Synthetic Liposomes and Natural Erythrocyte-Based Carriers. *Int. J. Mol. Sci.* **2021**, *22*, 6914. [CrossRef]
50. Haritoglou, C.; Priglinger, S.; Gandorfer, A.; Welge-Lussen, U.; Kampik, A. Histology of the Vitreoretinal Interface after Indocyanine Green Staining of the ILM, with Illumination Using a Halogen and Xenon Light Source. *Investig. Opthalmology Vis. Sci.* **2005**, *46*, 1468–1472. [CrossRef]

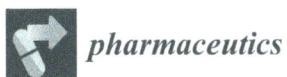

Article

Linoleic Acid-Based Transferosomes for Topical Ocular Delivery of Cyclosporine A

Onyinye Uwaezuoke [1], Lisa C. Du Toit [1], Pradeep Kumar [1], Naseer Ally [2] and Yahya E. Choonara [1,*]

[1] Wits Advanced Drug Delivery Platform Research Unit, Department of Pharmacy and Pharmacology, School of Therapeutic Sciences, Faculty of Health Sciences, University of the Witwatersrand, 7 York Road, Parktown, Johannesburg 2193, South Africa

[2] Department of Neurosciences, Division of Ophthalmology, University of the Witwatersrand, 7 York Road, Parktown, Johannesburg 2193, South Africa

* Correspondence: yahya.choonara@wits.ac.za; Tel.: +27-11-717-2274

Abstract: Delivering high-molecular-weight hydrophobic peptides, such as cyclosporine A, across the corneal epithelium remains a challenge that is complicated by other physio-anatomical ocular structures that limit the ocular bioavailability of such peptides. Transferosomes have previously been used to improve transdermal permeability, and have the potential for improving the ocular corneal permeability of applicable drugs. In this study, transferosomes for the potential ocular delivery of cyclosporine A were investigated. Linoleic acid was evaluated for its effect on the stability of the transferosomes and was substituted for a portion of the cholesterol in the vesicles. Additionally, Span® 80 and Tween® 80 were evaluated for their effect on transferosome flexibility and toxicity to ocular cells as edge activators. Attenuated Total Reflectance–Fourier Transform Infrared spectroscopy (ATF-FTIR), differential scanning calorimetry (DSC), and dynamic light scattering (DLS) were used to evaluate the physicochemical parameters of the blank and the cyclosporine A-loaded transferosomes. Cyclosporine A release and corneal permeability were studied in vitro and in a New Zealand albino rabbit corneal model, respectively. The linoleic acid contributed to improved stability and the nano-size of the transferosomes. The Tween®-based formulation was preferred on the basis of a more favorable toxicity profile, as the difference in their corneal permeability was not significant. There was an initial burst release of cyclosporine A in the first 24 h that plateaued over one week. The Tween®-based formulation had a flux of 0.78 µg/cm^2/h. The prepared transferosomes demonstrated biocompatibility in the ocular cell line, adequately encapsulated cyclosporine A, ensured the corneal permeability of the enclosed drug, and were stable over the period of investigation of 4 months at −20 °C.

Keywords: topical ocular drug delivery; transferosomes; linoleic acid; cyclosporine A; nanoparticle drug-delivery systems

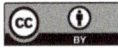

1. Introduction

Topical ocular delivery is fraught with numerous challenges, arising mainly from the physio-anatomical barriers posed by ocular structures in their normal physiological line of duty [1]. A formidable barrier to topically applied substances is regularly presented by the corneal epithelium, barely permitting the passage of low molecular weight substances by diffusion [2]. The corneal epithelial cells allow the passage of lipophilic drugs that then is barred by the corneal stroma, which is hydrophilic [3]. In addition, the paracellular passage of substances is heavily challenged by the tight junctions presented by the cornea [4]. Consequently, the drive to deliver drugs across the cornea via topical ocular formulations is a continuing venture. There is also the additional challenge of increasing the time that such formulations stay on the ocular surface. This surface residence time is shortened by the blink reflex, as well as the constant flow of the tear film. Various colloidal systems, such as polymeric micelles [5], nanoparticles [6] nanocapsules [7], microemulsions [8] and vesicular systems, have been explored to overcome many of these challenges. Among these, vesicular systems such as liposomes have stood out, overcoming the polarity issues associated with many of the new chemical entities (and which limit their passage through many biological membranes) and bringing biocompatibility, extended release, reduced systemic side-effects, and improved ocular biodistribution to topical ocular delivery [9].

Many of the ocular conditions require the topical application of medicaments for their treatment. Among these, the most frequently occurring are dry eye syndrome (keratoconjunctivitis sicca), keratoconus, and keratitis [10]. Cyclosporine A (CysA) is a strong immune suppressive oligopeptide with 11 amino acid residues that has found use in many inflammatory conditions of the eye, such as non-infectious uveitis and vernal keratoconjunctivitis corneal healing [11]. Even though the systemic administration of CysA, which was the initial mode of administration for ocular interventions, achieves high concentrations in ocular tissues, the high incidence and level of side effects arising from such a systemic administration is driving the search for topical formulations that could achieve the same therapeutic concentrations in the ocular tissues [12]. Unfortunately, the high molecular weight (1202.6 Da), strong hydrophobicity (Log P lies between 1.4 and 3 depending on the solvent), and the presence of formidable barriers leaves little room for flexibility in terms of formulation maneuvers to achieve the optimum availability in ocular tissues from topical applications [11,13]. Nevertheless, various nanoplatforms have been explored for overcoming some of these issues with the physicochemical properties of CysA. Many of these platforms utilized excipients, to enable the solubilization and stabilization of CysA, some of which may be contraindicated in the disease conditions which these formulations are intended to treat, as a result of the additional disruptions brought about on the corneal surface [5,14]. Allergan Inc., USA (now AbbVie) was the first company to push a nanoemulsion formulation of CysA to the market. Most of the other marketed CysA topical drops are micellar solutions in which various surfactants, alcohols, co-solvents, and even some excipients that have been shown to be harmful to ocular health, were used. One such excipient is EDTA, which is employed for the solubilization of CysA [4,15].

Transferosomes were introduced three decades ago to further expound the capabilities of the liposomal systems though directed to improve the delivery via the stratum corneum of the skin [16]. Transferosomes as ultra-elastic lipid vesicles have, since inception, been exploited in transdermal delivery for their exceptional permeability and the deformability properties imparted to the bilayer of regular vesicles, due to the presence of edge activators, such as Tween® 80, Span® 80, and sodium cholate [17]. Transferosomes are currently being deployed to improve the permeability of the stratum corneum to a variety of drugs. The success of transferosomes as a transdermal delivery system has been attributed partly to the osmotic gradient that exists across the outer and inner skin layers, and partly to the ability of transferosomes to deform while passing pores that are much smaller than them. This understanding and the existence of similar gradients across the corneal epithelium and stroma suggest that the same possibilities may exist for the permeation of large molecules across the tight junctions of the eye cornea. One major challenge that may deter the use of transferosomes in the corneal drug delivery has to do with the possible toxicity of the surfactants employed as the edge activators to ocular cells and therefore, requires a careful selection of, and delicate balance between, the edge activators and their use level. A major challenge in dry eye disease is the instability in the tear film as a result of suboptimal tear volume and function [10]. While CysA has a strong stimulating effect on tear fluid production, the excipients that will adequately stabilize the produced tear fluid are still lacking in many commercial formulations. As a result of these considerations, linoleic acid was introduced as a vesicle component to complement the pharmacological action of cyclosporine A in the treatment of the targeted ocular condition. Linoleic acid is an essential fatty acid that has been shown to stabilize the tear film when applied topically [18], and could therefore contribute to the therapeutic experience in patients with dry eye syndrome, in whom tear film stability is a major challenge contributing to the discomfort from the disease [19]. Daull and co-workers [13] had earlier concluded, after reviewing many formulations of cyclosporine A currently on the market, that the vehicle carrier in cyclosporine A topical formulations could contribute to a significantly improved performance.

The benefits of transferosomes that have chronicled its application in transdermal delivery underscore their potential in topical ocular delivery. Thus far, no study has explored the possibility of transferosomes in ocular applications; hence, in this investigation, a topical transferosomal formulation was proposed and explored as an alternative topical formulation for CysA, particularly in the treatment of dry eye disease. In this investigation, transferosomes, which are generally composed of phospholipids and an edge activator as a membrane-softening agent, were formulated. Both Tween® 80 and Span® 80 were selected for investigation, based on their demonstrated efficacy in facilitating the deformability of the transferosomes. The additional challenge of tear film stability that accompanies and complicates ocular conditions, such as dry eye, informed the decision to include linoleic acid in the formulation. Linoleic acid has been found to have a stabilizing effect on tear film. In addition, linoleic acid can contribute to permeation enhancement as a fatty acid since other fatty acids, such as oleic acid, have demonstrated potential as permeation enhancers in dermal formulations [20]. Additionally, linoleic acid was explored for its effect on stabilizing the lipid bilayer of the transferosome, thereby acting as both an excipient and an active ingredient. Spectroscopic methods were used to characterize and confirm the inclusion of CysA in the form of transferosomes. Further physicochemical parameters, such as size and zeta potential, were studied, as well as the biocompatibility in an ocular cell line. In addition, the ex vivo corneal permeability of the developed transferosomes were assessed, employing rabbit corneal tissue.

2. Materials and Methods

2.1. Materials

The cyclosporine A was purchased from LEAP pharma (DLD Scientific, South Africa). The Tween® 80, Span® 80, linoleic acid, soy phosphatidylcholine, cholesterol, and the MTT assay kit were purchased from Sigma-Aldrich (St. Louis, MO, USA). The ultrapure water (Milli Q, water, Sigma-Aldrich, Burlington, MA, USA) was used. All of the other solvents were obtained and used without further purification.

2.2. Preparation of the Transferosomes

The thin film method was employed in the preparation of blank and CysA-loaded transferosomes, as depicted in Scheme 1 using the formulation variables outlined in Table 1. The lipids, cholesterol, and linoleic acid were dissolved in an appropriate volume of chloroform–methanol solution, mixed in a ratio of 3:1. For the CysA-loaded transferosome, the cyclosporine was added in the film-forming solution. The resulting solution was evaporated in a rotary shaker (Rotavapor1 RII, Büchi Labortechnik AG, Flawil, Switzerland) to obtain a thin film which was subsequently hydrated using either a Tween® or Span® solution constituted in artificial tear fluid (ATF) of pH 7.4. The concentration of the Tween® or Span® solution was varied, as shown in Table 1 and incorporated either as part of the hydrating fluid or as part of the lipid film. The resulting multilamellar vesicles were ultrasonicated for 5 min in ice using a probe sonicator (Sonics Vibra cell, Newtown, CT, USA) set at a 20 s on and 5 s off cycle, and an amplitude of 50%. The obtained nanovesicles were subsequently lyophilized (Freezone 12 freeze drier, Labonco, Kansas City, KS, USA) and characterized appropriately. A 2% sucrose solution was used as a cryoprotectant. The effect of the linoleic acid inclusion on the physicochemical characteristics of the transferosomes was also evaluated by preparing Tween® 80-based transferosomes, with and without linoleic acid.

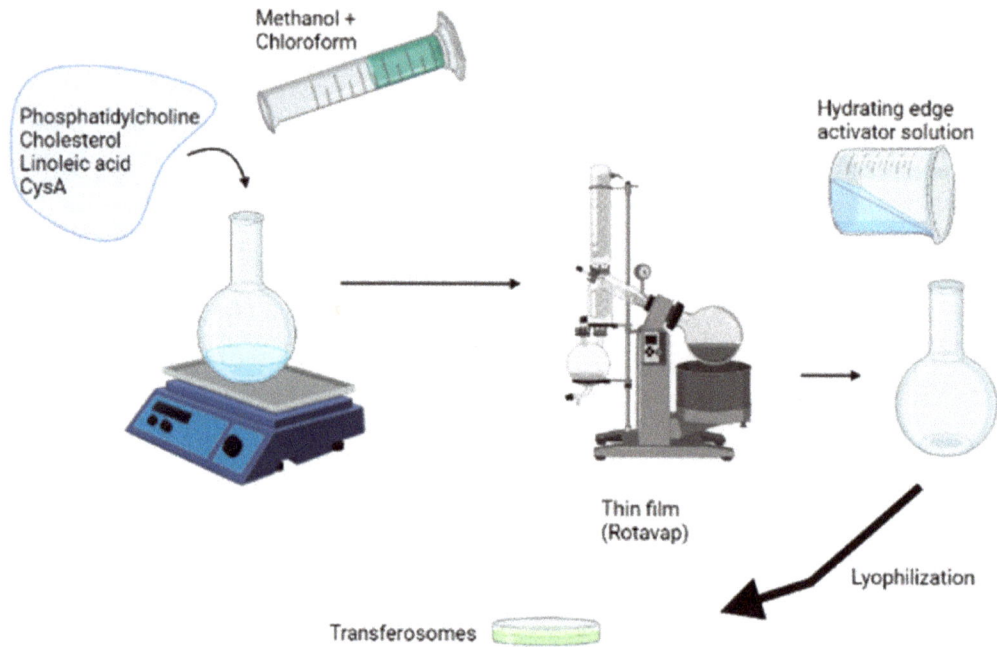

Scheme 1. Formulation of the transferosomes.

Table 1. Composition of transferosomes.

Component	Composition	Function
Soy Lecithin	180 mg	Lipid
Cholesterol	20 mg	Lipid
Linoleic acid	20 mg	Stabilizer/moisturizer
Tween® 80	1–2% v/v	Edge activator
Span® 80	1–2% v/v	Edge activator
CysA	60 mg	Active ingredient
Sucrose	2% w/v	Cryoprotectant

2.3. Characterization of the Transferosomes

The size, zeta potential, and polydispersity index of the prepared transferosomes were determined in triplicate, using dynamic light scattering (DLS) on the ZetaSizer NanoZS (Malvern Instruments, Malvern, UK). These measurements were undertaken shortly after sonication and after 4 months of storage at −20 °C in a freezer (GL I472QPZX, LG Korea) [21].

A FEI Tecnai T12 transmission electron microscope (TEM, Hillsboro, OR, USA) and the ZEISS Sigma 300 VP with a ZEISS 'smart SEM' software (Field Emission Scanning Electron Microscope, SEM, FEI, Orlando, FL, USA) were used to characterize the morphology of the transferosomes. A dispersion of the lyophilized transferosomes was prepared in deionized water to a concentration of 0.5 mg/mL and dropped on a copper grid. The excess was dabbed with a filter paper and the dispersion allowed to dry. The grid was subsequently covered by a drop of 2% v/v phosphotungstic acid and imaged with the FEI Tecnai T12 transmission electron microscope. For the SEM imaging, a drop of the dispersion was dropped onto a two-sided carbon tape mounted on an aluminum stub. The dispersion was dried, and sputter-coated with gold/palladium before imaging.

Differential scanning calorimetry (DSC) was undertaken (Mettler Toledo, DSC, STARe System, Swchwerzenback, ZH, Switzerland) to study the heat transitions in both the CysA-loaded and unloaded vesicles.

Attenuated Total Reflectance–Fourier Transform Infrared spectroscopy was undertaken on a Perkin Elmer Spectrum 2000 ATR-FTIR spectrometer (PerkinElmer 100, Llantrisant, Wales, UK), fitted with a single-reflection diamond. A MIRTGS detector was used to study the surface transitions and functional groups on both the cyclosporine A-loaded and unloaded transferosomes.

The stability of the transferosomes was assessed by storing lyophilized transferosomes at a representative storage temperature of $-20\ °C$ over a period of 4 months. At specified time intervals, the size distribution, polydispersity index, and zeta potential of the samples were measured.

The elasticity of the transferosomes was studied, using a modified method as applied by Jain and coworkers [22]. An appropriate amount of the lyophilized transferosomes was dispersed in artificial tear fluid (ATF) to formulate a stock suspension that was diluted appropriately before analysis. The stock suspension (one part) was diluted with nine parts of ATF and the particle size determined. Subsequently, 1 mL of the diluted system was extruded through a 100 nm polycarbonate filter. The volume extruded was noted, as well as the hydrodynamic size of the extruded dispersion. The extrusion process was repeated five times.

2.4. Encapsulation Efficiency and In Vitro Drug Release from Cyclosporine A-Loaded Transferosomes

The direct method was employed in determining the quantity of the drug encapsulated in the transferosomes [23]. To this end, a dispersion of the lyophilized drug-loaded transferosomes was prepared in ATF and the absorbance read at a wavelength of 207 nm on an IMPLEN NanoPhotometer®, (Implen GmbH, Munchen, Germany) The concentration was subsequently determined from a standard calibration curve of cyclosporine A, prepared using methanol: ATF (9:1) solution as solvent. The encapsulation efficiency (EE%) was subsequently calculated, using Equation (1):

$$\text{EE\%} = \frac{Actual\ amount\ of\ drug\ entrapped\ in\ the\ transferosome}{Amount\ of\ drug\ incoporated\ in\ the\ transferosome} \times 100 \qquad (1)$$

In a similar process, the drug release from the transferosomes was determined, using a modified USP dissolution apparatus, commonly applied as an in vitro drug release test for colloidal drug carriers [24]. Briefly, one end of a glass tube (open at both ends) was covered with dialysis tubing (12,000–14,000 MWCO), which had initially been equilibrated in ATF at 37 °C. The prepared transferosome dispersion in ATF (1 mL) was introduced from the other open end and suspended in 100 mL of ATF of pH 7.4 as the dissolution medium. The dissolution medium was stirred at 50 rpm and maintained at $37\ °C \pm 1\ °C$. At scheduled time intervals, a 1 mL sample was withdrawn from the dissolution medium and replaced with an equivalent volume of ATF and the drug content subsequently calculated from the absorbance reading acquired from the Implen NanoPhotometer™ (Implen GmbH, Munchen Germany).

2.5. Ex Vivo Corneal Permeability of the Transferosomes

The corneal permeability of the formulations was determined, using the cornea from New Zealand albino rabbits. The rabbits were selected because the size of the rabbits' cornea is similar to that of humans. The eyes of the rabbits were enucleated, and the cornea removed accompanied by about 3 mm of scleral tissue. These were immediately rinsed with ATF and wrapped with film to prevent dehydration. Subsequently, they were stored at 4 °C until used within 4 h of harvest [4,25]. The permeability study was undertaken in a Franz diffusion cell (PermeGear Inc., Bethlehem, PA, USA) with three cells. The cornea was used as the separating membrane between the donor and receptor chamber (enclosed in silicon rings) with the epithelial surface facing upward to the donor chamber. The receptor chamber was filled with 12 mL of degassed ATF, stirred at 60 rpm, and the system temperature maintained at 36 °C by means of a circulating water bath. A transferosomal dispersion in ATF was made and 1 mL introduced into the donor chamber. At 3, 6, and 24 h, 0.4 mL was withdrawn from the receptor chamber and replaced with an equal volume of degassed ATF. These were subsequently analyzed and the amount of drug that had passed through was determined from the cyclosporine A calibration curve.

2.6. Cytotoxicity Studies of the Transferosomes in Human Retinal Epithelial Primary Cell Line

The MTT, (3-[4,5-dimethylthiazol-2-yl]-2,5-diphenyltetrazolium bromide), assay to determine the cytotoxicity of the transferosomes was carried out using an ocular cell line, human retinal epithelial primary (HREP) cells. The HREP cells were grown in DMEM: HAM's F12 (50:50) medium supplemented with 10% FBS and 1% penicillin/streptomycin. The cells were grown until they were 80 to 90% (about 48 h incubation) confluent in an incubator set at a temperature of 37 °C with 5% CO_2. Thereafter, the cells were detached using 2 mL of 1% trypsin. The cells were thereafter seeded in two 96-well plates at a cell density of 40,000 cells per plate for the HREP cells and further incubated for 24 h. The plates were thereafter treated with 10 µL of a 5 mg/mL transferosome dispersion. After the treatment, the plates were incubated at a temperature of 37 °C with 5% CO_2. At 24 and 48 h, respectively, each well plate was treated with 10 µL of (3-[4,5-dimethylthiazol-2-yl]-2,5-diphenyltetrazolium bromide) (MTT) at a final concentration of 5 mg/mL. Each plate was further incubated for 4 h in a humidified atmosphere at 37 °C and 5–6% CO_2. A solubilization reagent (100 µL) was then added and the plate allowed to stand overnight in the incubator. The absorbance of the developed purple formazan crystals was then read in a VX3 microplate reader at 570 nm. The percent viability of the cells was subsequently calculated using Equation (2):

$$\% \; Viability = \frac{Absorbance\; of\; treated\; well - absorbance\; of\; blank}{Absorbance\; of\; control - absorbance\; of\; blank} \times 100 \qquad (2)$$

The ATF was used as the negative control, the 5-fluorouracil and DMSO were used as the positive controls, and the untreated wells were used as the blank.

2.7. Statistical Analysis

The continuous variables with a normal distribution, such as particle size, size distribution, zeta potential, etc., are reported as mean ± SD. Comparisons to establish the statistical significance where needed were undertaken using one way ANOVA and Student's *t*-test at $p = 0.05$. All of the statistical analyses were performed using Microsoft Excel 2016 (Microsoft Corp., Redmond, WA, USA) and GraphPad by Dotmatics (Boston, MA, USA).

3. Results

3.1. Formulation and Characterization of the Transferosomes

The hydrodynamic diameter, polydispersity index, and zeta potential transferosomes prepared using 1% v/v Span® 80 or Tween® 80, together with linoleic acid, are displayed in Table 2. During preliminary studies, the concentration of the surfactants employed was varied between 1% v/v and 2% v/v to establish a compromise between toxicity, and elasticity/deformability. A concentration of 1% v/v of Span® 80 or Tween® 80 was employed in the ensuing investigations, based on the ability to form stable, deformable transferosomes of adequately low toxicity. The results displayed in Table 2 indicate that the hydrodynamic diameter of the transferosomes formed using the Span 80® was higher than that formed by the Tween 80®. Contrary to the norm, loading CysA seemed to yield smaller sized transferosomes. Most of the studies report an increase in the size of vesicles after drug loading.

Table 2. Size distribution and polydispersity of blank and CysA-loaded transferosomes.

Parameter	Non-Lyophilized Tween® 1%		Lyophilized Tween® 1%		Non-Lyophilized Span® 1%		Lyophilized Span® 1%	
	Loaded	Blank	Loaded	Blank	Loaded	Blank	Loaded	Blank
Size (nm)	64.68 ± 0.14	69.33 ± 0.31	183.67 ± 0.62	243.01 ± 1.61	104.87 ± 0.8	159.37 ± 0.63	246.5 ± 3.09	315.7 ± 4.41
Polydispersity index	0.209 ± 0.005	0.223 ± 0.004	0.367 ± 0.01	0.388 ± 0.01	0.127 ± 0.01	0.244 ± 0.01	0.305 ± 0.02	0.388 ± 0.05
Zeta potential (mV)	−18.9 ± 1.6	−26.23 ± 1.3	−24.43 ± 2.88	−20.2 ± 2.90	−35.5 ± 1.26	−43.6 ± 4.29	−24.77 ± 0.58	−35.5 ± 3.05

Lyophilization had a potentially stabilizing effect on all of the vesicles. This is evident from the results of the zeta potential, which depict the magnitude of charges that tend to cause repulsion between two vesicles in close proximity. The values above +30 mV and below −30 mV are considered acceptable for the stability of the colloids [26]. Even though the zeta potentials for all of the formulations were initially within an acceptable range, they all somewhat increased after lyophilization. The nanovesicles, by default, are prone to membrane destabilization that result from the double effect of environmental factors, such as moisture, oxygen, and the presence of large quantities of unsaturated fatty acids in an aqueous environment [27]. Lyophilization, which is often employed as one of the methods to limit this form of instability, can fracture the delicate vesicle membrane as a result of the effect of ice crystals. The stabilization can, therefore, be the result of an intricate interplay between the concentration and type of cryoprotectants used and the fracturing effect of lyophilization [28]. For Tween® 1% formulations, the stabilization effect is noted in the form of a favorable shift from a value of −18.9 ± 1.6 to −24.43 ± 2.88 for the CysA-loaded formulation.

To study the effect of linoleic acid, the preliminary formulations were prepared with and without linoleic acid. In all of the formulations studied, the zeta potential and, thus, the stability to aggregation was improved by the addition of linoleic acid both for the CysA-loaded and blank Tween® 80 transferosomes. The size of the transferosomes was also comparatively reduced. The results from a representative lyophilized Tween® 80 1% v/v CysA-loaded formulation are shown in Table 3. The two-tailed p-value for size and the zeta potential comparison between the representative formulations determined by GraphPad were less than 0.0001 and 0.0002, respectively, thus notably significant.

Table 3. Effect of incorporation of linoleic acid on the stability of transferosomes.

Formulation	Size (nm)	Polydispersity Index	Zeta Potential (mV)
With Linoleic acid	175.33 ± 1.60	0.319 ± 0.32	−23.4 ± 1.00
Without Linoleic acid	200.17 ± 1.20	0.382 ± 0.01	−15.71 ± 0.17

3.2. Physicochemical Characterization of the Transferosomes

Fourier-transform infrared spectroscopy is usually used to study and characterize the nature of functional groups occurring at molecular surfaces. The results displayed in Figure 1 depict the FTIR fingerprints for pure CysA, blank transferosomes, and CysA-loaded transferosomes. The FTIR of both the blank and CysA-loaded transferosomes are identical, showing the same band intensities for identified functional groups occurring at the same wave numbers. None of the characteristic bands for CysA could be detected in the CysA-loaded transferosomes. This confirms the encapsulation of CysA within the transferosome vesicles and that no new bonds were formed when CysA was loaded into the transferosomes [29].

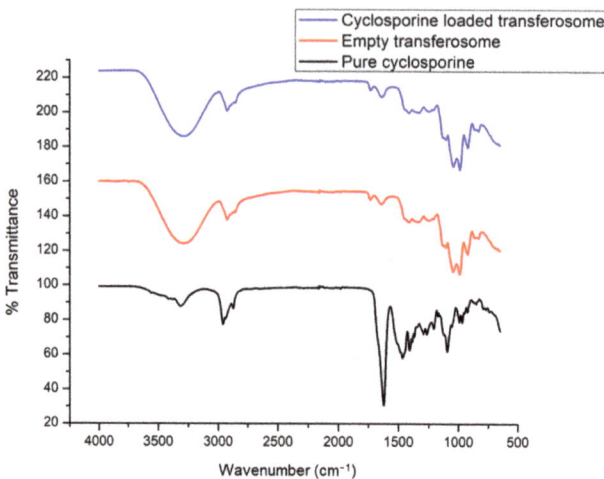

Figure 1. FTIR analysis of drug-free and drug-loaded transferosomes.

Figure 2 depicts the thermograms derived from the differential scanning calorimetric analysis performed on pure CysA, the unloaded transferosomes prepared with and without linoleic acid, and the transferosomes loaded with CysA. DSC was applied to characterize the thermal transitions between phases that occur in materials, resulting from temperature changes as directed by heat flow. The thermogram of bilayers of pure lipids generally depicts the transition temperature at which the lipid transforms from gel to a liquid crystalline phase [30].

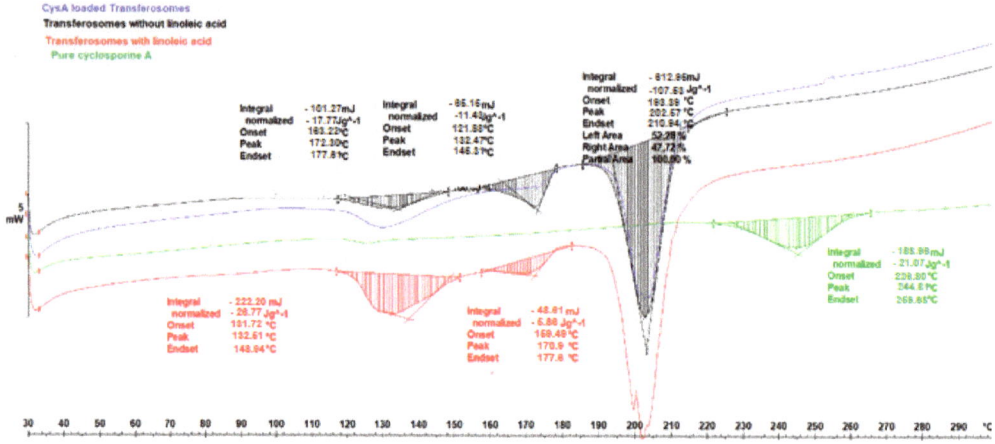

Figure 2. Differential scanning calorimetry of pure CysA, drug-free (with and without linoleic acid), and CysA-loaded transferosomes.

In Figure 2 the thermal transitions occurring in the lipid vesicles prepared in this study are evident. These vesicles were cryo-protected with a 2% sucrose solution before being lyophilized. The exothermic peaks that occurred at ~132 °C in all of the transferosomes represented the glass transition temperature. In the melting peaks occurring at 170.97 °C and 172.50 °C, respectively, for the transferosomes with and without linoleic acid; there was a slight depression in the melting temperature with respect to the transferosomes without linoleic acid. Londoño and co-workers [31] studied the thermal transitions in soy phosphatidylcholine-based ethosomes and observed peaks at 187.5 °C, which they attributed to the interdigitation of lipid chains that represents the presence of crystalline structures through which the heat flux is constant. The peaks, observed between 170.97 °C and 172.50 °C for the vesicles in the current study, can thus be attributed to such interdigitation of the vesicle chains. The melting endotherm for pure CysA in this study was found at ~130 °C (the melting point is reported as 148–151 °C [32]) and the decomposition started at 226.80 °C. These peaks, however, disappeared completely from the thermogram of the CysA-loaded transferosome, thus indicating the efficacy and stability of the encapsulation process. Similar observations were previously reported [29].

The representative SEM images shown in Figure 3 confirm the poly-dispersed nature of the prepared transferosomes obtained during DLS size analysis. The approach employed for the incorporation of the edge activators was explored for the possible effects on the morphology of the transferosomes. The morphology of the transferosomes prepared with Span® 80 as part of the hydrating fluid is shown in Figure 3a. The stabilizing effect of CysA loading into the transferosomes (Figure 3b) is noted as more uniformly distributed spheres of smaller diameters when compared with the blank. This effect corroborated the reduction in the hydrodynamic size with CysA loading, observed following the DLS size analysis. While Figure 3c represents the transferosomes prepared via the incorporation of Tween® 80 as a constituent of the hydration fluid, Figure 3d depicts the morphology of the CysA-loaded Tween® 80 transferosomes, resulting from incorporating the edge activator, Tween® 80, into the film-forming solution. Apart from a visually imperceptible difference in the size, the morphology is the same. This indicates that the method of incorporation of the edge activator had a minimal impact on the size and size distribution. A representative image of the morphology of the lyophilized samples is depicted in Figure 3e. The effect of lyophilization and the cryoprotectant used were obvious, as the spheres developed an elongated shape. This morphology was also observed in the TEM images obtained for the lyophilized samples prepared with Tween® 80.

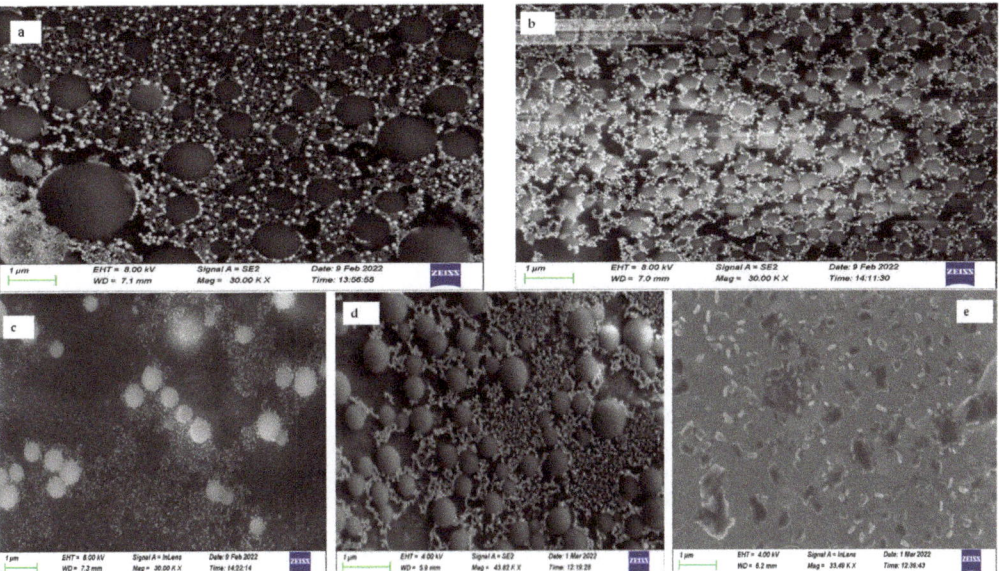

Figure 3. SEM images of transferosomes reflecting the impact of drug loading on the polydispersity and size for. (**a**) blank Span® transferosomes; (**b**) CysA-loaded Span® transferosomes; (**c**) blank Tween® transferosomes; (**d**) CysA-loaded Tween® transferosomes; and (**e**) lyophilized Tween® transferosomes. Scale bar represents 1 µm.

The TEM images depicted in Figure 4 were obtained from the lyophilized samples reconstituted in PBS and dried on a copper grid. The images highlight the spherical nature of the transferosomes. The mean sizes, determined from an analysis of the TEM images for the drug-loaded Span® 80 transferosomes, were about 200 nm, while the sizes of the blanks were in the range of 300 to 400 nm. The TEM-determined sizes for the blank Tween® 80 transferosomes were between 100 and 150 nm for the lyophilized samples, while that of the drug-loaded un-lyophilized sample was in the range of 100 nm. The TEM images in Figure 4 corroborate the morphology observed from the SEM. The samples also showed a somewhat elongated morphology approaching cuboids for the non-lyophilized Tween® samples, as observed in the SEM images.

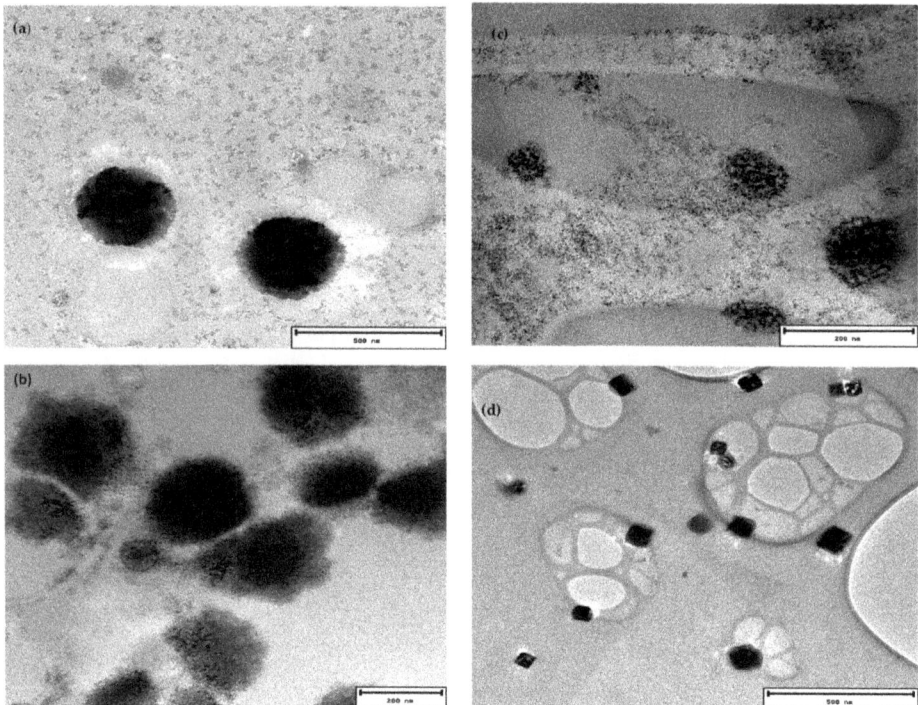

Figure 4. TEM images of lyophilized (**a**) blank Span 80® transferosomes; (**b**) CysA-loaded Span 80®; (**c**) blank Tween 80® transferosomes; and (**d**) un-lyophilized Tween 80® transferosomes. The scale bars for (**a,d**) are 500 nm, while those for (**b,c**) are 200 nm.

Table 4 shows the results of the stability evaluations obtained from the representative Tween®-based transferosome samples. The differences in the size, size distribution, and zeta potential were statistically different, but all in favor of stability. Even though the average hydrodynamic size of the transferosomes was smaller at the beginning, the polydispersity index was high, showing a high variability in the size distribution. The presence of polydisperse vesicles could have resulted from the method of vesicle formation, since the thin film method is known for the production of multilamellar vesicles [26].

Table 4. Stability profile of transferosomes.

Time (Months)	Size (nm)	Polydispersity Index	Zeta Potential (mV)
0	76.91 ± 0.81	0.504 ± 0.005	−15.93 ± 0.69
4	113.17 ± 1.11	0.277 ± 0.003	−12.7 ± 1.85

This trend was later reversed, however, evident in the presence of more uniformly distributed larger spheres, that could be due to the effect of annealing that results from the reassembly into bigger vesicles following the disruption in the lamellar membrane by the ice crystals during freezing [33]. The contributions of drug loading towards stability were also observed in terms of increased zeta potential values (-19.07 ± 1.22 mV) when compared to the blank vesicles. This corresponds with previous investigations involving lipid nanocapsules [34].

The results of the flexibility studies undertaken with both blank and CysA-loaded transferosomes are shown in Table 5. Jain and coworkers [22] had previously established the inverse relationship that exists between the volume reduction after extrusion and flexibility. Even though the percentage reduction in size for the drug-loaded vesicles was high, these results represent some degree of fluidity when the molecular size cut-off of the polycarbonate membrane (100 μm) used in the extrusion is considered. Statistically significant differences were obtained ($p < 0.05$) when the means of the percent decrease in the size of the blank and drug-loaded vesicles were compared, indicating that the CysA-loaded vesicles were in a more fluid state than the blank vesicles for both of the surfactants studied. The size and stability of the lipid vesicles were shown to depend on membrane packing, and this in turn depends on the interaction of the proteins and peptide molecules with the lipid bilayer [24]. Likewise, the blank vesicles based on Tween® 80 were more deformable than those based on Span® 80 for the blank vesicles based on consideration of the percent decrease in the size of vesicles. This observation is further confirmed by the volume reduction result, which showed a statistically insignificant difference. On the other hand, the difference in size reduction between the CysA-loaded transferosomes based on Tween 80® and those based on Span 80® were statistically not significant. This observation may have serious implications for the contributions of the drug to the membrane stability and fluidity, as was also observed from the dynamic light scattering experiments.

Table 5. Flexibility analysis of transferosomes.

Formulation	Size before Extrusion (nm)	Size after Extrusion (nm)	% Decrease in Size	Volume Loss (%)
Blank Span® 80	315.77 ± 4.41	140.07 ± 2.08	55.60 ± 0.78	8 ± 1.58
CysA-loaded Span® 80	246.57 ± 3.65	158.8 ± 0.59	35.72 ± 1.38	13 ± 1.05
Blank Tween® 80	243.07 ± 1.61	132.77 ± 0.37	45.37 ± 0.25	6 ± 2.02
CysA-loaded Tween® 80	183.17 ± 0.62	120.13 ± 0.90	34.42 ± 0.34	14 ± 1.02

3.3. Ocular Cytocompatibility of Transferosomes

In order to evaluate the safety of use of the prepared transferosomes in the eye, a toxicity assay was undertaken in a human retinal epithelial primary cell line (HREP). This cell line was selected because of the very high sensitivity of retinal epithelial cells to exogenous substances. The viability of the cells tested with 3.5 mg/mL stock dispersions of the transferosomes hydrated with surfactant concentrations of 1% v/v were similar to the viability of the negative control, as displayed in Figure 5. The % viability of the Tween®-based transferosomes was higher than the % viability of the Span®-based transferosomes at all of the concentrations tested. The viability of the HREP cells to the blank transferosomes was, likewise, similar to the viability of the CysA-loaded transferosomes. Figure 6 shows the morphology of the HREP cells treated with the dispersions of the Span® 80 and Tween® 80-based transferosomes. The morphology of the cells reflects the environment in which the cells are growing. The abnormalities in the morphology can thus be a stress response to the toxic elements in the growth medium [35]. The morphology of the cells shown in Figure 6 was normal and thus confirms the safety of the transferosomes. Therefore, at the concentrations evaluated, the transferosomes formulated in this study can safely be applied to ocular cells.

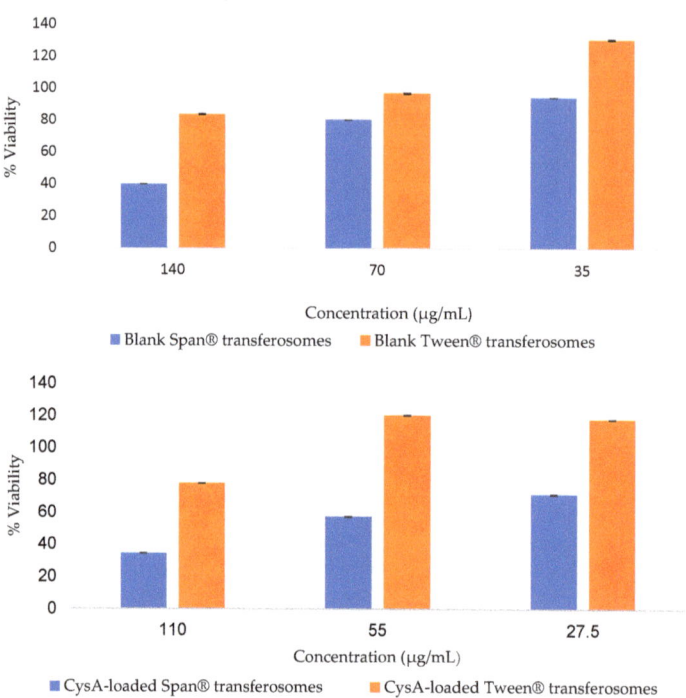

Figure 5. Viability of HREP cells against CysA-loaded transferosomes and blank transferosomes.

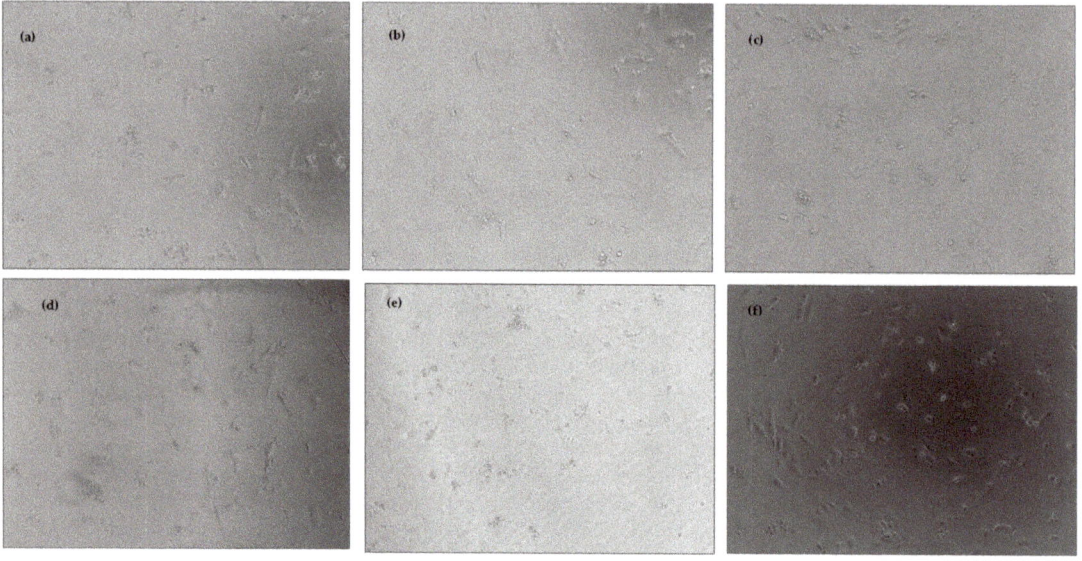

Figure 6. Morphology of HREP cells treated with (**a**) CysA-loaded Span® transferosomes; (**b**) blank Span® transferosomes; (**c**) blank Tween® transferosomes; (**d**) CysA-loaded Tween® transferosomes; (**e**) ATF; and (**f**) before treatment.

3.4. Encapsulation Efficiency and In Vitro Release Profile of CysA from Loaded Transferosomes Prepared with Tween® 80

The encapsulation efficiency is a measure of the amount of drug loaded into the vesicles and represents the ability of the nanocarriers to encapsulate the enclosed drug. The encapsulation efficiency obtained from the transferosomes prepared using Tween® 80 included in the hydrating fluid was 52.05% ± 2.06%, while that obtained when the Tween® was included in the lipid film former before evaporation was 44.06% ± 3.01%. The edge activators were incorporated using two different approaches to delineate the effect of the incorporation method on the properties of the formed transferosomes. The EE% obtained by including the Tween® 80 in the hydrating fluid was much higher than that from the alternate method. Increasing the cholesterol content, which is important for maintaining the rigidity and hence, the stability of the vesicles, has been shown to decrease the inclusion of CysA into the phospholipid membrane [36]. Additionally, CysA has been shown to partly partition between the aqueous core and the phospholipid membrane [37].

The in vitro release profile (Figure 7a) of the transferosomes was obtained for the Tween®-based formulation since it had a more favorable toxicity profile. In vitro release studies have variously been applied as an indication of the potential performance of a delivery system in vivo [38]. The release of CysA was initially rapid with over 15% of the loaded drug being released in the first 24 h. After this phase, there was a steady gradual increase over the next 72 h up to the time the release study was terminated. Other investigators have made similar observations with regards to the drug release behavior from other vesicle-based delivery systems [39]. The release data were fitted to different dissolution models and the Korsmeyer–Peppas model, which describes the release mechanism from polymeric systems, was selected as the best fit, based on the Akaike Information Criterion (AIC) and the Model Selection Criterion (MSC). The calculated Korsmeyer–Peppas constant, Kkp, was 4.106 while the n factor for the release data was 0.36, signifying that a Non-Fickian diffusion was the release mechanism from the transferosomes [35]. Figure 7b shows the predicted and the observed release data after fitting into the Korsmeyer–Peppas model.

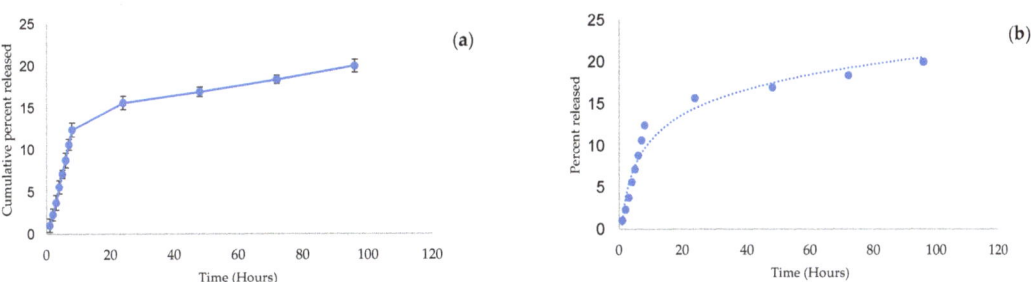

Figure 7. Release profile from transferosomes: (**a**) In vitro release of CysA from transferosomes; (**b**) The predicted release profile based on the Korsmeyer–Peppas model.

3.5. Ex Vivo Corneal Permeability and Flux across Rabbits' Cornea

Figure 8 shows the results of the corneal permeability studies represented as the cumulative amount of CysA diffusing per unit area plotted against time. In this study, the cumulative amount diffused per unit area increased over time during the 24 h period of investigation. The values were higher for the Tween® based formulation, though the similarity factor between the permeability profiles of the two formulations was close (F2 = 69.05). Agarwal and colleagues [40] similarly determined the permeability of CysA across the rabbit cornea, though using formulations based on semi-fluorinated alkanes. According to their study, the best formulation based on perfluorobutylpentane demonstrated a cumulative CysA permeation of 15 µg/g of the cornea over a 4-h period. Even though this is similar to the value obtained in this study for the Tween® 80 formulation, the volatility of the semi-fluoroalkanes used as a solubilizer in their formulation can lead to precipitation of the dissolved drug. According to Fick's laws of diffusion, that govern the transport of molecules across the corneal surface, the flux across the cornea depends upon the concentration gradient across the corneal barrier and the diffusion or permeability coefficient [41]. The maximum flux is usually determined from the slope of the curve for the cumulative amount permeated/unit area versus the time for the formulations not enclosed in reservoirs. The slope of the linear part of the curve for the Tween®- and Span®-based transferosome formulations were 0.78 µg/cm^2/h and 0.912 µg/cm^2/h, respectively, which represents the flux. The Span® 80 transferosomes had a higher flux than the Tween® formulation, even though the cumulative amount permeated per unit time for the Tween® was initially higher. A higher flux from Span® formulation indicates that, over time and at a steady state, the Span® formulation will enable the permeation of higher quantities of CysA. Despite the higher flux from the Span® formulation, the Tween® formulation may still be preferred, considering that this difference in flux is not significant ($p > 0.05$). In addition, the Tween® formulation had a more favorable toxicity profile.

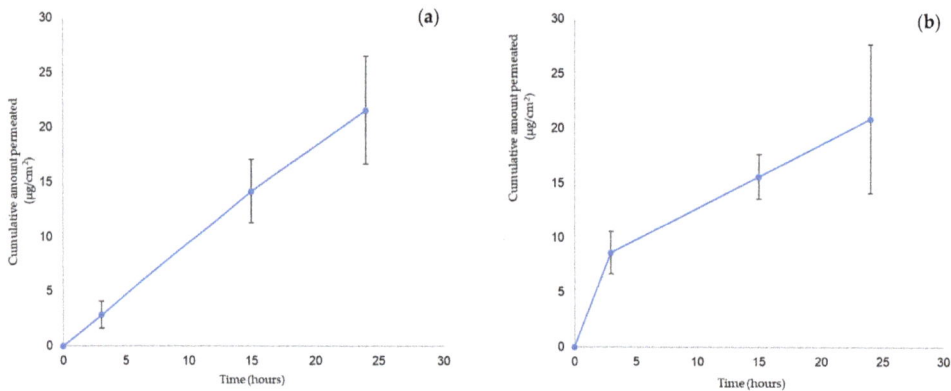

Figure 8. Corneal permeability of the transferosomes prepared with 1% of the edge activators (**a**) Span® 80 transferosomes; (**b**) Tween® 80 transferosomes.

4. Discussion

The hydrodynamic diameters obtained in this study are congruent with those observed in previous studies [42]. The linoleic acid was incorporated to replace a portion of the cholesterol as part of the lipid concentration for the membrane stabilization. Cholesterol is known to contribute to the membrane thickness and hence the increased size of the vesicles [43]. The replacement of a part of the cholesterol with linoleic acid and the CysA-loading that improves membrane fluidity all contributed to a reduction in the hydrodynamic size of the prepared transferosomes. Most of the studies report an increase in the size of the vesicles after drug loading. Shen and co-workers reported a slight decrease in the size of paclitaxel-loaded micelles, although this decrease was not consistent across all of their formulations [44]. The reduction in size observed in this study may have resulted from an effect of the CysA on the membrane packing. The defects in the lipid membrane are an important factor modulating the binding of different peripheral proteins [45], that in turn affects fluidity, and membrane thickness [46]. Pezeshky and co-workers [47] described the effect of cholesterol, for example, on the size of vesicles after 30 days of storage. The membrane thickness has been identified as one parameter that affects the size of vesicles [46]. According to Huang and co-workers, an increase in the membrane thickness leads to an increase in the vesicle size [48]. It can be inferred that CysA, being hydrophobic, is loaded into the lipid bilayer and facilitates the compact packing that reduces the thickness of the membrane, and therefore the vesicles size. The level of surfactants incorporated into ophthalmic products is critical for both the ocular cell toxicity and formulation stability. In transferosomes, an additional demand is placed on the surfactant for effective flexibility and deformability. The transferosomes enable the effective deposition of the contained drug at the site of physiological action possessing the potential to migrate through orifices smaller than their size. Tween® 80 was selected because it has found use in ophthalmic products on the market due to its acceptable safety profile.

For the soy phosphatidylcholine employed in this investigation, the phase transition temperature was previously determined to be 58.1 °C in other studies [31]. Shalaev and Steponkus [49] had earlier studied the influence of sugar concentration and hydration states in DOPE-based vesicles and found that both the presence of sucrose and hydration states modified the phase transition temperature. In addition, they found that the physical state of the sugar matrix at the transition point affected the temperature of the transition and that the depression of the transition temperature for lipid vesicles always occurred if the glass transition temperature of the sugar is higher than that of the lipid used [49]. The peaks observed between 170.97 °C and 172.50 °C for the vesicles can thus be attributed to such an interdigitation of the vesicle chains. The melting endotherm for pure CysA was found at ~130 °C and the decomposition started at 226.80 °C. These peaks disappeared completely from the thermogram of the CysA-loaded transferosomes, thus indicating the efficacy and stability of the encapsulation process. Wagh and colleagues [29] made a similar observation while working with CysA nanoparticles prepared with PLGA and Eudragit 100®. The melting peak that appeared in the thermogram of CysA completely disappeared from the thermogram of the optimized formulation, signifying the efficacy of the encapsulation process.

The size measurements from TEM varied slightly from the DLS-determined sizes. The dehydration process may have accounted for the slight disparity in size obtained from the DLS, TEM, and SEM, as observed by Carreras and co-workers [50].

The dissolution of pure CysA was discussed and characterized in other investigations, where the poor solubility of CysA was demonstrated. For example, Dubey et al. [51] compared the drug release profiles for the CysA/micelle incorporated nanofibers with that from the corresponding quantity of pure crystalline CysA, which highlighted that there was a complete release of CysA from the nanofiber after 14 min, whereas there was negligible dissolution of the pure drug [52]. Nano-systems, such as those discussed by Dubey et al. [52] and presented herein, serve to improve the dissolution rate of the poorly soluble CysA through various mechanisms (i.e., solubilization, high surface area, improved wetting, and molecular dispersion of the drug); however, the transferosome system also serves to control the release of the drug, thus providing effective CysA levels for an extended period.

The studies that quantitate the amount of CysA released from topical formulations are limited. Most of the studies generally focus on the efficacy of CysA in the ocular condition being targeted for treatment. One study, however, evaluated the blood concentrations of CysA following the topical application of the usually administered topical doses of 0.05% and 0.1% [52]. Although the ocular concentrations of CysA were not measured, the study established that, at these doses, the 0.05% formulation was below the limit of detection while only 5.5% of the population treated with the 0.1% formulation showed detectable levels of CysA in the blood. Another study evaluated the corneal penetration of CysA from polymeric micelles in a Lewis and Brown Norway rat model [5]. The corneal CysA levels in the transplanted and healthy rats were 11710 ± 7530 ng/g and 6470 ± 1730 ng/g of tissue, respectively, and implied a superior corneal penetration performance to both a CysA oily solution and normal saline. A similar study compared a CysA micellar formulation with an emulsion formulation [23]. In their study, and over a 7-day period, 78.36% and 88.87% were released, respectively, from the emulsion and micellar formulation in vitro. The pharmacokinetic profile showed that both of the formulations displayed a similar bioavailability, but with significantly different elimination profiles, resulting in a slower elimination from the micelles. The micellar formulation was thus shown to contribute to maintaining the presence of CysA over a longer period. Even though the current transferosomal formulation presented in this investigation exhibited similar drug delivery profiles, their safety profile was improved, which was also a result of the exclusion of the toxic solvents.

The corneal epithelium has been identified as the strongest barrier limiting the passage of topically applied drugs to molecules less than 500 Da and various nano-systems have been explored to overcome this barrier. The contributions of these nano-systems towards overcoming the corneal epithelial barrier have mainly been based on the size advantage. However, evidence is also emerging to underscore the nature of the components of the nano-system viz-à-viz their interaction with the epithelial layer [7], such as interactions with the cholesterol and lipid components of the corneal epithelium, rendering it more permeable to exogenous substances [53].

5. Conclusions

The potential for the ocular delivery of CysA using transferosomes was explored in this investigation. The toxicity of the developed transferosomes, which is of major concern, was within acceptable limits. The transferosomes showed potential for sustaining the release of the incorporated CysA in vitro over the time period investigated in this study. The possible interaction of the loaded drug with the lipid membrane, as well as the presence of linoleic acid, may have contributed to the stabilizing effect on the size of the transferosomes over time. The corneal permeability and flux from the Span® and Tween® formulations were similar. A future assessment of the in vivo performance of the developed transferosomes, in terms of toxicity and therapeutic efficacy, is proposed.

Author Contributions: Conceptualization, Y.E.C., O.U., N.A. and P.K.; methodology, O.U., L.C.D.T., P.K., N.A. and Y.E.C.; validation, O.U. and L.C.D.T.; formal analysis, O.U., L.C.D.T. and P.K.; investigation, O.U.; resources, Y.E.C.; data curation, O.U.; writing—original draft preparation, O.U.; writing—review and editing, L.C.D.T.; supervision, Y.E.C., N.A. and P.K.; project administration, Y.E.C.; funding acquisition, Y.E.C. All authors have read and agreed to the published version of the manuscript.

Funding: This research was funded by Prof. Choonara's National Research Foundation of South Africa Research Chair Initiative Grant (Grant number: 64814).

Institutional Review Board Statement: The study was conducted in accordance with the Declaration of Helsinki and approved by the Animal Research Ethics Committee of the University of the Witwatersrand. (2021-07-03C, July 2021).

Informed Consent Statement: Not applicable.

Data Availability Statement: Not applicable.

Conflicts of Interest: The authors declare no conflict of interest.

References

1. Uwaezuoke, O.J.; Kumar, P.; Pillay, V.; Choonara, Y.E. Fouling in ocular devices: Implications for drug delivery, bioactive surface immobilization, and biomaterial design. *Drug Deliv. Transl. Res.* **2021**, *11*, 1903–1923. [CrossRef] [PubMed]
2. Mun, E.A.; Morrison, P.W.J.; Williams, A.C.; Khutoryanskiy, V.V. On the Barrier Properties of the Cornea: A Microscopy Study of the Penetration of Fluorescently Labeled Nanoparticles, Polymers, and Sodium Fluorescein. *Mol. Pharm.* **2014**, *11*, 3556–3564. [CrossRef] [PubMed]
3. Grass, G.M.; Robinson, J.R. Mechanisms of corneal drug penetration. I: In vivo and in vitro kinetics. *J. Pharm. Sci.* **1988**, *77*, 3–14. [CrossRef] [PubMed]
4. Ramsay, E.; del Amo, E.M.; Toropainen, E.; Tengvall-Unadike, U.; Ranta, V.-P.; Urtti, A.; Ruponen, M. Corneal and conjunctival drug permeability: Systematic comparison and pharmacokinetic impact in the eye. *Eur. J. Pharm. Sci.* **2018**, *119*, 83–89. [CrossRef] [PubMed]
5. Di Tommaso, C.; Bourges, J.-L.; Valamanesh, F.; Trubitsyn, G.; Torriglia, A.; Jeanny, J.-C.; Behar-Cohen, F.; Gurny, R.; Möller, M. Novel micelle carriers for cyclosporin A topical ocular delivery: In vivo cornea penetration, ocular distribution and efficacy studies. *Eur. J. Pharm. Biopharm.* **2012**, *81*, 257–264. [CrossRef]
6. Sharma, R.; Ahuja, M.; Kaur, H. Thiolated pectin nanoparticles: Preparation, characterization and ex vivo corneal permeation study. *Carbohydr. Polym.* **2012**, *87*, 1606–1610. [CrossRef]

7. Calvo, P.; Vila-Jato, J.L.; Alonso, M.J. Evaluation of cationic polymer-coated nanocapsules as ocular drug carriers. *Int. J. Pharm.* **1997**, *153*, 41–50. [CrossRef]
8. Ibrahim, M.M.; Maria, D.N.; Wang, X.; Simpson, R.N.; Hollingsworth, T.J.; Jablonski, M.M. Enhanced Corneal Penetration of a Poorly Permeable Drug Using Bioadhesive Multiple Microemulsion Technology. *Pharmaceutics* **2020**, *12*, 704. [CrossRef]
9. Urtti, A.; Salminen, L. Minimizing systemic absorption of topically administered ophthalmic drugs. *Surv. Ophthalmol.* **1993**, *37*, 435–456. [CrossRef]
10. Moiseev, R.V.; Morrison, P.W.J.; Steele, F.; Khutoryanskiy, V.V. Penetration Enhancers in Ocular Drug Delivery. *Pharmaceutics* **2019**, *11*, 321. [CrossRef]
11. Lallemand, F.; Schmitt, M.; Bourges, J.-L.; Gurny, R.; Benita, S.; Garrigue, J.-S. Cyclosporine A delivery to the eye: A comprehensive review of academic and industrial efforts. *Eur. J. Pharm. Biopharm.* **2017**, *117*, 14–28. [CrossRef] [PubMed]
12. Utine, C.A.; Stern, M.; Akpek, E.K. Clinical Review: Topical Ophthalmic Use of Cyclosporin A. *Ocul. Immunol. Inflamm.* **2010**, *18*, 352–361. [CrossRef] [PubMed]
13. Daull, P.; Baudouin, C.; Liang, H.; Feraille, L.; Barabino, S.; Garrigue, J.-S. Review of Preclinical Outcomes of a Topical Cationic Emulsion of Cyclosporine A for the Treatment of Ocular Surface Diseases. *Ocul. Immunol. Inflamm.* **2021**, 1–11. [CrossRef]
14. Jumelle, C.; Gholizadeh, S.; Annabi, N.; Dana, R. Advances and limitations of drug delivery systems formulated as eye drops. *J. Control. Release* **2020**, *321*, 1–22. [CrossRef]
15. Burstein, N.L. Corneal cytotoxicity of topically applied drugs, vehicles and preservatives. *Surv. Ophthalmol.* **1980**, *25*, 15–30. [CrossRef]
16. Cevc, G.; Blume, G. Lipid vesicles penetrate into intact skin owing to the transdermal osmotic gradients and hydration force. *Biochim. Biophys. Acta BBA-Biomembr.* **1992**, *1104*, 226–232. [CrossRef]
17. Opatha, S.A.T.; Titapiwatanakun, V.; Chutoprapat, R. Transfersomes: A Promising Nanoencapsulation Technique for Transdermal Drug Delivery. *Pharmaceutics* **2020**, *12*, 855. [CrossRef]
18. Mudgil, P. Evaluation of use of essential fatty acids in topical ophthalmic preparations for dry eye. *Ocul. Surf.* **2020**, *18*, 74–79. [CrossRef]
19. Yokoi, N.; Uchino, M.; Uchino, Y.; Dogru, M.; Kawashima, M.; Komuro, A.; Sonomura, Y.; Kato, H.; Tsubota, K.; Kinoshita, S. Importance of tear film instability in dry eye disease in office workers using visual display terminals: The Osaka study. *Am. J. Ophthalmol.* **2015**, *159*, 748–754. [CrossRef]
20. Hashmat, D.; Shoaib, M.H.; Ali, F.R.; Siddiqui, F. Lornoxicam controlled release transdermal gel patch: Design, characterization and optimization using co-solvents as penetration enhancers. *PLoS ONE* **2020**, *15*, e0228908. [CrossRef]
21. Sydykov, B.; Oldenhof, H.; Sieme, H.; Wolkers, W.F. Storage stability of liposomes stored at elevated subzero temperatures in DMSO/sucrose mixtures. *PLoS ONE* **2018**, *13*, e0199867. [CrossRef] [PubMed]
22. Jain, S.; Jain, P.; Umamaheshwari, R.B.; Jain, N.K. Transfersomes—A Novel Vesicular Carrier for Enhanced Transdermal Delivery: Development, Characterization, and Performance Evaluation. *Drug Dev. Ind. Pharm.* **2003**, *29*, 1013–1026. [CrossRef] [PubMed]
23. Yu, Y.; Chen, D.; Li, Y.; Yang, W.; Tu, J.; Shen, Y. Improving the topical ocular pharmacokinetics of lyophilized cyclosporine A-loaded micelles: Formulation, in vitro and in vivo studies. *Drug Deliv.* **2018**, *25*, 888–899. [CrossRef] [PubMed]
24. Abdel-Mottaleb, M.M.A.; Lamprecht, A. Standardized in vitro drug release test for colloidal drug carriers using modified USP dissolution apparatus I. *Drug Dev. Ind. Pharm.* **2011**, *37*, 178–184. [CrossRef]
25. Development of a Convenient Ex Vivo Model for the Study of the Transcorneal Permeation of Drugs: Histological and Permeability Evaluation-Pescina-2015-Journal of Pharmaceutical Sciences-Wiley Online Library. Available online: https://onlinelibrary.wiley.com/doi/full/10.1002/jps.24231 (accessed on 11 November 2020).
26. Danaei, M.; Kalantari, M.; Raji, M.; Samareh Fekri, H.; Saber, R.; Asnani, G.P.; Mortazavi, S.M.; Mozafari, M.R.; Rasti, B.; Taheriazam, A. Probing nanoliposomes using single particle analytical techniques: Effect of excipients, solvents, phase transition and zeta potential. *Heliyon* **2018**, *4*, e01088. [CrossRef]
27. Yang, E.; Yu, H.; Choi, S.; Park, K.-M.; Jung, H.-S.; Chang, P.-S. Controlled rate slow freezing with lyoprotective agent to retain the integrity of lipid nanovesicles during lyophilization. *Sci. Rep.* **2021**, *11*, 24354. [CrossRef]
28. Almalik, A.; Alradwan, I.; Kalam, M.A.; Alshamsan, A. Effect of cryoprotection on particle size stability and preservation of chitosan nanoparticles with and without hyaluronate or alginate coating. *Saudi Pharm. J. SPJ* **2017**, *25*, 861–867. [CrossRef]
29. Wagh, V.D.; Apar, D.U. Cyclosporine A Loaded PLGA Nanoparticles for Dry Eye Disease: In Vitro Characterization Studies. *J. Nanotechnol.* **2014**, *2014*, e683153. [CrossRef]
30. Demetzos, C. Differential Scanning Calorimetry (DSC): A Tool to Study the Thermal Behavior of Lipid Bilayers and Liposomal Stability. *J. Liposome Res.* **2008**, *18*, 159–173. [CrossRef]
31. Londoño, C.A.; Rojas, J.; Yarce, C.J.; Salamanca, C.H. Design of Prototype Formulations for In Vitro Dermal Delivery of the Natural Antioxidant Ferulic Acid Based on Ethosomal Colloidal Systems. *Cosmetics* **2019**, *6*, 5. [CrossRef]
32. The Merck Index: An Encyclopedia of Chemicals, Drugs, and Biologicals (Book, 2006) [WorldCat.org]. Available online: https://www.worldcat.org/title/merck-index-an-encyclopedia-of-chemicals-drugs-and-biologicals/oclc/70882070 (accessed on 16 June 2022).
33. Gonzalez Gomez, A.; Syed, S.; Marshall, K.; Hosseinidoust, Z. Liposomal Nanovesicles for Efficient Encapsulation of Staphylococcal Antibiotics. *ACS Omega* **2019**, *4*, 10866–10876. [CrossRef] [PubMed]

34. Urimi, D.; Widenbring, R.; Pérez García, R.O.; Gedda, L.; Edwards, K.; Loftsson, T.; Schipper, N. Formulation development and upscaling of lipid nanocapsules as a drug delivery system for a novel cyclic GMP analogue intended for retinal drug delivery. *Int. J. Pharm.* **2021**, *602*, 120640. [CrossRef] [PubMed]
35. Sassine, J.; Sousa, J.; Lalk, M.; Daniel, R.A.; Vollmer, W. Cell morphology maintenance in Bacillus subtilis through balanced peptidoglycan synthesis and hydrolysis. *Sci. Rep.* **2020**, *10*, 17910. [CrossRef]
36. Ouyang, C.; Choice, E.; Holland, J.; Meloche, M.; Madden, T.D. Liposomal cyclosporine. Characterization of drug incorporation and interbilayer exchange. *Transplantation* **1995**, *60*, 999–1006. [CrossRef] [PubMed]
37. Czogalla, A. Oral cyclosporine A—The current picture of its liposomal and other delivery systems. *Cell. Mol. Biol. Lett.* **2008**, *14*, 139–152. [CrossRef] [PubMed]
38. du Toit, L.C.; Carmichael, T.; Govender, T.; Kumar, P.; Choonara, Y.E.; Pillay, V. In vitro, in vivo, and in silico evaluation of the bioresponsive behavior of an intelligent intraocular implant. *Pharm. Res.* **2014**, *31*, 607–634. [CrossRef]
39. Shashidhar, G.M.; Manohar, B. Nanocharacterization of liposomes for the encapsulation of water soluble compounds from Cordyceps sinensis CS1197 by a supercritical gas anti-solvent technique. *RSC Adv.* **2018**, *8*, 34634–34649. [CrossRef]
40. Agarwal, P.; Scherer, D.; Günther, B.; Rupenthal, I.D. Semifluorinated alkane based systems for enhanced corneal penetration of poorly soluble drugs. *Int. J. Pharm.* **2018**, *538*, 119–129. [CrossRef]
41. Alkilani, A.Z.; McCrudden, M.T.C.; Donnelly, R.F. Transdermal Drug Delivery: Innovative Pharmaceutical Developments Based on Disruption of the Barrier Properties of the Stratum Corneum. *Pharmaceutics* **2015**, *7*, 438–470. [CrossRef]
42. Ahad, A.; Al-Saleh, A.A.; Al-Mohizea, A.M.; Al-Jenoobi, F.I.; Raish, M.; Yassin, A.E.B.; Alam, M.A. Formulation and characterization of novel soft nanovesicles for enhanced transdermal delivery of eprosartan mesylate. *Saudi Pharm. J.* **2017**, *25*, 1040–1046. [CrossRef]
43. Nakhaei, P.; Margiana, R.; Bokov, D.O.; Abdelbasset, W.K.; Jadidi Kouhbanani, M.A.; Varma, R.S.; Marofi, F.; Jarahian, M.; Beheshtkhoo, N. Liposomes: Structure, Biomedical Applications, and Stability Parameters With Emphasis on Cholesterol. *Front. Bioeng. Biotechnol.* **2021**, *9*, 705886. [CrossRef] [PubMed]
44. Shen, Y.; Tang, H.; Zhan, Y.; Van Kirk, E.A.; Murdoch, W.J. Degradable Poly(β-amino ester) nanoparticles for cancer cytoplasmic drug delivery. *Nanomed. Nanotechnol. Biol. Med.* **2009**, *5*, 192–201. [CrossRef] [PubMed]
45. Tripathy, M.; Thangamani, S.; Srivastava, A. Three-Dimensional Packing Defects in Lipid Membrane as a Function of Membrane Order. *J. Chem. Theory Comput.* **2020**, *16*, 7800–7816. [CrossRef] [PubMed]
46. Huang, C.; Quinn, D.; Sadovsky, Y.; Suresh, S.; Hsia, K.J. Formation and size distribution of self-assembled vesicles. *Proc. Natl. Acad. Sci. USA* **2017**, *114*, 2910–2915. [CrossRef] [PubMed]
47. Pezeshky, A.; Ghanbarzadeh, B.; Hamishehkar, H.; Moghadam, M.; Babazadeh, A. Vitamin A palmitate-bearing nanoliposomes: Preparation and characterization. *Food Biosci.* **2016**, *13*, 49–55. [CrossRef]
48. Huang, Y.; Tao, Q.; Hou, D.; Hu, S.; Tian, S.; Chen, Y.; Gui, R.; Yang, L.; Wang, Y. A Novel Ion-Exchange Carrier Based upon Liposome-Encapsulated Montmorillonite for Ophthalmic Delivery of Betaxolol Hydrochloride. Available online: https://www.dovepress.com/a-novel-ion-exchange-carrier-based-upon-liposome-encapsulated--montmor-peer-reviewed-article-IJN (accessed on 27 March 2018).
49. Shalaev, E.Y.; Steponkus, P.L. Phase behavior and glass transition of 1,2-dioleoylphosphatidylethanolamine (DOPE) dehydrated in the presence of sucrose. *Biochim. Biophys. Acta BBA-Biomembr.* **2001**, *1514*, 100–116. [CrossRef]
50. Carreras, J.J.; Tapia-Ramirez, W.E.; Sala, A.; Guillot, A.J.; Garrigues, T.M.; Melero, A. Ultraflexible lipid vesicles allow topical absorption of cyclosporin A. *Drug Deliv. Transl. Res.* **2020**, *10*, 486–497. [CrossRef]
51. Dubey, P.; Barker, S.A.; Craig, D.Q.M. Design and Characterization of Cyclosporine A-Loaded Nanofibers for Enhanced Drug Dissolution. *ACS Omega* **2020**, *5*, 1003–1013. [CrossRef]
52. Small, D.S.; Acheampong, A.; Reis, B.; Stern, K.; Stewart, W.; Berdy, G.; Epstein, R.; Foerster, R.; Forstot, L.; Tang-Liu, D.D.-S. Blood concentrations of cyclosporin a during long-term treatment with cyclosporin a ophthalmic emulsions in patients with moderate to severe dry eye disease. *J. Ocul. Pharmacol. Ther. Off. J. Assoc. Ocul. Pharmacol. Ther.* **2002**, *18*, 411–418. [CrossRef]
53. Morrison, P.W.J.; Connon, C.J.; Khutoryanskiy, V.V. Cyclodextrin-Mediated Enhancement of Riboflavin Solubility and Corneal Permeability. *Mol. Pharm.* **2013**, *10*, 756–762. [CrossRef]

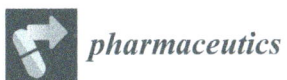

Article

Ciprofloxacin-Loaded Zein/Hyaluronic Acid Nanoparticles for Ocular Mucosa Delivery

Telma A. Jacinto [1,†], Breno Oliveira [1,†], Sónia P. Miguel [1,2], Maximiano P. Ribeiro [1,2] and Paula Coutinho [1,2,*]

1. CPIRN-UDI/IPG, Centro de Potencial e Inovação em Recursos Naturais, Unidade de Investigação para o Desenvolvimento do Interior do Instituto Politécnico da Guarda, Avenida Dr. Francisco de Sá Carneiro, No. 50, 6300-559 Guarda, Portugal; telmajacinto@ipg.pt (T.A.J.); brennofcb@hotmail.com (B.O.); spmiguel@ipg.pt (S.P.M.); mribeiro@ipg.pt (M.P.R.)
2. CICS-UBI, Centro de Investigação em Ciências da Saúde, Universidade da Beira Interior, Avenida Infante D. Henrique, 6200-506 Covilhã, Portugal
* Correspondence: coutinho@ipg.pt
† These authors contributed equally to this work.

Abstract: Bacterial conjunctivitis is a worldwide problem that, if untreated, can lead to severe complications, such as visual impairment and blindness. Topical administration of ciprofloxacin is one of the most common treatments for this infection; however, topical therapeutic delivery to the eye is quite challenging. To tackle this, nanomedicine presents several advantages compared to conventional ophthalmic dosage forms. Herein, the flash nanoprecipitation technique was applied to produce zein and hyaluronic acid nanoparticles loaded with ciprofloxacin (ZeinCPX_HA NPs). ZeinCPX_HA NPs exhibited a hydrodynamic diameter of <200 nm and polydispersity index of <0.3, suitable for ocular drug delivery. In addition, the freeze-drying of the nanoparticles was achieved by using mannitol as a cryoprotectant, allowing their resuspension in water without modifying the physicochemical properties. Moreover, the biocompatibility of nanoparticles was confirmed by in vitro assays. Furthermore, a high encapsulation efficiency was achieved, and a release profile with an initial burst was followed by a prolonged release of ciprofloxacin up to 24 h. Overall, the obtained results suggest ZeinCPX_HA NPs as an alternative to the common topical dosage forms available on the market to treat conjunctivitis.

Keywords: flash nanoprecipitation; conjunctivitis; nanoparticles; zein; hyaluronic acid; ciprofloxacin

Citation: Jacinto, T.A.; Oliveira, B.; Miguel, S.P.; Ribeiro, M.P.; Coutinho, P. Ciprofloxacin-Loaded Zein/Hyaluronic Acid Nanoparticles for Ocular Mucosa Delivery. *Pharmaceutics* 2022, 14, 1557. https://doi.org/10.3390/pharmaceutics14081557

Academic Editors: Hugo Almeida and Ana Catarina Silva

Received: 30 June 2022
Accepted: 24 July 2022
Published: 27 July 2022

Publisher's Note: MDPI stays neutral with regard to jurisdictional claims in published maps and institutional affiliations.

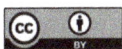

Copyright: © 2022 by the authors. Licensee MDPI, Basel, Switzerland. This article is an open access article distributed under the terms and conditions of the Creative Commons Attribution (CC BY) license (https://creativecommons.org/licenses/by/4.0/).

1. Introduction

Conjunctivitis affects many people worldwide and consists of the inflammation and swelling of the conjunctival tissue, as well as dilation of the blood vessels, ocular discharge, and discomfort. Conjunctivitis can be divided into four main groups based on the etiology: bacterial, viral, allergic, and irritant [1,2]. Bacterial conjunctivitis is the second-most common infectious conjunctivitis and is more frequent in children [3]. Further, bacterial conjunctivitis is one of the most common ophthalmic diseases in developed countries [4]. Several bacterial are etiological agents of conjunctivitis, the most common of which being *Streptococcus pneumoniae*, *Haemophilus influenza*, *Moraxella catarrhalis*, and *Staphylococcus aureus*; the last is more common in adults [5]. Ciprofloxacin (CPX) is one of the most-used antibiotics in the treatment of bacterial conjunctivitis [6], and is a broad-spectrum antibiotic that belongs to a class of antibiotics designed by fluoroquinolones [7]. Fluoroquinolones have excellent antibacterial effects against Gram-negative and many Gram-positive bacteria [8]. Nevertheless, commercial CPX eye drop solutions have an acidic pH, which causes local burning and itching [9,10]. Furthermore, the low solubility of CPX under ocular physiological conditions (pH ≈ 7) leads to a lower drug bioavailability [9].

Up to the present, topical dosage forms were elected as a less invasive administration route to the ocular mucosa. However, obstacles such as tear fluid production and the corneal barrier limit drug bioavailability. To tackle this challenge, researchers have proposed nanoparticles (NPs)-based systems for treating ocular infections, as reviewed by Liu et al. [11]. These systems can increase the retention time of the drugs on the ocular surface and protect them from enzymatic degradation, while simultaneously contributing to the decrease of the drug concentration administered to assure the therapeutic effect [12–14]. In addition, other authors demonstrated that by incorporating drugs into NPs, there is an enhancement of corneal permeability [11,15]. Hence, flash nanoprecipitation (FNP) is a simple and effective approach to producing NPs with high drug-encapsulation efficiency (EE) [16]. The FNP technique is based on a rapid mixing that creates high-supersaturation conditions, leading to the precipitation and encapsulation of both hydrophobic and hydrophilic drugs into polymeric NPs [16–18]. Several studies demonstrated that FNP allows the encapsulation of hydrophobic and hydrophilic drugs with high EE, as we have previously reported [18,19].

Herein, ZeinCPX_HA NPs were prepared using the FNP technique. Zein is a water-insoluble protein extracted from corn and is generally recognized as safe (GRAS) by the FDA [20]. In fact, zein has been widely explored in biomedical applications, namely in the field of pharmaceuticals, due to its physicochemical and biological properties [21]. Further, zein has been widely applied as a drug carrier due to its biocompatibility and amphiphilic nature which promote the self-assembly process [18,22–24] and the encapsulation of poorly water-soluble compounds [25]. On the other hand, hyaluronic acid (HA) is a polysaccharide selected due to its mucoadhesive character so that it will increase the pre-corneal residence of the drug [26]. Therefore, the pre-corneal clearance will be reduced by using HA, and consequently, a higher cellular interaction and ocular bioavailability will be attained [27]. Moreover, HA is a ligand for the CD44 receptor, which is present in the human cornea and conjunctiva. Under some pathological and inflammatory conditions, the CD44 receptor number increases, prompting the interaction with HA [28–31].

To the best of our knowledge, this is the first report of ZeinCPX_HA NPs produced by FNP. In the first instance, the polymer ratio (zein and HA) and cryoprotectants (glucose and mannitol) were optimized to obtain stable lyophilized NPs suitable for ocular drug delivery. These cryoprotectants can act as protective agents during freezing due to an increase in the surface tension of the water molecules, and can also work as cryoprotectants by preventing stress during the drying phase [32,33].

Thus, the main purpose of this study was to develop biocompatible polymeric NPs suitable for CPX ocular delivery with enhanced bioavailability and stability under long-term storage.

2. Materials and Methods

2.1. Materials

Dulbecco's Modified Eagle Medium/Nutrient Mixture F-12 (DMEM-F12), phosphate-buffered saline (PBS) solution, 3-(4,5-Dimethylthiazol-2-yl)-2,5-diphenyltetrazolium bromide (MTT), trypsin, D(-)-Glucose, and high-performance liquid chromatography (HPLC) grade ciprofloxacin 98% were acquired from Sigma-Aldrich (Lisboa, Portugal). Ethanol (99.9%), glacial acetic acid, D(-)-Mannitol, dimethyl sulfoxide (DMSO) $\geq$ 99.9%, and HPLC-gradient grade acetonitrile were purchased from VWR Chemicals (Radnor, PA, USA). Normal human dermal fibroblasts (NHDFs) were purchased from PromoCell (Labclinics, S.A., Barcelona, Spain). Hydrochloric acid (HCl) was bought from Panreac (Barcelona, Spain). HPLC-grade ortho-phosphoric acid was acquired from Fisher Scientific (Oeiras, Portugal). Hyaluronic acid (MW: 1.0–2.0 Million Da) was purchased from Carbosynth (Bershire, UK). Zein (purified) was obtained from Acros Organics (Waltham, MA, USA). Fetal bovine serum (FBS) was obtained from Biowest (Riverside, MO, USA). Cell culture T-flasks were supplied by Orange Scientific (Braine-l'Alleud, Belgium). Ultrapure water was obtained by using a Q-POD® dispenser (Merck Millipore, Burlington, MA, USA) (0.22 µm filtered; 18.2 MΩ/cm at 25 °C). Sodium bicarbonate $\geq$ 99% and ethanol were acquired from

José Manuel Gomes dos Santos, LDA (Odivelas, Portugal). Sodium chloride 99.5% and potassium chloride $\geq$ 99.5% were purchased from Honeywell Fluka (Charlotte, NC, USA).

2.2. Production of the Zein and HA-Based NPs

The production of the Zein_HA NPs was achieved by the FNP technique using a confined impinging jets mixer (CIJM), which was produced at Fablab-IPG according to the model described by Han et al. [34]. Zein and HA (with pH $\approx$ 7) solutions were prepared, under agitation, in ethanol (80% v/v) and ultrapure water, respectively. Before mixing, the concentration of the zein solution was set at 2.5 and 5 mg/mL and the HA solution was set to 1 and 2.5 mg/mL. Briefly, the solution of zein (2.5 mL) was mixed against an equal volume of the HA solution. The NPs were collected in a solution of 45 mL of ultrapure water (pH $\approx$ 11).

2.3. Screening of Cryoprotectants

It is well documented that the long-term storage of the NPs is preferable under dried solid forms to liquid forms [35]. This way, glucose and mannitol (5 and 10% w/v) were added to the NPs solution before the freeze-drying process. Briefly, 1 mL of NPs solution with or without cryoprotectant (in a 1:1 ratio) were placed into glass vials and frozen at $-80\,^\circ$C for 12 h. Then the samples were lyophilized for 24 h in a Telstar LyoQuest $-85\,^\circ$C (Telstar, Madrid, Spain) operating a condenser at $-67\,^\circ$C and pressures below 0.05 mbar and lyophilized. After lyophilization, NPs were rehydrated by adding ultrapure water and left under static conditions for 10 min at room temperature before being fully reconstituted by manual shaking.

To evaluate the protective effect exerted by the cryoprotectants (5 and 10% w/v), the redispersibility index (RDI) was calculated according to the following Equation (1) [36]:

$$\text{RDI (\%)} = \frac{D}{D_0} \times 100 \quad (1)$$

where D is the rehydrated NPs hydrodynamic diameter (Dh), and D_0 is the Dh of fresh NPs. RDI values close or equal to 100% mean that samples can be appropriately resuspended.

2.4. Characterization of the NPs

2.4.1. Particle Dh, Zeta Potential and Polydispersity Index (PDI) Measurements

Zein_HA NPs' Dh, zeta potential, and PDI were determined by dynamic light scattering (DLS) using Zetasizer Nano ZS (Malvern Instruments, Malvern, UK). These parameters were also assessed for fresh and rehydrated NPs at room temperature.

2.4.2. Fourier Transform Infrared (FTIR) Analysis

The FTIR spectra of the lyophilized NPs, drug, polymers, and cryoprotectant were acquired on a Nicolet iS10 spectrometer, with a 4 cm^{-1} spectral resolution from 500 to 4000 cm^{-1} and 128 scans per run (Thermo Scientific Inc., Waltham, MA, USA).

2.4.3. Thermogravimetric (TGA) and Differential Scanning Calorimetry (DSC) Analysis

TGA and DSC analyses were carried out on a STA 7200 Hitachi® (Fukuoka, Japan). Briefly, both freeze-dried NPs formulations were heated up to 400 $^\circ$C, at a heating rate of 10 $^\circ$C/min under nitrogen atmosphere (20 mL/min).

2.5. Production of ZeinCPX_HA NPs and Stability Studies

The production of ZeinCPX_HA NPs was performed by following the methodology described in Section 2.2, where the CPX (4 mg/mL in 0.1 N HCl) was dissolved in the zein solution in a volume ratio of 1:10 (CPX and zein). Then, the characterization of ZeinCPX_HA NPs was conducted by using the same procedures outlined in Section 2.4.

Further, the stability studies were performed on both NPs (Zein_HA NPs and ZeinCPX_HA NPs). Briefly, NPs were rehydrated, after lyophilization, by adding ultrapure water and left under static conditions for 10 min at room temperature (22 ± 2 °C) before being fully reconstituted by manual shaking. Then, the lyophilized NPs were stored at room temperature for 28 days, redispersed in ultrapure water every 7 days and characterized as described in Section 2.4. Additionally, the RDI of the ZeinCPX_HA NPs was also calculated according to Equation (1) of Section 2.3.

2.6. Encapsulation Efficiency and Loading Capacity

The EE and drug loading (DL) of CPX into the NPs were assessed in the supernatant after centrifuging the NPs (4000× g; 10 min), using a 10 kDa Amicon® Ultra-2 Centrifugal Filter Device (Merck Millipore, Darmstadt, Germany). Then, the CPX was quantified by HPLC as previously described by [37]. The chromatographic analysis was performed using an UltiMate 3000 HPLC chromatography device (Thermo Scientific, Waltham, MA, USA) with a column C18 (Acclaim™ 120 Reversed-Phase Columns C18, 5 µm, 4.6 × 150 mm, Thermo Scientific, Waltham, MA, USA) at a temperature of 40 °C. The mobile phase consisted of 0.025 M ortho-phosphoric acid and acetonitrile (87:13 v/v) with a flow rate of 0.9 mL/min, and the injection volume was 20 µL. The run time cycle was completed in 20 min. CPX was detected at 278 nm with a retention time of ≈11 min. All experiments were carried out in triplicate. The standard calibration curve was obtained (y = 2.5253x − 0.707; R^2 = 0.9993).

The EE was calculated by using the following Equation (2)

$$EE\ (\%) = \frac{A_1 - A_2}{A_1} \times 100 \tag{2}$$

where A_1 is the total amount of CPX added into NPs and A_2 is the amount of drug in the supernatant.

The DL was determined using the following Equation (3)

$$DL\ (\%) = \frac{\text{Weight of the drug in NPs}}{\text{Weight of the NPs}} \times 100 \tag{3}$$

2.7. In Vitro Drug Release of CPX-Loaded NPs

The in vitro release of CPX from lyophilized NPs was performed in simulated tear fluid (STF), which contains 0.22 g of sodium bicarbonate, 0.68 g of sodium chloride, 0.008 g of calcium chloride dehydrate, and 0.14 g of potassium chloride, dissolved in 100 mL of distilled deionized water to mimic ocular physiological conditions [38,39]. In brief, ZeinCPX_HA NPs were immersed in STF (pH 7.4) at 600 mg/mL, and then 1 mL was collected in microcentrifuge tubes at different time points for 24 h, under continuous agitation at 37 °C. At precise time points (0, 1 h 30 min, 2 h 30 min, 4 h 30 min, 6 h 30 min, 8 h 30 min and 24 h), the corresponding microcentrifuge tube was centrifuged (4000× g, 10 min, 25 °C) through a 10 kDa Amicon® Ultra-2 Centrifugal Filter Device (Merck Millipore, Darmstadt, Germany), and the CPX remaining in the supernatant was quantified by HPLC-UV (Thermo Scientific, Waltham, MA, USA). All experiments were performed in triplicate. Zein_HA NPs without CPX were used as a control.

Furthermore, the drug-release kinetics displayed by the NPs was also characterized by applying the zero-order Equation (4), first-order Equation (5), Peppas–Korsmeyer Equation (6) and Higuchi model Equation (7):

$$\text{Zero order: } D_t = D_0 + k_0 t \tag{4}$$

$$\text{First order: } \log C = \log C_0 - \frac{K_t}{2.303} \tag{5}$$

$$\text{Korsmeyer-Peppas: } \frac{M_t}{M_\infty} = K t^n \tag{6}$$

$$\text{Higuchi: } Q_t = K_H\, t^{1/2} \tag{7}$$

where D_t is the amount of drug released at time t, D_0 is the initial drug amount in the solution, and k_0 is the constant release rate. C_0 is the initial drug concentration, K is the first-order rate constant. M_t is the cumulative amount of drug released at time t, M∞ is the initial drug loading, K is a constant characteristic of the drug-polymer system, and n is the diffusion exponent, indicating the release mechanism. Q_t is the amount of drug dissolved in time t, and K_H is the Higuchi dissolution constant.

2.8. Biocompatibility Assay

The biocompatibility of both NPs (with and without CPX) was assessed on normal human dermal fibroblasts (NHDF) cells by the MTT assay, according to the ISO 10993-5 *"Biological evaluation of medical devices—Part 5: Tests for in vitro cytotoxicity"*. Briefly, NHDF cells were seeded in 96-wells plates (6000 cells/well) and maintained in DMEM-F12 medium supplemented with 10% FBS and 1% penicillin–streptomycin–amphotericin B at 37 °C in 5% CO_2 humidified atmosphere. After 24 h of incubation, the culture medium was replaced by NPs solutions cryopreserved with 5% of mannitol (with and without CPX) at different concentrations (12.5, 25, 50, 100 and 125 mg/mL). Following 24 h of incubation, the medium in each cell was replaced by a mixture of 50 µL of MTT solution (5 mg/mL) and incubated for 4 h at 37 °C and 5% CO_2. Then, the MTT solution was removed, and cells were treated with 100 µL of DMSO (0.04 N) for 30 min. Afterwards, the absorbance of the wells (n = 5) was determined at 570 nm using a microplate reader (Thermo Scientific Multiskan GO UV/Vis microplate spectrophotometer, Waltham, MA, USA). Cells incubated with ethanol (96%) were used as a positive control (K^+), whereas untreated cells were used as negative control (K^-).

3. Results and Discussion

3.1. Effect of Polymers' Concentration on Their Properties

NPs produced with lower concentrations of HA and zein resulted in smaller NPs with low PDI (Table 1).

Table 1. Dh and PDI of the NPs with different polymer concentrations. Data are presented as mean ± SD (n = 3).

Polymers	Dh (nm)	PDI
HA (2.5 mg/mL) + Zein (2.5 mg/mL)	146.1 ± 7.4	0.523 ± 0.019
HA (2.5 mg/mL) + Zein (5 mg/mL)	230.3 ± 15.1	0.853 ± 0.056
HA (1 mg/mL) + Zein (2.5 mg/mL)	86 ± 14	0.21 ± 0.07

When zein and HA had a concentration of 5 and 2.5 mg/mL, respectively, the produced NPs had a Dh higher than 200 nm, which is unsuitable to permeate the mucus [40]. On the other hand, when zein concentration decreased to 2.5 mg/mL the resulting NPs had a lower Dh, but with a PDI over 0.5. So, the NPs produced with 1 mg/mL of HA and 2.5 mg/mL of zein, presented the most suitable Dh and PDI, being selected for subsequent analysis.

3.2. Selection of the Cryoprotectant

The freeze-drying process was conducted to evaluate the stability of the nanosystem for long-term storage. The lyophilization process strongly affected the Dh and PDI of Zein_HA NPs, as shown in Figure 1. As for, glucose and mannitol were used at different concentrations (5 and 10% *w/v*) as cryoprotectants.

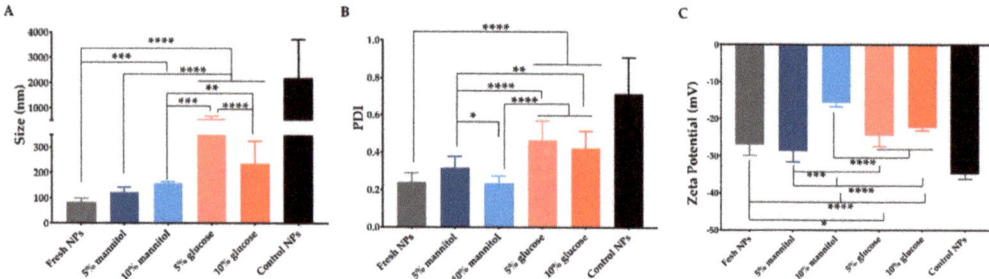

Figure 1. Evaluation of the physicochemical properties of Zein_HA NPs with and without cryoprotectants. Data are presented as mean ± standard deviation ($n > 3$), * < p = 0.05, ** < p = 0.01, *** < p = 0.001, **** p < 0.0001.

As shown in Figure 1, the addition of cryoprotectant affected the NPs physicochemical properties, namely Dh, PDI and zeta potential. The use of mannitol at 5% w/v does not affect the physicochemical properties; however, the Dh of the Zein_HA NPs increased from ≈86 nm to ≈160 nm after using the mannitol at 10% w/v, whereas when used glucose as a cryoprotectant, the Dh increased to ≈589 nm and ≈236 nm at 5 and 10% w/v, respectively. These results are in accordance with the findings presented by Wang et al., where the authors also denoted an increase in the NPs after lyophilization [41]. Further, results show that NPs cryoprotected with mannitol resulted in NPs with a Dh, PDI, and zeta potential more similar to the fresh NPs. In light of these findings, the RDI values were calculated for mannitol at 5 and 10% since these cryoprotectants did not affect the Dh and PDI of Zein_HA NPs (Table 2).

Table 2. RDI of the Zein_HA NPs after lyophilization with different cryoprotectants. Data are presented as mean ± standard deviation (n = 3).

Cryoprotectant	RDI (%)
Mannitol 5%	116 ± 32
Mannitol 10%	187 ± 72

The RDI obtained for mannitol at 5 and 10% was 116 ± 32 and 187 ± 72%, respectively. Taking into account the results obtained, the Zein_HA NPs produced and freeze-dried with mannitol at 5% were selected for the subsequent studies. This result is in accordance with those previously obtained for cryoprotected zein NPs [36]. Moreover, Gagliadri et al. demonstrated that the protective effect of mannitol on zein NPs could be related to its physicochemical properties, which can prevent Maillard reactions that commonly occur when subjected to freeze-drying [25]. Additionally, Feng et al. suggest using mannitol once it crystalizes around the NPs, forming a protective shell and ultimately preventing aggregation [42].

3.3. Characterization of NPs Incorporating CPX

Initially, the successful production of both NPs was also confirmed by FTIR analysis after the freeze-drying process (Figure 2).

The FTIR spectrum of zein is in line with previous reports, exhibiting its characteristic peaks at 3292 cm^{-1} (–OH stretching), 1643 cm^{-1} (C–O stretching and C–N stretching, amide I), and 1515 cm^{-1} (C–N stretching and N–H bending, amide II) [43–45]. The HA spectrum displays its characteristic peaks at 3200–3650 cm^{-1} (O–H stretching), 2900 cm^{-1} (CH$_2$ vibration), 1607 cm^{-1} (carboxyl group in the glucuronic unit), and 1035 cm^{-1} (C–O–C stretching) [43,46,47]. The typical band of CPX was displayed at 1612 cm^{-1} (vibration of phenyl structure conjugated to –COOH), 1282 cm^{-1} (C–F bond stretching), 3044, and 2844 cm^{-1} (C–H stretching from the phenyl ring) [48–50]. In turn, mannitol FTIR spectrum presents its characteristic peaks between 3386 and 2902 cm^{-1} (O–H and C–H stretching vibration) and at 1417, 1280, and 1077 cm^{-1} [51].

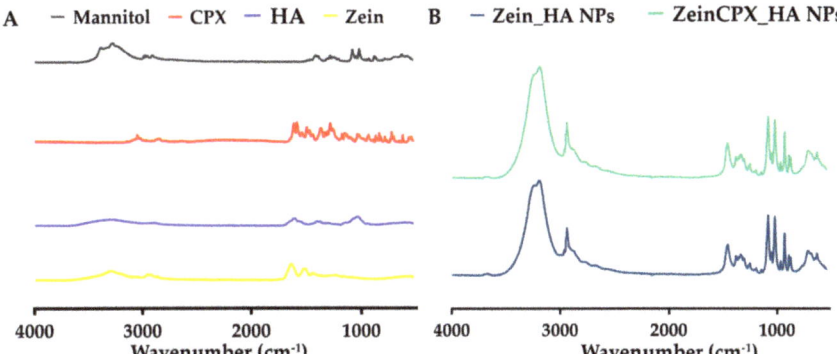

Figure 2. FTIR spectra of the NPs and raw materials: (**A**) spectra of the raw materials (zein, HA, CPX, and mannitol) used for the production and lyophilization of the NPs; (**B**) spectra of the Zein_HA NPs and ZeinCPX_HA NPs.

The FTIR spectrum of ZeinCPX_HA NPs displays high similarity with the Zein_HA NPs spectrum, without relevant peak shifts or new peaks. According to Cacicedo et al., this can be due to the low ratio of CPX in NPs compared to the polymers and cryoprotectants, or the overlap of peaks between CPX and the other compounds [52]. Concerning the presence of both polymers in the NPs, there was a slight shift in the NPs spectra from 3292 cm^{-1} (zein) and 3200–3650 cm^1 (HA) to 3186 cm^{-1}.

As shown in Figure 3A, the TGA thermogram representing HA weight loss exhibits a water loss of about 12% up to 220 °C, in the second step occurs a weight loss of approximately of 55.2% at 220–280 °C due to the polysaccharide degradation, and at the end there is a linear weight loss of close to 10% up to 400 °C [53,54]. CPX TGA thermogram (Figure S1) presents a significant weight loss at 250–450 °C, which is in accordance with the melting point of ≈280–290 °C presented in the DSC thermogram (Figure S2).

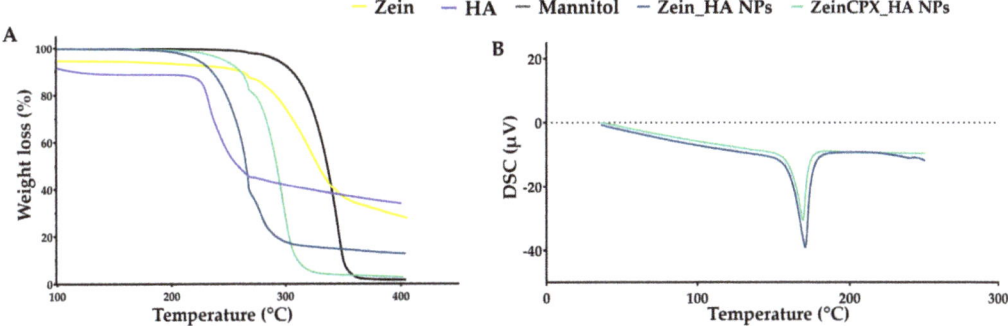

Figure 3. TGA (**A**) and DSC (**B**) analysis of the raw materials (zein, HA and mannitol), Zein_HA NPs and ZeinCPX_HA NPs.

Regarding zein, it presents two decomposition steps. The first step of about 9% weight loss occurs due to the water loss between 100–250 °C. The second step shows a weight loss of 79%, at 250–500 °C due to the degradation of peptide bounds [55]. On the DSC thermogram (Figure S2), zein endothermic peak is 115 °C. As for mannitol, TGA thermogram revealed a weight loss of higher than 90% between 250–400 °C, and regarding the DSC thermogram (Figure S2) mannitol endothermic peak registered at 170 °C [56].

The Zein_HA NPs exhibit a weight loss of −84.1% at 200–320 °C. On the other hand, ZeinCPX_HA NPs have a weight loss of 96% at 199–340 °C; this slight shift can be due the encapsulation of CPX. As shown on the DSC thermogram, Zein_HA NPs and ZeinCPX_HA NPs present an endothermic peak at 165.5 °C and 163 °C, respectively. The endothermic peak of CPX does not appear in the ZeinCPX_HA NPs, so CPX can be dispersed in amorphous state, which can enhance the solubility of the drug and consequently, their bioavailability [57,58].

Ocular drug delivery is challenging due to physiological barriers, limitations associated with conventional ocular therapy (i.e., blurred vision and frequent administration), and NPs' properties, such as Dh, charge, and hydrophilicity. It is extremely important to overcome the challenges mentioned above [59–61]. The Dh of the fresh NPs suffered a significant increase upon the encapsulation of CPX from 86 ± 14 nm to 109 ± 10.2 nm, as shown in Figure 4. This increment can be due to the incorporation of the drug, which is in accordance with other authors' findings. For instance, Nunes et al. demonstrated that the Dh of zein NPs increased from 129 ± 3 nm to 141 ± 7 nm, with the augment of resveratrol loading [20]. Ye et al. also reported an increase in the Dh of polysaccharide/zein NPs after the encapsulation of doxorubicin [44]. The Dh of ZeinCPX_HA NPs is suitable for ocular drug delivery, given that NPs with Dhs between 50 and 200 nm can permeate through the ocular mucous [40]. Furthermore, the incorporation of HA is expected to improve the cellular uptake by ophthalmic cells, as described by Apaolaza et al. for HA-coated gold NPs [62]. In addition, HA is present in the eye constitution [63,64] and described as promising mucoadhesive polymer for ocular drug delivery systems development [65,66]. Thus, this mucoadhesiveness property results on an increase of drug ocular residence time [63,67].

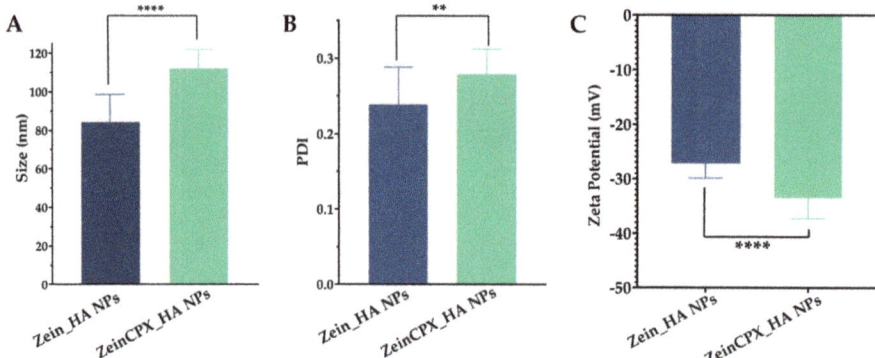

Figure 4. Evaluation of morphological properties of Zein_HA NPs and ZeinCPX_HA NPs: determination of the hydrodynamic diameter values (**A**), PDI (**B**), and zeta potential (**C**). Data are presented as mean ± standard deviation, $n = 5$, ** $< p = 0.01$, **** $p < 0.0001$.

Moreover, PDI is another crucial characteristic in assessing the successful production of NPs, indicating the formulations' homogeneity [68]. There was a slight increase in the PDI (from 0.21 ± 0.07 to 0.27 ± 0.03) after the loading with CPX; however, it remains below 0.3, which indicates that ZeinCPX_HA NPs are monodisperse.

The surface charge of the NPs also plays an important role in the stability and cell interaction. The ZeinCPX_HA NPs presented a zeta potential of −33 ± 4.2, which is considered suitable for achieving colloidal stability [69]. Since ocular mucosa has an anionic character, HA can bind to the negatively charged mucin in the corneal and conjunctival epithelium [27].

Next, the stability of lyophilized NPs with 5% mannitol was evaluated for 28 days, as shown in Figure 5.

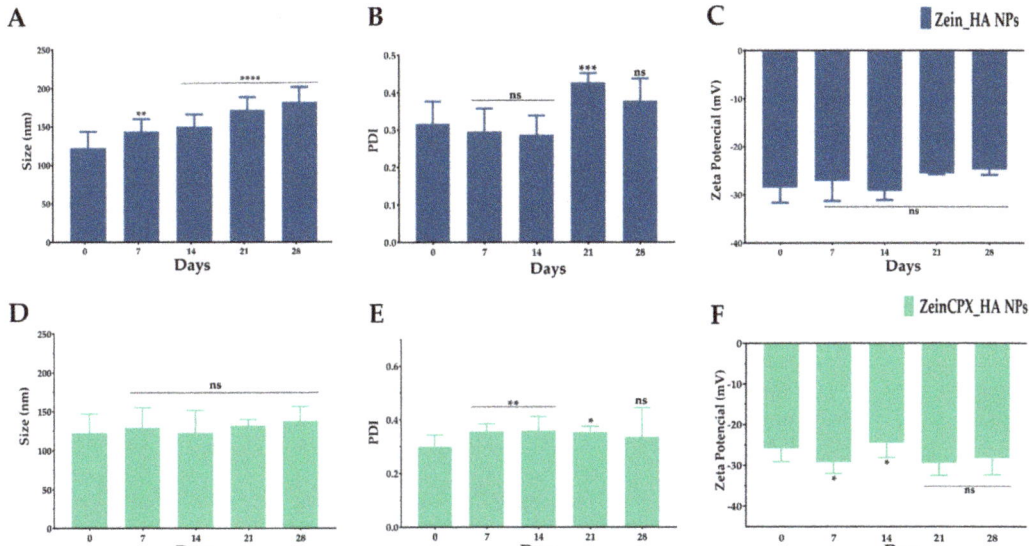

Figure 5. Stability of Zein_HA NPs (**A–C**) and ZeinCPX_HA NPs (**D–F**), after lyophilization, for 28 days. Data are presented as mean ± standard deviation, $n = 5$, ns $p > 0.05$, * $< p = 0.05$, ** $< p = 0.01$, *** $p < 0.001$, **** $< p = 0.0001$, values marked with asterisks are statistically different from Day 0 (immediate re-hydration of the NPs upon lyophilization).

During the 28 days, the Dh of ZeinCPX_HA NPs remained stable, and the PDI of both NPs did not suffer significant differences.

Furthermore, during the 28 days, there were no changes in the zeta potential of Zein_HA NPs and ZeinCPX_HA NPs, which means that the nano-formulations are chemically stable [51]. Besides, the obtained zeta potential values are close to −30 mV, so according to the literature, nano-formulations with zeta potential values more than +30 mV and less than −30 mV are considered stable [70].

Moreover, the RDI values were also calculated, corroborating the efficiency of the NPs reconstitution, given that the RDI value of the ZeinCPX_HA NPs was $92 \pm 13\%$.

3.4. Encapsulation Efficiency and Drug Loading

In the clinic, the concentration of ciprofloxacin on eye drops used for topical treatment of ocular infections is around 3000 mg/L. This treatment implies the administration of 1–2 drops every 15–30 min (initially) in acute infections and 1–2 drops application 6 times per day, or more, in severe conditions [71–73]. On the other hand, the incorporation of ciprofloxacin into polymeric drug delivery system will allow to decrease the drug concentration to be used, and will assure a controlled drug release and a prolonged therapeutic effect, as has been demonstrated by Günday et al. for ciprofloxacin-loaded poly(DL-lactide-co-glycolide) NPs with a CPX concentration of 20 µg/mL [74]. This CPX concentration was incorporated into ZeinCPX_HA NPs, with an EE of $69 \pm 5\%$ and a loading content of $3.7 \pm 1.4\%$, indicating that CPX was successfully encapsulated through the FNP technique. To the best of our knowledge, this is the first report on encapsulating CPX into zein nanosystems. Fu et al. (2009) obtained an EE between 4.97% and 8.29% and a drug loading ranging from 0.87 to 2.41%, when encapsulating CPX (2 to 5 mg/mL) into zein (8 to 20 mg/mL) microspheres [75]. Furthermore, the EE of ZeinCPX_HA NPs is in line with other studies with polymeric NPs, which reported an EE of CPX ranging between 51.8 and 82.7% [74,76,77]. For CPX-loaded PLGA and PEG NPs produced by nanoprecipitation, there was an EE of $25 \pm 9\%$ and a loading rate of $3.6 \pm 1.3\%$ [78]. Additionally, Xu et al., reported low EE of CPX in PLA-DEX NPs (1.1 ± 0.04% (CPX at 4 mg/mL) and a mass loading of 8.45 ± 0.31%) in PLGA-PEG NPs the EE was 1.35 ± 0.07% with a loading of 10.79 ± 0.59% [79]. Furthermore, the encapsulation of other lipophilic compounds into zein NPs is comprehended between 47.80 and 98% [18,24,80–83].

3.5. CPX Release Profile from ZeinCPX_HA NPs

After assessing the drug encapsulation and loading, the in vitro release of CPX from lyophilized ZeinCPX_HA NPs was studied in STF. As shown in Figure 6, the release profile of CPX displays an initial burst release in the first 1 h and 30 min of incubation, followed by a prolonged release for at least 24 h. This initial burst release can be due to the hydrophilic nature of HA, which rapidly dissolves in STF and releases the drug [84]. Then, the decrease of the released drug can be attributed to the CPX entrapment in the hydrophobic core (zein) of the ZeinCPX_HA NPs [22,85]. This is in accordance with previous reports on improved ability of nanosystems for ocular drug delivery; however, a formulation providing a sustained release for CPX is not available as commercial dosage form. This was already discussed in a comparative analysis of commercial topical dosage forms (e.g., 0.3% CPX-hydrochloride Ciloxan® drop, Alcon Laboratories Inc., Fort Worth, TX, USA) with drug release carriers, highlighting that: (i) the MIC of CPX incorporated into liposomal formulations was lower, and with an increased antibacterial effect; (ii) the ocular bioavailability of CPX was improved in comparison with Ciloxan® ophthalmic drops; and (iii) the drug residence time on corneal surface was improved by the surface properties of the nanosystem [10].

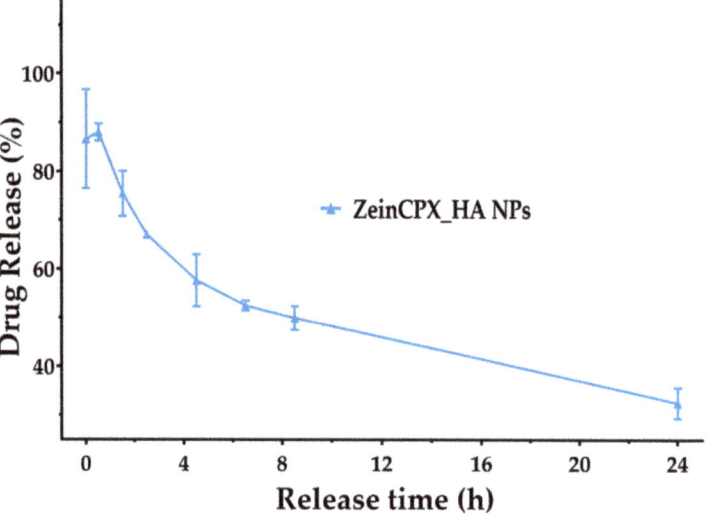

Figure 6. Release profile of ZeinCPX_HA NPs in STF at 37 °C, pH = 7.4 for 24 h (non-cumulative). Results are presented as mean ± SEM (n = 3).

Furthermore, applying mathematical models also assessed the kinetics of CPX release. The release of CPX by the NPs follows Korsmeyer–Peppas kinetic model (R^2 = 0.9505 and n < 0.43), since this model presents the correlation coefficient (R^2) closer to 1 (Table 3). The coefficient value was acquired by plotting the log of the percentage of drug release versus log time [84]. The Korsmeyer–Peppas results also indicated that the CPX release occurs due to a Fickian diffusion process ($n \leq 0.45$), resulting from the swelling of the polymeric matrix [19,86,87].

Table 3. Regression coefficients of mathematical models fitted to the release of CPX from ZeinCPX_HA NPs.

Mathematical Model	R^2	n
Zero order	0.7657	-
First order	0.5791	-
Higuchi	0.9269	-
Korsmeye–Peppas	0.9505	0.2635

3.6. Characterization of NPs' Biological Properties

The biocompatibility of both NPs (with and without CPX) was confirmed on NHDF cells (Figure 7). NHDF cells were used as a cell model, given that these cells are constituents of the subepithelial layer of the conjunctiva [88]. Additionally, these cells recruit neutrophils and monocytes at an early stage of infection regardless of the type of microorganism [89].

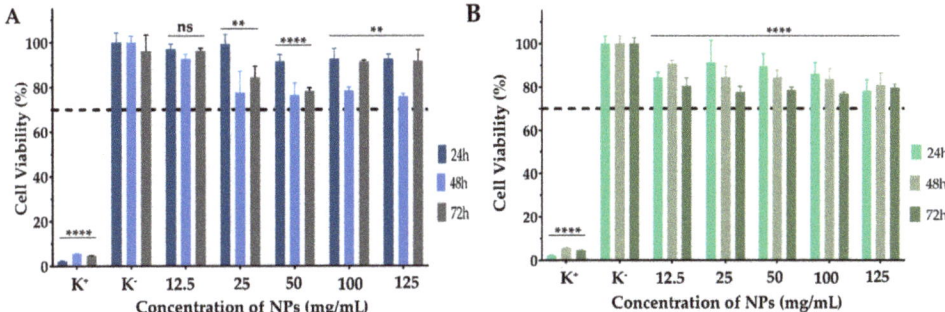

Figure 7. Characterization of the biocompatibility of (A) Zein_HA NPs cryoprotected with 5% mannitol and (B) ZeinCPX_HA cryoprotected with 5% mannitol NPs in contact with NHDF cells during 24 h, 48 h and 72 h. Data are presented as mean ± SEM, $n = 5$, ns—not statistically significant, ** $< p = 0.001$, **** $< p = 0.0001$, values marked with asterisks are statistically different from the mean of K^-.

Our results demonstrated that the NPs are biocompatible, which is expected considering the reported results in other studies for zein and HA NPs. Our results demonstrated that the NPs are biocompatible, which was expected considering the reported results in other studies for zein and HA NPs, as well as their approval by the FDA and wide application in the pharmaceutical field [20,21,44,46]. Furthermore, HA is widely employed in commercial dosage forms for ocular disorders treatment, such as Healon®, Amvisc®, Provisc® and AMO Vitrax® [26]. These results highlighted that the ZeinCPX_HA NPs could act as a drug delivery system. However, in further studies assuring the translation potential of this formulation, additional assays (preclinical and clinical evaluation) would be extremely important to assure a complete characterization of this new therapeutic system for clinics.

4. Conclusions

In this study, zein and hyaluronic acid were used for the first time to produce nanoparticles by the flash nanoprecipitation technique aimed to encapsulate ciprofloxacin to work as a topical drug delivery system to treat ocular mucosa disorders, such as bacterial conjunctivitis. The obtained results demonstrate that the nanoparticles cryoprotected with 5% mannitol were stable upon the freeze-drying process, as corroborated by the RDI, size, PDI, and zeta potential values.

Overall, our results support the application of ZeinCPX_HA NPs as a possible alternative to the current antibacterial topical dosage forms available on the market to treat conjunctivitis. In the future, the investigation of antibacterial and ex vivo assays can be achieved to evaluate further the potential of these nanosystems for translation to the clinical management of bacterial conjunctivitis.

Supplementary Materials: The following supporting information can be downloaded at: https://www.mdpi.com/article/10.3390/pharmaceutics14081557/s1, Figure S1: TGA analysis of ciprofloxacin; Figure S2: DSC thermograms of zein (A), hyaluronic acid (B), ciprofloxacin (C) and mannitol (D).

Author Contributions: T.A.J.: data curation, formal analysis, investigation, writing—original draft. B.O.: data curation, formal analysis, investigation, writing—original draft. S.P.M.: data curation, formal analysis, investigation, methodology, writing—review and editing. M.P.R.: resources, methodology, validation, funding acquisition. P.C.: conceptualization, data curation, formal analysis, funding acquisition, investigation, methodology, project administration, supervision, writing—review and editing. All authors have read and agreed to the published version of the manuscript.

Funding: This work was supported by the projects Programa Operacional Regional do Centro (CENTRO-04-3559-FSE-000162), within the European Social Fund (ESF), and 0633_BIOIMPACE_4_A co-financed by European Union/ERDF, ESF, European Regional Development Fund (ERDF) under the Interreg V-A Spain–Portugal (POCTEP) during the 2014–2020 program.

Institutional Review Board Statement: Not applicable.

Informed Consent Statement: Not applicable.

Data Availability Statement: No new data were created or analyzed in this study. Data sharing is not applicable to this article.

Acknowledgments: The authors gratefully acknowledge to Rosa Santos and Ana Gonçalves from Coficab, Portugal for the technical support on the TGA and DSC analysis.

Conflicts of Interest: The authors declare no conflict of interest.

References

1. Haq, A.; Wardak, H.; Kraski, N. Infective Conjunctivitis—Its Pathogenesis, Management and Complications. In *Common Eye Infections*; Chaudhry, I.A., Ed.; IntechOpen: London, UK, 2013. [CrossRef]
2. Azari, A.A.; Arabi, A. Conjunctivitis: A Systematic Review. *J. Ophthalmic Vis. Res.* **2020**, *15*, 372–395. [CrossRef] [PubMed]
3. Watson, S.; Cabrera-Aguas, M.; Khoo, P. Common eye infections. *Aust. Prescr.* **2018**, *41*, 67–72. [CrossRef] [PubMed]
4. Benitez-del-Castillo, J.; Verboven, Y.; Stroman, D.; Kodjikian, L. The Role of Topical Moxifloxacin, a New Antibacterial in Europe, in the Treatment of Bacterial Conjunctivitis. *Clin. Drug Investig.* **2011**, *31*, 543–557. [CrossRef] [PubMed]
5. Pippin, M.M.; Le, J.K. Bacterial Conjunctivitis. Available online: https://www.ncbi.nlm.nih.gov/books/NBK546683/ (accessed on 18 June 2022).
6. Alharbi, W.S.; Hosny, K.M. Development and optimization of ocular in situ gels loaded with ciprofloxacin cubic liquid crystalline nanoparticles. *J. Drug Deliv. Sci. Technol.* **2020**, *57*, 101710. [CrossRef]
7. Pham, T.D.M.; Ziora, Z.M.; Blaskovich, M.A.T. Quinolone antibiotics. *Medchemcomm* **2019**, *10*, 1719–1739. [CrossRef]
8. Zhanel, G.G.; Walkty, A.; Vercaigne, L.; Karlowsky, J.A.; Embil, J.; Gin, A.S.; Hoban, D.J. The new fluoroquinolones: A critical review. *Can. J. Infect. Dis.* **1999**, *10*, 207–238. [CrossRef]
9. Taha, E.I.; El-Anazi, M.H.; El-Bagory, I.M.; Bayomi, M.A. Design of liposomal colloidal systems for ocular delivery of ciprofloxacin. *Saudi Pharm. J.* **2014**, *22*, 231–239. [CrossRef]
10. Al-Joufi, F.A.; Salem-Bekhit, M.M.; Taha, E.I.; Ibrahim, M.A.; Muharram, M.M.; Alshehri, S.; Ghoneim, M.M.; Shakeel, F. Enhancing Ocular Bioavailability of Ciprofloxacin Using Colloidal Lipid-Based Carrier for the Management of Post-Surgical Infection. *Molecules* **2022**, *27*, 733. [CrossRef]
11. Liu, D.; Lian, Y.; Fang, Q.; Liu, L.; Zhang, J.; Li, J. Hyaluronic-acid-modified lipid-polymer hybrid nanoparticles as an efficient ocular delivery platform for moxifloxacin hydrochloride. *Int. J. Biol. Macromol.* **2018**, *116*, 1026–1036. [CrossRef]
12. Meza-Rios, A.; Navarro-Partida, J.; Armendariz-Borunda, J.; Santos, A. Therapies Based on Nanoparticles for Eye Drug Delivery. *Ophthalmol. Ther.* **2020**, *9*, 1–14. [CrossRef]
13. Omerović, N.; Vranić, E. Application of nanoparticles in ocular drug delivery systems. *Health Technol.* **2020**, *10*, 61–78. [CrossRef]
14. Vaneev, A.; Tikhomirova, V.; Chesnokova, N.; Popova, E.; Beznos, O.; Kost, O.; Klyachko, N. Nanotechnology for Topical Drug Delivery to the Anterior Segment of the Eye. *Int. J. Mol. Sci.* **2021**, *22*, 12368. [CrossRef]
15. Ban, J.; Zhang, Y.; Huang, X.; Deng, G.; Hou, D.; Chen, Y.; Lu, Z. Corneal permeation properties of a charged lipid nanoparticle carrier containing dexamethasone. *Int. J. Nanomed.* **2017**, *12*, 1329–1339. [CrossRef]
16. Massella, D.; Celasco, E.; Salaün, F.; Ferri, A.; Barresi, A.A. Overcoming the Limits of Flash Nanoprecipitation: Effective Loading of Hydrophilic Drug into Polymeric Nanoparticles with Controlled Structure. *Polymers* **2018**, *10*, 1092. [CrossRef]

17. Pustulka, K.M.; Wohl, A.R.; Lee, H.S.; Michel, A.R.; Han, J.; Hoye, T.R.; McCormick, A.V.; Panyam, J.; Macosko, C.W. Flash Nanoprecipitation: Particle Structure and Stability. *Mol. Pharm.* **2013**, *10*, 4367–4377. [CrossRef]
18. Loureiro, J.; Miguel, S.P.; Seabra, I.J.; Ribeiro, M.P.; Coutinho, P. Single-Step Self-Assembly of Zein–Honey–Chitosan Nanoparticles for Hydrophilic Drug Incorporation by Flash Nanoprecipitation. *Pharmaceutics* **2022**, *14*, 920. [CrossRef]
19. Miguel, S.P.; Loureiro, J.; Ribeiro, M.P.; Coutinho, P. Osmundea sp. macroalgal polysaccharide-based nanoparticles produced by flash nanocomplexation technique. *Int. J. Biol. Macromol.* **2022**, *204*, 9–18. [CrossRef]
20. Nunes, R.; Baião, A.; Monteiro, D.; das Neves, J.; Sarmento, B. Zein nanoparticles as low-cost, safe, and effective carriers to improve the oral bioavailability of resveratrol. *Drug Deliv. Transl. Res.* **2020**, *10*, 826–837. [CrossRef]
21. Corradini, E.; Curti, P.S.; Meniqueti, A.B.; Martins, A.F.; Rubira, A.F.; Muniz, E.C. Recent advances in food-packing, pharmaceutical and biomedical applications of zein and zein-based materials. *Int. J. Mol. Sci.* **2014**, *15*, 22438–22470. [CrossRef]
22. Yu, X.; Wu, H.; Hu, H.; Dong, Z.; Dang, Y.; Qi, Q.; Wang, Y.; Du, S.; Lu, Y. Zein nanoparticles as nontoxic delivery system for maytansine in the treatment of non-small cell lung cancer. *Drug Deliv.* **2020**, *27*, 100–109. [CrossRef]
23. Dong, F.; Padua, G.W.; Wang, Y. Controlled formation of hydrophobic surfaces by self-assembly of an amphiphilic natural protein from aqueous solutions. *Soft Matter* **2013**, *9*, 5933–5941. [CrossRef]
24. Rodrigues, D.A.; Miguel, S.P.; Loureiro, J.; Ribeiro, M.; Roque, F.; Coutinho, P. Oromucosal Alginate Films with Zein Nanoparticles as a Novel Delivery System for Digoxin. *Pharmaceutics* **2021**, *13*, 2030. [CrossRef]
25. Gagliardi, A.; Voci, S.; Salvatici, M.C.; Fresta, M.; Cosco, D. Brij-stabilized zein nanoparticles as potential drug carriers. *Colloids Surf. B Biointerfaces* **2021**, *201*, 111647. [CrossRef]
26. Dubashynskaya, N.; Poshina, D.; Raik, S.; Urtti, A.; Skorik, Y.A. Polysaccharides in Ocular Drug Delivery. *Pharmaceutics* **2020**, *12*, 22. [CrossRef]
27. Zhang, X.; Wei, D.; Xu, Y.; Zhu, Q. Hyaluronic acid in ocular drug delivery. *Carbohydr. Polym.* **2021**, *264*, 118006. [CrossRef] [PubMed]
28. Kim, D.J.; Jung, M.-Y.; Pak, H.-J.; Park, J.-H.; Kim, M.; Chuck, R.S.; Park, C.Y. Development of a novel hyaluronic acid membrane for the treatment of ocular surface diseases. *Sci. Rep.* **2021**, *11*, 2351. [CrossRef] [PubMed]
29. Aragona, P.; Papa, V.; Micali, A.; Santocono, M.; Milazzo, G. Long term treatment with sodium hyaluronate-containing artificial tears reduces ocular surface damage in patients with dry eye. *Br. J. Ophthalmol.* **2002**, *86*, 181–184. [CrossRef] [PubMed]
30. Entwistle, J.; Hall, C.L.; Turley, E.A. HA receptors: Regulators of signalling to the cytoskeleton. *J. Cell. Biochem.* **1996**, *61*, 569–577. [CrossRef]
31. Kalam, M.A. The potential application of hyaluronic acid coated chitosan nanoparticles in ocular delivery of dexamethasone. *Int. J. Biol. Macromol.* **2016**, *89*, 559–568. [CrossRef]
32. Butreddy, A.; Dudhipala, N.; Janga, K.Y.; Gaddam, R.P. Lyophilization of Small-Molecule Injectables: An Industry Perspective on Formulation Development, Process Optimization, Scale-Up Challenges, and Drug Product Quality Attributes. *AAPS PharmSciTech* **2020**, *21*, 252. [CrossRef]
33. Rayaprolu, B.M.; Strawser, J.J.; Anyarambhatla, G. Excipients in parenteral formulations: Selection considerations and effective utilization with small molecules and biologics. *Drug Dev. Ind. Pharm.* **2018**, *44*, 1565–1571. [CrossRef]
34. Han, J.; Zhu, Z.; Qian, H.; Wohl, A.R.; Beaman, C.J.; Hoye, T.R.; Macosko, C.W. A simple confined impingement jets mixer for flash nanoprecipitation. *J. Pharm. Sci.* **2012**, *101*, 4018–4023. [CrossRef]
35. Hong, D.Y.; Lee, J.-S.; Lee, H.G. Chitosan/poly-γ-glutamic acid nanoparticles improve the solubility of lutein. *Int. J. Biol. Macromol.* **2016**, *85*, 9–15. [CrossRef]
36. Voci, S.; Gagliardi, A.; Salvatici, M.C.; Fresta, M.; Cosco, D. Influence of the Dispersion Medium and Cryoprotectants on the Physico-Chemical Features of Gliadin- and Zein-Based Nanoparticles. *Pharmaceutics* **2022**, *14*, 332. [CrossRef]
37. Ministério da Saúde, I. *Farmacopeia Portuguesa 9*; Instituto Nacional da Farmacia e do Medicamento: Ponta Delgada, Portugal, 2008.
38. Liu, Y.; Liu, J.; Zhang, X.; Zhang, R.; Huang, Y.; Wu, C. In Situ Gelling Gelrite/Alginate Formulations as Vehicles for Ophthalmic Drug Delivery. *AAPS PharmSciTech* **2010**, *11*, 610–620. [CrossRef]
39. Paulsson, M.; Hägerström, H.; Edsman, K. Rheological studies of the gelation of deacetylated gellan gum (Gelrite®) in physiological conditions. *Eur. J. Pharm. Sci.* **1999**, *9*, 99–105. [CrossRef]
40. Dave, R.S.; Goostrey, T.C.; Ziolkowska, M.; Czerny-Holownia, S.; Hoare, T.; Sheardown, H. Ocular drug delivery to the anterior segment using nanocarriers: A mucoadhesive/mucopenetrative perspective. *J. Control Release* **2021**, *336*, 71–88. [CrossRef]
41. Wang, L.; Ma, Y.; Gu, Y.; Liu, Y.; Zhao, J.; Yan, B.; Wang, Y. Cryoprotectant choice and analyses of freeze-drying drug suspension of nanoparticles with functional stabilisers. *J. Microencapsul.* **2018**, *35*, 241–248. [CrossRef]
42. Feng, J.; Zhang, Y.; McManus, S.A.; Qian, R.; Ristroph, K.D.; Ramachandruni, H.; Gong, K.; White, C.E.; Rawal, A.; Prud'homme, R.K. Amorphous nanoparticles by self-assembly: Processing for controlled release of hydrophobic molecules. *Soft Matter* **2019**, *15*, 2400–2410. [CrossRef]
43. Figueira, D.R.; Miguel, S.P.; de Sá, K.D.; Correia, I.J. Production and characterization of polycaprolactone-hyaluronic acid/chitosan-zein electrospun bilayer nanofibrous membrane for tissue regeneration. *Int. J. Biol. Macromol.* **2016**, *93*, 1100–1110. [CrossRef]
44. Ye, W.; Zhang, G.; Liu, X.; Ren, Q.; Huang, F.; Yan, Y. Fabrication of polysaccharide-stabilized zein nanoparticles by flash nanoprecipitation for doxorubicin sustained release. *J. Drug Deliv. Sci. Technol.* **2022**, *70*, 103183. [CrossRef]

45. Yuan, Y.; Li, H.; Liu, C.; Zhu, J.; Xu, Y.; Zhang, S.; Fan, M.; Zhang, D.; Zhang, Y.; Zhang, Z.; et al. Fabrication of stable zein nanoparticles by chondroitin sulfate deposition based on antisolvent precipitation method. *Int. J. Biol. Macromol.* **2019**, *139*, 30–39. [CrossRef] [PubMed]
46. Jacinto, T.A.; Rodrigues, C.F.; Moreira, A.F.; Miguel, S.P.; Costa, E.C.; Ferreira, P.; Correia, I.J. Hyaluronic acid and vitamin E polyethylene glycol succinate functionalized gold-core silica shell nanorods for cancer targeted photothermal therapy. *Colloids Surf. B Biointerfaces* **2020**, *188*, 110778. [CrossRef]
47. Sakulwech, S.; Lourith, N.; Ruktanonchai, U.; Kanlayaavattanakul, M. Preparation and characterization of nanoparticles from quaternized cyclodextrin-grafted chitosan associated with hyaluronic acid for cosmetics. *Asian J. Pharm. Sci.* **2018**, *13*, 498–504. [CrossRef]
48. Demirci, S.; Celebioglu, A.; Aytac, Z.; Uyar, T. pH-responsive nanofibers with controlled drug release properties. *Polym. Chem.* **2014**, *5*, 2050–2056. [CrossRef]
49. Devanand Venkatasubbu, G.; Ramasamy, S.; Ramakrishnan, V.; Kumar, J. Nanocrystalline hydroxyapatite and zinc-doped hydroxyapatite as carrier material for controlled delivery of ciprofloxacin. *3 Biotech* **2011**, *1*, 173–186. [CrossRef]
50. Wang, Q.; Dong, Z.; Du, Y.; Kennedy, J.F. Controlled release of ciprofloxacin hydrochloride from chitosan/polyethylene glycol blend films. *Carbohydr. Polym.* **2007**, *69*, 336–343. [CrossRef]
51. Ibrahim, A.H.; Rosqvist, E.; Smått, J.-H.; Ibrahim, H.M.; Ismael, H.R.; Afouna, M.I.; Samy, A.M.; Rosenholm, J.M. Formulation and optimization of lyophilized nanosuspension tablets to improve the physicochemical properties and provide immediate release of silymarin. *Int. J. Pharm.* **2019**, *563*, 217–227. [CrossRef]
52. Cacicedo, M.L.; Pacheco, G.; Islan, G.A.; Alvarez, V.A.; Barud, H.S.; Castro, G.R. Chitosan-bacterial cellulose patch of ciprofloxacin for wound dressing: Preparation and characterization studies. *Int. J. Biol. Macromol.* **2020**, *147*, 1136–1145. [CrossRef]
53. Ahire, J.J.; Robertson, D.; Neveling, D.P.; van Reenen, A.J.; Dicks, L.M.T. Hyaluronic acid-coated poly(d,l-lactide) (PDLLA) nanofibers prepared by electrospinning and coating. *RSC Adv.* **2016**, *6*, 34791–34796. [CrossRef]
54. Dhayanandamoorthy, Y.; Antoniraj, M.G.; Kandregula, C.A.B.; Kandasamy, R. Aerosolized hyaluronic acid decorated, ferulic acid loaded chitosan nanoparticle: A promising asthma control strategy. *Int. J. Pharm.* **2020**, *591*, 119958. [CrossRef]
55. Acevedo, F.; Hermosilla, J.; Sanhueza, C.; Mora-Lagos, B.; Fuentes, I.; Rubilar, M.; Concheiro, A.; Alvarez-Lorenzo, C. Gallic acid loaded PEO-core/zein-shell nanofibers for chemopreventive action on gallbladder cancer cells. *Eur. J. Pharm. Sci.* **2018**, *119*, 49–61. [CrossRef]
56. Abate, M.; Scotti, L.; Nele, V.; Caraglia, M.; Biondi, M.; De Rosa, G.; Leonetti, C.; Campani, V.; Zappavigna, S.; Porru, M. Hybrid Self-Assembling Nanoparticles Encapsulating Zoledronic Acid: A Strategy for Fostering Their Clinical Use. *Int. J. Mol. Sci.* **2022**, *23*, 5138.
57. Liu, J.; Grohganz, H.; Löbmann, K.; Rades, T.; Hempel, N.-J. Co-Amorphous Drug Formulations in Numbers: Recent Advances in Co-Amorphous Drug Formulations with Focus on Co-Formability, Molar Ratio, Preparation Methods, Physical Stability, In Vitro and In Vivo Performance, and New Formulation Strategies. *Pharmaceutics* **2021**, *13*, 389.
58. Stewart, A.M.; Grass, M.E. Practical Approach to Modeling the Impact of Amorphous Drug Nanoparticles on the Oral Absorption of Poorly Soluble Drugs. *Mol. Pharm.* **2020**, *17*, 180–189. [CrossRef]
59. Gorantla, S.; Rapalli, V.K.; Waghule, T.; Singh, P.P.; Dubey, S.K.; Saha, R.N.; Singhvi, G. Nanocarriers for ocular drug delivery: Current status and translational opportunity. *RSC Adv.* **2020**, *10*, 27835–27855. [CrossRef]
60. Mohamed, H.B.; Attia Shafie, M.A.; Mekkawy, A.I. Chitosan Nanoparticles for Meloxicam Ocular Delivery: Development, In Vitro Characterization, and In Vivo Evaluation in a Rabbit Eye Model. *Pharmaceutics* **2022**, *14*, 893. [CrossRef]
61. Saraiva, S.M.; Castro-López, V.; Pañeda, C.; Alonso, M.J. Synthetic nanocarriers for the delivery of polynucleotides to the eye. *Eur. J. Pharm. Sci.* **2017**, *103*, 5–18. [CrossRef]
62. Apaolaza, P.S.; Busch, M.; Asin-Prieto, E.; Peynshaert, K.; Rathod, R.; Remaut, K.; Dünker, N.; Göpferich, A. Hyaluronic acid coating of gold nanoparticles for intraocular drug delivery: Evaluation of the surface properties and effect on their distribution. *Exp. Eye Res.* **2020**, *198*, 108151. [CrossRef]
63. Jin, Y.; Ubonvan, T.; Kim, D.-D. Hyaluronic Acid in Drug Delivery Systems. *J. Pharm. Investig.* **2010**, *40*, 33–43.
64. Widjaja, L.K.; Bora, M.; Chan, P.N.P.H.; Lipik, V.; Wong, T.T.L.; Venkatraman, S.S. Hyaluronic acid-based nanocomposite hydrogels for ocular drug delivery applications. *J. Biomed. Mater. Res. Part A* **2014**, *102*, 3056–3065. [CrossRef]
65. Bongiovì, F.; Di Prima, G.; Palumbo, F.S.; Licciardi, M.; Pitarresi, G.; Giammona, G. Hyaluronic Acid-Based Micelles as Ocular Platform to Modulate the Loading, Release, and Corneal Permeation of Corticosteroids. *Macromol. Biosci.* **2017**, *17*, 1700261. [CrossRef]
66. Ricci, F.; Racaniello, G.F.; Lopedota, A.; Laquintana, V.; Arduino, I.; Lopalco, A.; Cutrignelli, A.; Franco, M.; Sigurdsson, H.H.; Denora, N. Chitosan/sulfobutylether-β-cyclodextrin based nanoparticles coated with thiolated hyaluronic acid for indomethacin ophthalmic delivery. *Int. J. Pharm.* **2022**, *622*, 121905. [CrossRef]
67. Zeng, W.; Li, Q.; Wan, T.; Liu, C.; Pan, W.; Wu, Z.; Zhang, G.; Pan, J.; Qin, M.; Lin, Y.; et al. Hyaluronic acid-coated niosomes facilitate tacrolimus ocular delivery: Mucoadhesion, precorneal retention, aqueous humor pharmacokinetics, and transcorneal permeability. *Colloids Surf. B Biointerfaces* **2016**, *141*, 28–35. [CrossRef]
68. Abdellatif, A.A.H.; El-Telbany, D.F.A.; Zayed, G.; Al-Sawahli, M.M. Hydrogel Containing PEG-Coated Fluconazole Nanoparticles with Enhanced Solubility and Antifungal Activity. *J. Pharm. Innov.* **2019**, *14*, 112–122. [CrossRef]

69. Joseph, E.; Singhvi, G. Chapter 4—Multifunctional nanocrystals for cancer therapy: A potential nanocarrier. In *Nanomaterials for Drug Delivery and Therapy*; Grumezescu, A.M., Ed.; William Andrew Publishing: Norwich, NY, USA, 2019; pp. 91–116.
70. Khorrami, S.; Zarrabi, A.; Khaleghi, M.; Danaei, M.; Mozafari, M.R. Selective cytotoxicity of green synthesized silver nanoparticles against the MCF-7 tumor cell line and their enhanced antioxidant and antimicrobial properties. *Int. J. Nanomed.* **2018**, *13*, 8013–8024. [CrossRef]
71. Campoli-Richards, D.M.; Monk, J.P.; Price, A.; Benfield, P.; Todd, P.A.; Ward, A. Ciprofloxacin. A review of its antibacterial activity, pharmacokinetic properties and therapeutic use. *Drugs* **1988**, *35*, 373–447. [CrossRef] [PubMed]
72. Leigue, L.; Montiani-Ferreira, F.; Moore, B.A. Antimicrobial susceptibility and minimal inhibitory concentration of Pseudomonas aeruginosa isolated from septic ocular surface disease in different animal species. *Open Vet. J.* **2016**, *6*, 215–222. [CrossRef] [PubMed]
73. Mundada, A.S.; Shrikhande, B.K. Formulation and evaluation of ciprofloxacin hydrochloride soluble ocular drug insert. *Curr. Eye Res.* **2008**, *33*, 469–475. [CrossRef]
74. Günday, C.; Anand, S.; Gencer, H.B.; Munafò, S.; Moroni, L.; Fusco, A.; Donnarumma, G.; Ricci, C.; Hatir, P.C.; Türeli, N.G.; et al. Ciprofloxacin-loaded polymeric nanoparticles incorporated electrospun fibers for drug delivery in tissue engineering applications. *Drug Deliv. Transl. Res.* **2020**, *10*, 706–720. [CrossRef] [PubMed]
75. Fu, J.-X.; Wang, H.-J.; Zhou, Y.-Q.; Wang, J.-Y. Antibacterial activity of ciprofloxacin-loaded zein microsphere films. *Mater. Sci. Eng. C* **2009**, *29*, 1161–1166. [CrossRef]
76. Arafa, M.G.; Mousa, H.A.; Afifi, N.N. Preparation of PLGA-chitosan based nanocarriers for enhancing antibacterial effect of ciprofloxacin in root canal infection. *Drug Deliv.* **2020**, *27*, 26–39. [CrossRef]
77. Patel, K.K.; Tripathi, M.; Pandey, N.; Agrawal, A.K.; Gade, S.; Anjum, M.M.; Tilak, R.; Singh, S. Alginate lyase immobilized chitosan nanoparticles of ciprofloxacin for the improved antimicrobial activity against the biofilm associated mucoid P. aeruginosa infection in cystic fibrosis. *Int. J. Pharm.* **2019**, *563*, 30–42. [CrossRef]
78. Gheffar, C.; Le, H.; Jouenne, T.; Schaumann, A.; Corbière, A.; Vaudry, D.; LeCerf, D.; Karakasyan, C. Antibacterial Activity of Ciprofloxacin-Loaded Poly(lactic-co-glycolic acid)-Nanoparticles Against Staphylococcus aureus. *Part. Part. Syst. Charact.* **2021**, *38*, 2000253. [CrossRef]
79. Xu, J.; Chen, Y.; Jiang, X.; Gui, Z.; Zhang, L. Development of Hydrophilic Drug Encapsulation and Controlled Release Using a Modified Nanoprecipitation Method. *Processes* **2019**, *7*, 331. [CrossRef]
80. Brotons-Canto, A.; González-Navarro, C.J.; Gil, A.G.; Asin-Prieto, E.; Saiz, M.J.; Llabrés, J.M. Zein Nanoparticles Improve the Oral Bioavailability of Curcumin in Wistar Rats. *Pharmaceutics* **2021**, *13*, 361. [CrossRef]
81. Ghalei, S.; Asadi, H.; Ghalei, B. Zein nanoparticle-embedded electrospun PVA nanofibers as wound dressing for topical delivery of anti-inflammatory diclofenac. *J. Appl. Polym. Sci.* **2018**, *135*, 46643. [CrossRef]
82. Lin, M.; Fang, S.; Zhao, X.; Liang, X.; Wu, D. Natamycin-loaded zein nanoparticles stabilized by carboxymethyl chitosan: Evaluation of colloidal/chemical performance and application in postharvest treatments. *Food Hydrocoll.* **2020**, *106*, 105871. [CrossRef]
83. Reboredo, C.; González-Navarro, C.J.; Martínez-López, A.L.; Martínez-Ohárriz, C.; Sarmento, B.; Irache, J.M. Zein-Based Nanoparticles as Oral Carriers for Insulin Delivery. *Pharmaceutics* **2022**, *14*, 39. [CrossRef]
84. Saraswathy, K.; Agarwal, G.; Srivastava, A. Hyaluronic acid microneedles-laden collagen cryogel plugs for ocular drug delivery. *J. Appl. Polym. Sci.* **2020**, *137*, 49285. [CrossRef]
85. Sabra, S.A.; Elzoghby, A.O.; Sheweita, S.A.; Haroun, M.; Helmy, M.W.; Eldemellawy, M.A.; Xia, Y.; Goodale, D.; Allan, A.L.; Rohani, S. Self-assembled amphiphilic zein-lactoferrin micelles for tumor targeted co-delivery of rapamycin and wogonin to breast cancer. *Eur. J. Pharm. Biopharm.* **2018**, *128*, 156–169. [CrossRef] [PubMed]
86. Kim, A.R.; Lee, S.L.; Park, S.N. Properties and in vitro drug release of pH- and temperature-sensitive double cross-linked interpenetrating polymer network hydrogels based on hyaluronic acid/poly (N-isopropylacrylamide) for transdermal delivery of luteolin. *Int. J. Biol. Macromol.* **2018**, *118*, 731–740. [CrossRef] [PubMed]
87. Miguel, S.P.; Simões, D.; Moreira, A.F.; Sequeira, R.S.; Correia, I.J. Production and characterization of electrospun silk fibroin based asymmetric membranes for wound dressing applications. *Int. J. Biol. Macromol.* **2019**, *121*, 524–535. [CrossRef] [PubMed]
88. Labib, B.A.; Chigbu, D.I. Therapeutic Targets in Allergic Conjunctivitis. *Pharmaceuticals* **2022**, *15*, 547. [CrossRef]
89. Fukuda, K. Corneal fibroblasts: Function and markers. *Exp. Eye Res.* **2020**, *200*, 108229. [CrossRef]

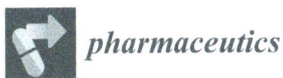

Article

Physicochemical and Stability Evaluation of Topical Niosomal Encapsulating Fosinopril/γ-Cyclodextrin Complex for Ocular Delivery

Hay Marn Hnin [1], Einar Stefánsson [2], Thorsteinn Loftsson [3], Rathapon Asasutjarit [4], Dusadee Charnvanich [1] and Phatsawee Jansook [1,*]

1. Faculty of Pharmaceutical Sciences, Chulalongkorn University, 254 Phyathai Road, Pathumwan, Bangkok 10330, Thailand; haymarn793@gmail.com (H.M.H.); dusadee.v@chula.ac.th (D.C.)
2. Department of Ophthalmology, Faculty of Medicine, National University Hospital, University of Iceland, Landspitalinn, IS-101 Reykjavik, Iceland; einarste@landspitali.is
3. Faculty of Pharmaceutical Sciences, University of Iceland, Hofsvallagata 53, IS-107 Reykjavik, Iceland; thorstlo@hi.is
4. Faculty of Pharmacy, Thammasat University, 99 Moo 18 Paholyothin Road, Klong Luang, Rangsit 12120, Thailand; rathapon@tu.ac.th
* Correspondence: phatsawee.j@chula.ac.th; Tel.: +66-2-218-8273

Abstract: This study aimed to develop a chemically stable niosomal eye drop containing fosinopril (FOS) for lowering intraocular pressure. The effects of cyclodextrin (CD), surfactant types and membrane stabilizer/charged inducers on physiochemical and chemical properties of niosome were evaluated. The pH value, average particle size, size distribution and zeta potentials were within the acceptable range. All niosomal formulations were shown to be slightly hypertonic with low viscosity. Span® 60/dicetyl phosphate niosomes in the presence and absence of γCD were selected as the optimum formulations according to their high %entrapment efficiency and negative zeta potential values as well as controlled release profile. According to ex vivo permeation study, the obtained lowest flux and apparent permeability coefficient values confirmed that FOS/γCD complex was encapsulated within the inner aqueous core of niosome and could be able to protect FOS from its hydrolytic degradation. The in vitro cytotoxicity revealed that niosome entrapped FOS or FOS/γCD formulations were moderate irritation to the eyes. Furthermore, FOS-loaded niosomal preparations exhibited good physical and chemical stabilities especially of those in the presence of γCD, for at least three months under the storage condition of 2–8 °C.

Keywords: cyclodextrin; ophthalmic; fosinopril sodium; niosomes; encapsulation; stabilization

Citation: Hnin, H.M.; Stefánsson, E.; Loftsson, T.; Asasutjarit, R.; Charnvanich, D.; Jansook, P. Physicochemical and Stability Evaluation of Topical Niosomal Encapsulating Fosinopril/γ-Cyclodextrin Complex for Ocular Delivery. *Pharmaceutics* **2022**, *14*, 1147. https://doi.org/10.3390/pharmaceutics14061147

Academic Editors: Ana Catarina Silva and Hugo Almeida

Received: 27 April 2022
Accepted: 26 May 2022
Published: 27 May 2022

Publisher's Note: MDPI stays neutral with regard to jurisdictional claims in published maps and institutional affiliations.

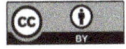

Copyright: © 2022 by the authors. Licensee MDPI, Basel, Switzerland. This article is an open access article distributed under the terms and conditions of the Creative Commons Attribution (CC BY) license (https://creativecommons.org/licenses/by/4.0/).

1. Introduction

Glaucoma is a multifactorial long term ocular neuropathy, which is associated with a progressive loss of visual field, structural abnormalities of retinal nerve fiber and cupping of the optic nerve head [1,2]. Recently, it has become the second leading cause of blindness worldwide after cataracts [3]. It was estimated that the primary open angle glaucoma cases in adult population will be risen up to 79.76 million in 2040 [4]. Many predictors for glaucoma have been identified, including age, positive family history, race, myopia and exfoliation syndrome [5]. Currently, intraocular pressure (IOP) is a major known risk factor for glaucoma. To lower IOP, treatment options involve oral and topical medications, laser therapy and surgical operation. Effective drug therapies include the drugs that reduce the rate of aqueous humor production and/or enhance its drainage. Several classes of drugs are available in managing long-term treatment of glaucoma, such as prostaglandin analogues, carbonic anhydrase inhibitors, α-adrenergic agonists, β-adrenergic blockers, and cholinergic agonists [1,2].

Angiotensin-converting enzyme (ACE) inhibitors have recently received attention as a new class of drug possessing the ability to lower IOP to treat glaucoma [6–8]. ACE is responsible for the conversion of the biologically inactive angiotensin I to the potent vasopressor, angiotensin II as well as the breakdown of bradykinin. Inhibition of ACE leads to the accumulation of bradykinin and promote the synthesis of prostaglandins, which could in turn lower IOP by increasing the uveoscleral outflow [9]. They also have a beneficial effect on retarding the progression of diabetic retinopathy in type II diabetic patients [10,11]. Moreover, ACE inhibitors showed beneficial effect in age-related macular degeneration [12]. Of these, fosinopril (FOS), the ester prodrug of fosinoprilat, and the first orally active phosphorus-containing ACE inhibitor, is an interesting compound to be used for lowering IOP. However, hydrolysis degradation of FOS was found in all conditions, i.e., acidic, basic and neutral, whereas the greater extent in basic condition [13]. Our previous study reported that the application of γ-cyclodextrin (γCD) as an inclusion complex could be able to enhance the solubility and chemical stability of FOS in aqueous solution [14].

Recently, colloidal drug delivery has been introduced as an alternative formulation approach for problematic drug candidates. Numerous colloidal carriers such as liposomes, niosomes, nanoparticles, microemulsions and micelles have been developed, which are applicable not only to solving the problems of poor solubility and stability but also to providing specific drug targeting, optimizing drug release properties and reducing toxicity [15]. As a vesicular carrier, niosome has gained attention because of its advantages including: (i) enhanced solubility and permeability; (ii) improved chemical stability; (iii) simple and cost-effective fabrication and (iv) low toxicity and high compatibility because of their nonionic nature [16].

Niosomes are nonionic surfactant vesicles, rising from the self-assembly of nonionic amphiphiles in aqueous media. The spherical shaped niosomes are capable of entrapping lipophilic molecules within the lipid bilayer by interacting with alkyl chains of nonionic surfactants, whereas hydrophilic drug molecules are located within an aqueous core by interacting with polar head groups of nonionic surfactants [17,18]. Numerous studies have reported the successful use of niosomes as ocular drug delivery carriers [19–23]. Vesicular delivery systems used in ophthalmic applications offer targeting at the site of action, improving chemical stability of encapsulated drugs and providing controlled release action at the corneal surface [24,25]. Vyas et al. (1998) reported that the ocular bioavailability of niosome entrapped water-soluble drugs, i.e., timolol maleate, increased as compared with timolol maleate solution [19]. This can be explained in that surfactants behave as penetration enhancers by removing the mucus layer and breaking junctional complexes [26].

In this study, niosomal eye drop preparations containing FOS alone or FOS/γCD inclusion complex were developed. The combined strategies, i.e., CD inclusion complex incorporated into a niosomal vesicle was applied to increase the chemical stability and to provide controlled drug release action. The physicochemical and chemical properties of niosomal formulations were evaluated. In addition, in vitro release, ex vivo permeation, in vitro cytotoxicity, and physical and chemical stability studies were also determined.

2. Materials and Methods

2.1. Materials

Fosinopril sodium (FOS) was purchased from Dideu Industries Group, Ltd. (Shaanxi, China). γ-Cyclodextrin (γCD) was purchased from Cyclolab (Budapest, Hungary). Polyoxyethylene 10 stearyl ether (Brij® 76) was distributed by The East Asiatic Public Company Ltd., (Bangkok, Thailand). Sorbitan monostearate (Span® 60) and poly-24-oxyethylene cholesteryl ether (Solulan® C-24, SC24) were kindly donated by Chemico Inter Corporation Ltd. (Bangkok, Thailand). Cholesterol, dicetyl phosphate (DCP) and stearylamine (STA) were received from Sigma-Aldrich (St. Louis, MO, USA), ethylenediamine tetra-acetic acid disodium salt (EDTA) and sodium metabisulfite (Na-MS) from Ajax Finechem Pty Ltd. (Taren Point, Australia). Semi-permeable cellophane membranes (SpectaPor®, molecular weight cut-off (MWCO) 12–14,000 Da) were obtained from Spectrum Europe (Breda, The Netherlands). All other chemicals used were of analytical reagent grade purity. Milli-Q (Millipore, Billerica, MA, USA) water was used to prepare all solutions.

2.2. Preparation of Niosomal Formulations Containing FOS

Niosome was prepared using thin-film hydration method. The niosome formulations were composed of nonionic surfactant, cholesterol, and membrane stabilizer/charged inducer at the mole ratio of 47.5: 47.5: 5. This ratio was optimized and shown to possess relatively good physicochemical characteristics obtained from blank niosome preparations. The total lipid composition was prepared at 100 µM in 5 mL of hydration medium (10 mM phosphate-buffered saline (pH 7.4) containing 1% (w/v) FOS, 0.1% (w/v) EDTA and 0.1% (w/v) Na-MS). The surfactants used in this study included Span® 60 and Brij® 76. Nonionic SC24 was used as a steric stabilizer, while positively charged STA and negatively charged DCP were used to provide the electrostatic stabilization of vesicles. Briefly, accurately weighed amounts of nonionic surfactant, cholesterol and membrane stabilizer/charge inducer were dissolved in 10 mL of chloroform in a 1 L round-bottom flask. The lipid mixture was slowly evaporated under reduced pressure at 40 °C using a rotary evaporator (Rotavapor R-200, BÜCHI Labortechnik AG, Flawil, Switzerland) with a constant rotation speed. The flask was partially immersed in a water bath and evaporated until a dried thin film appeared on the inner wall of the flask. Then, the formulation was kept in a desiccator under vacuum for 2 h to ensure the total removal of trace solvents. After that, dried lipid film was hydrated with 5 mL of hydration medium with and without 5% (w/v) γCD. Our previous work reported that EDTA and Na-MS are powerful antioxidants to protect FOS degradation [14]. The hydration of dried film was carried out by rotating the flask in a water bath at 60 °C for 30 min using a rotavapor under normal pressure. The size reduction was made by sonicating in an ultrasonic bath (GT sonic, GT SONIC Technology Park, Guangdong, China) at 60 °C for 30 min. To complete annealing and partition of the drug between the lipid bilayer and the aqueous phase, the formulation was left overnight at room temperature and then stored at 4 °C until subjected to analysis. The compositions of niosome formulae are shown in Table 1.

Table 1. Compositions of FOS-loaded niosomal formulations.

Formulation [a]	Span® 60-Niosome						Brij® 76-Niosome					
	Sp-SC24	Sp-DCP	Sp-STA	Sp-SC24+γCD	Sp-DCP+γCD	Sp-STA+γCD	Br-SC24	Br-DCP	Br-STA	Br-SC24+γCD	Br-DCP+γCD	Br-STA+γCD
	Ingredients in organic phase (µM) [b]											
Span® 60	47.5	47.5	47.5	47.5	47.5	47.5	-	-	-	-	-	-
Brij® 76	-	-	-	-	-	-	47.5	47.5	47.5	47.5	47.5	47.5
Cholesterol	47.5	47.5	47.5	47.5	47.5	47.5	47.5	47.5	47.5	47.5	47.5	47.5
SC24	5	-	-	5	-	-	5	-	-	5	-	-
DCP	-	5	-	-	5	-	-	5	-	-	5	-
STA	-	-	5	-	-	5	-	-	5	-	-	5
	Ingredients in aqueous phase (% w/v) [c]											
FOS	1	1	1	1	1	1	1	1	1	1	1	1
γCD	-	-	-	5	5	5	-	-	-	5	5	5

[a] SC24, Solulan®C24; DCP, dicetylphosphate; STA, stearylamine; FOS, fosinopril sodium, [b] solubilized in 10 mL of chloroform, [c] solubilized in 5 mL of phosphate-buffered saline pH 7.4 containing 0.1% (w/v) EDTA and 0.1% (w/v) sodium metabisulfite.

2.3. Physicochemical and Chemical Characterizations

2.3.1. Osmolality, pH and Viscosity Determination

The pH values of all formulations were measured using a pH meter (SevenCompact S220-Micro, Mettler Toledo, Gießen, Germany) at 25 °C. The viscosity was determined by viscometer (Sine-wave Vibro SV-10, A&D Company, Limited, Tokyo, Japan) using the tuning-fork vibration method with frequency of 30 Hz at 25 °C and 34 °C. The osmolality was determined by osmometer (OSMOMAT 3000 basic, Gonotec GmbH, Berlin, Germany) at room temperature using the freezing point depression principle. All measurements were determined in triplicate.

2.3.2. Particle Size, Size Distribution, and Zeta Potential

The particle size, size distribution and zeta potential of FOS-loaded niosome formulations were measured using the dynamic light scattering (DLS) technique (Zetasizer ™ Nano ZS with software, Version 7.11, Malvern, UK). The measurements were carried out at a scattering angle of 180° and a temperature of 25 °C, a medium viscosity of 0.8872 mPa.s and a medium refractive index of 1.330. The concentration of niosome preparation was 20 µM. The particle size distribution was expressed as polydispersity (PDI). The particle size, size distribution and zeta potential were automatically calculated and analyzed using the software included within the system. Each measurement was performed in triplicate.

2.3.3. Determining Drug Content and Entrapment Efficiency (EE)

The FOS was quantitatively determined using a reversed-phase HPLC component system from Agilent 1260 Infinity II consisting of a liquid chromatography pump (quaternary pump, G7111A), diode array UV-Vis detector (DAD, G7115A), auto sampler (G7129A) with Chem Station Software, Version E.02.02 and Phenomenex Kinetex 5 µm C18 reverse-phase column (150 × 4.6 mm) with C18 guard cartridge column MG II 5 µm, 4 × 10 mm. The HPLC conditions were as described below. The mobile phase comprised aqueous solution containing 1% (v/v) tetrahydrofuran and 0.05% (v/v) phosphoric acid: acetonitrile (30:70 volume ratio); a flow rate of 0.9 mL/min; wavelength of 205 nm; injection volume of 20 µL; column oven temperature of 40 °C; and run time of 6 min. The analytical method validation was performed to satisfy the validation criteria.

Total FOS content in niosomal preparation was determined by dissolving 100 µL of the sample in 10 mL of methanol:water (50:50 v/v). After proper dilution, the solution was filtered through a 0.45 µm nylon filter and analyzed using HPLC. To determine the percentage of EE (%EE), the sample was ultra-centrifuged (CP100NX, Hitachi Koki Co., Ltd., Tokyo, Japan) at 18,000 rpm at 4 °C for 1 h. Then, the content of unentrapped drug in the supernatant was diluted with methanol: water (50:50 v/v) and quantified by HPLC. All samples were performed in triplicate. The %EE was calculated as Equation (1):

$$\%EE = \frac{(D_t - D_s)}{D_t} \times 100 \qquad (1)$$

where D_t is the total FOS content and D_s is the FOS content in the supernatant.

2.3.4. Transmission Electron Microscopy (TEM) Analysis

The morphologic examinations of selected FOS-loaded niosomes with or without γCD were performed using the TEM technique. Initially, the sample was placed on a formvar-coated grid. After blotting the grid with a filter paper, the grid was transferred onto a drop of negative stain. Aqueous 1% phosphotungstic acid solution was used as a negative stain. The sample was air dried at room temperature and finally the samples were examined by TEM (Model JEM-2100F, JEOL, Peabody, MA, USA).

2.4. In Vitro Release Study

The in vitro release study was performed using a modified Franz diffusion cell apparatus consisting of donor and receptor chambers (NK Laboratories Co., Ltd., Bangkok, Thailand). These two chambers were separated by a semipermeable membrane (MWCO 12,000–14,000 Da). The membrane was presoaked overnight in the receptor phase consisting of phosphate-buffered saline (PBS, pH 7.4). The receptor phase was degassed to remove dissolved air before being placed in the receptor chamber. The sample (1.5 mL) of each niosomal formulation was placed in the donor chamber. The receptor phase was continuously stirred at 150 rpm throughout the experiment and a controlled temperature was maintained at 34 ± 1 °C by a thermostated circulating bath (GRANT W6, Akribis Scientific Limited, Cheshire, UK). A 150 µL aliquot of the receptor medium was withdrawn at timed intervals and replaced immediately with an equal volume of fresh receptor phase.

The FOS content in the receptor medium was determined using HPLC and the amount of cumulative drug release was calculated. Each formulation was performed in triplicate.

2.5. Ex Vivo Permeation Study

The ex vivo permeation study was performed across the cornea and sclera of porcine eyes obtained within 4 h after the death of pigs from a slaughterhouse. In this study, the cornea and sclera were dissected from porcine eyes and replaced with the semipermeable cellophane membrane as previously described in in vitro release study. The selected FOS-loaded Span® 60-niosomal formulations and an aqueous saturated solution of FOS/γCD complex used as a control were conducted at least in triplicate. The FOS content in the receptor phase at timed intervals was determined using HPLC. The steady state flux was calculated as the slope of linear section of the amount of drug in the receptor chamber (q) versus time (t) profiles, and the apparent permeability coefficient (P_{app}) was calculated from the flux (J) according to Equation (2):

$$J = \frac{dq}{A \cdot dt} = P_{app} \cdot C_d \qquad (2)$$

where A is the surface area of the mounted membrane (1.7 cm^2) and C_d is the initial concentration of the drug in the donor chamber.

2.6. Cell Viability and Short Time Exposure (STE) Test

In vitro cytotoxicity test was determined using the methylthiazolyl-diphenyl-tetrazolium bromide (MTT) assay [27,28]. Briefly, the niosomal formulations containing FOS without and with γCD (Sp-DCP and Sp-DCP+γCD, respectively) including their respective blank samples, i.e., B-Sp-DCP and B-Sp-DCP+γCD were evaluated for their toxicity to the rabbit corneal fibroblasts, i.e., the SIRC (rabbit corneal cell line) cells (CCL-60; ATCC, Manassas, VA, USA). Each sample was diluted to the concentration of 0.5, 1, 2, 5 and 10% (v/v) of the test samples by a complete medium that contained Eagle's Minimum Essential Medium and fetal bovine serum (FBS). FOS concentrations in the tested samples ranged from 0.005 to 0.1% w/v. The cells were cultured in the complete medium and maintained at 37 °C under 5% CO$_2$ atmosphere. They were seeded in 96-well plates with a density of 1×10^5 cells/well/100 µL and incubated for 24 h. Thereafter, each test sample (100 µL) was added to the well. The cells were incubated for 24 h and washed twice with PBS (pH 7.4) at the end of incubation period. MTT solution in PBS (pH 7.4) was added to each well and incubated for 4 h. The formazan crystals were dissolved using 0.04 M HCl in isopropanol (100 µL/well). The optical density (OD) of each well was measured at 570 nm by a microplate reader (Fluostar Omega, BMG Labtech, Ortenberg, Germany). The experiments were performed in four replications, and cell viability (CV) was calculated following Equation (3). The test samples were considered to be toxic to the cells if the CV (%) was less than 70%.

$$CV(\%) = \frac{OD_{sample}}{OD_{control}} \times 100 \qquad (3)$$

where the OD_{sample} and $OD_{control}$ are an OD of the media from the wells containing the SIRC cells incubated with the samples and MTT solution, and an OD of media from the wells containing the cells incubated with MTT solution without the samples, respectively.

The eye irritation potential of those test samples was further evaluated based on the MTT reduction assay [29]. The in vitro eye irritation test was performed according to the procedure of the STE test proposed by Takahashi et al. (2008) [30]. The CV of SIRC cells was determined after they were exposed to 200 µL of either 5% or 0.05% of the test samples dispersed in normal saline for 5 min. The eye irritation potential from the STE test was scored following the criteria for STE irritation scoring. Then, the obtained scores from the 5% and the 0.05% tests were summed up to rank the eye irritation potential. The total scores were ranked as 1, 2 and 3, defined as minimal ocular irritant, moderate ocular irritant, and severe ocular irritant, respectively.

2.7. Physical and Chemical Stability Studies

To investigate the effect of γCD on stability of FOS in niosomal vesicles, selected optimal FOS-loaded niosomal formulations (in the presence and absence of γCD) and aqueous solution of FOS/γCD complex (as a control) were evaluated using the ongoing stability program following International Conference on Harmonization (ICH) guidelines [31]. The samples were stored in tightly closed glass vials at 4 °C, long term condition (30 ± 2 °C, 75 ± 5% relative humidity (RH)) and accelerated condition (40 ± 2 °C, 75 ± 5% RH). Physical appearance was assessed, and formulations were analyzed with respect to pH, particle size and size distribution, zeta potential and the FOS content at timed intervals of 0, 1, 3 and 6 months.

2.8. Statistical Analysis

All quantitative data were presented as means ± standard deviation (SD). The data were statistically calculated using one-way ANOVA (SPSS Software, Version 16.0, SPSS Inc., Chicago, IL, USA). The $p < 0.05$ was considered statistically significant.

3. Results and Discussion

3.1. Physicochemical and Chemical Characterizations of Niosomal Formulations Containing FOS

3.1.1. Osmolality, pH and Viscosity

Table 2 shows the osmolality, pH and viscosity values of FOS-loaded niosomal formulations. The pH values of all formulations were in the range of 6.7 to 7.2, which was acceptable and very close to the ideal pH for the eye drop, i.e., 7.2 ± 0.2 [32]. The slightly lower pH values were found by adding γCD but without significance ($p > 0.05$). All niosomal preparations were at a low viscosity of about 1 to 2 mPa.s. The low viscosity preparation is expected to easily spread on the eye surface and not affect the vision, and it is unlikely to cause any lacrimation or blurredness [33]. Conversely, due to the absence of viscosity-inducing agents, instillation of eye drops may be required several times a day. As expected, the viscosity measured at 34 °C was slightly lower than that measured at 25 °C [34]. All formulations were slightly hypertonic and beyond the acceptable values (within 260 to 330 mOsm/kg). Due to the osmotic property of CDs, osmolality was found to be higher in preparations containing γCD. However, hypertonic eye drops are better tolerated than hypotonic eye drops and they also provide short term discomfort due to dilution with lachrymal fluid taking place rapidly after administration [35].

Table 2. Osmolality, pH and viscosity values of the FOS-loaded niosomal formulations ($n = 3$, mean ± SD).

Formulation	pH	Osmolality (mOsm/kg)	Viscosity (mPa.s)	
			25 ± 1 °C	34 ± 1 °C
Span® 60-Niosome				
Sp-SC24	7.02 ± 0.05	358 ± 5	1.48 ± 0.01	1.18 ± 0.01
Sp-DCP	6.73 ± 0.04	364 ± 6	1.81 ± 0.02	1.30 ± 0.01
Sp-STA	7.26 ± 0.03	366 ± 8	1.38 ± 0.02	1.12 ± 0.01
Sp-SC24+γCD	6.83 ± 0.03	372 ± 5	1.76 ± 0.02	1.50 ± 0.01
Sp-DCP+γCD	6.70 ± 0.03	374 ± 6	1.98 ± 0.02	1.72 ± 0.02
Sp-STA+γCD	6.75 ± 0.01	382 ± 5	1.75 ± 0.01	1.52 ± 0.01
Brij® 76-Niosome				
Br-SC24	6.91 ± 0.01	346 ± 6	1.43 ± 0.01	1.21 ± 0.01
Br-DCP	6.95 ± 0.01	354 ± 8	1.64 ± 0.02	1.34 ± 0.01
Br-STA	7.22 ± 0.03	359 ± 10	1.41 ± 0.01	1.15 ± 0.01
Br-SC24+γCD	6.87 ± 0.02	364 ± 8	1.68 ± 0.02	1.34 ± 0.02
Br-DCP+γCD	6.78 ± 0.08	378 ± 3	1.86 ± 0.01	1.56 ± 0.01
Br-STA+γCD	6.86 ± 0.05	379 ± 9	1.65 ± 0.02	1.38 ± 0.01

3.1.2. Particle Size, Size Distribution and Zeta Potential

The particle size and size distribution of FOS-loaded niosomal formulations measured by DLS technique are shown in Table 3. The average particle size was found to range from 190 to 270 nm, and PDI values were found between 0.1 and 0.5. This demonstrated polydisperse sample with heterogenous population of particles. In lipid-based nanoparticles, a PDI value of 0.3 and below indicates a homogenous population and is considered to be an acceptable nanocarrier for drug delivery systems [36]. Thus, further steps in the manufacturing process, such as extrusion or high-pressure homogenization, may be necessary to lower the PDI values for monodispersed systems. In most cases, the size of niosomes with Span® 60 (HLB 4.7) were larger than those of Brij® 76 (HLB 12.4). Vesicle size is generally known to be directly dependent on HLB value of the surfactant used where higher HLB produces larger size vesicles [37–40]. However, several studies have inversely reported that lower HLB values produce larger size vesicles [22,41,42]. This discrepancy is probably due to differing preparation methods, differing physiochemical properties of loaded drugs and the effect of membrane additives.

Table 3. Mean particle size, size distribution, zeta potential and %EE of FOS-loaded niosomal formulations (n = 3, mean ± SD).

Formulation	Z-Average (d.nm)	Size Distribution (PDI)	Zeta Potential (mV)	%EE
Sp-SC24	245.1 ± 5.02	0.46 ± 0.03	−32.70 ± 1.64	21.34 ± 0.42
Sp-DCP	262.4 ± 5.00	0.45 ± 0.01	−37.70 ± 1.15	28.68 ± 0.77
Sp-STA	250.4 ± 6.31	0.35 ± 0.03	−15.43 ± 1.46	9.20 ± 0.30
Sp-SC24+γCD	198.0 ± 4.50	0.52 ± 0.01	−20.27 ± 0.67	25.99 ± 0.78
Sp-DCP+γCD	246.8 ± 3.71	0.42 ± 0.01	−27.17 ± 1.63	34.43 ± 0.80
Sp-STA+γCD	229.1 ± 5.16	0.36 ± 0.06	−13.40 ± 1.91	11.30 ± 0.85
Br-SC24	257.2 ± 4.29	0.32 ± 0.01	−24.30 ± 2.01	10.70 ± 0.27
Br-DCP	212.0 ± 0.72	0.36 ± 0.03	−34.97 ± 0.35	12.94 ± 0.57
Br-STA	214.8 ± 4.01	0.37 ± 0.02	−7.41 ± 0.40	7.73 ± 0.97
Br-SC24+γCD	246.0 ± 0.96	0.11 ± 0.02	−21.20 ± 1.04	12.58 ± 0.85
Br-DCP+γCD	200.0 ± 1.87	0.32 ± 0.01	−23.73 ± 1.97	14.02 ± 0.10
Br-STA+γCD	211.6 ± 1.52	0.34 ± 0.05	−6.94 ± 0.43	8.09 ± 0.80

The addition of a membrane charge was observed to influence particle size (Table 3). Incorporating DCP in Span® 60-niosome, i.e., Sp-DCP, produced relatively larger average particle sizes than those of STA followed by SC24 (Sp-STA and Sp-SC24, respectively). This could be explained by the similar charge of DCP, Span® 60 and cholesterol head groups producing electrostatic repulsion among them, decreasing membrane curvature; and therefore, increasing particle size [43]. In contrast, in the case of Brij® 76, vesicle size was found in the trend of SC24 > STA > DCP. This might be due to differences in the accommodating ability of surfactants among the membrane additives. Incorporating SC24 in hydrophilic Brij® 76 surfactant led to increased membrane permeability and interstitial spaces between the bilayer membranes due to its bulky structures with long and highly hydrophilic poly-24-oxyethylene chains, resulting in increased in size [44].

Compared with the formulations with or without γCD, the preparations containing γCD displayed smaller mean particle size than those of the corresponding pure FOS-loaded niosomes. CDs form hydrophobic interactions with a hydrophobic tail as well as hydrogen bonding with the polar head group of nonionic surfactants [45]. Therefore, the complexation of CD with hydrophobic tails of surfactants resulted in lower packing density of incorporated surfactant and thereby decreased membrane thickness [46]. Additionally, the adsorption of γCD on surface modified niosomes also decreased vesicle size. This was due to CD interacting with polar head groups of surfactants through hydrogen bonding, leading to increased area of the polar head groups at the interphase as well as altering the radius of the curvature [47].

All FOS niosomal formulations exhibited negative zeta-potential values (Table 3). This might have been due to free hydroxyl groups present in cholesterol and surfactant molecules [48]. Because of the contribution of a negative charge due to ionization of the acidic (–HPO$_4$) group by DCP, it produced a higher negative zeta potential value. The resultant electrostatic repulsion was likely to account for reducing the tendency of niosome aggregation. Conversely, STA introduced a positive charge via the protonation of the basic-NH$_2$ group which adsorbed on the surface of niosome and exhibited lower negative zeta potential values through charge neutralization than the uncharged one, i.e., SC24 [49]. SC24 has no net charge and does not provide additional ions in dispersion media. It enhances membrane physical stability by providing steric stabilization [17]. It has been concluded that the highest negative zeta potential obtained by adding DCP could be of great importance to increase the stability and restraining niosomal dispersions from coalescence and aggregation during storage. Regarding niosomal formulations in the presence of γCD, lower zeta potential values were observed than those observed for corresponding nonCD-based niosomes. This was due to CD acting as a shell on the surface charge of niosome by hydrogen bond formation between the hydrophilic head group of surfactants with hydroxy groups on the exterior of CD [46,47,50,51].

3.1.3. %EE of FOS-Loaded Niosomal Formulations

Lipophilic drugs are well known to be preferentially taken up by niosome compared with hydrophilic ones due to higher partitioning through the lipid phase of the vesicles [52]. The %EE values of 21 to 35% were obtained in Span® 60-niosomes, which were relatively superior to those prepared with Brij® 76 (Table 3). This might have been due to the lower HLB value of Span® 60 (HLB 4.7) in contrast to Brij® 76 (HLB 12.4). In addition, Span® 60 has a higher transition temperature (Tc), i.e., 53 °C, compared with Brij® 76 (34 °C) [53]. The surfactant with higher Tc usually forms less leaky vesicles; and thus, results in higher drug entrapment of water-soluble solutes [23,38].

The effect of stabilizer on %EE was found in the trend of DCP > SC24 > STA. The presence of double hydrocarbon chains in DCP imparted a greater packing of the bilayer membrane resulting in higher %EE. Due to the presence of highly hydrophilic poly-24-oxyethylene chains of SC24, the membrane becomes more flexible and permeable; thus decreasing %EE [44]. The lowest %EE by STA could be explained by an electrostatic induced chain tilt which subsequently changes the lateral packing of the bilayers [54]. This result was similar to the observation of the rupture of vesicles by the aggregation and fusion of vesicles under the polarized light microscope (data not shown).

According to our knowledge base, few studies have reported CD inclusion complex in niosome vesicles [47,55–60]. Our data results have shown that %EE of FOS increased when incorporating the FOS/γCD inclusion complex in niosomal preparations. This finding was similar to related reports [58,61]. The higher %EE in niosome containing γCD might have been because CD forms hydrogen bonds interacting with the polar head group of nonionic surfactants. The stronger the hydrogen binding intensity, the greater %EE was obtained [45,62]. Moreover, complexation of free CD with hydrophobic tails of surfactants creates a more internal aqueous space by decreasing membrane thickness [46,47]. However, all niosomal formulations have poor %EE of FOS (<40%). Remote loading method and changes to the formulation variables (i.e., surfactant/cholesterol ratio and their concentrations, buffer molarity and pH, hydration time, etc.) can be applied to optimize %EE. Due to the lower %EE of Brij® 76-niosomes (stabilized by SC24 and DCP) and the evidence of the particle aggregation with the lowest %EE among the groups in all niosomes using STA as stabilizer, these formulations were excluded from further studies.

3.1.4. TEM Analysis

The TEM micrographs of FOS-loaded Span® 60-niosomes are shown in Figure 1. It demonstrated that the vesicles were well identified and presented in a nearly spherical shape. TEM images of niosomal formulations in the presence of γCD showed smaller particle size which corresponded to those determined by DLS measurement (Table 3). It has been observed that the small white spots distributed in niosome were stabilized by SC24 in the presence and absence of γCD (Figure 1a,c). Interestingly, in the case of DCP in the presence of γCD (Sp-DCP+γCD), the larger internal aqueous core was detected (Figure 1d) when compared with the one without γCD (Sp-DCP) (Figure 1b). The wider the hydrophilic core of niosome, the more capacity it could accommodate, including both hydrophilic drugs and water-soluble drug/CD complexes. Therefore, TEM micrographs showed a good correlation with the higher %EE of FOS-loaded Span® 60/DCP niosome containing γCD (Table 3).

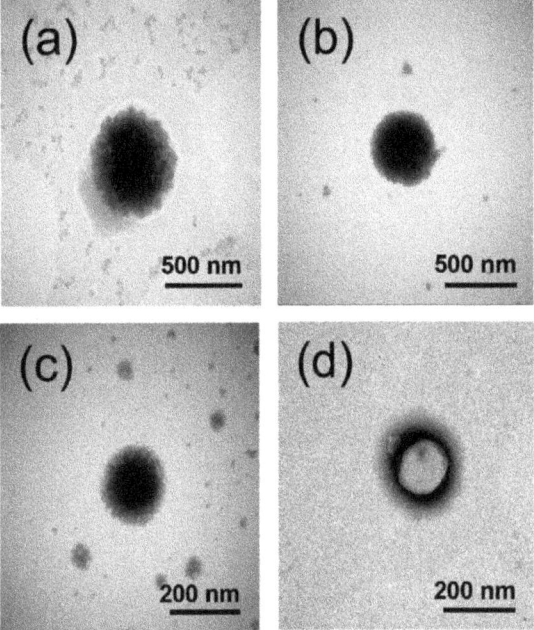

Figure 1. TEM micrographs of FOS-loaded Span® 60-niosomes (**a**) Sp-SC24; (**b**) Sp-DCP; (**c**) Sp-SC24+γCD and (**d**) Sp-DCP+γCD.

3.2. In Vitro Release Study

The in vitro release profiles of selected FOS-loaded Span® 60-niosomes are shown in Figure 2. Notably, a more controlled release manner was obtained from FOS-loaded niosomes stabilized by DCP than that obtained from those stabilized by SC24. Due to the parallel alignment of double hydrocarbon chains of DCP to the hydrocarbon chains of Span® 60 as well as its parallel orientation of polar phosphate groups to the polar heads of Span® 60, DCP provided more packing and filling in of any irregularities through the bilayer membrane. Such enhancement in the packing properties could render less membrane permeability to the entrapped water-soluble molecules and retard the drug release [44]. In both cases, FOS/γCD complexes that were entrapped niosomal formulations showed slower release rates than those of only FOS-loaded niosomes. Similar results have been reported with methotrexate where niosome with drug/βCD inclusion complexes produced relatively slower release pattern of the entrapped drug compared with both free drug incorporated niosome and drug/CD complex preparation [61]. Sheena et al. (1997) compared the release profiles of pilocarpine/βCD loaded and nonCD-based niosomal preparations. The result revealed that βCD-based niosomal formulations showed slower and more sustained release than that of conventional niosomes [58].

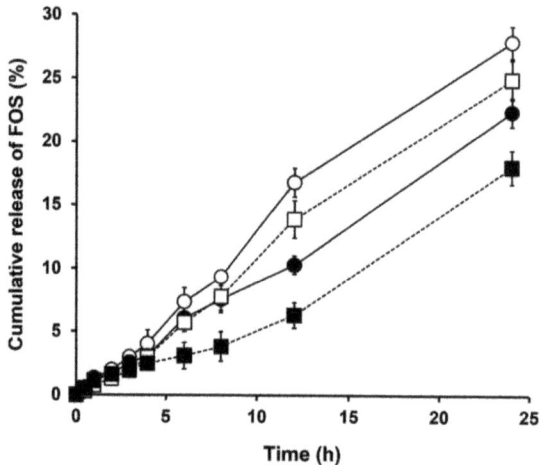

Figure 2. The release profiles of FOS-loaded Span® 60-niosomes through semipermeable membrane with MWCO 12,000–14,000 Da; (○) Sp-SC24; (□) Sp-DCP; (●) Sp-SC24+γCD and (■) Sp-DCP+γCD.

An important issue in evaluating reduced IOP among patients with glaucoma is 24 h control [63]. The more controlled release pattern of FOS niosomal preparation provides greater benefit for targeted glaucoma treatment. In contrast, the slow drug release may affect the insufficient therapeutic drug level in the ocular tissues. Niosomes have been investigated to enhance the poorly absorbed drug molecules by binding to the corneal surface and improving the contact time, thereby increasing the ocular bioavailability of drugs. To evaluate the FOS permeation through the ocular membranes, the optimum formulations, i.e., Sp-DCP and Sp-DCP+γCD were selected for further ex vivo permeation and stability studies.

3.3. Ex Vivo Permeation Study

The flux and P_{app} values of FOS-loaded Span®/DCP niosomal preparations in the presence and absence of γCD including aqueous solution containing FOS/γCD complex are displayed in Table 4. Notably, P_{app} level through sclera was higher than that of the cornea in all tested preparations. This might be due to the loose structural matrix and less complicated tissue layer of sclera [64,65]. According to the literature, the permeability of sclera is approximately 10 times greater than that of the cornea [66]. Thus, the scleral route is an alternative pathway to deliver drugs in both anterior and posterior segments of the eye. Loch et al. (2012) showed that the P_{app} values of ciprofloxacin, timolol and lidocaine for sclera are higher than those for the cornea [67]. Ahmed and Patton (1985) also revealed that intraocular penetration of a large molecule weight, i.e., insulin across the sclera was higher than those through the cornea [68].

Table 4. Flux and apparent permeation coefficient (P_{app}) of FOS-loaded Span® 60/DCP niosomal formulations in the presence and absence of γCD and aqueous FOS/γCD complex solution, through porcine cornea or sclera ($n = 4$, Mean ± SD).

Formulation	Cornea		Sclera	
	Flux ± S.D. ($\mu g h^{-1} cm^{-2}$)	P_{app} ± S.D. ($\times 10^{-6} cm s^{-1}$)	Flux ± S.D. ($\mu g h^{-1} cm^{-2}$)	P_{app} ± S.D. ($\times 10^{-6} cm s^{-1}$)
Sp-DCP	31.086 ± 6.32	0.920 ± 0.18	40.066 ± 40.35	1.155 ± 0.11
Sp-DCP+γCD	22.843 ± 7.95	0.635 ± 0.21	33.092 ± 2.38	0.927 ± 0.08
FOS/γCD complex	62.794 ± 6.23 [a]	1.870 ± 0.18 [a]	86.762 ± 5.25 [a]	2.583 ± 0.16 [a]

[a] Statistically significant difference compared with FOS-loaded niosomal formulations ($p < 0.05$).

In both cases of cornea and sclera, the flux and P_{app} values of FOS from niosomal preparations were significantly lower than those for the FOS/γCD complex preparation ($p < 0.05$) (Table 4). As expected, the FOS-loaded niosomes exhibited a more controlled drug release manner than that of the FOS/γCD complex preparation because the free drug or drug/CD inclusion complex had to be diffused from the inner aqueous core of the niosome through the lipid bilayer and then permeated through the membrane [69]. It has been supported and confirmed that FOS molecules in both free and inclusion complex forms were deposited in the inner core of niosomes. Regarding the effect of CD incorporated in niosomal formulations, both flux and P_{app} of niosome containing γCD (Sp-DCP+γCD) were lower than those without γCD (Sp-DCP). Again, it has been emphasized that most FOS molecules were included in the γCD cavity as inclusion complexes and were localized in the inner core of the niosome, i.e., high %EE. In addition, CD forms a strong hydrogen bonding interaction with the polar head group of nonionic surfactants, resulting in lower flux and P_{app} values of FOS-loaded niosome containing γCD.

3.4. Cell Viability and STE Test

Figure 3 shows the viability (%) of SIRC cells against the concentrations of unloaded and FOS-loaded Span® 60/DCP niosomal formulations. As expected, the test samples at high concentrations were toxic to the SIRC cells. However, unloaded FOS Sp-DCP niosomes (blank) were safer than other formulations because the cell viability of the SIRC cells was greater than 70% at the entire concentrations around 5 to 0.5% *v/v*. Further, the others were safe to the SIRC cells at a concentration around 0.5% *v/v* only.

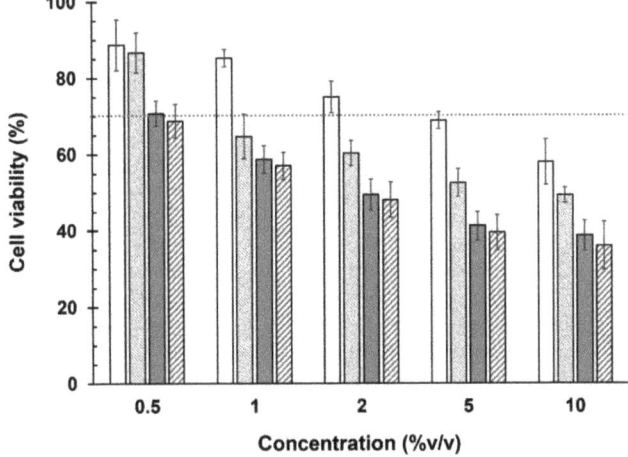

Figure 3. In vitro cytotoxicity test of FOS-loaded niosomal formulations, (▮) Sp-DCP and (▨) Sp-DCP+γCD, and, (☐) blank Sp-DCP and (▥) blank Sp-DCP+γCD, at various concentrations in the SIRC cells ($n = 4$, mean ± SD).

The in vitro irritation test was further evaluated. The STE test could provide representative information to the animal testing that involves the Draize test in rabbits [30]. The %CV of SIRC cells after exposure to 5% and 0.05% concentrations of niosomal formulation with loaded and unloaded FOS for 5 min are shown in Table 5. Notably, the total scores of eye irritation potential of both niosomal formulations entrapped FOS or FOS/γCD and their respective blank formulations were equal to 2. Thus, these formulations were defined as a moderate ocular irritant. On the other hand, this result demonstrated that FOS-loaded niosomal preparations could be conditionally accepted as safe for ophthalmic use. These observations might be due to the hyperosmolar solutions of the eye drop preparations.

Table 5. Scores obtained from the short time exposure (STE) test of the test samples.

Concentration of the Test Samples	Test Samples	%CV of the SIRC Cells	Criteria for Scoring	Obtained Scores
(I) 5%	(1) Blank Sp-DCP	67 ± 5	If CV >70%: scored 0	1
	(2) Blank Sp-DCP + γCD	63 ± 3	If CV ≤ 70%: scored 1	1
	(3) Sp-DCP	52 ± 4		1
	(4) Sp-DCP + γCD	47 ± 4		1
(II) 0.05%	(1) Blank Sp-DCP	87 ± 6	If CV >70%: scored 1 If CV ≤ 70%: scored 2	1
	(2) Blank Sp-DCP + γCD	85 ± 4		1
	(3) Sp-DCP	83 ± 4		1
	(4) Sp-DCP + γCD	81 ± 2		1
	Total score (I and II)		(1) Blank Sp-DCP	2
			(2) Blank Sp-DCP+γCD	2
			(3) Sp-DCP	2
			(4) Sp-DCP+γCD	2

3.5. Physical and Chemical Stability Studies of FOS

The pH, particle size, size distribution, zeta potential and percent drug content were used as the parameters to evaluate the stability of FOS in niosomal formulations. In this study, two selected formulations, i.e., FOS-loaded Span® 60/DCP niosomal formulations in the presence and absence of γCD were evaluated, and the aqueous solution of FOS/γCD complex was used as a control. The physical stability, i.e., pH, mean particle size, size distribution and zeta potential, of FOS after storage at 4 °C, in long term and accelerated conditions at various time intervals is shown in Tables S1 and S2.

In the case of the aqueous solution of the FOS/γCD complex, the pH value slightly decreased at 4 °C but more obviously at higher temperatures. The particle size was significantly increased at all storage conditions and PDI values were out of specification at 30 and 40 °C. The zeta potential values also decreased under all conditions and significantly decreased at storage condition at 40 °C. It was concluded that FOS in the complexing aqueous medium exhibited low physical stability, especially the particle size growth upon storing for six months.

After storing for six months at 4 °C, a slightly decreased pH was found in both niosomal formulations; however, at higher storage temperatures of 30 and 40 °C, significantly reduced pH was detected ($p < 0.05$). This might have been due to a progressive increase in the hydrolysis of fatty acid in niosome with increasing temperature [70]. Regarding vesicle sizes and size distribution, both FOS-loaded niosomes had no appreciable changes at 4 °C, indicating a good physical stability. As expected, larger differences in these parameters were observed at higher temperatures of 30 and 40 °C. The particle size was exponentially increased and the PDI values were out of specification at 30 and 40 °C (PDI > 0.7) over the six-month period. The aggregation or fusion of vesicles generally occurred as molecular mobility increased and transformed to larger ones [71,72]. While particle size and size distributions indicate stability for particle-based formulations, %EE is considered as a stability-indicating parameter for this study in direct comparison to its non-particulate counterparts. Decreasing zeta potential values were found in all storage conditions but more significantly at higher temperatures. This lower zeta potential directly correlated to lower electrostatic repulsion and as a result, aggregation or fusion of vesicles resulted in increased particle size.

According to the six-month chemical stability data (Table 6), the drug content was significantly decreased in the aqueous solution consisting of the FOS/γCD complex representing 51, 8 and 3% at 4, 30 and 40 °C, respectively. Notably, FOS could not withstand an aqueous solution containing γCD. On the other hand, the CD inclusion complex was insufficient to enhance the chemical stability of FOS. We have found that the niosomal preparations revealed greater chemical stability than nonvesicular preparations, i.e., aqueous solutions containing the FOS/γCD complex at all storage conditions. Regarding the effect of γCD on chemical stability of FOS in niosome, Sp-DCP+γCD niosome showed relatively greater stability than Sp-DCP niosome at all storage temperatures. Under the refrigerated condition of 4 °C, 92% of FOS remained in Sp-DCP+γCD niosome, whereas only 88% remained in Sp-DCP niosome after storing for six months. Incorporating γCD as FOS/γCD complex in niosome showed relatively more stability than in that without CD.

Table 6. Total FOS content (%) of FOS-loaded niosomal preparations and FOS/γCD complex storage at 4 °C, 30 ± 2 °C (75 ± 5% RH) and 40 ± 2 °C (75 ± 5% RH) for 0, 1, 3 and 6 months (n = 3, mean ± SD) The % FOS content was calculated based on 100% as initial drug content at 0 month.

Time (Month)	Formulations		
	Sp-DCP	Sp-DCP+γCD	FOS/γCD Complex
	5 ± 3 °C		
1 Month	97.95 ± 0.70	98.44 ± 0.64	81.09 ± 0.92
3 Months	93.72 ± 0.73	95.21 ± 0.39	73.84 ± 0.68
6 Months	88.33 ± 0.54	92.75 ± 0.83	51.10 ± 1.18
	30 ± 2 °C (65 ± 5% RH)		
1 Month	93.32 ± 0.53	95.13 ± 0.86	28.72 ± 0.30
3 Months	83.40 ± 0.78	87.37 ± 0.57	20.94 ± 0.73
6 Months	17.17 ± 0.59	23.67 ± 0.57	8.49 ± 0.70
	40 ± 2 °C (75 ± 5% RH)		
1 Month	46.09 ± 0.88	56.34 ± 0.82	19.95 ± 0.60
3 Months	27.88 ± 0.71	36.70 ± 1.08	12.26 ± 0.36
6 Months	7.75 ± 0.83	10.68 ± 1.06	3.59 ± 0.70

From the overall data results, the proposed drawings of FOS-loaded niosomes are shown in Figure 4. Niosomal platform could protect chemically unstable drug molecule, FOS by entrapping its inner the aqueous core. Additionally, the effect of γCD inclusion complex formation is the predominant factor to provide higher %EE of FOS in niosomal formulations by preventing the drug degradation via hydrolysis and consequently enhances the chemical stability of FOS in aqueous solution.

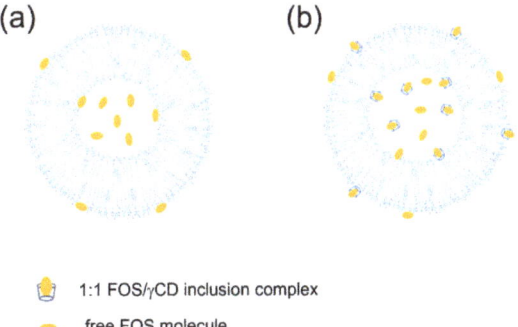

1:1 FOS/γCD inclusion complex
free FOS molecule

Figure 4. Proposed drawing of (**a**) FOS-loaded niosomes and (**b**) FOS/γCD loaded noisome.

4. Conclusions

To enhance the chemical stability of FOS in aqueous solution, niosomal formulations were developed. The effects of CD, surfactant type and membrane stabilizer/charged inducers on physiochemical and chemical properties of niosome were characterized. The average particle size was detected within the nanometer range and PDI values were within an acceptable range. The slow permeation rate of FOS through excised porcine cornea and sclera was obtained in γCD-loaded Span® 60/DCP niosomal formulation. The chemical stability of FOS in the formation of γCD inclusion complex could not withstand the aqueous solution. Niosomal preparations with moderate irritation could prevent FOS degradation and they exhibited physical and chemical stability for at least three months at 4 °C. The optimum formulation to enhance the chemical stability of FOS consisted of FOS/γCD complex loaded niosome. To increase the shelf-file of the FOS niosomal formulation, the conversion to lyophilized powder for reconstitution is considered for further studies. Our studies successfully investigated the preformulation and ophthalmic formulation development of FOS. However, to demonstrate a clinically viable formulation, the in vivo pharmacokinetic in rabbit eye was considered for future perspective studies.

Supplementary Materials: The following supporting information can be downloaded at: https://www.mdpi.com/article/10.3390/pharmaceutics14061147/s1, Table S1: pH and zeta potential values of FOS niosomal preparation and FOS/γCD complex storage at 4 °C, 30 $\pm$ 2 °C (75 $\pm$ 5% RH) and 40 $\pm$ 2 °C (75 $\pm$ 5% RH) for 0, 1, 3 and 6 months; Table S2: Average particle size and size distribution (PDI) of FOS niosomal preparation and FOS/γCD complex storage at 4 °C, 30 $\pm$ 2 °C (75 $\pm$ 5% RH) and 40 $\pm$ 2 °C (75 $\pm$ 5% RH) for 0, 1, 3 and 6 months.

Author Contributions: Conceptualization, P.J.; investigation, H.M.H. and R.A.; resources, D.C. and E.S.; writing—original draft preparation, H.M.H. and P.J.; writing—review and editing, P.J. and T.L.; supervision, T.L. All authors have read and agreed to the published version of the manuscript.

Funding: This work was financially supported by the European Union's Eurostar Program under project No. PREVIN E11008 and by The Second Century Fund (C2F), Chulalongkorn University.

Institutional Review Board Statement: Not applicable.

Informed Consent Statement: Not applicable.

Data Availability Statement: Not applicable.

Conflicts of Interest: The authors declare no conflict of interest.

References

1. Sugrue, M.F. The pharmacology of antiglaucoma drugs. *Pharmacol. Ther.* **1989**, *43*, 91–138. [CrossRef]
2. Alward, W.L.M. Medical management of glaucoma. *N. Engl. J. Med.* **1998**, *339*, 1298–1307. [CrossRef] [PubMed]
3. Quigley, H.A.; Broman, A.T. The number of people with glaucoma worldwide in 2010 and 2020. *Br. J. Ophthalmol.* **2006**, *90*, 262–267. [CrossRef] [PubMed]
4. Tham, Y.C.; Li, X.; Wong, T.Y.; Quigley, H.A.; Aung, T.; Cheng, C.Y. Global prevalence of glaucoma and projections of glaucoma burden through 2040: A systematic review and meta-analysis. *Ophthalmology* **2014**, *121*, 2081–2090. [CrossRef]
5. Kwon, Y.H.; Fingert, J.H.; Kuehn, M.H.; Alward, W.L. Primary open-angle glaucoma. *N. Engl. J. Med.* **2009**, *360*, 1113–1124. [CrossRef]
6. Costagliola, C.; Di Benedetto, R.; De Caprio, L.; Verde, R.; Mastropasqua, L. Effect of oral captopril (SQ 14225) on intraocular pressure in man. *Eur. J. Ophthalmol.* **1995**, *5*, 19–25. [CrossRef]
7. Mehta, A.; Iyer, L.; Parmar, S.; Shah, G.; Goyal, R. Oculohypotensive effect of perindopril in acute and chronic models of glaucoma in rabbits. *Can. J. Physiol. Pharmacol.* **2010**, *88*, 595–600. [CrossRef]
8. Loftsson, T.; Thorisdóttir, S.; Fridriksdóttir, H.; Stefánsson, E. Enalaprilat and enalapril maleate eyedrops lower intraocular pressure in rabbits. *Acta Ophthalmol.* **2010**, *88*, 337–341. [CrossRef]
9. Lotti, V.J.; Pawlowski, N. Prostaglandins mediate the ocular hypotensive action of the angiotensin converting enzyme inhibitor MK-422 (enalaprilat) in African green monkeys. *J. Ocul. Pharmacol. Ther.* **1990**, *6*, 1–7. [CrossRef]
10. Rachmani, R.; Lidar, M.; Levy, Z.; Ravid, M. Effect of enalapril on the incidence of retinopathy in normotensive patients with type 2 diabetes. *Eur. J. Intern. Med.* **2000**, *11*, 48–50. [CrossRef]
11. Manschot, S.M.; Gispen, W.H.; Kappelle, L.J.; Biessels, G.J. Nerve conduction velocity and evoked potential latencies in streptozotocin-diabetic rats: Effects of treatment with an angiotensin converting enzyme inhibitor. *Diabetes/Metab. Res. Rev.* **2003**, *19*, 469–477. [CrossRef]
12. Choudhary, R.; Kapoor, M.S.; Singh, A.; Bodakhe, S.H. Therapeutic targets of renin-angiotensin system in ocular disorders. *J. Curr. Ophthalmol.* **2017**, *29*, 7–16. [CrossRef]
13. Narayanam, M.; Singh, S. Characterization of stress degradation products of fosinopril by using LC-MS/TOF, MSn and on-line H/D exchange. *J. Pharm. Biomed. Anal.* **2014**, *92*, 135–143. [CrossRef]
14. Hnin, H.M.; Stefánsson, E.; Loftsson, T.; Rungrotmongkol, T.; Jansook, P. Angiotensin converting enzyme inhibitors/cyclodextrin inclusion complexes: Solution and solid-state characterizations and their thermal stability. *J. Incl. Phenom. Macrocycl. Chem.* **2022**, *102*, 347–358. [CrossRef]
15. Boyd, B.J. Past and future evolution in colloidal drug delivery systems. *Expert Opin. Drug Deliv.* **2008**, *5*, 69–85. [CrossRef]
16. Moghassemi, S.; Hadjizadeh, A. Nano-niosomes as nanoscale drug delivery systems: An illustrated review. *J. Control. Release* **2014**, *185*, 22–36. [CrossRef]
17. Uchegbu, I.F.; Vyas, S.P. Non-ionic surfactant based vesicles (niosomes) in drug delivery. *Int. J. Pharm.* **1998**, *172*, 33–70. [CrossRef]

18. Carafa, M.; Santucci, E.; Alhaique, F.; Coviello, T.; Murtas, E.; Riccieri, F.M.; Lucania, G.; Torrisi, M.R. Preparation and properties of new unilamellar non-ionic/ionic surfactant vesicles. *Int. J. Pharm.* **1998**, *160*, 51–59. [CrossRef]
19. Vyas, S.; Mysore, N.; Jaitely, V.; Venkatesan, N. Discoidal niosome based controlled ocular delivery of timolol maleate. *Die Pharm.* **1998**, *53*, 466–469.
20. Abdelbary, G.; El-gendy, N. Niosome-encapsulated gentamicin for ophthalmic controlled delivery. *AAPS PharmSciTech* **2008**, *9*, 740–747. [CrossRef]
21. Saettone, M.; Perini, G.; Carafa, M.; Santucci, E.; Alhaique, F. Non-ionic surfactant vesicles as ophthalmic carriers for cyclopentolate. A preliminary evaluation. *STP Pharma Sci.* **1996**, *6*, 94–98.
22. Guinedi, A.S.; Mortada, N.D.; Mansour, S.; Hathout, R.M. Preparation and evaluation of reverse-phase evaporation and multilamellar niosomes as ophthalmic carriers of acetazolamide. *Int. J. Pharm.* **2005**, *306*, 71–82. [CrossRef]
23. Abdelkader, H.; Wu, Z.; Al-Kassas, R.; Alany, R.G. Niosomes and discomes for ocular delivery of naltrexone hydrochloride: Morphological, rheological, spreading properties and photo-protective effects. *Int. J. Pharm.* **2012**, *433*, 142–148. [CrossRef]
24. Kaur, I.P.; Garg, A.; Singla, A.K.; Aggarwal, D. Vesicular systems in ocular drug delivery: An overview. *Int. J. Pharm.* **2004**, *269*, 1–14. [CrossRef]
25. Jain, S.; Jain, V.; Mahajan, S. Lipid based vesicular drug delivery systems. *Adv. Pharm.* **2014**, *2014*, 574673. [CrossRef]
26. Kaur, I.P.; Smitha, R. Penetration enhancers and ocular bioadhesives: Two new avenues for ophthalmic drug delivery. *Drug Dev. Ind. Pharm.* **2002**, *28*, 353–369. [CrossRef]
27. Manconi, M.; Manca, M.L.; Valenti, D.; Escribano, E.; Hillaireau, H.; Fadda, A.M.; Fattal, E. Chitosan and hyaluronan coated liposomes for pulmonary administration of curcumin. *Int. J. Pharm.* **2017**, *525*, 203–210. [CrossRef]
28. Asasutjarit, R.; Managit, C.; Phanaksri, T.; Treesuppharat, W.; Fuongfuchat, A. Formulation development and in vitro evaluation of transferrin-conjugated liposomes as a carrier of ganciclovir targeting the retina. *Int. J. Pharm.* **2020**, *577*, 119084. [CrossRef]
29. Asasutjarit, R.; Theerachayanan, T.; Kewsuwan, P.; Veeranondha, S.; Fuongfuchat, A.; Ritthidej, G.C. Gamma sterilization of diclofenac sodium loaded- N-trimethyl chitosan nanoparticles for ophthalmic use. *Carbohydr. Polym.* **2017**, *157*, 603–612. [CrossRef]
30. Takahashi, Y.; Koike, M.; Honda, H.; Ito, Y.; Sakaguchi, H.; Suzuki, H.; Nishiyama, N. Development of the short time exposure (STE) test: An in vitro eye irritation test using SIRC cells. *Toxicol. Vitr.* **2008**, *22*, 760–770. [CrossRef]
31. ICH. *Stability Testing of New Drug Substances and Products (Q1AR2)*; European Medicines Agency: Amsterdam, The Netherlands, 2003.
32. Mathis, G.A. *Clinical Ophthalmic Pharmacology and Therapeutics: Ocular Drug Delivery. Veterinary Ophthalmology*; Lippincott Williams & Wilkins: Orlando, FL, USA, 1999; pp. 291–297.
33. Yasin, M.N.; Hussain, S.; Malik, F.; Hameed, A.; Sultan, T.; Qureshi, F.; Riaz, H.; Perveen, G.; Wajid, A. Preparation and characterization of chloramphenicol niosomes and comparison with chloramphenicol eye drops (0.5% w/v) in experimental conjunctivitis in albino rabbits. *Pak. J. Pharm. Sci.* **2012**, *25*, 117–121. [PubMed]
34. Frisch, D.; Eyring, H.; Kincaid, J.F. Pressure and temperature effects on the viscosity of liquids. *J. Appl. Phys.* **1940**, *11*, 75–80. [CrossRef]
35. Kramer, I.; Haber, M.; Duis, A. Formulation requirements for the ophthalmic use of antiseptics. *Dev. Ophthalmol.* **2002**, *33*, 85–116.
36. Danaei, M.; Dehghankhold, M.; Ataei, S.; Hasanzadeh Davarani, F.; Javanmard, R.; Dokhani, A.; Khorasani, S.; Mozafari, M.R. Impact of Particle Size and Polydispersity Index on the Clinical Applications of Lipidic Nanocarrier Systems. *Pharmaceutics* **2018**, *10*, 57. [CrossRef] [PubMed]
37. Suwakul, W.; Ongpipattanakul, B.; Vardhanabhuti, N. Preparation and characterization of propylthiouracil niosomes. *J. Liposome Res.* **2006**, *16*, 391–401. [CrossRef] [PubMed]
38. Yoshioka, T.; Sternberg, B.; Florence, A.T. Preparation and properties of vesicles (niosomes) of sorbitan monoesters (Span 20, 40, 60 and 80) and a sorbitan triester (Span 85). *Int. J. Pharm.* **1994**, *105*, 1–6. [CrossRef]
39. Ruckmani, K.; Jayakar, B.; Ghosal, S.K. Nonionic surfactant vesicles (niosomes) of cytarabine hydrochloride for effective treatment of leukemias: Encapsulation, storage, and In vitro release. *Drug Dev. Ind. Pharm.* **2000**, *26*, 217–222. [CrossRef]
40. Khazaeli, P.; Pardakhty, A.; Shoorabi, H. Caffeine-loaded niosomes: Characterization and in vitro release studies. *Drug Deliv.* **2007**, *14*, 447–452. [CrossRef]
41. Manconi, M.; Sinico, C.; Valenti, D.; Loy, G.; Fadda, A.M. Niosomes as carriers for tretinoin. I. Preparation and properties. *Int. J. Pharm.* **2002**, *234*, 237–248. [CrossRef]
42. Tabbakhian, M.; Tavakoli, N.; Jaafari, M.R.; Daneshamouz, S. Enhancement of follicular delivery of finasteride by liposomes and niosomes: 1. In vitro permeation and in vivo deposition studies using hamster flank and ear models. *Int. J. Pharm.* **2006**, *323*, 1–10. [CrossRef]
43. Hasan, A.A. Design and in vitro characterization of small unilamellar niosomes as ophthalmic carrier of dorzolamide hydrochloride. *Pharm. Dev. Tech.* **2014**, *19*, 748–754. [CrossRef]
44. Abdelkader, H.; Ismail, S.; Kamal, A.; Alany, R.G. Design and evaluation of controlled-release niosomes and discomes for naltrexone hydrochloride ocular delivery. *J. Pharm. Sci.* **2011**, *100*, 1833–1846. [CrossRef]
45. Valente, A.J.; Söderman, O. The formation of host–guest complexes between surfactants and cyclodextrins. *Adv. Colloid Interface Sci.* **2014**, *205*, 156–176. [CrossRef]
46. Tsianou, M.; Fajalia, A.I. Cyclodextrins and surfactants in aqueous solution above the critical micelle concentration: Where are the cyclodextrins located? *Langmuir* **2014**, *30*, 13754–13764. [CrossRef]

47. Machado, N.D.; Silva, O.F.; de Rossi, R.H.; Fernández, M.A. Cyclodextrin modified niosomes to encapsulate hydrophilic compounds. *RSC Adv.* **2018**, *8*, 29909–29916. [CrossRef]
48. Zubairu, Y.; Negi, L.M.; Iqbal, Z.; Talegaonkar, S. Design and development of novel bioadhesive niosomal formulation for the transcorneal delivery of anti-infective agent: In-vitro and ex-vivo investigations. *Asian J. Pharm. Sci.* **2015**, *10*, 322–330. [CrossRef]
49. Junyaprasert, V.B.; Teeranachaideekul, V.; Supaperm, T. Effect of charged and non-ionic membrane additives on physicochemical properties and stability of niosomes. *AAPS PharmSciTech* **2008**, *9*, 851. [CrossRef]
50. Silva, O.F.; Correa, N.M.; Silber, J.J.; de Rossi, R.H.; Fernández, M.A. Supramolecular assemblies obtained by mixing different cyclodextrins and AOT or BHDC reverse micelles. *Langmuir* **2014**, *30*, 3354–3362. [CrossRef]
51. Zhou, C.; Cheng, X.; Zhao, Q.; Yan, Y.; Wang, J.; Huang, J. Self-assembly of nonionic surfactant tween 20@2β-CD inclusion complexes in dilute solution. *Langmuir* **2013**, *29*, 13175–13182. [CrossRef]
52. Essa, E.A. Effect of formulation and processing variables on the particle size of sorbitan monopalmitate niosomes. *Asian J. Pharm.* **2010**, *4*, 227–233. [CrossRef]
53. Balakrishnan, P.; Shanmugam, S.; Lee, W.S.; Lee, W.M.; Kim, J.O.; Oh, D.H.; Kim, D.-D.; Kim, J.S.; Yoo, B.K.; Choi, H.-G.; et al. Formulation and in vitro assessment of minoxidil niosomes for enhanced skin delivery. *Int. J. Pharm.* **2009**, *377*, 1–8. [CrossRef]
54. Jaehnig, F.; Harlos, K.; Vogel, H.; Eibl, H. Electrostatic interactions at charged lipid membranes. Electrostatically induced tilt. *Biochemistry* **1979**, *18*, 1459–1468. [CrossRef]
55. Chi, L.; Wu, D.; Li, Z.; Zhang, M.; Liu, H.; Wang, C.; Gui, S.; Geng, M.; Li, H.; Zhang, J. Modified release and improved stability of unstable BCS II drug by using cyclodextrin complex as carrier to remotely load drug into niosomes. *Mol. Pharm.* **2016**, *13*, 113–124. [CrossRef]
56. Marianecci, C.; Rinaldi, F.; Esposito, S.; Di Marzio, L.; Carafa, M. Niosomes encapsulating ibuprofen-cyclodextrin complexes: Preparation and characterization. *Curr. Drug Targets* **2013**, *14*, 1070–1078. [CrossRef]
57. Paul, B.K.; Ghosh, N.; Mondal, R.; Mukherjee, S. Contrasting effects of salt and temperature on niosome-bound norharmane: Direct evidence for positive heat capacity change in the niosome: β-cyclodextrin interaction. *J. Phys. Chem. B* **2016**, *120*, 4091–4101. [CrossRef]
58. Sheena, I.; Singh, U.; Aithal, K.; Udupa, N. Pilocarpine β-cyclodextrin complexation and niosomal entrapment. *Pharm. Sci.* **1997**, *3*, 383–386.
59. Oommen, E.; Shenoy, B.D.; Udupa, N.; Kamath, R.; Devi, P.U. Antitumour efficacy of cyclodextrin-complexed and niosome-encapsulated plumbagin in mice bearing melanoma B16F1. *Pharm. Pharmacol. Commun.* **1999**, *5*, 281–285. [CrossRef]
60. D'souza, S.; Ray, J.; Pandey, S.; Udupa, N. Absorption of ciprofloxacin and norfloxacin when administered as niosome-encapsulated inclusion complexes. *J. Pharm. Pharmacol.* **1997**, *49*, 145–149. [CrossRef] [PubMed]
61. Oommen, E.; Tiwari, S.B.; Udupa, N.; Kamath, R.; Devi, P.U. Niosome entrapped β-cyclodextrin methotrexate complex as a drug delivery system. *Indian J. Pharmacol.* **1999**, *31*, 279–284.
62. Hao, Y.-M.; Li, K. Entrapment and release difference resulting from hydrogen bonding interactions in niosome. *Int. J. Pharm.* **2011**, *403*, 245–253. [CrossRef] [PubMed]
63. Wax, M.B.; Camras, C.B.; Fiscella, R.G.; Girkin, C.; Singh, K.; Weinreb, R.N. Emerging perspectives in glaucoma: Optimizing 24-hour control of intraocular pressure. *Am. J. Ophthalmol.* **2002**, *133*, S1–S10. [CrossRef]
64. Barar, J.; Javadzadeh, A.R.; Omidi, Y. Ocular novel drug delivery: Impacts of membranes and barriers. *Expert Opin. Drug Deliv.* **2008**, *5*, 567–581. [CrossRef]
65. Loftsson, T.; Sigurđsson, H.H.; Konráđsdóttir, F.; Gísladóttir, S.; Jansook, P.; Stefánsson, E. Topical drug delivery to the posterior segment of the eye: Anatomical and physiological considerations. *Die Pharm.* **2008**, *63*, 171–179. [CrossRef]
66. Hämäläinen, K.M.; Kananen, K.; Auriola, S.; Kontturi, K.; Urtti, A. Characterization of paracellular and aqueous penetration routes in cornea, conjunctiva, and sclera. *Investig. Ophthalmol. Vis. Sci.* **1997**, *38*, 627–634.
67. Loch, C.; Zakelj, S.; Kristl, A.; Nagel, S.; Guthoff, R.; Weitschies, W.; Seidlitz, A. Determination of permeability coefficients of ophthalmic drugs through different layers of porcine, rabbit and bovine eyes. *Eur. J. Pharm. Sci.* **2012**, *47*, 131–138. [CrossRef]
68. Ahmed, I.; Patton, T.F. Importance of the noncorneal absorption route in topical ophthalmic drug delivery. *Investig. Ophthalmol. Vis. Sci.* **1985**, *26*, 584–587.
69. Gharib, R.; Greige-Gerges, H.; Fourmentin, S.; Charcosset, C.; Auezova, L. Liposomes incorporating cyclodextrin–drug inclusion complexes: Current state of knowledge. *Carbohydr. Polym.* **2015**, *129*, 175–186. [CrossRef]
70. Bates, T.R.; Nightingale, C.H.; Dixon, E. Kinetics of hydrolysis of polyoxyethylene (20) sorbitan fatty acid ester surfactants. *J. Pharm. Pharmacol.* **1973**, *25*, 470–477. [CrossRef]
71. Kopermsub, P.; Mayen, V.; Warin, C. Potential use of niosomes for encapsulation of nisin and EDTA and their antibacterial activity enhancement. *Food Res. Int.* **2011**, *44*, 605–612. [CrossRef]
72. Khan, M.I.; Madni, A.; Peltonen, L. Development and in-vitro characterization of sorbitan monolaurate and poloxamer 184 based niosomes for oral delivery of diacerein. *Eur. J. Pharm. Sci.* **2016**, *95*, 88–95. [CrossRef]

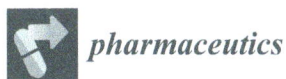

Review

Recent Progress in Chitosan-Based Nanomedicine for Its Ocular Application in Glaucoma

Hassan A. Albarqi [1], Anuj Garg [2], Mohammad Zaki Ahmad [1], Abdulsalam A. Alqahtani [1], Ismail A. Walbi [3] and Javed Ahmad [1,*]

1 Department of Pharmaceutics, College of Pharmacy, Najran University, Najran 11001, Saudi Arabia
2 Institute of Pharmaceutical Research, GLA University, Mathura 281406, India
3 Department of Clinical Pharmacy, College of Pharmacy, Najran University, Najran 11001, Saudi Arabia
* Correspondence: jahmad18@gmail.com or jaahmed@nu.edu.sa

Abstract: Glaucoma is a degenerative, chronic ocular disease that causes irreversible vision loss. The major symptom of glaucoma is high intraocular pressure, which happens when the flow of aqueous humor between the front and back of the eye is blocked. Glaucoma therapy is challenging because of the low bioavailability of drugs from conventional ocular drug delivery systems such as eye drops, ointments, and gels. The low bioavailability of antiglaucoma agents could be due to the precorneal and corneal barriers as well as the low biopharmaceutical attributes of the drugs. These limitations can be overcome by employing nanoparticulate drug delivery systems. Over the last decade, there has been a lot of interest in chitosan-based nanoparticulate systems to overcome the limitations (such as poor residence time, low corneal permeability, etc.) associated with conventional ocular pharmaceutical products. Therefore, the main aim of the present manuscript is to review the recent research work involving the chitosan-based nanoparticulate system to treat glaucoma. It discusses the significance of the chitosan-based nanoparticulate system, which provides mucoadhesion to improve the residence time of drugs and their ocular bioavailability. Furthermore, different types of chitosan-based nanoparticulate systems are also discussed, namely nanoparticles of chitosan core only, nanoparticles coated with chitosan, and hybrid nanoparticles of chitosan. The manuscript also provides a critical analysis of contemporary research related to the impact of this chitosan-based nanomedicine on the corneal permeability, ocular bioavailability, and therapeutic performance of loaded antiglaucoma agents.

Keywords: glaucoma; chitosan; nanoparticles; mucoadhesion; ocular bioavailability; therapeutic efficacy

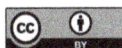

1. Introduction

Glaucoma is a degenerative disease that requires lifetime drug treatment and can be acute or chronic [1]. A blockage in the flow of aqueous humor between the front and back of the eye causes intraocular pressure to rise quickly, retinal degeneration, and optic neuropathy, all of which are signs of acute glaucoma [2,3]. If left untreated, acute glaucoma can cause permanent vision loss within hours or days. Acute glaucoma is more severe and causes serious visual loss in three times as many people as chronic glaucoma does, even though the former is more common (23.4 vs. 52.7 million occurrences in 2020) [4]. The schematic illustration in Figure 1 represents the pathophysiology of glaucoma. It illustrates the normal mechanism of ocular fluid production and drainage channels for its normal flow compared to the obstruction of flow drainage leading to an increase in intraocular pressure (IOP), ultimately affecting the vision due to optic nerve damage. The ocular fluid is produced in the posterior chamber of the eyes at the ciliary body behind the iris and flows through the anterior chamber of the eye to ultimately come out through the uveoscleral pathway. The rise in IOP and oxidative stress in the glaucoma-conditioned eye finally led to damage to retinal ganglion cells and optical nerves [4,5]. Neurovascular dysfunction and neuroinflammation of the eye have also been implicated in the pathogenesis of glaucoma. It is very well reported that oxidative stress and choroidal vascular dysfunction are mainly involved in the pathogenesis of age-related macular degeneration [2,3]. In addition, the poor bioavailability of presently marketed medications necessitates frequent doses and low patient compliance, putting the vision of patients at further risk. Ninety percent of commercial ocular drugs are available as eye drops, which is a simple and effective way to administer a drug. However, corneal permeability limits the absorption, bioavailability, and therapeutic activity of ocular drugs [6]. Ocular barriers, such as the precorneal, corneal, and conjunctival layers, limit drug diffusion in ocular tissues. The precorneal barriers include blinking reflexes, lacrimal turnover, nasolacrimal drainage, efflux transporters, and drug metabolism by lysozymes present in tears. Furthermore, ocular absorption of drugs is poor due to drug binding to or repulsion from the conjunctiva and tight junctional complexes in the corneal epithelium [7]. In recent years, several novel ocular drug delivery systems were investigated utilizing nanotechnology-mediated drug delivery strategies to overcome the pre-corneal and corneal barriers to enhance the ocular absorption and hence therapeutic efficacy of drugs [8,9].

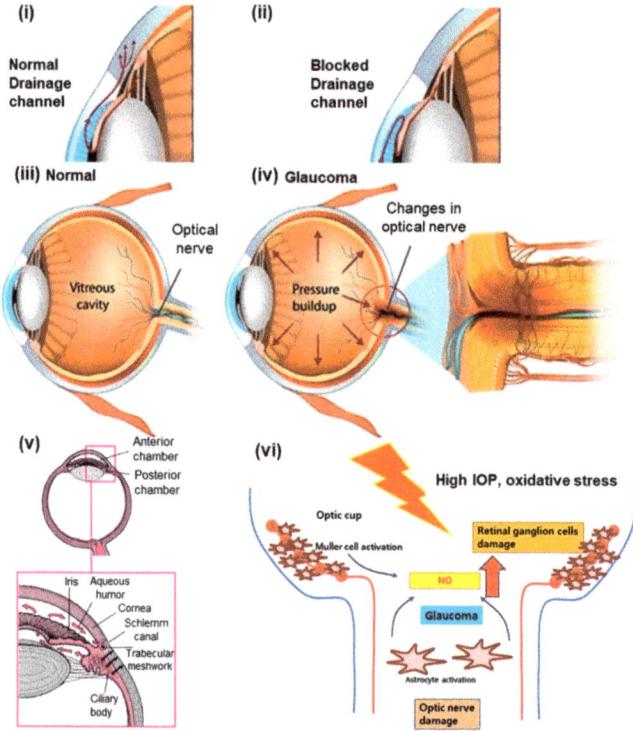

Figure 1. Schematic illustration presenting the pathophysiology of the eye in glaucoma compared to normal eyes. (**i**) Normal drainage channel in healthy eye. (**ii**) Blocked drainage channel in glaucoma. (**iii**) Normal IOP in a vitreous cavity and normal optical nerve in a healthy eye. (**iv**) Rise in IOP in a vitreous cavity and changes in the optical nerve in glaucoma. (**v**) Ocular fluid is produced in a posterior chamber at the ciliary body behind the iris and flows through the anterior chamber of the eye to ultimately come out through the uveoscleral pathway (highlighted by the black arrow). (**vi**) Rise in IOP and oxidative stress in the glaucoma-conditioned eye finally led to damage to retinal ganglion cells and optical nerves. Reproduced from Patel et al. [10], Elsevier, 2022.

Nanotechnology-mediated drug delivery approaches involved the delivery of loaded therapeutics employing nano drug carriers of polymeric, lipidic, inorganic, and biological origin [11,12]. Nano drug carriers prepared from the polymer entail a nanoparticulate system of natural/synthetic origin and are biodegradable/nonbiodegradable in nature such as chitosan, poly lactic-co-glycolic acid (PLGA), polycaprolactone (PCL), etc. [13,14]. Nano drug carriers prepared from lipids are nanoparticulate/nanovesicular systems of natural/synthetic lipids of a biodegradable/nonbiodegradable nature such as phospholipid (lecithins), stearic acid, glycerol monostearate, compritol®, etc. [15,16]. Furthermore, nano drug carriers prepared from inorganic materials are a nanoparticulate system of metallic/nonmetallic origin such as gold, silver, mesoporous silica, carbon, etc. [17,18]. Similarly, erythrocytes (red blood cells) are also utilized as drug carriers for the administration of loaded therapeutics in a biological system to achieve efficacy in different disease conditions [19,20]. Among the various drug carrier systems utilized to improve disease conditions in glaucoma, chitosan is a nanomaterial widely explored for ocular drug administration, particularly in the management of glaucoma [21,22]. The specific characteristics of chitosan (such as mucoadhesion to the cornea, biodegradability in nature, antimicrobial properties, etc.) [23] make it a promising nanomaterial to design a nanomedicine for ocular drug delivery in the management of glaucoma (Schematic illustration in Figure 2). The comparative advantages of nanotechnology-mediated ocular drug delivery with respect to conventional ocular drug delivery are summarized in Table 1.

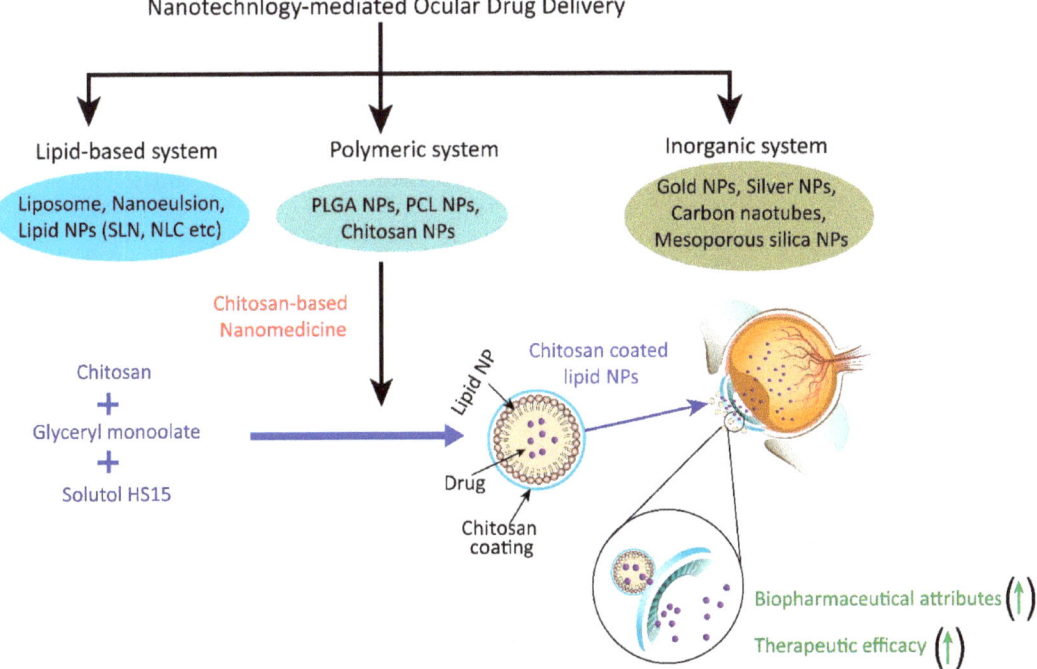

Figure 2. Nanotechnology-mediated drug delivery approach particularly regarding a chitosan-based nanomedicine employed to improve the biopharmaceutical attributes and therapeutic efficacy of a loaded drug in glaucoma. (↑) indicates improvement/increase.

Table 1. Comparative advantages of nanotechnology-mediated ocular drug delivery in respect to conventional ocular drug delivery.

Conventional Ocular Drug Delivery	Nanotechnology-Mediated Ocular Drug Delivery
Limited aqueous solubility	Improved aqueous solubility
Limited ocular/corneal permeability	Improved ocular/corneal permeability
Immediate effects	Sustained/prolong effects
Nonspecific	Specific
Low bioavailability and intersubject variability	Improved bioavailability and minimized intersubject variability
Limited drug efficacy	Improved drug efficacy
Possibility of untoward effects	Minimized possibility of untoward effects

The present manuscript provides a detailed discussion of the recent advancement of chitosan-based nanomedicine for its utilization to improve the efficacy of loaded therapeutics in better glaucoma management. The manuscript also discusses the significance of chitosan-based nanomedicine for its ocular delivery in glaucoma along with main emphasis on recent research carried out in the last 2 years in this area.

2. Significance of Chitosan-Based Nanomedicine to Overcome Drug Delivery Challenges in Glaucoma

Chitosan is a biodegradable natural polymer that has been investigated extensively due to its strong mucoadhesive qualities [24]. The drug's mucoadhesion and retention time on the ocular surface are enhanced by the ionic interactions enabled by its positively charged nature with the anionic ocular mucosa [25]. As a result, a chitosan-based nanoparticulate system can lessen the number of ocular injections required and boost long-term patient compliance [26]. Chitosan improves permeability by relaxing the tight connections between cells [27]. Furthermore, it is produced from crustacean exoskeletons and fungal cell walls via deacetylation, so its production cost is low and its ecological impact is minimal. Chitosan, in particular, demonstrates remarkable swelling behaviors in a variety of physiological environments, making it a potentially useful platform for research into stimuli-responsive biological delivery systems.

In recent times, mucoadhesive nanoparticulate systems particularly, chitosan-based nanomedicines, have been widely explored for their specific characteristics (illustrated in Figure 3) in terms of their ocular application to overcome the challenges of ophthalmic drug delivery. It is interesting to note that chitosan immune-modulating capabilities minimize specific inflammatory responses through intracellular signaling pathways (cGAS-STING, and NLRP3) [24]. This signify the possible role of chitosan in the treatment of age-related diseases and its effect on inflammatory cytokines.

The chitosan-based nanomedicine is helpful in protecting loaded therapeutics from unintended drug release, degradation/instability, and making it easier to cross through different ocular barriers (illustrated in Figure 4) in drug absorption [6].

Chitosan-based nanomedicine has a wide utility in biomedical applications including therapeutic, diagnostic, and theranostic purposes in different disease conditions [28]. The literature survey using the keywords "chitosan" and "ocular drug delivery" in the SCOPUS database indicated exponential growth in publications during the last 20 years (1993–2022) as shown in Figure 5.

Furthermore, the analysis of the results showed that out of nearly 4500 publications in the last 20 years, more than 1100 publications had been added to the SCOPUS database in just these two years. Therefore, in the present review, the research papers in these two years that explored chitosan for the ocular delivery of drugs, particularly in the management of glaucoma, were discussed in detail. The different types of chitosan-based nanomedicine employed for ocular drug delivery are discussed in the subsequent section.

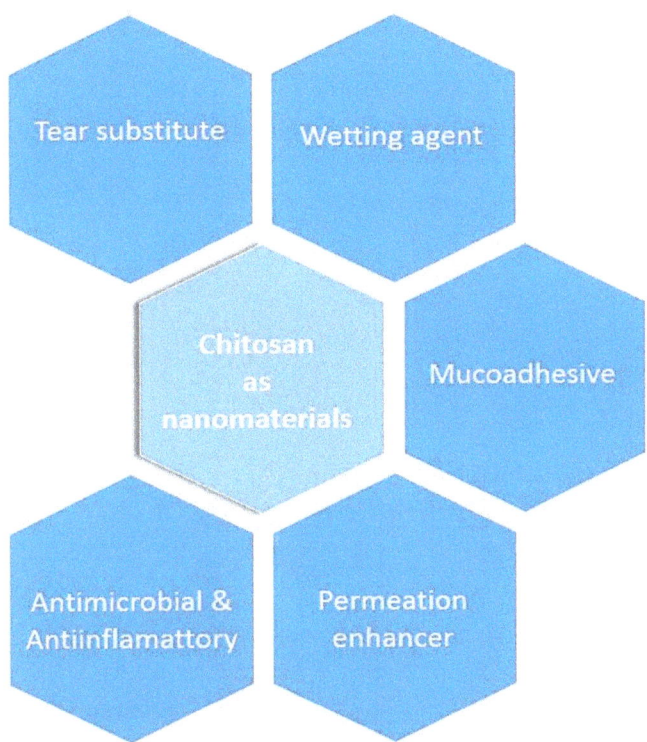

Figure 3. The characteristics that make chitosan a nanomaterial and a promising candidate for nanotechnology-mediated ocular drug delivery in glaucoma.

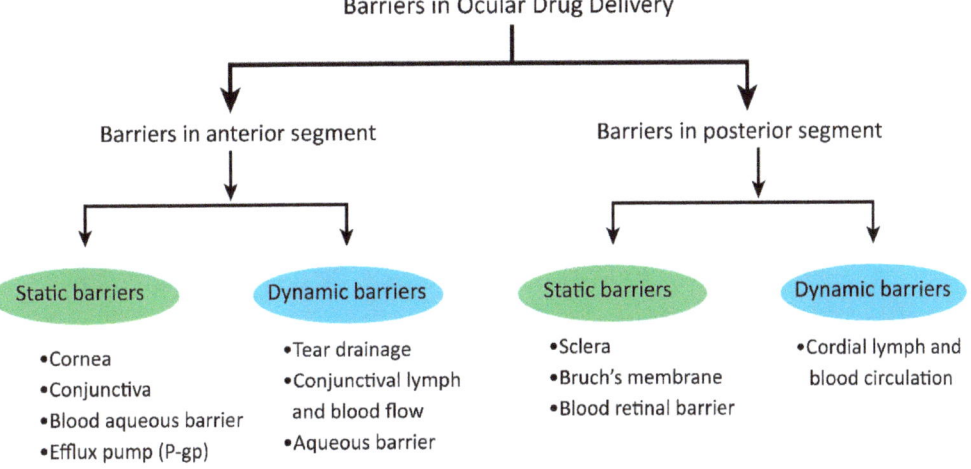

Figure 4. Different barriers in ocular drug delivery for glaucoma pose challenges in ocular bioavailability.

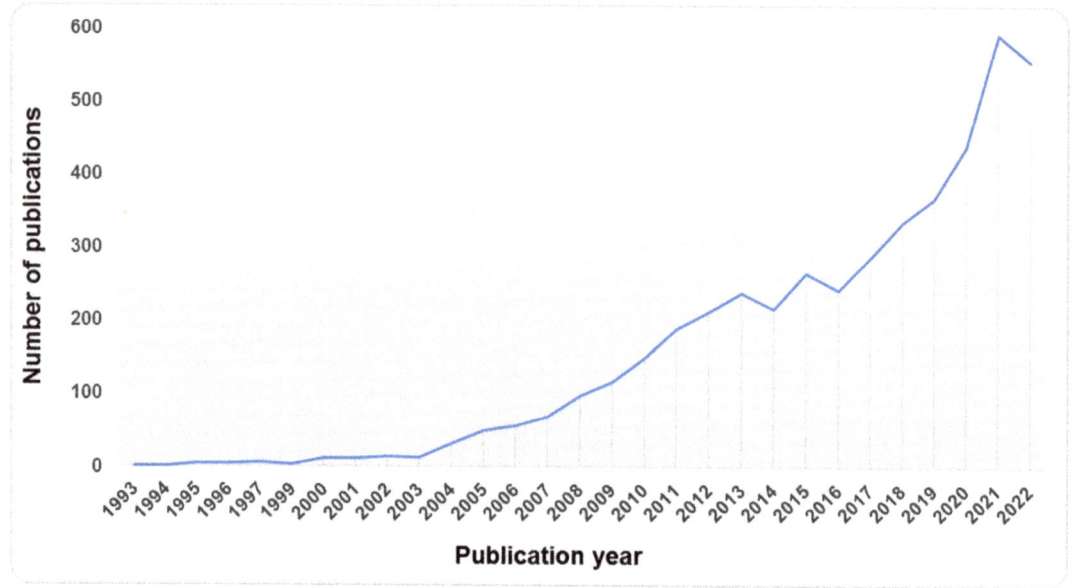

Figure 5. Graph depicts the number of publications in the concerning year published after using keywords "chitosan" and "ocular drug delivery" in the SCOPUS database.

3. Different Types of Chitosan-Based Nanomedicine for Ocular Application

Different types of chitosan-based nanomedicines (such as chitosan NPs, chitosan-coated NPs, and chitosan-based hybrid NPs) have been widely explored in recent years for their ocular applications in glaucoma (Illustrated in Figure 6).

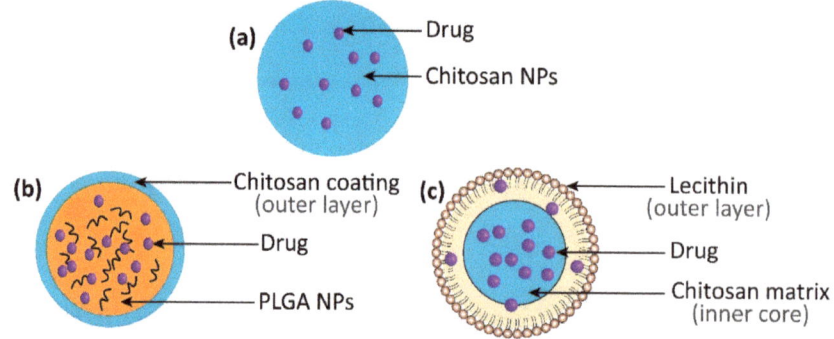

Figure 6. Different types of chitosan-based nanomedicines. (**a**) Chitosan NPs. (**b**) Chitosan-coated NPs. (**c**) Chitosan-based hybrid NPs.

The different characteristics of the chitosan polymer such as molecular weight and deacetylation degree impacted the mucoadhesion to ocular tissues [29]. It is reported in the literature that increasing the chitosan deacetylation degree from 60.7% to 98.5% leads to slower degradation, low drug entrapment, and prolonged drug release profile [30]. Furthermore, chitosan oligosaccharide coated NPs help to delay the clearance of ocular formulation and significantly enhance the AUC of a loaded drug due to improved transcorneal penetration compared to noncoated NPs [31]. The detail related to different types of chitosan-based nanomedicines are discussed in the subsequent section.

3.1. Chitosan Nanoparticles

The chitosan nanoparticles are fabricated by ionic or covalent crosslinking, emulsification, precipitation, or combinations thereof [32]. It is a convenient carrier for drugs and is bioactive. Recently, Mohamed et al. fabricated meloxicam-loaded chitosan nanoparticles using the "polyelectrolyte complexation" method [33]. Chitosan (0.25–0.5% w/v) was first dissolved in an aqueous acetic acid solution (0.5–1% v/v), and the pH was adjusted to 4.7 using a molar solution of sodium hydroxide. Meloxicam particles were then dissolved in either a tripolyphosphate aqueous solution (0.25% w/v) or PEG 400 (100% v/v). Meloxicam-loaded chitosan nanoparticles can be produced spontaneously by adding meloxicam solution drop by drop to a magnetically agitated chitosan solution (10 mL) for 30 min, followed by probe sonication for 10 min.

In another investigation, Ricci et al. prepared chitosan nanoparticles containing indomethacin by the "ionotropic gelation" method [34]. The amine group of chitosan, which has a positive charge, reacts with the sulfonic group of sulfobutyl ether cyclodextrin complexed with indomethacin. The chitosan nanoparticles were stabilized by polysorbate 80 (0.5% w/v) as a nonionic stabilizer. Furthermore, the prepared nanoparticles were coated with a thiolated derivative of low molecular weight hyaluronic acid. It was also reported in an earlier investigation [35]. The significance of this investigation is that only a small amount of the drug was lost during nano-encapsulation.

3.2. Chitosan Coated Nanoformulation System

A chitosan coated nanoformulation system was designed by the coating of chitosan over different nanoparticulate-based drug delivery systems such as liposomes, inorganic, polymeric, and lipidic nanoparticles to impart additional physicochemical characteristics (such as improving the residence time, corneal penetration, and ultimately ocular bioavailability of loaded therapeutics) for ocular drug delivery [36,37]. Recently, Badran et al. prepared metoprolol-loaded liposomes coated with chitosan for ocular application [38]. The metoprolol-loaded liposomes were added dropwise to the chitosan solution at different concentrations (0.25–1% w/v) in an equivalent volume under probe ultrasonication for 3 min, and the resulting suspension was kept on a magnetic stirrer for 2 h at an ambient temperature to achieve successful coating. The study indicated that increasing the amount of chitosan enhanced the vesicle size of liposomes. Moreover, the zeta potential of metoprolol-loaded liposomes was found to change from negative to positive after coating with chitosan. In addition, it was found that the positive charge increased upon increasing the amount of chitosan from 0.25% w/v to 1% w/v. The change in size morphology of metoprolol-loaded deformable liposome and metoprolol-loaded chitosan-coated deformable liposome was examined through transmission electron microscopy (TEM) and shown in Figure 7.

The positive charge could be attributed to the presence of an amine group on chitosan molecules [39]. In another investigation, pilocarpine-loaded ceria nanocapsules were modified with chitosan of different amination levels [40]. Amination levels are critical and may affect the pH-responsive release because free amine groups on the chitosan backbone considerably affect the swelling behavior of chitosan [41].

Ceria nanocapsules werechosen as the carriers for drug delivery because they have a huge cavity inside that can load a significant amount of drugs. It also has strong bioactive properties that help to reduce inflammation, which is a major risk factor for acute glaucoma [42,43]. The rate at which pilocarpine is released from ceria nanocapsules is controlled by the acetylation and deacetylation of the functional chitosan coatings with acetic anhydride and sodium hydroxide, respectively. The surface of the ceria nanocapsule was modified with chitosan using a conjugation method. Briefly, the ends of "phosphonate polyethylene glycol with a carboxylic acid group" can be added to the surface of nanoceria materials so that they can bond with chitosan. Phosphonate groups have a high affinity for cerium surfaces, whereas COOH groups can chemically conjugate with amino groups on the chitosan backbone. The study showed that higher levels of amination can lead to more positive charges on the surface, likely because there are more amino groups [44]. Similarly, chitosan-coated tetrandrine containing bovine serum albumin nanoparticles were formulated and optimized for the concentration of BSA, chitosan, glutaraldehyde, and pH to achieve the desired physiochemical properties for the effective treatment of ocular glaucoma [45]. At pH levels above the isoelectric point (pH > 5) of bovine serum albumin, the net charge of a developed nanoparticle is very negative. This causes molecules and smaller nanoparticles to stick together minimally. The study found that as glutaraldehyde decreased from 8% to 4%, particle size and the polydispersity index decreased significantly, while the zeta potential increased. The coating of chitosan on the nanoparticle is meant to enhance ocular residence and transcorneal penetration of the drug with poor aqueous solubility. The developed system caused the drug to be released over a longer period. Compared to tetrandrine suspension, drug release was much slower in the case of albumin nanoparticles. The drug release was further suppressed by the chitosan coating on albumin nanoparticles. However, the drug release differential between the chitosan-coated albumin nanoparticles and the uncoated albumin nanoparticles disappeared in the later phase, possibly because of water uptake and swelling of the chitosan coat over time [46,47].

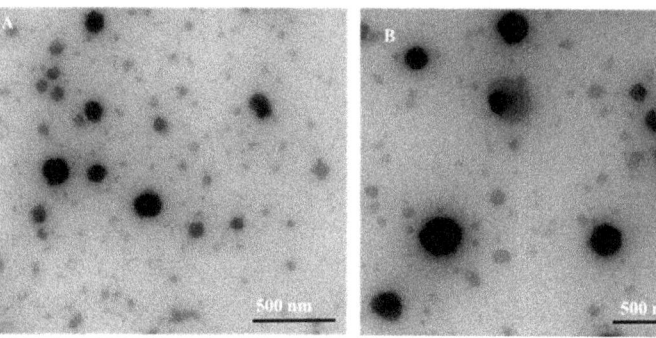

Figure 7. TEM image of (**A**) metoprolol-loaded deformable liposome and (**B**) metoprolol-loaded chitosan coated deformable liposome. Reproduced from Badran et al. [38].

3.3. Chitosan-Based Hybrid Nanoparticles

Chitosan-based hybrid nanoparticles may be prepared by a single step emulsion-sonication process employing a combination of polymers such as polycaprolactone, hyaluronic acid, polylactic-co-glycolic acid, etc., for ocular drug delivery [48,49]. Recently, Silva et al. prepared epoetin-β loaded chitosan-based hybrid nanoparticles in combination with a hyaluronic acid polymer to improve their mucoadhesion and residence time in the ocular tissues to improve their ocular absorption [50]. Epoetin-β, which is a recombinant form of human epoetin, was chosen as the active ingredient because it might protect and repair nerve cells, which could help to treat glaucoma. Ionotropic gelation was used to make hybrid nanoparticles using different hyaluronic acids. Out of six hyaluronic acids with different molecular weights (50–3000 kDa), one is in crystal form, and another is eye-grade hyaluronic acid. Further research is being conducted on nanoparticles with particle sizes of less than 300 nm, zeta potentials around +30 mV, and a low polydispersity index. It was observed that the high molecular weight hyaluronic acid had the highest entrapment efficiency (39.9 ± 0.6%) and drug loading (18.1 ± 0.3%), respectively. In another investigation, using a quality-by-design (QbD) approach and the ionotropic gelation process, Saha et al. created resveratrol-loaded mucoadhesive lecithin/chitosan hybrid nanoparticles. These nanoparticles were mucoadhesive [51]. Lecithin-chitosan hybrid nanoparticles were made by combining negatively charged lecithin with positively charged chitosan and allowing them to interact with each other to design a hybrid nanoparticulate system. The study utilized poloxamer 407 to dissolve chitosan, while resveratrol was dispersed in an ethanolic solution of lecithin. Subsequently, the alcoholic solution of resveratrol was rapidly injected into the aqueous chitosan-poloxamer 407 solutions under continuous stirring at 1500 rpm to develop chitosan-based hybrid nanoparticles. Chitosan-based hybrid nanoparticles are prepared for various therapeutics including melatonin [52], quercetin [53], insulin [54], diflucortolone valerate [55], and paclitaxel [56].

Different types of chitosan-based nanomedicines (such as chitosan nanoparticles, mucoadhesive chitosan-coated nano drug delivery systems, chitosan-based hybrid nano drug delivery systems, etc.) were explored for ocular applications to improve the biopharmaceutical attributes (such as aqueous solubility, corneal permeability, drug stability, and ocular pharmacokinetic, etc.) and pharmacodynamics performance of loaded therapeutics in glaucoma. The contemporary research carried out in this area in recent times is discussed in a subsequent section.

4. Chitosan-Based Nanomedicine for Ocular Application in Glaucoma: Contemporary Research

4.1. Improvement in Biopharmaceutical Attributes of Loaded Drugs

Chitosan-based nano formulation systems were investigated for various drugs to improve corneal penetration and residence time on the cornea, thus leading to enhanced ocular bioavailability of antiglaucoma drugs and improving their therapeutic efficacy [57–59]. One of the recently published investigations reported that the negatively charged mucus layer on the surface of the eye interacts with cationic chitosan-coated ceria nanocapsules through electrostatic forces [60]. This makes the ceria nanocapsules more resistant to tears and blinks, which means they remain adhered on the cornea surface for a longer period. Chitosan-coated ceria nanocapsules with strong amination diminish negative charges of mucin. The tight connections can be opened with the help of chitosan coatings, as proposed by Nguyen et al. [40], and this ability can be improved by raising the amination level of chitosan. Immunofluorescence labeling of ZO-1 in SIRC cells was used to examine the amination level's effect on opening the epithelial tight junctions in chitosan-coated ceria nanocapsules. ZO-1 is a crucial cytoplasmic protein involved in membrane activities; it can connect to transmembrane barrier proteins and stabilize tight junctions. At the edges of the SIRC cells, there was a distinct arrangement of ZO-1 in both the control and ceria nanocapsule groups, which showed that Ce-NCs could not open the tight junctions (Figure 8).

As shown in Figure 6, the ZO-1 patterns changed in response to the amination levels of the chitosan coatings for the groups that were treated with low (L), medium (M), and high (H) levels of amination. Chitosan-coated ceria nanocapsules lost pattern integrity and cellular boundaries as amination increased. The result shows that coatings made of chitosan can help ceria nanocapsules to open tight junctions. Furthermore, the ability to open the tight junctions can be increased by adding more amination levels. This study also indicated that the pilocarpine concentrations in the anterior chamber of the eye for the group treated with chitosan-coated ceria nanocapsules with varying amination levels (6.14 ± 2.14 (L), 12.56 ± 1.21 (M), and 25.72 ± 1.68 (H) μg/mL, respectively) were observed to be significantly higher compared to conventional eye drop formulations (0.93 ± 0.64 μg/mL) and the group treated with pilocarpine-loaded ceria nanocapsules (0.58 ± 0.71 μg/mL). The results suggest that the absorption of pilocarpine in the aqueous humor can be enhanced 44-fold by utilizing the chitosan covering with the highest amination level [40].

Tetrandrine shows promise as a prospective glaucoma therapy [61]. However, its restricted ocular bioavailability is a result of its poor aqueous solubility. After 6 h, merely 2.21 ± 0.7% of the tetrandrine suspension had penetrated the cornea. The apparent permeability coefficient for tetrandrine-loaded albumin nanoparticles increased by a factor of 2.3, and the amount of tetrandrine that was able to pass through the membrane increased to 4.72 ± 0.29%. Furthermore, chitosan coating of albumin nanoparticles showed a significant increase (11-fold and 5-fold) in the percentage of tetrandrine permeated compared to tetrandrine suspension and tetrandrine-loaded albumin nanoparticles, respectively. The developed system helps to improve (4-fold and 1.7-fold) the apparent permeability coefficient compared to tetrandrine suspension and tetrandrine-loaded albumin nanoparticles, respectively. The study also indicated a two-times increase in ocular bioavailability of tetrandrine from developed chitosan-coated albumin nanoparticles compared to tetrandrine suspension and tetrandrine-loaded albumin nanoparticles [45]. In another study, trimethyl chitosan-coated lipid nanoparticles significantly prolonged the residence of tetrandrine in tears and enhanced ocular absorption as compared to tetrandrine solution [62]. In addition, when compared to a pure drug solution, the area under the curve (AUC), elimination half-life, and mean residence time (MRT) of the developed system were increased by 2, 3, and 1.67-fold, respectively.

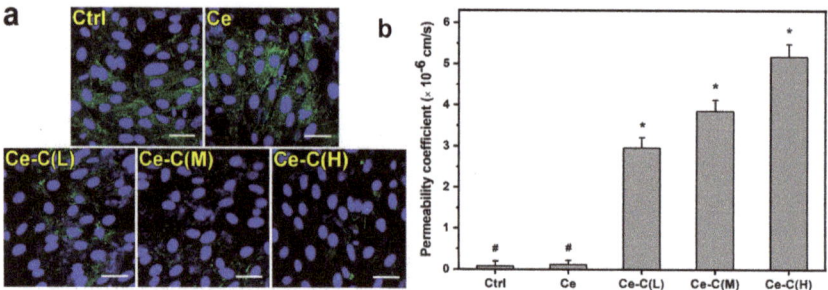

Figure 8. In vitro corneal permeability characteristics. (**a**) CLSM images of SIRC cell layers immunofluorescently stained with DAPI (blue fluorescence) and ZO-1 (green fluorescence) after incubation (for 4 h) with ceria nanocapsule (Ce) and chitosan-coated ceria nanocapsules with varying amination levels [Ce-C(L), Ce-C(M), Ce-C(H)). Ctrl: without test materials. (**b**) The permeability coefficient of ceria nanocapsules and chitosan-coated ceria nanocapsules (Ce) with varying amination levels [Ce-C(L), Ce-C(M), Ce-C(H)]. Ctrl: without test materials. Reproduced from Nguyen et al. [40], Elsevier, 2023. * $p < 0.05$ verses all groups; # $p < 0.05$ verses Ce-C(L), Ce-C(M), and Ce-C(H) groups.

In another investigation, Badran et al. indicated the enhanced penetration of metoprolol from the chitosan-coated flexible liposomes [38]. The enhanced permeability of metoprolol from liposomes could be due to the nanoscale dimension and flexible membrane of liposomes due to the presence of Tween 80 [63]. Furthermore, the cationic nature of chitosan on the liposome surface provided electrostatic interactions and hydrogen bonding with mucin on the ocular surface [64,65]. Hence, it demonstrated better permeation across the cornea compared to uncoated liposomes. In addition, chitosan coating over the surface of various nanodrug carriers was shown to promote corneal permeability by relaxing intracellular or tight connections between corneal epithelial cells [64]. Contemporary research related to chitosan-based nanomedicine utilized to increase the biopharmaceutical qualities of loaded drugs for glaucoma is summarized in Table 2.

Table 2. Chitosan-based nanomedicine utilized to improve the biopharmaceutical attributes of loaded therapeutics.

Type of Nanomedicine	Therapeutics	Composition	Biopharmaceutical Attributes	Ref.
Chitosan-coated NPs	Metoprolol	Chitosan, phosphatidylcholine, cholesterol	- Developed system exhibited extended drug release and significant mucin mucoadhesion resulting in an increase in residence time after ocular administration. - It has shown a 4.4-fold increase in ocular permeability compared to pure metoprolol.	[38]

Table 2. Cont.

Type of Nanomedicine	Therapeutics	Composition	Biopharmaceutical Attributes	Ref.
Chitosan-coated NPs	Pilocarpine	Chitosan, silica, ethylene glycol, cerium nitrate	- High amination level of chitosan is helpful to enhance the corneal permeability of the developed system by 43-fold compared to medium and low amination levels. - Developed system exhibited a sustained drug release profile.	[40]
Chitosan-coated NPs	Tetrandrine	Chitosan, bovine serum albumin, glutaraldehyde	- Developed system exhibited sustained drug release (19.65% in 2 h) compared to the tetrandrine suspension (35.6% in 2 h). - Corneal permeation profile of the developed system was 23.79% compared to 2.21% for the tetrandrine suspension after 6 h. - Developed system has shown a two-times increase in ocular bioavailability in rabbits compared to the tetrandrine suspension.	[45]
Chitosan-coated NPs	Tetrandrine	Chitosan, glyceryl monooleate, poloxamer 407, kolliphor® HS 15	- Trimethyl chitosan-based hybrid systems exhibited sustained drug release and improvement in pharmacokinetic parameters ($AUC_{0 \to \infty}$, $T_{1/2}$, $MRT_{0 \to \infty}$) compared to the tetrandrine solution.	[62]
Chitosan-based hybrid NPs	Latanoprost	Chitosan, hyaluronic acid, sodium tripolyphosphate	- The developed system may enhance the retention time on the corneal and conjunctiva of loaded therapeutics.	[66]
Chitosan-based hybrid NPs	Epoetin beta (EPOβ)	Chitosan and hyaluronic acid	- Developed system efficiently delivered EPOβ to the retina after administration through the subconjunctival route in immunofluorescence investigation in rats.	[67]
Chitosan-based hybrid NPs	Dorzolamide	Chitosan, polycaprolactone, polyvinyl alcohol	- Developed system exhibited a significant improvement in mucoadhesion to the cornea and an enhancement in permeation across goat cornea compared to dorzolamide solution as a control.	[68]
Chitosan-based hybrid NPs	Brinzolamide	Chitosan, pectin, Tween 80	- Developed system exhibited extended drug release for 8 h and a significant increase in corneal permeability compared to the marketed product.	[69]

4.2. Improvement in the Therapeutic Efficacy of Loaded Drugs

Acute glaucoma is often caused by inflammation, and nanoceria is very good at reducing inflammation [70]. Recently, the impact of chitosan coating on the anti-inflammatory characteristics of ceria nanocapsules was investigated [40]. Previous research has shown that this nanoparticulate system helps to remove the free radicals and reduce the generation of inflammatory cytokines such as TNF-α, IL-6, and MCP-1 [71–73]. This makes them potent anti-inflammatory agents. LPS control intracellular signaling pathways and were used to cause inflammation [74]. The mitogen-activated protein kinase (MAPK) signaling process can control inflammation by boosting the levels of specific mediators such as Interleukin-6 and Prostaglandin E2, which are common in glaucoma [75,76]. The study showed similar levels of these biomarkers in ceria nanocapsules and chitosan-coated ceria nanocapsules. The investigation also reported that the functionalization of the nanoceria did not affect its ability to fight inflammation. The pharmacological effectiveness of chitosan-coated ceria nanocapsules containing pilocarpine was evaluated in an acute glaucoma model in rabbits. Pilocarpine was used because it makes the ciliary muscles tighten and the pupils constrict, which ultimately lowers the intraocular pressure (IOP) [77]. Notably, the investigation demonstrated that chitosan-coated ceria nanocapsules composed of high amination levels exhibit significant improvements in reducing intraocular pressure in comparison to the marketed pharmaceutical formulation (eye drops of pilocarpine) and uncoated ceria nanocapsules. The drug release profile was maintained for an extended period of time in all chitosan-based formulations. However, only the chitosan-coated ceria nanocapsule with a high amination level was able to reduce and maintain healthy IOP. This is due to the exceptional ability of high-amination chitosan-coated ceria nanocapsules to penetrate the corneal epithelium and lead to improved ocular absorption.

Li et al. found in their investigation that tetrandrine can protect ganglionic cells in the retina from the damage caused by ischemia [61]. Research has shown that tetrandrine, at a concentration of 0.3%, reduces intraocular pressure in hypertensive rats. Tetrandrine at a topical dosage of 0.3% was shown to be effective in reducing intraocular pressure [78]. IOP was reduced by tetrandrine suspensions in the period of 0.5–4 h, with a maximum decrease of 25.1 ± 3.8% at 4 h, although this effect was short-lived, perhaps because the drug was rapidly removed from the corneal surface [59]. Tetrandrine-loaded albumin nanoparticles are helpful to reduce the IOP by 26.1 ± 1.08% after 4 h of ocular administration similar to tetrandrine suspension, while chitosan-coated albumin nanoparticles are more helpful to reduce the IOP compared to the tetrandrine suspension and uncoated albumin nanoparticle. Figure 9 presents the reduction in IOP of the eye of a rabbit after a single instillation of tetrandrine suspension, a tetrandrine-loaded uncoated albumin nanoparticle, and/or a tetrandrine-loaded chitosan-coated albumin nanoparticle. It showed a successful reduction in IOP after the instillation of all three types of ocular formulation but the chitosan-coated nano formulation system was more effective in the reduction of IOP compared to other ocular formulations.

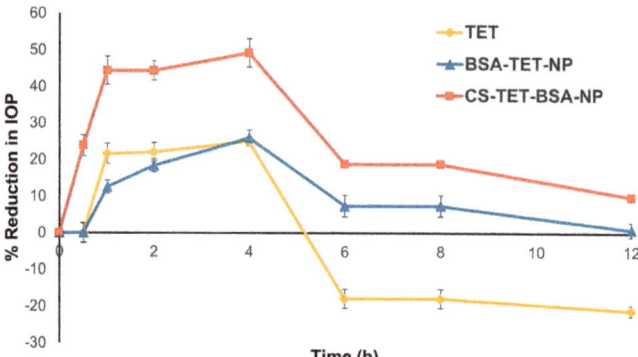

Figure 9. Illustration showed the results of antiglaucoma activity of different treatment investigations (TET: Tetrandrine suspension; TET-BSA-NPs: Tetrandrine loaded bovine serum albumin nanoparticles; CS-TET-BSA-NPs: Chitosan-coated bovine serum albumin nanoparticles containing tetrandrine). It highlights that the coating of chitosan over the bovine serum albumin nanoparticles is further helpful to reduce the IOP in rabbit glaucoma model compared to bovine serum albumin nanoparticles and tetrandrine suspension. Reproduced from Radwan et al. [45], Informa UK Limited, 2022.

As shown in Figure 9, the chitosan-coated nano formulation system is helpful to reduce the IOP by 49.35 ± 2.13% after 4 h of ocular administration. It was observed that the developed delivery system remains effective until 8 h after the ocular administration. It might be because chitosan interactions with mucin facilitate nanoparticle binding to the corneal membrane, extension of the corneal absorption of the drug, and ultimately improvement of the ocular efficacy of loaded therapeutics [79].

In another investigation, Badran et al. evaluated the lowering effect of plain metoprolol, metoprolol encapsulated liposome, and chitosan-coated liposome containing metoprolol on IOP using rabbits as an animal model [38]. The IOP-lowering impact of metoprolol was not fully evident after 1 h of metoprolol-loaded in situ gel instillation, but it was observed after 2, 3, 4, and 5 h following ocular application. In contrast, metoprolol-encapsulated uncoated and coated liposomes incorporated in in situ gels reduced IOP within the first hour after ocular application. Its impact lasted longer than that of a plain metoprolol-loaded in situ gel system. This investigation is in accordance with the previous investigation who reported that metoprolol ophthalmic gels extended the ocular residence time for >5 h [80]. After 6 h of ocular application, chitosan-coated metoprolol containing liposome incorporated in an situ gel system showed a 73.6 ± 4.13% decrease in IOP while metoprolol containing liposome incorporated in an situ gel system showed a 62.3 ± 6.28% decrease in IOP. Moreover, metoprolol-containing in situ gel systems showed only a 54.7 ± 3.15% reduction in IOP after 6 h of ocular application. This sustained effect on lowering IOP is the consequence of the greater corneal permeability of metoprolol upon administration of a chitosan-coated liposome formulation, which may result in increased contact duration and drug retention. Similarly, coating of glyco–chitosan on enalaprilat containing calcium phosphate nanoparticles significantly lowered the IOP for a longer period compared to the pure enalaprilat. The developed enalaprilat nanoparticulate system had a much greater influence on IOP. This effect could be due to the higher zeta potential of glycol–chitosan coated calcium phosphate nanoparticles, which impart a greater affinity towards negatively charged ocular corneal cells and hence provide better penetration [81]. Recently, Rubennicia et al. investigated the IOP lowering effect of latanoprost containing the chitosan–hyaluronic acid hybrid system in albino rats and compared its effect to the latanoprost alone [66]. The study indicated that the developed chitosan-based hybrid system has a significant improvement in the IOP lowering effect compared to that of plain latanoprost.

The neuroprotective effects of epoetin-β in glaucoma are encouraging. Silva et al. prepared a chitosan–hyaluronic acid hybrid system containing epoetin-β to improve their ocular bioavailability through increased mucoadhesion and prolonged residence in the ocular tissues [50]. The study evaluated the possibility of delivering epoetin-β to the ocular tissues through subconjunctival administration. The study found that the designed system could transport epoetin-β to the retina effectively. It was concluded that chitosan-based nanomedicine is thought to be safe for the in vivo system and could be a promising approach to treat retinopathy, such as glaucoma-related optic nerve degeneration. Radwan et al. proved in their investigation that chitosan coating over the nanoformulation system (such as bovine serum albumin nanoparticles) is helpful in further reducing the ocular irritation potential of the nanoformulation system (Illustrated in Figure 10) [45].

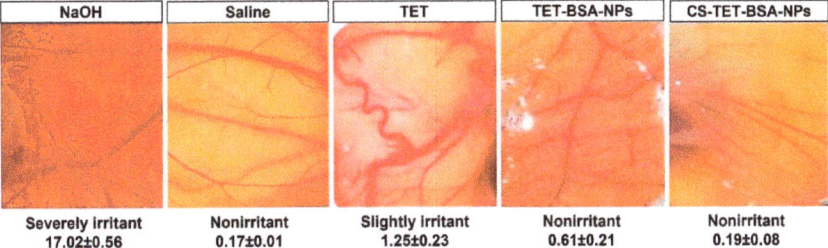

Figure 10. Illustration showed results of the hen's egg test-chorioallantoic membrane (HET-CAM) investigation after different treatments (TET: Tetrandrine suspension; TET-BSA-NPs: Tetrandrine loaded bovine serum albumin nanoparticles; CS-TET-BSA-NPs: Chitosan-coated bovine serum albumin nanoparticles containing tetrandrine). It highlights that the coating of chitosan over the bovine serum albumin nanoparticles is further helpful to reduce the ocular irritation index value compared to bovine serum albumin nanoparticles and tetrandrine suspension. Reproduced from Radwan et al. [45], Informa UK Limited, 2022.

The summary of current research on chitosan-based nanomedicines used to augment the therapeutic efficacy of loaded drugs for the management of glaucoma is presented in Table 3.

Table 3. Chitosan-based nanomedicine utilized to improve the pharmacodynamics performance of loaded therapeutics.

Type of Nanomedicine	Therapeutics	In Vivo Model	Pharmacodynamics Performance	Ref.
Chitosan-coated NPs	Metoprolol	Albino rabbits	Developed system exhibited a 73.6% decrease in IOP compared to a 54.7% decrease in IOP by the pure drug in a thermosensitive in situ gel after 6 h of ocular administration.	[38]
Chitosan-coated NPs	Pilocarpine	Acute glaucoma rabbit model	Developed system highly effective in decreasing the extremely high IOP (92 mmHg) to a normal level (20 mmHg) until 4 h of instillation.	[40]
Chitosan-coated NPs	Tetrandrine	Rabbits	Developed system exhibited a 49.35% decrease in IOP compared to a 25.1% decrease in IOP by a pure drug after 4 h of ocular administration.	[45]
Chitosan-based hybrid NPs	Latanoprost	Normotensive albino rabbits	A developed system is more effective in reducing the IOP than by a drug alone. IOP reduction during the treatment period was 27.3% by the developed chitosan-based system compared to 19.3% and 20.3% for the plain latanoprost and marketed product (Xalatan), respectively.	[66]
Chitosan-based hybrid NPs	Brinzolamide	Albino rabbits	Developed system exhibited significant improvement in % decrease in IOP and prolonged IOP lowering effect compared to the marketed product.	[69]
Chitosan-based hybrid NPs	Enalaprilat	Normotensive rabbits	Chitosan-calcium phosphate hybrid system exhibited a significant decrease in IOP after single instillation compared to enalaprilat in solution.	[81]

5. Conclusions

The chitosan-based nanoparticulate system indicated promising results in enhancing the biopharmaceutical attributes of various ocular therapeutics through the loosening of tight junctions present on the corneal epithelium. The chitosan nanoparticles or nanoparticles coated with chitosan showed a prolonged release of the drug and also offered mucoadhesion, which helped to augment the residence time of loaded therapeutics in different regions of the ocular tissues. The current review concluded that the chitosan nanoparticles and chitosan coating over different vesicular carrier systems (such as liposomes, micelles, and nanoemulsions) and nanoparticles showing advanced biocompatibility with chitosan, such as mesoporous silica nanoparticles [82], hypercrosslinked polymers [83], and polypeptides [84], have a significant impact to improve the residence time, corneal penetration, and ultimately ocular bioavailability of loaded therapeutics. Moreover, the research showed a significant improvement in the antiglaucoma activity of loaded therapeutics employing chitosan-based nanomedicine in preclinical investigations. However, the literature reveals that the clinical performance of chitosan-based nanomedicines through ocular drug delivery for glaucoma has yet to be addressed in detail. Furthermore, the safety perspectives of the chitosan-based nanomedicine in glaucoma should also be addressed systematically in future studies as it could increase the accumulation of the drug in the ocular tissues for a prolonged period, which could also increase the chances of therapeutic/adverse effects. In-depth molecular mechanisms of chitosan-coated NPs as anti-inflammatories to reduce neuroinflammation should be elucidated in future studies. In addition, ideal physicochemical characteristics (such as the molecular weight, degree of deacetylation, and level of amination) of chitosan being a nanomaterial for drug delivery in glaucoma should also be elucidated in future studies.

Funding: This work was funded by the Deanship of Scientific Research at Najran University, Saudi Arabia, under the Research Collaboration Funding program grant code (NU/RC/MRC/11/4).

Institutional Review Board Statement: Not applicable.

Informed Consent Statement: Not applicable.

Data Availability Statement: Not applicable.

Acknowledgments: The authors are thankful to the Deanship of Scientific Research at Najran University for funding this work under the Research Collaboration Funding program grant code (NU/RC/MRC/11/4).

Conflicts of Interest: The authors declare no conflict of interest.

References

1. Wagner, I.V.; Stewart, M.W.; Dorairaj, S.K. Updates on the Diagnosis and Management of Glaucoma. *Mayo Clin. Proc. Innov. Qual. Outcomes* **2022**, *6*, 618–635. [CrossRef] [PubMed]
2. Zhu, X.; Zeng, W.; Wu, S.; Chen, X.; Zheng, T.; Ke, M. Measurement of retinal changes in primary acute angle closure Glaucoma under different durations of symptoms. *J. Ophthalmol.* **2019**, *2019*, 540983. [CrossRef] [PubMed]
3. Almasieh, M.; Wilson, A.M.; Morquette, B.; Vargas JL, C.; Di Polo, A. The molecular basis of retinal ganglion cell death in glaucoma. *Prog. Retin. Eye Res.* **2012**, *31*, 152–181. [CrossRef] [PubMed]
4. Kumara, B.N.; Shambhu, R.; Prasad, K.S. Why chitosan could be apt candidate for glaucoma drug delivery–An overview. *Int. J. Biol. Macromol.* **2021**, *176*, 47–65. [CrossRef]
5. Sim, R.H.; Sirasanagandla, S.R.; Das, S.; Teoh, S.L. Treatment of glaucoma with natural products and their mechanism of action: An update. *Nutrients* **2022**, *14*, 534. [CrossRef]
6. Wadhwa, A.; Jadhav, C.; Yadav, K.S. Bimatoprost: Promising novel drug delivery systems in treatment of glaucoma. *J. Drug Deliv. Sci. Technol.* **2022**, *69*, 103156. [CrossRef]
7. Bachu, R.D.; Chowdhury, P.; Al-Saedi, Z.H.; Karla, P.K.; Boddu, S.H. Ocular drug delivery barriers—Role of nanocarriers in the treatment of anterior segment ocular diseases. *Pharmaceutics* **2018**, *10*, 28. [CrossRef]
8. Lanier, O.L.; Manfre, M.G.; Bailey, C.; Liu, Z.; Sparks, Z.; Kulkarni, S.; Chauhan, A. Review of approaches for increasing ophthalmic bioavailability for eye drop formulations. *AAPS Pharmscitech* **2021**, *22*, 107. [CrossRef]
9. Gómez-Garzón, M.; Martínez-Ceballos, M.A.; Gómez-López, A.; Rojas-Villarraga, A. Application of nanotechnology in ophthalmology: Where are we? *Charact. Appl. Nanomater.* **2022**, *5*, 66–78. [CrossRef]
10. Patel, K.D.; Silva, L.B.; Park, Y.; Shakouri, T.; Keskin-Erdogan, Z.; Sawadkar, P.; Kim, H.W. Recent advances in drug delivery systems for glaucoma treatment. *Mater. Today Nano* **2022**, *18*, 100178. [CrossRef]
11. Sahu, T.; Ratre, Y.K.; Chauhan, S.; Bhaskar LV, K.S.; Nair, M.P.; Verma, H.K. Nanotechnology based drug delivery system: Current strategies and emerging therapeutic potential for medical science. *J. Drug Deliv. Sci. Technol.* **2021**, *63*, 102487. [CrossRef]
12. Khiev, D.; Mohamed, Z.A.; Vichare, R.; Paulson, R.; Bhatia, S.; Mohapatra, S.; Biswal, M.R. Emerging nano-formulations and nanomedicines applications for ocular drug delivery. *Nanomaterials* **2021**, *11*, 173. [CrossRef]
13. Jain, A.; Prajapati, S.K.; Kumari, A.; Mody, N.; Bajpai, M. Engineered nanosponges as versatile biodegradable carriers: An insight. *J. Drug Deliv. Sci. Technol.* **2020**, *57*, 101643. [CrossRef]
14. Sur, R.; Rathore, A.; Dave, V.; Reddy, K.R.; Chouhan, R.S.; Sadhu, V. Recent developments in functionalized polymer nanoparticles for efficient drug delivery system. *Nano-Struct. Nano-Objects* **2019**, *20*, 100397. [CrossRef]
15. Buse, J.; El-Aneed, A. Properties, engineering and applications of lipid-based nanoparticle drug-delivery systems: Current research and advances. *Nanomedicine* **2010**, *5*, 1237–1260. [CrossRef]
16. Kraft, J.C.; Freeling, J.P.; Wang, Z.; Ho, R.J. Emerging research and clinical development trends of liposome and lipid nanoparticle drug delivery systems. *J. Pharm. Sci.* **2014**, *103*, 29–52. [CrossRef]
17. Ojea-Jimenez, I.; Comenge, J.; Garcia-Fernandez, L.; Megson, Z.A.; Casals, E.; Puntes, V.F. Engineered inorganic nanoparticles for drug delivery applications. *Curr. Drug Metab.* **2013**, *14*, 518–530. [CrossRef]
18. Vaneev, A.; Tikhomirova, V.; Chesnokova, N.; Popova, E.; Beznos, O.; Kost, O.; Klyachko, N. Nanotechnology for topical drug delivery to the anterior segment of the eye. *Int. J. Mol. Sci.* **2021**, *22*, 12368. [CrossRef]
19. Han, X.; Wang, C.; Liu, Z. Red blood cells as smart delivery systems. *Bioconj. Chem.* **2018**, *29*, 852–860. [CrossRef]
20. Li, Y.; Raza, F.; Liu, Y.; Wei, Y.; Rong, R.; Zheng, M.; Qiu, M. Clinical progress and advanced research of red blood cells based drug delivery system. *Biomaterials* **2021**, *279*, 121202. [CrossRef]
21. Bernkop-Schnürch, A.; Dünnhaupt, S. Chitosan-based drug delivery systems. *Eur. J. Pharm. Biopharm.* **2012**, *81*, 463–469. [CrossRef] [PubMed]
22. Irimia, T.; Ghica, M.V.; Popa, L.; Anuța, V.; Arsene, A.L.; Dinu-Pîrvu, C.E. Strategies for improving ocular drug bioavailability and corneal wound healing with chitosan-based delivery systems. *Polymers* **2018**, *10*, 1221. [CrossRef] [PubMed]
23. Burhan, A.M.; Klahan, B.; Cummins, W.; Andrés-Guerrero, V.; Byrne, M.E.; O'reilly, N.J.; Hughes, H. Posterior segment ophthalmic drug delivery: Role of muco-adhesion with a special focus on chitosan. *Pharmaceutics* **2021**, *13*, 1685. [CrossRef] [PubMed]
24. Fong, D.; Hoemann, C.D. Chitosan immunomodulatory properties: Perspectives on the impact of structural properties and dosage. *Future Sci. OA* **2018**, *4*, FSO225. [CrossRef]
25. Hamedi, H.; Moradi, S.; Hudson, S.M.; Tonelli, A.E.; King, M.W. Chitosan based bioadhesives for biomedical applications: A review. *Carbohydr. Polym.* **2022**, *282*, 119100. [CrossRef]
26. Silva, B.; São Braz, B.; Delgado, E.; Gonçalves, L. Colloidal nanosystems with mucoadhesive properties designed for ocular topical delivery. *Int. J. Pharm.* **2021**, *606*, 120873. [CrossRef]

27. Sun, X.; Sheng, Y.; Li, K.; Sai, S.; Feng, J.; Li, Y.; Tian, B. Mucoadhesive phenylboronic acid conjugated chitosan oligosaccharide-vitamin E copolymer for topical ocular delivery of voriconazole: Synthesis, in vitro/vivo evaluation, and mechanism. *Acta Biomater.* **2022**, *138*, 193–207. [CrossRef]
28. Jhaveri, J.; Raichura, Z.; Khan, T.; Momin, M.; Omri, A. Chitosan nanoparticles-insight into properties, functionalization and applications in drug delivery and theranostics. *Molecules* **2021**, *26*, 272. [CrossRef]
29. Zamboulis, A.; Nanaki, S.; Michailidou, G.; Koumentakou, I.; Lazaridou, M.; Ainali, N.M.; Bikiaris, D.N. Chitosan and its derivatives for ocular delivery formulations: Recent advances and developments. *Polymers* **2020**, *12*, 1519. [CrossRef]
30. Luo, L.J.; Huang, C.C.; Chen, H.C.; Lai, J.Y.; Matsusaki, M. Effect of deacetylation degree on controlled pilocarpine release from injectable chitosan-g-poly (N-isopropylacrylamide) carriers. *Carbohydr. Polym.* **2018**, *197*, 375–384. [CrossRef]
31. Luo, Q.; Zhao, J.; Zhang, X.; Pan, W. Nanostructured lipid carrier (NLC) coated with Chitosan Oligosaccharides and its potential use in ocular drug delivery system. *Int. J. Pharm.* **2011**, *403*, 185–191. [CrossRef]
32. Yanat, M.; Schroën, K. Preparation methods and applications of chitosan nanoparticles; with an outlook toward reinforcement of biodegradable packaging. *React. Funct. Polym.* **2021**, *161*, 104849. [CrossRef]
33. Mohamed, H.B.; Attia Shafie, M.A.; Mekkawy, A.I. Chitosan Nanoparticles for Meloxicam Ocular Delivery: Development, In Vitro Characterization, and In Vivo Evaluation in a Rabbit Eye Model. *Pharmaceutics* **2022**, *14*, 893. [CrossRef]
34. Ricci, F.; Racaniello, G.F.; Lopedota, A.; Laquintana, V.; Arduino, I.; Lopalco, A.; Denora, N. Chitosan/sulfobutylether-β-cyclodextrin based nanoparticles coated with thiolated hyaluronic acid for indomethacin ophthalmic delivery. *Int. J. Pharm.* **2022**, *622*, 121905. [CrossRef]
35. Kalam, M.A. Development of chitosan nanoparticles coated with hyaluronic acid for topical ocular delivery of dexamethasone. *Int. J. Biol. Macromol.* **2016**, *89*, 127–136. [CrossRef]
36. Nagarwal, R.C.; Kumar, R.; Pandit, J.K. Chitosan coated sodium alginate–chitosan nanoparticles loaded with 5-FU for ocular delivery: In vitro characterization and in vivo study in rabbit eye. *Eur. J. Pharm. Sci.* **2012**, *47*, 678–685. [CrossRef]
37. Wang, F.Z.; Zhang, M.W.; Zhang, D.S.; Huang, Y.; Chen, L.; Jiang, S.M.; Li, R. Preparation, optimization, and characterization of chitosan-coated solid lipid nanoparticles for ocular drug delivery. *J. Biomed. Res.* **2018**, *32*, 411.
38. Badran, M.M.; Alomrani, A.H.; Almomen, A.; Bin Jardan, Y.A.; Abou El Ela, A.E.S. Novel Metoprolol-Loaded Chitosan-Coated Deformable Liposomes in Thermosensitive In Situ Gels for the Management of Glaucoma: A Repurposing Approach. *Gels* **2022**, *8*, 635. [CrossRef]
39. Roy, S.; Goh, K.L.; Verma, C.; Dasgupta Ghosh, B.; Sharma, K.; Maji, P.K. A Facile Method for Processing Durable and Sustainable Superhydrophobic Chitosan-Based Coatings Derived from Waste Crab Shell. *ACS Sustain. Chem. Eng.* **2022**, *10*, 4694–4704. [CrossRef]
40. Nguyen, D.D.; Yao, C.H.; Lue, S.J.; Yang, C.J.; Su, Y.H.; Huang, C.C.; Lai, J.Y. Amination-mediated nano eye-drops with enhanced corneal permeability and effective burst release for acute glaucoma treatment. *Chem. Eng. J.* **2023**, *451*, 138620. [CrossRef]
41. Jiao, J.; Li, X.; Zhang, S.; Liu, J.; Di, D.; Zhang, Y.; Wang, S. Redox and pH dual-responsive PEG and chitosan-conjugated hollow mesoporous silica for controlled drug release. *Mater. Sci. Eng. C* **2016**, *67*, 26–33. [CrossRef] [PubMed]
42. Hirst, S.M.; Karakoti, A.S.; Tyler, R.D.; Sriranganathan, N.; Seal, S.; Reilly, C.M. Anti-inflammatory properties of cerium oxide nanoparticles. *Small* **2009**, *5*, 2848–2856. [CrossRef] [PubMed]
43. Chi, W.; Li, F.; Chen, H.; Wang, Y.; Zhu, Y.; Yang, X.; Zhuo, Y. Caspase-8 promotes NLRP1/NLRP3 inflammasome activation and IL-1β production in acute glaucoma. *Proc. Natl. Acad. Sci. USA* **2014**, *111*, 11181–11186. [CrossRef] [PubMed]
44. Richard, S.; Boucher, M.; Saric, A.; Herbet, A.; Lalatonne, Y.; Petit, P.X.; Motte, L. Optimization of pegylated iron oxide nanoplatforms for antibody coupling and bio-targeting. *J. Mater. Chem. B* **2017**, *5*, 2896–2907. [CrossRef]
45. Radwan SE, S.; El-Moslemany, R.M.; Mehanna, R.A.; Thabet, E.H.; Abdelfattah EZ, A.; El-Kamel, A. Chitosan-coated bovine serum albumin nanoparticles for topical tetrandrine delivery in glaucoma: In vitro and in vivo assessment. *Drug Deliv.* **2022**, *29*, 1150–1163. [CrossRef]
46. Raj, R.; Wairkar, S.; Sridhar, V.; Gaud, R. Pramipexole dihydrochloride loaded chitosan nanoparticles for nose to brain delivery: Development, characterization and in vivo anti-Parkinson activity. *Int. J. Biol. Macromol.* **2018**, *109*, 27–35. [CrossRef]
47. Piazzini, V.; Landucci, E.; D'Ambrosio, M.; Fasiolo, L.T.; Cinci, L.; Colombo, G.; Bergonzi, M.C. Chitosan coated human serum albumin nanoparticles: A promising strategy for nose-to-brain drug delivery. *Int. J. Biol. Macromol.* **2019**, *129*, 267–280. [CrossRef]
48. Khan, N.; Khanna, K.; Bhatnagar, A.; Ahmad, F.J.; Ali, A. Chitosan coated PLGA nanoparticles amplify the ocular hypotensive effect of forskolin: Statistical design, characterization and in vivo studies. *Int. J. Biol. Macromol.* **2018**, *116*, 648–663. [CrossRef]
49. Jiang, P.; Jacobs, K.M.; Ohr, M.P.; Swindle-Reilly, K.E. Chitosan–polycaprolactone core–shell microparticles for sustained delivery of bevacizumab. *Mol. Pharm.* **2020**, *17*, 2570–2584. [CrossRef]
50. Silva, B.; Marto, J.; São Braz, B.; Delgado, E.; Almeida, A.J.; Gonçalves, L. New nanoparticles for topical ocular delivery of erythropoietin. *Int. J. Pharm.* **2020**, *576*, 119020. [CrossRef]
51. Saha, M.; Saha, D.R.; Ulhosna, T.; Sharker, S.M.; Shohag, M.H.; Islam, M.S.; Reza, H.M. QbD based development of resveratrol-loaded mucoadhesive lecithin/chitosan nanoparticles for prolonged ocular drug delivery. *J. Drug Deliv. Sci. Technol.* **2021**, *63*, 102480. [CrossRef]
52. Hafner, A.; Lovrić, J.; Voinovich, D.; Filipović-Grčić, J. Melatonin-loaded lecithin/chitosan nanoparticles: Physicochemical characterisation and permeability through Caco-2 cell monolayers. *Int. J. Pharm.* **2009**, *381*, 205–213. [CrossRef]

53. Tan, Q.; Liu, W.; Guo, C.; Zhai, G. Preparation and evaluation of quercetin-loaded lecithin-chitosan nanoparticles for topical delivery. *Int. J. Nanomed.* **2011**, *6*, 1621.
54. Liu, L.; Zhou, C.; Xia, X.; Liu, Y. Self-assembled lecithin/chitosan nanoparticles for oral insulin delivery: Preparation and functional evaluation. *Int. J. Nanomed.* **2016**, *11*, 761. [CrossRef]
55. Özcan, İ.; Azizoğlu, E.; Şenyiğit, T.; Özyazıcı, M.; Özer, Ö. Enhanced dermal delivery of diflucortolone valerate using lecithin/chitosan nanoparticles: In-vitro and in-vivo evaluations. *Int. J. Nanomed.* **2013**, *8*, 461. [CrossRef]
56. Chu, X.Y.; Huang, W.; Wang, Y.L.; Meng, L.W.; Chen, L.Q.; Jin, M.J.; Gao, C.S. Improving antitumor outcomes for palliative intratumoral injection therapy through lecithin–chitosan nanoparticles loading paclitaxel–cholesterol complex. *Int. J. Nanomed.* **2019**, *14*, 689. [CrossRef]
57. Katiyar, S.; Pandit, J.; Mondal, R.S.; Mishra, A.K.; Chuttani, K.; Aqil, M.; Sultana, Y. In situ gelling dorzolamide loaded chitosan nanoparticles for the treatment of glaucoma. *Carbohydr. Polym.* **2014**, *102*, 117–124. [CrossRef]
58. Wadhwa, S.; Paliwal, R.; Paliwal, S.R.; Vyas, S.P. Hyaluronic acid modified chitosan nanoparticles for effective management of glaucoma: Development, characterization, and evaluation. *J. Drug Target.* **2010**, *18*, 292–302. [CrossRef]
59. Li, J.; Tian, S.; Tao, Q.; Zhao, Y.; Gui, R.; Yang, F.; Hou, D. Montmorillonite/chitosan nanoparticles as a novel controlled-release topical ophthalmic delivery system for the treatment of glaucoma. *Int. J. Nanomed.* **2018**, *13*, 3975. [CrossRef]
60. Abruzzo, A.; Giordani, B.; Miti, A.; Vitali, B.; Zuccheri, G.; Cerchiara, T.; Bigucci, F. Mucoadhesive and mucopenetrating chitosan nanoparticles for glycopeptide antibiotic administration. *Int. J. Pharm.* **2021**, *606*, 120874. [CrossRef]
61. Li, W.; Yang, C.; Lu, J.; Huang, P.; Barnstable, C.J.; Zhang, C.; Zhang, S.S. Tetrandrine protects mouse retinal ganglion cells from ischemic injury. *Drug Des. Dev. Ther.* **2014**, *8*, 327–339. [CrossRef] [PubMed]
62. Li, J.; Jin, X.; Zhang, L.; Yang, Y.; Liu, R.; Li, Z. Comparison of different chitosan lipid nanoparticles for improved ophthalmic tetrandrine delivery: Formulation, characterization, pharmacokinetic and molecular dynamics simulation. *J. Pharm. Sci.* **2020**, *109*, 3625–3635. [CrossRef] [PubMed]
63. Wenling, C.; Duohui, J.; Jiamou, L.; Yandao, G.; Nanming, Z.; Xiufang, Z. Effects of the degree of deacetylation on the physicochemical properties and Schwann cell affinity of chitosan films. *J. Biomater. Appl.* **2005**, *20*, 157–177. [CrossRef] [PubMed]
64. Gupta, K.C.; Jabrail, F.H. Effects of degree of deacetylation and cross-linking on physical characteristics, swelling and release behavior of chitosan microspheres. *Carbohydr. Polym.* **2006**, *66*, 43–54. [CrossRef]
65. Blanco, E.; Shen, H.; Ferrari, M. Principles of nanoparticle design for overcoming biological barriers to drug delivery. *Nat. Biotechnol.* **2015**, *33*, 941–951. [CrossRef]
66. Rubenicia AM, L.; Cubillan, L.D.; Sicam VA, D.; Macabeo AP, G.; Villaflores, O.B.; Castillo, A.L. Intraocular pressure reduction effect of 0.005% latanoprost eye drops in a hyaluronic acid-chitosan nanoparticle drug delivery system in albino rabbits. *Transl. Vis. Sci. Technol.* **2021**, *10*, 2. [CrossRef]
67. Silva, B.; Gonçalves, L.M.; Braz, B.S.; Delgado, E. Chitosan and Hyaluronic Acid Nanoparticles as Vehicles of Epoetin Beta for Subconjunctival Ocular Delivery. *Mar. Drugs* **2022**, *20*, 151. [CrossRef]
68. Shahab, M.S.; Rizwanullah, M.; Alshehri, S.; Imam, S.S. Optimization to development of chitosan decorated polycaprolactone nanoparticles for improved ocular delivery of dorzolamide: In vitro, ex vivo and toxicity assessments. *Int. J. Biol. Macromol.* **2020**, *163*, 2392–2404. [CrossRef]
69. Dubey, V.; Mohan, P.; Dangi, J.S.; Kesavan, K. Brinzolamide loaded chitosan-pectin mucoadhesive nanocapsules for management of glaucoma: Formulation, characterization and pharmacodynamic study. *Int. J. Biol. Macromol.* **2020**, *152*, 1224–1232. [CrossRef]
70. Kargozar, S.; Baino, F.; Hoseini, S.J.; Hamzehlou, S.; Darroudi, M.; Verdi, J.; Mozafari, M. Biomedical applications of nanoceria: New roles for an old player. *Nanomedicine* **2018**, *13*, 3051–3069. [CrossRef]
71. Kim, J.; Kim, H.Y.; Song, S.Y.; Go, S.H.; Sohn, H.S.; Baik, S.; Hyeon, T. Synergistic oxygen generation and reactive oxygen species scavenging by manganese ferrite/ceria co-decorated nanoparticles for rheumatoid arthritis treatment. *ACS Nano* **2019**, *13*, 3206–3217. [CrossRef]
72. Lese, I.; Graf, D.A.; Tsai, C.; Taddeo, A.; Matter, M.T.; Constantinescu, M.A.; Olariu, R. Bioactive nanoparticle-based formulations increase survival area of perforator flaps in a rat model. *PLoS ONE* **2018**, *13*, e0207802. [CrossRef]
73. Kalashnikova, I.; Chung, S.J.; Nafiujjaman, M.; Hill, M.L.; Siziba, M.E.; Contag, C.H.; Kim, T. Ceria-based nanotheranostic agent for rheumatoid arthritis. *Theranostics* **2020**, *10*, 11863. [CrossRef]
74. Lai, J.L.; Liu, Y.H.; Liu, C.; Qi, M.P.; Liu, R.N.; Zhu, X.F.; Hu, C.M. Indirubin inhibits LPS-induced inflammation via TLR4 abrogation mediated by the NF-kB and MAPK signaling pathways. *Inflammation* **2017**, *40*, 1–12. [CrossRef]
75. Lee, J.C.; Kassis, S.; Kumar, S.; Badger, A.; Adams, J.L. p38 mitogen-activated protein kinase inhibitors—Mechanisms and therapeutic potentials. *Pharmacol. Ther.* **1999**, *82*, 389–397. [CrossRef]
76. Doucette, L.P.; Walter, M.A. Prostaglandins in the eye: Function, expression, and roles in glaucoma. *Ophthalmic Genet.* **2017**, *38*, 108–116. [CrossRef]
77. Bensinger, R.; Shin, D.H.; Kass, M.A.; Podos, S.M.; Becker, B. Pilocarpine ocular inserts. *Investig. Ophthalmol. Vis. Sci.* **1976**, *15*, 1008–1010.
78. Huang, P.; Xu, Y.; Wei, R.; Li, H.; Tang, Y.; Liu, J.; Zhang, C. Efficacy of tetrandrine on lowering intraocular pressure in animal model with ocular hypertension. *J. Glaucoma* **2011**, *20*, 183–188. [CrossRef]
79. Abdelmonem, R.; Elhabal, S.F.; Abdelmalak, N.S.; El-Nabarawi, M.A.; Teaima, M.H. Formulation and characterization of acetazolamide/carvedilol niosomal gel for glaucoma treatment: In vitro, and in vivo study. *Pharmaceutics* **2021**, *13*, 221. [CrossRef]

80. Amal El Sayeh, F.; El Khatib, M.M. Formulation and evaluation of new long acting metoprolol tartrate ophthalmic gels. *Saudi Pharm. J.* **2014**, *22*, 555–563.
81. Popova, E.V.; Tikhomirova, V.E.; Beznos, O.V.; Chesnokova, N.B.; Grigoriev, Y.V.; Klyachko, N.L.; Kost, O.A. Chitosan-covered calcium phosphate particles as a drug vehicle for delivery to the eye. *Nanomed. Nanotechnol. Biol. Med.* **2022**, *40*, 102493. [CrossRef] [PubMed]
82. Gounani, Z.; Asadollahi, M.A.; Pedersen, J.N.; Lyngsø, J.; Pedersen, J.S.; Arpanaei, A.; Meyer, R.L. *Mesoporous silica* nanoparticles carrying multiple antibiotics provide enhanced synergistic effect and improved biocompatibility. *Colloids Surf. B Biointerfaces* **2019**, *175*, 498–508. [CrossRef] [PubMed]
83. Song, W.; Zhang, M.; Huang, X.; Chen, B.; Ding, Y.; Zhang, Y.; Kim, I. Smart l-borneol-loaded hierarchical hollow polymer nanospheres with antipollution and antibacterial capabilities. *Mater. Today Chem.* **2022**, *26*, 101252. [CrossRef]
84. Zhang, Y.; Song, W.; Lu, Y.; Xu, Y.; Wang, C.; Yu, D.G.; Kim, I. Recent advances in poly (α-L-glutamic acid)-based nanomaterials for drug delivery. *Biomolecules* **2022**, *12*, 636. [CrossRef]

Disclaimer/Publisher's Note: The statements, opinions and data contained in all publications are solely those of the individual author(s) and contributor(s) and not of MDPI and/or the editor(s). MDPI and/or the editor(s) disclaim responsibility for any injury to people or property resulting from any ideas, methods, instructions or products referred to in the content.

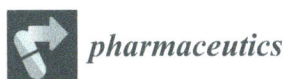

Review
Ocular Delivery of Therapeutic Proteins: A Review

Divyesh H. Shastri [1,*], Ana Catarina Silva [2,3,4] and Hugo Almeida [3,4,5]

1. Department of Pharmaceutics & Pharmaceutical Technology, K.B. Institute of Pharmaceutical Education and Research, Kadi Sarva Vishwavidyalaya, Sarva Vidyalaya Kelavani Mandal, Gandhinagar 382016, India
2. FP-I3ID (Instituto de Investigação, Inovação e Desenvolvimento), FP-BHS (Biomedical and Health Sciences Research Unit), Faculty of Health Sciences, University Fernando Pessoa, 4249-004 Porto, Portugal
3. UCIBIO (Research Unit on Applied Molecular Biosciences), REQUIMTE (Rede de Química e Tecnologia), MEDTECH (Medicines and Healthcare Products), Laboratory of Pharmaceutical Technology, Department of Drug Sciences, Faculty of Pharmacy, University of Porto, 4050-313 Porto, Portugal
4. Associate Laboratory i4HB-Institute for Health and Bioeconomy, Faculty of Pharmacy, University of Porto, 4050-313 Porto, Portugal
5. Mesosystem Investigação & Investimentos by Spinpark, Barco, 4805-017 Guimarães, Portugal
* Correspondence: divyeshshastri@gmail.com

Abstract: Therapeutic proteins, including monoclonal antibodies, single chain variable fragment (ScFv), crystallizable fragment (Fc), and fragment antigen binding (Fab), have accounted for one-third of all drugs on the world market. In particular, these medicines have been widely used in ocular therapies in the treatment of various diseases, such as age-related macular degeneration, corneal neovascularization, diabetic retinopathy, and retinal vein occlusion. However, the formulation of these biomacromolecules is challenging due to their high molecular weight, complex structure, instability, short half-life, enzymatic degradation, and immunogenicity, which leads to the failure of therapies. Various efforts have been made to overcome the ocular barriers, providing effective delivery of therapeutic proteins, such as altering the protein structure or including it in new delivery systems. These strategies are not only cost-effective and beneficial to patients but have also been shown to allow for fewer drug side effects. In this review, we discuss several factors that affect the design of formulations and the delivery of therapeutic proteins to ocular tissues, such as the use of injectable micro/nanocarriers, hydrogels, implants, iontophoresis, cell-based therapy, and combination techniques. In addition, other approaches are briefly discussed, related to the structural modification of these proteins, improving their bioavailability in the posterior segments of the eye without affecting their stability. Future research should be conducted toward the development of more effective, stable, noninvasive, and cost-effective formulations for the ocular delivery of therapeutic proteins. In addition, more insights into preclinical to clinical translation are needed.

Keywords: ocular diseases; sustained ocular delivery; therapeutic proteins; barriers of corneal tissues; nanocarriers; microcarriers; cell-penetrating peptides; hydrogels

Citation: Shastri, D.H.; Silva, A.C.; Almeida, H. Ocular Delivery of Therapeutic Proteins: A Review. Pharmaceutics 2023, 15, 205. https://doi.org/10.3390/pharmaceutics15010205

Academic Editor: Monica M. Jablonski

Received: 27 November 2022
Revised: 25 December 2022
Accepted: 4 January 2023
Published: 6 January 2023

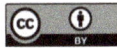

Copyright: © 2023 by the authors. Licensee MDPI, Basel, Switzerland. This article is an open access article distributed under the terms and conditions of the Creative Commons Attribution (CC BY) license (https://creativecommons.org/licenses/by/4.0/).

1. Introduction

Millions of people worldwide are affected by the diabetic retinopathy (DR), a neurodegenerative disorder of retina, which is one of the most common causes of blindness involving other complications, such as retinal vein occlusion (RVO) and corneal neovascularization (CNV) [1].

DR is caused by the damage of blood vessels at the back of the eye and does not show initial symptoms that lead to early DR or nonproliferative DR, where no new blood vessel growth occurs and patients have dilation of pre-existing capillaries, oedema, capillary occlusion, microaneurysms, and intraretinal neo-angiogenesis, leading to tortuous blood vessels formation [2]. Such proliferative vascular changes subsequently turned to severe-type damage to blood vessels and showed growth of fragile leaky blood vessels (neo-angiogenesis) in the retina called proliferative DR that leak a jelly-like substance, filling the center of the vitreous, leading to detachment of the retina from the back of the eye. Patients might observe black spot or floating strings in the vision, blurring or fluctuating vision, dark or empty areas in the vision, hemorrhage in the vitreous, and glaucoma, leading to gradual weakening of the vision [1–3].

A common cause of vision loss in older people is age-related macular degeneration (AMD), in which patients show degeneration of the retinal pigment epithelial cells and choroidal neovascularization [3]. In dry AMD, the macula thins (atrophic) with age in some patients. In wet AMD, known as neo-vascular AMD, the new vessel growth is the major cause that occurs with abrupt onset of central RVO, leading to capillary occlusion and inducing tissue hypoxia, increasing vascular endothelial growth factor (VEGF) expression and resulting in retinal proliferation of new vessels [3–5]. Thus, researchers are investigating new therapies that involve the use of monoclonal antibodies, vascular growth factors, oligonucleotides, genes, and anti-VEGF agents (e.g., ranibizumab, bevacizumab, aflibercept), for the prevention of neo-angiogenesis and stabilization of vascular leakage and, thereby, reducing the oedema.

Several therapeutic proteins have recently been approved on the market for the treatment of ocular diseases (Table 1). Although many of these proteins have low molecular weight (<50 kDa) and short half-life, the physiological and anatomical barriers of the ocular tissues limit their efficacy when administered to the posterior segments of the eye. In addition, the ocular environment makes them unstable and inactive, leading to the failure of the treatment. Among the factors that contribute to this is the presence of proteolytic enzymes, such as trypsin, in the vitreous, which can increase with aging, resulting in degradation of injectable proteins Moreover, various static, dynamic, and metabolic barriers are responsible for short half-lives of therapeutic proteins [6,7].

Anti-VEGF delivery to the posterior segment of the eye by the intravitreal route is very painful, involving the use of a needle to penetrate the globe and release the drug into the vitreous. Moreover, repeated injections are required during the treatment, leading to increased further complications such as cataracts, retinal tears, endophthalmitis, and retinal detachment [7].

Thus, the research focus should be directed at reducing the dosing frequency (e.g., novel prolonged release formulations) and development of novel noninvasive methods or devices for drug administration (e.g., through nonparenteral routes). So far, researchers worldwide have investigated several strategies for the treatment of retinal diseases to minimize the limitations or gap within the current therapies involving therapeutic proteins, reducing patient administration pain while improving compliance. The use of depot formulations of injectable carriers containing drug-loaded micro- or nanoparticles, injectable in situ hydrogels, implants, and cell-based systems are among the most useful approaches to provide safe and sustained ocular delivery of therapeutic proteins [8]. These formulations can improve the ocular drug bioavailability and help reduce the frequency of drug administration, providing an increased drug residence time within the intraocular tissues and improving the treatment efficacy with good patient compliance. In addition, cell-based systems and cell-penetrating peptides (CPPs) are also offering good ocular bioavailability indicated from the phase III clinical trials on an anti-inflammatory peptide conjugated CPP delivery [9].

Ideal therapeutic protein ocular delivery systems should provide stable delivery of encapsulated proteins, sustained release, maintenance of effective concentrations at the target tissues, and minimal invasiveness with low systemic exposure. A usual practice is to combine technologies, such as injectable hydrogels containing nano- or microparticles, liposomes, or nanoparticles containing therapeutic proteins coated with bioadhesive polymers [8,9]. Advantages of sustained delivery of therapeutic protein formulations include improved patient compliance, adherence to chronic therapy, and local delivery with fewer side effects and a reduction in dosage and dosing frequency [10].

Table 1. Molecular characteristics of various antivascular endothelial growth factor (VEGF) antibodies and anti-VEGF agents.

Molecule	Structure	Type	K$_D$ VEGF165 (pM) Equilibrium Dissociation Constant	Molecular Weight M$_w$ (kDa)	Standard Dose (IVT) (mg/mL)	T$_{1/2}$ Vitreous (days)	Indication	Target	References
Brolucizumab		ScFv	1.6	26	6/0.005	2.94 to 13.4	DR, DME, nAMD	VEGF-A	[11]
Ranibizumab (Lucentis®)		Monoclonal antibody fragment (Fab)	46–172	48	0.5/0.005	1.4 to 7.19	DR, DME, AMD	All isoforms of VEGF-A	[12–15]
Aflibercept		Fc Fusion protein fused with VEFR 1 domain 2 and VEGFR 2 domain 3	0.49	97–115	2/0.005	1.5 to 5.5	DR, DME, AMD	VEGF-A, B and PlGF	[16,17]
Bevacizumab (Avastin®)		Monoclonal antibody	58–1100	149	1.25/0.005	4.3 to 11.67	DR, DME, AMD	All isoforms of VEGF-A	[18–25]
Abicipar pegol (Allergan®)		Akyrin repeat protein (recombinant protein) coupled with PEG	486 fM	34	2/0.005	>13	nAMD	VEGF-A$_{165}$	[26,27]
Faricimab		Monoclonal antibody	-	150	6/0.005	2.83	nAMD, DME	VEGF-A and Angiopoietin-2	[28,29]
Conbercept (Lumitin®, Sichuan)		Fc Fusion protein fused with VEFR 1 domain 2 and VEGFR 2 domain 3 & 4	0.5	143	0.5/0.005	4.24	AMD	VEGF-B and PlGF	[30]
Pegaptanib (Macugen®)		Aptamer (pegylated oligonucleotide)	200	40	0.3/0.009	12	DR, DME, nAMD	VEGF$_{165}$	[31–34]

Abbreviations: DR—Diabetic retinopathy, AMD—age-related macular degeneration, nAMD—neovascularization due to AMD, DME—diabetic macular edema, VEGF—vascular endothelial growth factor, PlGF—placenta growth factor.

Currently, great attention is being focused on the development of a more effective noninvasive, sustained drug delivery in the treatment of ocular disorders for the anterior and posterior segments of the eye.

In this review, we discuss the recent approaches for protein delivery to the ocular tissues with a view to increase the patient compliance by increasing bioavailability for longer duration with minor side effects. Different approaches, which include injectable micro/nanocarriers injectable hydrogels, ocular implants, iontophoresis, and periocular injections, are addressed, with a view to improve the ocular bioavailability and provide sustained release to the ocular tissues in posterior segments of the eye of therapeutic proteins.

2. Routes of Ocular Drug Administration

Achieving an efficient ocular bioavailability of different therapeutic proteins remains a challenge due to presence of multiple ocular barriers (Figure 1). Moreover, diseases such as age-related macular degeneration, diabetic retinopathy, and cytomegalovirus (CMV) retinitis require therapeutic proteins to be delivered to the back of the eye. Herein, static barriers (different layers of cornea, sclera, and retina including blood aqueous and blood–retinal barriers), dynamic barriers (choroidal and conjunctival blood flow, lymphatic clearance, and tear dilution), and efflux pumps, in combination, constitute a significant challenge for drug delivery to the posterior segment of the eye [35].

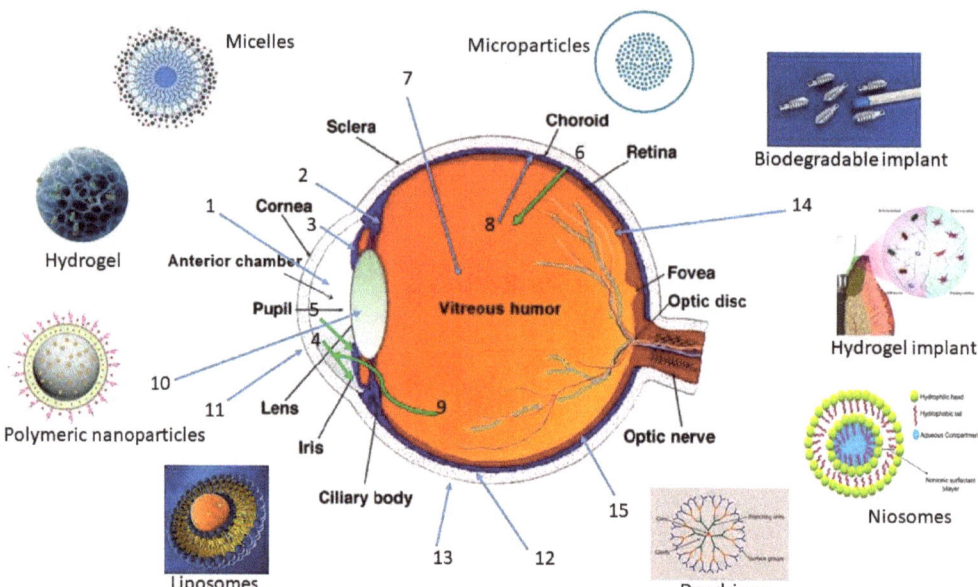

Figure 1. Schematic representation of various formulation approaches and routes of administration to the ocular tissues. 1. Transcorneal permeation into the anterior chamber, 2. Noncorneal drug permeation across conjunctiva to sclera into anterior uvea, 3. Drug distribution into anterior chamber from blood stream through blood aqueous barrier, 4. Drug elimination from anterior chamber by aqueous humor to trabecular meshwork and Schlemm's canal, 5. Elimination of drug from aqueous humor into systemic circulation across blood aqueous barrier, 6. Distribution of drug from blood into posterior segment across the blood retinal barrier, 7. Intravitreal route, 8. Drug elimination from vitreous via posterior route across blood retinal barrier, 9. Elimination of drug from vitreous via anterior route to posterior chamber, 10. Intracameral route, 11. Intrastromal route, 12. Subconjunctival route, 13. Subtenon route, 14. Suprachoroidal route, 15. Subretinal route.

The elimination of therapeutic proteins from the body is similar to the endogenous peptide molecules, i.e., enzymatic cleavage from liver, kidney, blood, and small intestine, although those that show enzymatic resistance can be eliminated via liver or kidney based on their lipophilicity. Only less than 1% of therapeutic proteins with molecular weight >4000 Da show undesirable immune response after administration, which led to the failure of some clinical trials [36].

Among the main barriers present in the eye that hinder the ocular delivery of therapeutics are static barriers and dynamic barriers. Static barriers include different layers of cornea, sclera and retina, and blood aqueous barriers (BAB) (Figure 2), while dynamic barriers comprise tear film, choroidal and conjunctival blood flow, and lymphatic clearance, which hinder the movement of drug molecules from the anterior part of the globe to the posterior tissues [36,37]. High selectivity of blood retinal barriers (BRB) limits the movement of topically instilled drugs to the posterior segment. Moreover, systemically administered drugs have to cross the blood ocular barriers, i.e., BAB and BRB, to reach the retina (Figure 2). The use of the systemic route for the delivery for ocular therapeutics has several limitations related to the need of high doses due to systemic metabolism and poor permeability across the BRB. Moreover, exposure to nontargeted organs may cause systemic toxicity and severe adverse effects [37].

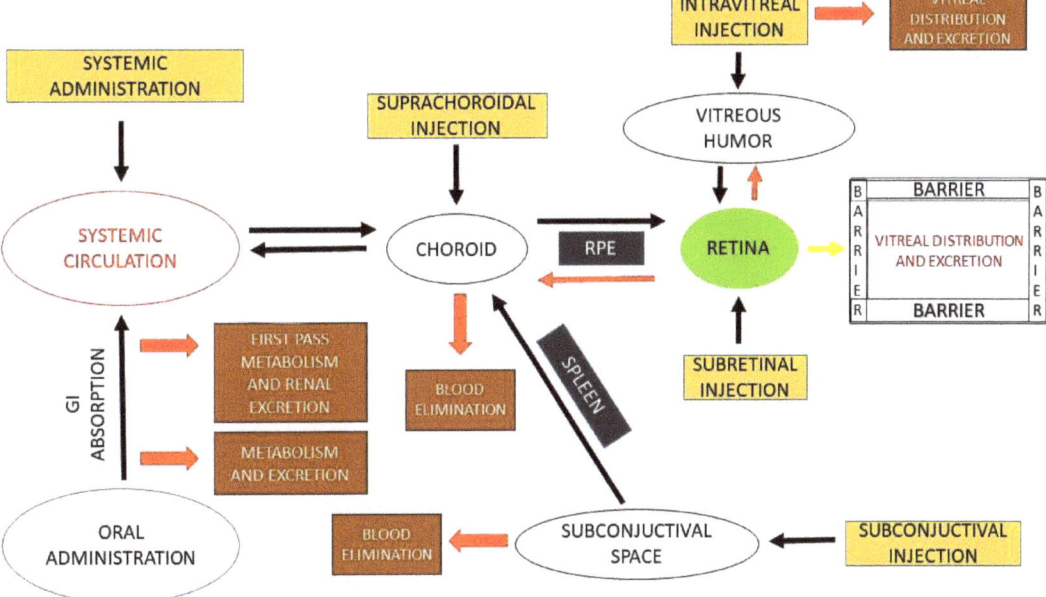

Figure 2. Different routes for ocular drug clearance/elimination.

The topical route is preferred for the delivery of drugs to the anterior chamber of the eye for the treatment of cataract, dry eye, and corneal and conjunctival inflammatory and infectious diseases [37]. The topical ocular delivery route is not commonly used for the delivery of therapeutic proteins for retinal tissues due to the presence of ocular barriers; only <5% of the instilled dose enters through anterior segment to the posterior segment via the tear film and cornea (epithelium, endothelium, and stroma) to the anterior chamber of the eye [8–10,38,39]. The extent of absorption of drug molecules from the corneal surface is severely limited by different physiological barriers, such as:

(1) Corneal epithelium that selectively inhibits the diffusion of hydrophilic and high molecular weight molecules such as proteins and peptides through the paracellular route, and it selectively prevents ion transport. Permeability of macromolecules is severely limited by the presence of tight junctions of the cornea and the lipophilic nature of the corneal epithelium.

(2) The endothelium, which is responsible for corneal hydration.

(3) Inner stroma, which presents a hydrophilic nature and inhibits the permeation of more lipophilic molecules [39,40].

These barriers protect the eyes from the entry of toxic entities and pathogenic substances and maintain homeostasis. Moreover, due to the high shear rate, tear turnover, and tear dilution, most (>95%) of the instilled dose is eliminated via the nasolacrimal duct to the gastrointestinal tract, leading to other systemic side effects (Figure 1). The presence of enzymes in the ciliary body digest the drug from the aqueous humor, and the corneal permeability is also limited depending on molecular size, surface charge, and hydrophilicity of drugs [41]. Large and hydrophilic drugs showed poor permeability compared to small and lipophilic peptides from the corneal epithelial tight junction (about 2 nm) [41]. Positively charged molecules can pass easily due to binding with the negatively charged corneal membrane [39].

Lipophilic drugs are distributed to corneal tissues via the transcorneal pathway (i.e., cornea > aqueous humor = iris = ciliary body > anterior sclera > lens), while hydrophilic drugs tend to move toward the posterior chamber via the conjunctival–sclera pathway. Large molecular drugs that show poor corneal permeability bypass the corneal epithelium penetration route and undergo noncorneal absorption [42]. Lipophilic peptides with molecular size >700 Da exhibit good membrane permeability [43,44].

2.1. Intraocular

Intraocular delivery involves delivery through injection or implants of sterile solutions or devices in the ocular tissues via (1) intravitreal, (2) subretinal, or (3) suprachoroidal routes.

(a) Intravitreal

The intravitreal route targets drugs to the retina, providing higher drug bioavailability directly into the posterior segment, avoiding several ocular barriers, and eliminating problems associated with systemic toxicities.

The vitreous has a mesh size of 500 nm that provides a loose barrier and allows diffusion and convection of large and small molecules as well as nanoparticles [45–47]. Molecular mobility in the vitreous also depends on the charge of the protein molecules, i.e., neutral and anionic molecules can diffuse more easily compared to cationic ones due to electrostatic interactions with the anionic hyaluronic acid polymer network in the vitreous [48]. Metabolic activity in the RPE determines the bioavailability of protein molecules injected intravitreally due to degradation by the presence of enzymes, i.e., cytochrome P450 and esterases [49]. PEGylation attachment of a high molecular weight hydrophilic moiety to the drug molecules, i.e., polyethylene glycol, either by covalent or noncovalent linkage or encapsulation in the nanoparticles, can dramatically reduce the enzymatic degradation [46].

Clearance observed between the posterior segment and anterior segment after intravitreal injection depends on the size, property, and concentration gradient. Molecules from the posterior segment diffuse to the inner limiting membrane (ILM) and finally reach to retina (Figure 2). The clearance efficiency also depends on penetration efficiency through the tight junction of RPE as the small and lipophilic ones can be transported easily compared to large and hydrophilic proteins [50]. From the retinal layer, the molecules pass through the choroidal blood vessels to the systemic circulation. Molecules that diffuse toward anterior side can be drained away into blood or lymphatic vessels via trabecular meshwork or Schlemm's canal [50].

(b) Subretinal

From subretinal injection, direct administration of molecules to the retina can be possible, so it is the most preferable and efficient route for the delivery of therapeutic proteins with low membrane permeability and of retinal gene therapy [51]. Drugs administered via this route to the inner layer of the retina are cleared via the anterior segment and not through choroidal vessels as RPE tight junctions limit the movement of drugs toward the outer layer of the retina and lead to damage to the RPE and retina (Figure 2) [52].

(c) Suprachoroidal

With the help of microneedles or cannulas, drugs can be administered via this route beneath the sclera into the suprachoroidal space, allowing the drug to be available at the choroidal site. Drug distribution is uneven due to restricted movement from ciliary arteries of the choroid. Moreover, due to high blood flow in the choroidal blood vessels, most of the administered drug is lost to the systemic circulation, which leads to short half-lives.

Macromolecules such as dextran of molecular weight 40 kDa have an experimental half-life of 3.6 h compared to 5.6 h obtained with a molecular weight of 250 kDa [52]. Bevacizumab (149 kDa) showed even greater half-life (7.9 h) indicating that, apart from molecular weight the charge, flexibility and lipophilicity can also affect the clearance [52]. Through rapid clearance, the particles containing therapeutic proteins form injectable implants with a long retention time that can last up to months. Thus, the suprachoroidal injections of implants containing therapeutics exhibit great scope for effective retinal delivery.

2.2. Periocular

It is a less invasive method where drugs are administered directly into the eye via injection into the subconjunctival, subtenon, peribulbar, retrobulbar, and posterior juxtascleral spaces, without any risk of cataract and endophthalmitis. Compared to the topical route, this route provides excellent drug bioavailability by avoiding corneal barriers. Injected drugs reach the posterior segment through the conjunctival sclera, but the bioavailability is much lower (0.1%) than that of the topical route (Figure 2) [53]. Drugs rapidly clearing (80–95%) into systemic circulation through choroidal vessels and multiple barriers between the retina and subconjunctival space leads to poor bioavailability. This route is less invasive and eliminates the drug permeation through sclera. Moreover, in the case of retinal diseases, for drug administration in large volumes, this route is preferred due to the high volume of the injection (100–500 µL) compared with the suprachoroidal route (50–200 µL) [54].

3. Ocular Barriers and Approaches to Ocular Administration
3.1. Ocular Barriers

Ocular distribution of protein therapeutics to the eye depends on several factors such as membrane permeability, ocular elimination, nontarget binding, and degradation by proteolytic enzymes. Membrane permeability and ocular elimination closely depend on their size, surface charge, and hydrophilicity and lipophilicity [55]. However, complexity of the ocular tissues in deciding parameters for ocular pharmacokinetics is a major obstacle in the designing of an effective delivery system for therapeutic proteins due to the presence of various ocular barriers.

3.1.1. Tissue Conditions

Collagen fibers from the hydrophilic stroma also limit the penetration of therapeutic proteins, which usually takes place via pinocytosis or endocytosis (active transport mechanism) [55,56]. The tight junctions present in the cornea, sclera, and retina significantly prevent the diffusion of hydrophilic large macromolecules [56,57]. The tight junctions in the conjunctival epithelium are usually wider than those in the corneal epithelium but are still unable to provide penetration of large molecules [58,59].

The vitreous humor is a highly viscous fluid-like gel composed of 98 to 99% w/v water content, salts, sugars, a network of collagen-type II fibrils with hyaluronan, glycosaminoglycan, and a wide array of proteins located in the posterior segment of the ocular globe [60]. Drugs administered intravitreally will have direct access to the vitreous cavity and retina and may take several hours to diffuse across the entire vitreous humor. The clearance of macromolecules from the vitreous cavity is very slow due to hindrance by RPE, whereas diffusion from the vitreous to the retina is restricted by ILM [61]. Because several other factors are involved such as initial dose, volume of distribution, and the rate of elimination [62,63], it also depends on size, surface charge, and characteristics of the macromolecules injected [64–67]. The vitreous can allow the diffusion of small, anionic macromolecules, restricting the bigger size or cationic macromolecules that exhibit non-diffusion kinetics and distribution profile. Molecules can be eliminated through anterior and/or posterior routes [], which is influenced primarily by volume of distribution and elimination half-life [63].

A large number of diseases uveitis, cytomegalovirus retinitis, and retinitis and proliferative vitreoretinopathy affect the ocular pharmacokinetics of various topically instilled molecules and their formulations. The diseased conditions produce certain physiological changes in the corneal stroma composed of collagen and water, leading to poor bioavailability of hydrophobic molecules [68]. Fungal keratitis involving chronic inflammation of corneal tissues leads to poor permeation [69]. To solve this problem, drugs are administered with a vehicle/emulsion to avoid evaporation of the limited natural tears in dry-eye patients, as well as the use of the iontophoretic technique to permeate the ionized molecules into ocular tissues.

BRB breakdown as well as choroidal and retinal neovascularization were observed in glaucoma, leading to blindness in a large population. Pharmacokinetic parameters need to be determined in such conditions using animal models to prove efficacy. In one study [70] of measuring the pharmacokinetic parameters, using healthy and diseased animal models, it was observed that the AUC and Cmax were significantly lower in diseased models compared to normal animal models due to BRB breakdown and exposure of drugs to ocular tissues. Therefore, dose calculation needs to be performed to avoid dose-related toxicity.

3.1.2. Physicochemical Characteristics of Drug Molecules

Various physicochemical parameters of macromolecules such as solubility, hydrophilicity/lipophilicity, molecular weight, size and shape, surface charge, and degree of ionization affect the selection of the route and rate of drug permeation through the cul-de-sac [71]. Small and lipophilic molecules can diffuse and distribute rapidly and largely through RPE, inner limiting membrane (ILM), and outer limiting membranes (OLM), exhibiting efficient distribution to (and even faster elimination from) ocular tissues. Large and lipophilic molecules have poor membrane permeability, showing relatively longer retention time at the site of injection with poor ocular tissue distributions [72,73]. For example, the particles with a size of 200 nm were found to be retained in the retinal tissues for two months after injection [72,73]. The vitreal clearance rate is rapid for smaller particles and can also be observed from their half-lives, i.e., particles of size 50 nm, 200 nm and 2 μm showed half-lives of 5.4 ± 0.8, 8.6 ± 0.7, and 10.1 ± 1.8 days, respectively [74].

Most of the therapeutic proteins have complex structure, large size with molecular weight > 1000 Da, and large hydrogen bonding donor/acceptor groups and show poor membrane permeability across the ocular tissues and barriers [75]. Human retinal tissues prevent the permeation of macromolecules of size > 76 kDa due to inner and outer plexiform layers. Macromolecules greater than 150 kDa cannot reach the inner retinal tissues, while molecules such as brolucizumab (smaller size) can penetrate the retina and choroid tissues more effectively than other anti-VEGF [57,76]. Brolucizumab showed 2.2-fold higher concentrations in the retinal tissues and 1.7-fold higher concentrations in RPE/choroid tissues than ranibizumab in rabbits [77]. These macromolecular proteins, when traversing through the choroid, may wash out through the choriocapillaris, leading to a reduction in therapeutic concentrations, and, due to the large complex molecular structure, may increase the risk of their degradation at the physiological environment of pH and temperature resulting into shorter half-lives. Macromolecules showed half-life in the range of days to a week (Table 1) in the vitreous humor, i.e., bevacizumab had a half-life of 4.32 days with a minimum concentration of 162 µg/mL in the vitreous [78]. Frequent intravitreal injections of ranibizumab 0.3–2.0 mg/eye biweekly or monthly is required to maintain the therapeutic levels as it showed vitreous elimination of 9 days and intrinsic systemic elimination half-life of 2 h, making it noncompliant and often associated with other complications such as cataract, retinal hemorrhage, and detachment and endophthalmitis [79,80]. One comparative study showed brolucizumab clearance from the ocular tissues with a mean terminal half-life of 56.8 ± 7.6 h; ranibizumab took 62 h, and aflibercept was cleared with a half-life of 53 h in the same model [81–83]. The rapid clearance is presumed to be due to smaller molecular size and absence of the Fc domain in the case of brolucizumab. Unlike aflibercept, which has full-length antibodies, leading to the conservation mechanism, molecules without the Fc region are more prone to degradation and do not show a cumulative effect even after multiple injections [84].

The surface charge being a complex and heterogenous property of amino acid sequence of the therapeutic proteins along with pH of the surroundings are important criteria to be considered. Deamination, isomerization, or post-translational modification of the therapeutic proteins in a particular environment lead to formation of charge variant species in a mixture of therapeutic proteins [85]. Most therapeutic proteins are found to be positively charged at an isoelectric point (pI) of 7–9, leading to charge interactions with other molecules and ocular membranes and showing good penetration compared to negatively charged proteins [85]. Although the undesired entrapment of the polymeric network of the vitreous (negatively charged) should not be ignored, positively charged molecules tend to remain clumped in the vitreous without diffusion, while anionic particles diffuse to the retina [86,87]. The effect of surface charge on the particles was studied on human serum albumin (HSA) and showed that anionic particles of size 114 nm with an overall zeta potential of −33.3 mV can easily diffuse through the vitreal collagen fibrils to the retina within 5 h after injection, while cationic particles of size 175.5 nm with mean zeta potential of +11.7 mV showed aggregation in the vitreous [87]. An inflammatory condition of the vitreous showed accelerated diffusion and clearance of HSA [88].

3.1.3. Viscosity and pH of the Formulation

Most of the protein formulations are available with high and variable viscosity as sustained release of therapeutic proteins for longer duration needs very high quantities to be injected in single-dose administration, which is often associated with high viscosity and difficulty of the syringe to handle the formulation and is not allowed by FDA. A high concentration of therapeutic proteins is very difficult to pass through an 18 mm, 27–30 G needle [89]. Use of viscosity builders required in the formulation of small molecules helps the proteins reach the anterior chamber of the eye in contrast to macromolecules, which helps provide sufficient viscosity to the formulation up to 20 cps, prolong the corneal residence time, enhance the transcorneal absorption into the anterior chamber, and thereby increase bioavailability [90].

pH and osmolarity play a vital role in the ocular therapeutics. For drug delivery to the anterior segment, maximum therapeutic benefits can be achieved when the pH of the formulation matches the lacrimal fluid. The pH of the formulation is a critical parameter that needs to be observed as proteins become denatured and unstable due to irreversible conformational changes at both high and low pH values. Apart from pH, the type and concentration of buffer used can also influence the protein degradation pathways, i.e., deamination, disulfide bond formation/exchange, isomerization, and fragmentation [91,92]. A weak acidic buffer is optimal for the storage of antibodies, i.e., adalimumab (pH 5.2), ranibizumab (pH 5.5), and bevacizumab (pH 6.2), below their isoelectric points (~8.3–8.8) for ocular treatments [93,94]. Though buffers play a crucial role in providing stability and preservation of macromolecules, their use must be carefully considered to avoid associated complications such as immunogenicity and local toxicity [95]. Buffers used also must be within the osmolarity range (280–300 mOsm/kg) to be compatible with ocular tissues as they also impair tonicity. Moreover, hypotonic solutions originate clouding and cause edema of the corneal tissues, while hypertonic solutions desiccate the corneal tissues in the anterior chamber [96]. Therefore, to facilitate protein delivery, proper understanding of the formulation pH and viscosity, selection of buffer system, and use of chemical chaperones are of the utmost importance. This helps to control the behavior and characteristics of the therapeutic proteins and also avoid protein misfolding [97,98].

3.1.4. Protein Binding

Protein binding shows less effect on ocular distribution of therapeutic proteins as the level of protein in the eye (0.5–1.5 mg/mL) is significantly less compared to that of plasma (60–80 mg/mL) [99,100]. Vasotide® administered in genetically modified mouse model showed significant reduction in retinal angiogenesis in AMD [101].

Intravitreally administered molecules required to cross the ILM to reach the retina after diffusion through the vitreous body, which contains a high-density extracellular matrix made up of collagen, laminin, and heparin sulphate proteoglycan (composition changes with age), affect the drug permeability [102]. Higher drug penetration was observed with high binding affinity to the extracellular matrix, which led to effective penetration to the ILM, making the drug available to the retina. For example, adeno-associated virus serotype-2 showed excellent transduction to the retina after intravitreal injection due to high heparin sulphate proteoglycan binding affinity, while other serotypes and modified serotypes failed to transfect (low affinity with proteoglycan) [103].

3.1.5. Enzymatic Degradation

Different metabolic pathways also cause the loss of therapeutic activity or inactivation of the macromolecules by protein denaturation, aggregation, precipitations, adsorption, and proteolytic degradation, denaturation by temperature, pH, salt or ionic concentrations, and complexations with enzymes/coenzymes. Enzymatic degradation by proteolytic enzymes depends on concentrations of the enzymes in the vitreous (levels may rise with age and tissue conditions) and on the hydrolytic enzymes and esterases in retina [104,105].

Structural changes in the active form of complex primary, tertiary, or quaternary structures of protein molecules or chemical modification lead to irreversible aggregation and finally inactivation. The main routes of drug administration and fate from ocular tissues are shown schematically in the Figures 1 and 2, respectively.

Peptides are highly susceptible to enzymatic degradation (proteolytic cleavage) [106]. The proteolytic cleavage and breakdown to small peptides leads to lower half-lives. The drug pharmacokinetic properties and thereby therapeutic efficacy can be achieved by improving bioavailability to the ocular tissues, and that can be achieved by chemical or physical modification of the molecules using various formulation strategies, i.e., coadministration, conjugation of functional moieties, particle formulation, encapsulation into implant or hydrogel, and chemical modification/substitutions. Proteolytic stabilization of macromolecules and membrane permeability can be achieved by a prodrug approach or using biological analogues [55,107,108]. Similarly, lipophilicity or hydrophobicity can also be increased by covalent conjugation with hydrophobic moiety or by noncovalent interactions with any hydrophobic compound. Solubility improvements can also be achieved using a conjugation with cyclodextrin and PEG, eliminating enzymatic degradation [39,40,56,75]. Thus, the pharmacokinetic properties of therapeutic proteins can be optimized, keeping in mind these changes must not affect their biological efficacy.

Therapeutic proteins need protection against enzymatic attack from the various proteolytic enzymes present in the vitreous such as matrix metalloproteinase and serine/cysteine protease. The level of enzyme concentration in the vitreous changes with the age and disease conditions, so the formulation targeted to the retinal diseases needs to be optimized against such enzymatic attack [109,110]. Use of D-form peptides or peptoid type has been shown to have good enzymatic resistance [111] in addition to chemical modifications at the N and C terminus; for example, C-terminal amidation or N-terminal acetylation will make the peptides more difficult to be recognized and targeted by the enzymatic attack [112,113]. Apart from proteolytic enzymes, certain metabolic enzymes such as cytochrome P450 reductases and lysosomal enzymes are also found in large amounts in the ocular tissues that maintain homeostasis and protect the ocular tissues [114–116]. Encapsulation of retinal drugs in a nanoparticulate system or implant matrix can improve the protection against the enzymatic degradation [117], as discussed later in formulation approaches.

3.2. Use of Penetration Enhancers

Different therapeutic approaches have been investigated for the improvement of drug bioavailability and providing sustained drug release to the corneal tissues. Bioavailability improvement to the anterior segment of the eye can be achieved by maximizing corneal absorption and reduction in precorneal drug loss, which can be achieved by using viscosity enhancers, penetration enhancers, and prodrug approaches [80–82].

The presence of tight junctions in the stratified epithelium allows only ions to be transported across the tissues, offering high resistance to therapeutic proteins; thus, the addition of absorption promotors or penetration enhancers can be more helpful to improve the permeability across the corneal tissues or membrane [53,81,118]. Permeation enhancers alter the integrity of the corneal epithelium, leading to the promotion of the corneal uptake and thus a rate-limiting step in the transport of macromolecules from the corneal tissues to the receptor site [82]. Inclusion of cetylpyridinium chloride [119], lasalocid [120], benzalkonium chloride [76], parabens [118], tween® 20, saponins [64], Brij® 35, Brij® 78, Brij® 98 ethylenediaminetetraacetic acid, bile salts [83], bile acids (such as sodium cholate, sodium taurocholate, sodium glycodeoxycholate, sodium taurodeoxycholate, taurocholic acid, chenodeoxycholic acid, and ursodeoxycholic acid), capric acid, azone, fusidic acid, hexamethylene lauramide, saponins [84], hexamethylene octanamide, and decyl methyl sulfoxide [121] in different formulations has shown a significant enhancement of corneal drug absorption. Moreover, the ability to catalyze the degradation of hyaluronic acid by hyaluronidase is also utilized since it has taken decades to improve the permeability across the ocular tissue barriers [122]. In the vitreous, hyaluronic acid provides a key role in maintaining structural integrity, volume expansion, and viscosity of the vitreous body [123]. Keeping in mind the associated toxicity and irritation, penetration enhancers should be used precisely and carefully.

4. Conjugation Approaches

Therapeutic proteins are very potent and offer advantages related to specific mechanisms of action. Despite these benefits, therapeutic proteins have shown several drawbacks, including high molecular weight, short half-lives, instability, and immunogenicity, which must be kept in mind when developing a delivery system. Among the several strategies discussed above, there are few conjugation approaches that are being used to improve the stability and overcome the limitations, called second-generation therapeutic proteins. Change in formulations (i.e., using liposomes and polymeric micro/nanoparticles) or change in the protein itself (i.e., changing the protein structure by attaching covalently some moiety to the protein molecule) are among the few conjugation approaches (Table 2). The covalent conjugation of therapeutic proteins with PEG, hyaluronan, lipid derivatives, and melanin are also better alternatives to modifying the protein moiety itself, as discussed below.

Table 2. Examples of different approaches used to improve the bioavailability of ocular therapeutic proteins.

Approaches	Remarks
Use of penetration enhancers	Increases corneal permeability.
Improve enzymatic resistance	Avoids degradation by enzymes present in ocular tissues.
Conjugation Approaches	
Conjugation with ligands	Tissue-specific delivery with minimal toxicity and minimal systemic exposures.
Conjugation with ligand, lipids, melanin, hyaluronan, and PEG	Improves half-lives or reduces immunogenicity, protects macromolecules, prevents proteolytic degradation, and provides long-term stability/stability. Improves membrane penetration.
Formulation Approaches	
Hydrogels	Protect molecules from degradation and provide long-term release.
Micro/Nanocarriers	Protect molecules from enzymatic degradation. Enhance permeation. Restrict drug release to the desired area of eye. Provide depot and prolonged retention of the formulation. Improve physical stability. Increase drug permeability.
Mucoadhesive polymeric system	Achieve site-specific drug delivery. Improves permeation.
Cell-Penetrating Peptides	Improve penetration overcoming ocular barriers and provide sustained release by preventing degradation and increasing the drug residence time.
Encapsulated Cell Technology	Enzyme protection, stability, long-term release.
Iontophoresis	Improves permeation, provides transfer of ionized molecules through biological membranes using low electric current to the ocular tissues.
Microneedles	Provide passive diffusion of therapeutics, overcoming the transport barriers of epithelial tissues, eliminating clearance by conjunctival mechanisms, and minimizing retinal damage.
Implants	Protect from degradation and provide depot with slow and sustained release at constant rate over extended period.

4.1. Conjugation with Ligands

Receptor-mediated drug delivery can be used for improvement in drug permeation at the target tissue with a high selectivity, specificity, and efficiency. Delivering therapeutic proteins to the ocular tissues with minimum systemic exposure or minimal toxicity is a great benefit obtained by using receptor/ligand-binding. It also enhances the membrane permeability of most biopharmaceuticals/macromolecules, making the intracellular delivery convenient by enhancing receptor/ligand mediated endocytosis. Few example, transferrin-receptor-specific monoclonal antibody on the surface of transgene-containing liposomes, when introduced into retina-specific drug delivery for CNV treatment, showed expression of transgenes throughout the RPE and multiple areas of ocular tissues [124]. Another study in which an RPE-specific drug delivery platform was used in AMD and vitreoretinopathy as a conjugate (in vitro) observed that CD44-specific RNA aptamer-FITC conjugates were efficiently taken up by the RPE-overexpressing CD44 receptors via a receptor-mediated endocytosis pathway [125].

4.2. Conjugation with Lipid Derivatives

Self-assembled peptides modulated via intermolecular (hydrophobic, hydrogen) interactions or conjugation with polymers can be used along with lipidic derivatives [126]. These self-assembled particles can be applied through intravitreal injection using 27–30 gauge needles, which is less invasive compared to those used in implants (25 G) [127,128].

4.3. Conjugation with Melanin

A macromolecule derived from tyrosine known as melanin, a polyanionic pigment, showed good affinity with most drugs, exhibiting high retention in ocular tissues [129]. Drugs bound to melanosomes (a form of melanin found in choroid and RPE) found in very high concentrations formed a reservoir and showed slow release over a longer duration, evidence of the good binding affinity of melanin with the drug and the intracellular permeability of drugs. Melanin bound to lipophilic pazopanib and GW771806 showed effective drug retention for several weeks in rat eyes with an ocular half-life of 18 days after a single oral dose of 100 mg/kg [130,131]. Thus, melanin drug binding can be used as a potential carrier for sustained release with extended half-life, facilitating delivery to the posterior segment via noninvasive topical or oral administration. Thus, this can be another potential strategy for delivering fast-eliminating peptides (anti-VEGF proteins), providing good ocular retention and prolonged therapeutic effect.

4.4. Conjugation with Hyaluronan

Apart from melanin binding, combining the hyaluronan-binding peptide with anti-VEGF is another approach in which an anti-VEGF protein, when combined with hyaluronan, results in high residence time with a longer sustained release in the vitreous, providing 3–4-fold longer therapeutic effect in corneal neovascularization tested in rabbits and monkeys [131]. These hyaluronan-binding peptides can be used as prodrugs with extended vitreous retention an alternative to frequent intravitreal injections.

4.5. Conjugation with Polyethylene Glycol

PEGylated peptides are more preferable for slow release and long retention time in the vitreous. Pegatinib, an anti-VEGF aptamer of RNA combined with high molecular weight PEG (40 kDa), showed prolonged retention due to high molecular size when applied in the treatment of neovascular age-related macular degeneration. Similar results were observed with PEGylated-complement C3 inhibitor-Pegcetacoplan [132]. The vitreous contains a high number of proteolytic enzymes, so ocular delivery of peptides needs protection against such enzymatic degradation for long-term delivery [49,133,134]. PEGylation can shield macromolecules such as peptides and genes and reduces the chances of enzymatic attack [135]. However, no studies have been reported so far for the proteolytic degradation and resistance of drugs in the vitreous. The use of the D-form of peptides instead of the L-form or chemical modification of the C and N terminus of peptides by amidation or acetylation increases the enzymatic resistance, as enzymes do not recognize the peptide [136]. Encapsulation of peptides in nanoparticles or implants can help in minimizing enzymatic degradation during delivery [137].

5. Formulation Approaches

Formulation approaches are based on providing sustained drug release to the anterior and posterior segments of the eye, which can be achieved by providing continuous and controlled delivery to the ocular tissues using hydrogels, micro- and nanocarriers, implants, inserts and some modern approaches as CPPs, encapsulated cell technology, iontophoresis, and microneedle formulations [138–142].

Table 2 shows examples of approaches used to improve the bioavailability of ocular therapeutic proteins, and Table 3 describes the most relevant results observed with different formulation approaches used to improve the ocular delivery of therapeutic proteins.

5.1. Hydrogels

One of the most promising categories of delivery systems for safe and sustained ocular delivery of therapeutic proteins that is gaining popularity is injectable hydrogels. They are aqueous, highly soft and elastic in nature, and have physicochemical similarities with ocular fluids, being adequate for intraocular use. Moreover, a mild crosslinking of polymers is enough to preserve the biological activity of therapeutic proteins in the hydrogels [143–145]. Hydrogels are preferable over other dosage forms for the delivery of proteins, peptides, and antibodies, as the formation of the hydrogel can occur at ambient temperature conditions. These systems can be administered in the vitreous cavity via injection through small gauge needle, as "in situ"-forming aqueous dispersion, which is turned immediately into gel in response to internal or external stimuli mediated by changes in the physiological environment, i.e., pH, temperature, ions, or enzymes [144]. The sol-gel phase transition occurs within seconds to minutes, entrapping and stabilizing the therapeutic proteins in an aqueous polymeric network [146–148]. Several in situ gelling polymeric systems prepared with hyaluronic acid, chitosan, poloxamer, HPMC, and polycaprolactone have exhibited safe use as depot systems in the ocular environment. After injection, the hydrogel forms a reservoir, allowing continuous release of loaded protein molecules over time, which restricts their mobility in the polymeric network after the sol-gel phase transition in the ocular tissues. The drug release occurs via different mechanisms from the reservoir, i.e., diffusion-controlled and degradation-controlled [149,150]. The hydrogel's properties can be modulated for setting the diffusion rate and permeability of entrapped molecules in the hydrogel by different process parameters, such as time, type and degree of crosslinking, and the polymers-to-crosslinker ratio. The level of crosslinking aids in determining the diffusion rate and mechanism of therapeutic proteins from the hydrogels. It also depends on the degree of polymer modification, molecular weight, concentration, density, and polymer architecture [151].

(a) Hydrogels

For decades, tremendous efforts have been made by the formulators to develop biocompatible, biodegradable, fast-gelling hydrogels to overcome challenges such as initial burst release, initial gel viscosity, hydrogel turbidity, crosslinking strategies, sterilization procedures, storage conditions and long-term intraocular stability and safety to facilitate their clinical translation. Many thermosensitive hydrogels become turbid on gelation at body temperature after administration. Moreover, the use of high concentrations in solutions/dispersions for the formulation of long-term depot hydrogels results in formulations too viscous to inject via 22–31 G needles [152–155].

An injectable hydrogel of PLGA in N-methyl pyrrolidone and sucrose acetate isobutyrate showed sustained release of proteins [147]. Polysaccharide crosslinked hydrogels exhibited sustained release of bevacizumab for three days with a low initial burst, while thermosensitive hydrogels exhibited sustained release of bevacizumab for 18 days [152]. Intravitreal administration of bevacizumab in situ gel of hyaluronic acid-vinyl sulfone and dextran-thiol (HA-VS/Dex-SH) showed controlled release of bevacizumab when tested using rabbit eye model [146,156,157]. In situ hydrogel of bevacizumab administered in a single injection intravitreally in a rabbit eye showed therapeutic concentration (>50 ng/mL) for up to six months with specific binding to VEGF measured using a specific quantification technique, i.e., ELISA assay, at different time intervals [157,158]. A hydrogel formulation with bevacizumab prepared with methoxy-poly(ethylene glycol)-block-poly(lactic-co-glycolic) acid crosslinked with 2,2-bis(2-oxazoline) showed sustained release up to one month using in vivo rabbit model without any cytotoxicity [159].

Another study using a thermosensitive hydrogel of triblock copolymer of poly(2-ethyl-2-oxazoline)-b-poly(e-caprolactone)-b-poly(2-ethyl-2-oxazoline) containing bevacizumab showed good biocompatibility even two months after intravitreal injection, exhibiting sustained release properties [160]. A silk hydrogel containing anti-VEGF therapeutics formulated using silk fibroin as the vehicle for delivery and bevacizumab-loaded hydrogel formulations showed sustained release for three months both in vitro and in vivo in Dutch-belted rabbit eyes when injected intravitreally [161].

A light-activated polycaprolactone dimethacrylate and hydroxyethyl methacrylate in situ hydrogel showed stable and sustained release of bevacizumab for up to four months [162].

A biodegradable thermosensitive poly(N-isopropyl)acrylamide hydrogel showed sustained release of insulin without retinal damage or any inflammatory reactions seven days after subconjunctival injection of the hydrogel [163]. Another study of subconjunctival injection of a biodegradable thermosensitive hydrogel prepared with triblock copolymer of PLGA and PEG containing ovalbumin protein showed 14 days of concentration of the drug in the sclera, choroid, and retina [164]. Bevacizumab released from poly(ethylene glycol)-poly-(serinol-hexamethylene urethane) thermal hydrogel after intravitreal injection in a rabbit eye was observed with sustained release up to nine weeks, which was 4- to 5-fold longer than that observed with free protein injections (2 weeks). The rheological studies conducted using phosphate-buffered saline exhibited a phase transition at 32 °C with maximum elastic modulus at 37 °C [165–167].

(b) Combined Hydrogel Systems

Today, nanoparticles have been combined with hydrogels to form a hybrid system for the controlled delivery of therapeutics, especially for localized application and to increase the therapeutic efficacy. Tremendous research has been carried out to show the efficacy of injectable nanocarriers for ocular delivery of therapeutics along with hydrogel systems. A thermo-gelling hydrogel for administration to the eye has been prepared by Cho et al. using thermosensitive hexanoyl glycol chitosan [168]. A nano formulation containing thermosensitive penta-block gelling copolymer for ocular delivery of therapeutic proteins was cited as the platform technology for the ocular delivery of therapeutic proteins via intravitreal injection providing continuous zero-order release without any side effects or potential toxicity associated with targeted ocular tissues [169]. An injectable thermosensitive poly(N-isopropyl acryl amide) hydrogel containing PLGA nanoparticles of protein (ranibizumab/aflibercept) showed an initial burst release followed by sustained release of ranibizumab (0.153 g/day) and aflibercept (0.065 g/day) for up to 196 days [170].

One comparative study of nanoparticles with a nanoparticulate thermoreversible hydrogel containing PLGA-PEG-PLGA polymers showed $1.53 \pm 11.1\%$ reduction in VEGF production in a human RPE cell line in plain drug nanoparticles in comparison with $43.5 \pm 3.9\%$ observed with nanoparticulate hydrogel formulation [171]. About 12 weeks of successful long-term in vitro release was observed when encapsulated macromolecules in nanoparticles dispersed in a thermosensitive hydrogel [169]. Overall, the injectable in situ gelling depot system has emerged as a novel and attractive tool for sustained and stable protein delivery to the segment of the eye for as little as a few weeks up to as long as several months.

5.2. Particulate Carrier Systems

5.2.1. Microcarriers

The most preferable and useful strategy to provide slow, sustained, and prolonged release of drugs is the use of injectable colloidal particulate scaffolds.

Microparticles are micron-sized carriers that carry active drug molecules and are usually suspended in a liquid media. Several polymeric microspheres are being developed for ocular delivery of therapeutic proteins, and few have reached early stages of clinical trials. The use of biodegradable or biocompatible polymers in the formulation of microparticles, i.e., poly(lactic-co-glycolic acid) (PLGA) [172], polyanhydrides [173], and cyclodextrins [174], eliminates the problems of generating toxic products. These non-toxic products generated can be eliminated easily from the systemic circulation and, thus, cleared safely from the ocular environment [172]. Nonetheless, it is too early to say that microspheres are providing sustained release of macromolecules, maintaining therapeutic levels for longer durations of up to a week or months in ocular tissues. The release of macromolecules from the microparticles is closely associated with the structural properties, surface charge, porosity, size and shape, degradation rate, entrapment efficiency, and molar ratio of the polymers used and the diffusion rate of macromolecules [175]. Additionally, the method of preparation requires caution to protect the structural integrity of protein molecules and preserve their biological activity [176,177].

PLGA microspheres containing pegatinib showed sustained release of up to 20 days when injected via the transscleral route and up to several weeks from intravitreal route [178,179]. Sustained release of ranibizumab (0.153 µg/day) and aflibercept (0.065 µg/day) for 196 days was observed after initial burst release of 22.2 ± 2.1 and 13.10 ± 0.5 µg, respectively, when suspended in poly(N-isopropylacrylamide) injectable thermosensitive hydrogel [180]. Moreover, various techniques have been used to control the degradation and burst release of macromolecules from the microspheres. Using hydrophobic ion-pairing complexation, biocompatible block copolymers that can sustain the drug release for up to three months using stimuli sensitive hydrogel (pH, temperature, enzyme, light, ultrasound, and multiresponsive)-based formulations for ocular delivery of therapeutics are the examples discussed in the final section of this review [181,182]. PLGA microspheres containing interferon-alpha (IFN-α) provide sustained release and antiproliferative efficacy [183,184]. PLGA microspheres with anti-VEGF aptamer EYE001 has been tested in humans and showed sustained release over a period of 20 days [178]. PEG-bevacizumab conjugate, bevacizumab encapsulated with PLGA, and free bevacizumab when studied for reduction in experimentally induced choroidal neovascularization (CNV) showed no significant difference between all three formulations [185]. Sustained release of polylactic acid microparticles with a diameter of 7.6 µm, encapsulating TG-0054 (a hydrophilic drug intended for neovascularization and related diseases) for up to 3 months, was observed in rabbit model. After 3 months, the drug level in the choroid-RPE, retina, and vitreous was similar to that after one month [185]. In another case, the intravitreal injection of the plain injection of the same drug showed low intraocular levels after one month, with no detectable levels after three months [186]. PLGA is a well-known choice for the preparation of microparticles but offers several drawbacks, including poor protein stability, ineffective loading, and fast release profile [22]. A "system-within-system" matrix has been developed to transport ranibizumab to the vitreous for the treatment of age-related macular degeneration [187]. Chitosan-based microparticles in PLGA originated the highest ranibizumab-loading percentage and release when examined along with ranibizumab nanoparticles. Additionally, chitosan-tripolyphosphate-hyaluronic acid microparticles demonstrated antiangiogenic activity owing to hyaluronic acid, which was an advantageous property but one that was regrettably offset by the quick disintegration of the matching PLGA microparticles [188].

5.2.2. Nanocarriers

Polymeric Nanoparticles

Polymeric nanocarriers are particles with dimensions between 10 nm and 1000 nm loaded with drug molecules dissolved, entrapped, encapsulated, or adsorbed in natural or synthetic polymers. According to the distribution of the drug molecules in the polymeric matrix, these nanocarriers are categorized as nanospheres (drug molecules are homogeneously dispersed or dissolved in the polymer matrix) and nanocapsules (drug molecules are in the core, which is covered by a polymeric shell) [138]. Injectable nanocarriers have potential for ocular delivery because they provide increased stability to the encapsulated molecules, good ocular residence time, and adherence, leading to excellent bioavailability in the ocular tissues [189–191].

Among the different routes for ocular delivery of therapeutic proteins via nanocarriers are topical, periocular, suprachoroidal, and intravitreal routes. As shown in Table 1, injectable polymeric nanoparticles play a significant role in delivering therapeutic proteins via the intravitreal route. More effective and long-term inhibition of corneal neovascularization was observed with intravitreally injected nanoparticles, as compared to other peptides [192–194]. The efficient corneal neovascularization inhibition may be due to enhanced pharmacokinetic properties, including prolonged retention time, formation of nanosized depots intravitreally, and avoidance of enzymatic degradation [192,193].

The polymers used provided several benefits such as chemical stability, biocompatibility, tunable degradability, and flexibility in designing the formulation. The polymeric nanoparticles exhibited light-scattering properties, which may cause clouding of the vitreous, loss of bioactivity, and low stability of therapeutic proteins, and need proper attention to the selection of the polymer matrix and nanoencapsulation technique for their delivery through the ocular route [194].

The parameter that determines the stability, particle size, surface charge, or zeta potential of the nanoparticles is the composition of the nanoparticles, i.e., lipidic or polymeric. In addition, this parameter does not affect only at the intravitreal level but also topically and subretinally. Moreover, the use of ligands is important before formulating injectable nanocarriers for the delivery of therapeutic proteins to the ocular tissues (see Figure 3).

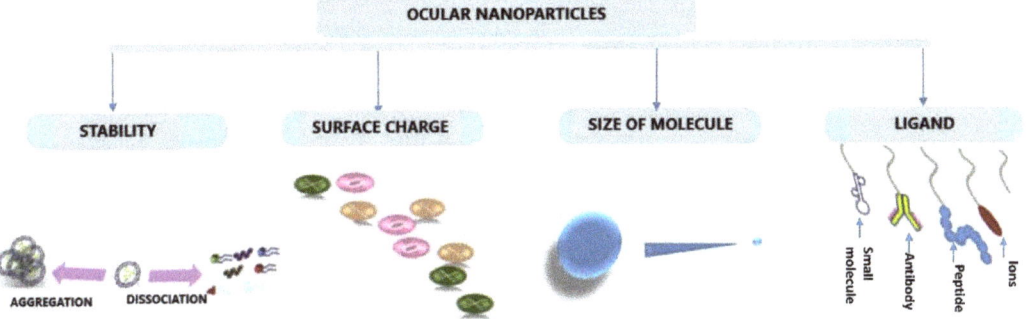

Figure 3. Characteristics of the ocular nanoparticles that affect their intraocular distribution and elimination.

A study related to ocular tissue distribution of nanoparticles with different surface modifications (positive and negative charges and PEGylated) using ex vivo bovine vitreous was carried out and showed that particles sized greater than 1000 nm can be used for sustained release of retinal drugs due to the slower clearance from the vitreous [45]. Moreover, high and hindered movements of negatively charged and PEGylated particles and marginal mobility of positively charged nanoparticles were observed. Positively charged particles of size around 200 nm showed marginal mobility when compared to negatively or PEGylated particles of size 500–1000 nm. The mobility of positively charged particles was also affected by the presence of negatively charged hyaluronic acid in the vitreous [195].

Surface charge of the nanoparticles needs to be considered for ocular penetration of therapeutics as higher diffusion in the vitreous was observed with negatively charged human serum albumin compared with positively charged [196]. Thus, negatively charged polymeric nanocarriers are more useful in delivering cationic therapeutic proteins as observed with the delivery of IgG containing gold nanoparticles to the retinal pigment epithelium and photoreceptor cells through subretinal injection [197].

Montmorillonite-chitosan nanoparticles loaded with Betaxolol developed for the treatment of glaucoma showed a positive surface charge of 29 ± 0.18 mV and mean size of 460 ± 0.6 nm and provided strong contact with the negatively charged mucin layer of the corneal membrane. Thus, it was concluded that the developed nanoparticles could provide drug release for longer duration with improved bioavailability [198].

Having the ability to provide sustained drug release, low cytotoxicity, and fewer side effects, PLGA, one of the most commonly used materials among the preferred synthetic or natural biodegradable polymers, has been studied extensively for ocular delivery of therapeutics [199]. For instance, PLGA nanoparticles loaded with dexamethasone after intravitreal injection in rabbits showed 50 days of sustained release with constant drug levels for more than 30 days with a mean concentration of 3.85 mg/L [200]. Based on the areas under the curve (AUC), the bioavailability of dexamethasone in the experimental group was found to be significantly (4.96, 4.15, and 6.35 times) higher than the control group injected with free dexamethasone solution [200].

Both hydrophobic and hydrophilic molecules can be loaded in PLGA nanoparticles [201]. For example, bovine serum albumin, a hydrophilic serum protein, was encapsulated with high efficiency using PLGA nanoparticles [202,203]; lysozyme and human pigment epithelium-derived factor beta 1 separately encapsulated in PLGA nanoparticles provided sustained release across 30 days [204]; in vitro sustained release of the antiangiogenic pigment epithelium-derived factor from PLGA nanoparticles was obtained over 40 days with 70% release within 10 days [205]. The vitreous concentration of bevacizumab was above 500 ng/mL for up to 8 weeks after intravitreal injection of PLGA nanoparticles in rabbits [206]. In the treatment of wet AMD using nano or microspheres of poly(ethylene glycol-b-poly(DL-lactic acid) as the delivery vehicle loaded with bevacizumab, a sustained release of up to 90 days was observed. Moreover, the drug/polymer ratio can be changed to control the drug release rate, and thus, the release rate and bioavailability can be improved as needed [207]. In the treatment of neovascular diseases, nanoparticle-mediated pathway control and expression of natural antiangiogenic factors were found to have significant therapeutic potential in which a proteolytic fragment plasminogen Kringle 5 was found to exhibit sustained angiogenic impact with reduced CNV regions and vascular leakage for two weeks, as observed in CNV models [208,209]. VLN, a low-density lipoprotein receptor extracellular domain, encapsulated in PLGA nanoparticles, exhibited excellent expression of VLN, both in cultured cells and the retina for up to 4 weeks [210]. Another study carried out for the treatment of AMD using anti-inflammatory and antiangiogenic drugs to retinal pigment epithelium showed an antiangiogenic effect for up to three weeks [211]. The PLGA nanoparticles were easily and effectively internalized by ARPE-19 cells via folate receptor-mediated endocytosis, forming a depot and thus providing the sustained effect by downregulating VEGF and upregulating pigment epithelium-derived factor [212]. Aflibercept-loaded PLGA nanoparticles showed 75% drug release in one week, and it has been concluded that it can be more patient-compliant compared to frequent intravitreal injection of plain aflibercept [213]. It was observed that the PLGA microparticles and polylactic acid nanoparticles showed sustained release of bevacizumab (of up to two months) intravitreally in rat model as compared to the effect (of up to two weeks) observed with plain bevacizumab solution when injected intravitreally in rat model [214]. Similarly, PLGA microparticles containing ranibizumab entrapped in chitosan-based nanoparticles for ocular delivery of ranibizumab showed quantifiable release of up to 12 days [215].

Micelles

A subclass of amphiphilic nanocarriers that self-assemble in an aqueous environment, producing supramolecular structures in the size range of 10 to 1000 nm known as micelles, has been studied extensively for delivery of small molecules to the ocular tissues [216]. They offer several advantages such as controlled release, reduced toxicity, high drug-loading capacity, and enhanced stability, with highly changeable surfaces, providing high patient compliance [216]. Micelles are prepared using different polymers such as Pluronic F127/F68, N-isopropyl acrylamide, polyhydroxy-ethyl-aspartamide, methoxy-poly(ethylene glycol)-poly(e-caprolactone), and poly(butylene oxide) [196]. Polymeric micelles provide excellent ocular residence time due to their mucoadhesive properties and, having nanosized range, are an excellent system for drugs with poor permeability. Thus, ocular delivery of therapeutics using polymeric micelles showed significant improvement in antiangiogenic therapy for retinal and choroidal vascular diseases and diabetic retinopathy. Anti-Flt1 peptide of GNQWFI, an antagonist for vascular endothelial growth factor (VEGFR1 or Flt1) receptor, (inhibits VEGFR1-mediated cell migration and tube formation), was chemically conjugated to tetra-n-butyl-ammonium modified hyaluronate via amide bond formation in dimethyl sulfoxide using benzotriazolel-1-yloxy-tris(dimethyl amino)phosphonium hexafluorophosphate successfully. It self-assembled itself to form micelle-like nanoparticles in an aqueous solution, showing significant reduction in retinal vascular permeability and deformation of the retinal vascular structure in diabetic retinopathy and effectively inhibiting the CNV in laser-induced CNV in rat model, and it increased the mean residence time of the macromolecule by more than two weeks [207]. Further encapsulation of this conjugated antagonist (anti-Flt1 peptide-HA conjugate) to genistein (tyrosine-specific protein kinase inhibitor) when used as combination therapy in corneal neovascularization showed sustained delivery of more than 24 h with an excellent inhibitory effect both on CNV and vascular hyper permeability [216].

Dendrimers

Dendrimers are branched nanosized polymeric carriers, which are layered like liposomes and used extensively for the delivery of ocular therapeutics. Compared to linear polymeric particles, they exhibit high concentrations of payloads of therapeutic proteins. They are monodispersed, having a tree-like architecture based on the polymers, i.e., polyamidoamiones, polyamides, poly (aryl ethers), polyesters, and carbohydrates [217]. The pattern of release, absorption, and elimination of the therapeutics are dependent on the surface charge and molecular weight of the dendrimers, i.e., absorption is at its maximum with cationic charge, and rapid clearance is observed with high molecular weight (>40 kDa) [218]. When using several copies of therapeutics, dendrimers are very useful in controlling the functionality by providing numerous functional groups, which hasten the stimuli responsive ability of dendrimers and help in targeting the connected components and providing binding strength of the ligand to the receptors [218]. A polyamidoamiones hydrogel containing a dendrimer was prepared by crosslinking stimuli-responsive acrylate groups using PEG–acrylate chains activated by UV light and was found to be highly mucoadhesive and nontoxic to the corneal epithelial cells, with high cellular uptake and enhanced corneal bovine transport [217]. Similarly, the polyamidoamiones/PLGA nanoparticulate dendrimer hydrogel was also found to be nontoxic, highly effective, and able to provide the sustained release of the drug on the ocular surface of a rabbit eye [219]. Use of proper conjugation techniques to design different dendrimer conjugates can help in understanding the mechanism of protein adsorption on the surface of dendrimers, also known as "protein corona", for the use as carriers in ocular delivery of therapeutics [218].

Lipid-Based Nanocarriers

Among the injectable colloidal drug delivery systems, the lipid-based nanocarriers are the more interesting and emerging systems also known as "nano-safe carrier systems" for delivering drugs to the ocular tissues due to their excellent biocompatibility, biodegradability, and ability to improve the bioavailability and thereby therapeutic efficacy.

(a) Solid Lipid Nanoparticles (SLNs) and Nanostructured Lipid Carriers (NLCs)

Solid lipid nanoparticles, nanostructured lipid carriers, and liposomes are promising approaches for the safe, sustained, and targeted delivery of therapeutic proteins in many locals, including the ocular tissues. These nanocarriers provide nontoxic, stable, controlled, scalable, and targeted delivery of therapeutic proteins [220]. For example, a sustained release and new synthesis of cytokines in corneal tissues with long-term anti-inflammatory effects can be achieved from p-IL10 containing solid lipid nanoparticles [221]. Recently, a lactoferrin-based nanostructured lipid carrier was evaluated for its stability, cytotoxicity, entrapment efficiency, loading capacity, ocular surface retention, surface charge, and morphology [222]. The results showed nanostructured lipid carriers with an average size around 119.45 ± 11.44 nm, a PDI value of 0.151 ± 0.045, and a surface charge of 17.50 ± 2.53 mV [208]. Moreover, regulated release of lactoferrin, high entrapment efficiency, and lipid content (up to 75%) can be achieved [222]. Nonetheless, more research work is required for understanding the use of solid lipid nanoparticles and nanostructured lipid carriers for the ocular delivery of therapeutics.

(b) Niosomes

There is another self-assembling, nonionic carrier system of lipid-based nanocarriers capable of encapsulating both lipophilic and hydrophilic molecules in their bilayered structured nanovesicles known as niosomes. They release the drug independent of pH, resulting in enhanced ocular bioavailability. Though, similar to liposomes, they are biodegradable, biocompatible, nontoxic, nonimmunogenic, and have good chemical stability, the efficacy of the niosomes as carriers for protein delivery to ocular tissues is still under investigation [223]. Discosomes, another modified version of niosomes, are an excellent strategy for ocular delivery. They are prepared using nonionic surfactants, with a size range of 12–16 nm, and prevent systemic drainage and, thus, improve the ocular residence time; however, they are nonbiodegradable and nonbiocompatible in nature [223]. Persistent protein expression after transfection of pDNA containing niosomes intravitreally for at least one month after injection was found to provide protection against enzymatic digestion and broad surface transfection in inner layer of retina with no cytotoxicity [224].

(c) Liposomes

Liposomes are very small nano- or microsized vesicles containing one or more concentric amphiphilic lipid bilayers and are nontoxic, biodegradable, and biocompatible [225]. The surface charge of the liposomes is very important as positively charged liposomes can make intimate contact with the corneal (negatively charged) and conjunctival surfaces compared to neutral or negatively charged liposomes [226,227]. Bevacizumab-containing liposomes were prepared from PC-PS (cholesterol) to be 100 nm in size using the dehydration–rehydration technique and were coated with annexin successfully for intravitreal administration [226]. The highest transfection effect was observed in low quantities of plasmid DNA in liposomes, with the peak level being reached within 3 days after intravitreal injection of pDNA containing liposomes [228]. In another study, sustained release in the vitreous and retina–choroid from intravitreal injections of liposomal oligonucleotides showed a protective effect against enzymatic degradation [229]. Significant improvement in mean residence time of bevacizumab after intravitreal injection of liposomes [230] and sustained release of bevacizumab from the liposomes were observed for up to 42 days after intravitreal injection [221]. Significantly reduced inflammation with prolonged protection of peptides of up to 14 days in vivo after intravitreal injection of vasoactive intestinal peptide-containing liposomes was also observed [225].

5.3. Microbubbles Technology

A new ocular delivery technology using the microbubble, a stimuli-responsive intelligent polymeric carrier system easily converted to nanoscale microbubble vesicles in the presence of stimuli such as pH, temperature, and magnetic field, was found to deliver the therapeutic proteins effectively to the anterior as well as posterior segments of the eye [231].

5.4. Nanofibers and Amphiphiles

Self-assembling peptide nanofibers and peptide amphiphiles are also under investigation for use as carriers for ocular delivery of therapeutics. After subconjunctival injection, nanofibers containing LPPR peptide bind to VEGFR1 and NRP1 and significantly inhibit endothelial cell proliferation and cell migration; in addition, abnormal capillary synthesis showed a significant reduction (81.3%) in corneal neovascularization in 14 days in rat as compared to bevacizumab (51.2%), justifying its efficiency to cure angiogenesis-related diseases [232–235].

5.5. Nanowafers

A tiny, transparent circular disc-type or rectangular membrane-shaped nanoreservoir type known as a nanowafer is applied easily with the fingertips and is synthesized using different polymers (e.g., polyvinyl pyrrolidone, carboxymethyl cellulose, hydroxypropylmethylcellulose, and polyvinyl alcohol) and provides sustained release for a few hours to several days as it remains on the ocular surface for a long period of time [236]. Axitinib nanowafers were tested in ocular burn-induced murine model and observed for inhibitory effects on CNV in mouse model. The results were compared with twice-daily axitinib eye drops (0.1% w/v) and showed that corneal treatment with nanowafers significantly reduced the proliferation of limbal blood vessels as compared with the corneal treatment with the conventional axitinib eye drops. From the reverse transcriptase polymerase chain reaction study, it was found that the Axi-nanowafer is more effective in downregulating the drug target proteins, i.e., vascular endothelial growth factor (A, R1 and R2), PDGFR-A, and bFGF, compared to that of the conventional eye drop treatment. Thus, once-a-day axitinib nanowafers are more effective than twice-a-day conventional eye drops [236].

5.6. Cell-Penetrating Peptides

With excellent membrane modulating ability, cell-penetrating peptides are widely used as penetration enhancers to overcome ocular junction barriers and provide effective drug delivery to ocular tissues. These compounds consist of natural and synthetic amino acid sequences, which facilitate the delivery of peptides, proteins, and genes to intracellular ocular tissues [237,238]. Involving noninvasive or minimally invasive treatments capable of crossing biological membranes, the use of cell-penetrating peptides for ocular delivery has gained increasing attention these days.

Quick translocation of the conjugated protein molecules through the cell membranes into mammalian cells using CPPs as nanocarriers is possible through energy-dependent pinocytosis/endocytosis/direct translocation, which make this an effective strategy for the ocular delivery of therapeutic proteins [238]. CPPs can be integrated within the dosage form, providing sustained release by preventing degradation and increasing the drug residence time.

Intravitreal injection of bevacizumab linked to CPPs (5(6)-carboxyfluorescein-RRRRRR-COOH) with anti-VEGF, topical bevacizumab-CPP with anti-VEGF (twice daily), or dexamethasone gavage (every day) for 10 days revealed a significant reduction in corneal neovascularization areas in all mice for all with in vivo and ex vivo rabbit model [239].

Low cytotoxicity and enhanced permeability of CPPs were reported by Liu et al. [240], who studied the uptake, permeability, and toxicity of various CPPs on human epithelial cells including transactivating transcriptional activator (TAT), penetratin, poly (arginine), low molecular weight protamine, and poly (serine). All the CPPs showed efficient membrane permeability of topically delivered drugs to the posterior segments [240]. In another study, researchers found that the penetratin showed the most efficient distribution of peptides in both anterior and posterior segments of eye as compared to all other CPPs, indicated from significantly higher concentrations of penetratin-conjugated polyarginine (R8) in corneal epithelium and the retina for up to six hours [241]. Topical administration of bevacizumab/ranibizumab conjugated with polyarginine (R6) in a rat eye showed effective concentration of a drug in the retina/vitreous and aqueous humor, which indicated that CPP-conjugated macromolecules showed significantly higher penetration through corneal epithelium and RPE cells, providing effective therapeutic treatment in CNV mouse model [242,243].

Fibroblast growth factor (FGF) administered topically after conjugation with TAT showed effective concentration in the retina for up to 8 h [244]. Similarly, endostatin, an antiangiogenetic protein in conjugation with TAT (22 kDa), when administered topically in mouse eyes, showed significant protein expression resulting in inhibition of CNV [245]. PLGA nanoparticles loaded with macromolecules with TAT linked in the surface showed an excellent efficient delivery in the posterior segment after topical administration [244].

Poor serum stability and toxicity from the CPPs of nonhuman origin were observed in a study performed with CPPs of human and nonhuman origin to overcome immunogenicity [238]. Proteolytic enzymes metabolize noncovalent constraints rapidly, while covalent constraints are proteolyzed by crosslinking with disulfides and amides [246]. Thus, the stability can be improved by increasing the binding affinity of peptides with antibodies using different crosslinks, i.e., lactam, triazole, or thioether group at the helix of peptides [246,247]. The confirmational stabilization of long-chain helix using macrocyclic bridging features or mutagenesis can also be utilized to improve the hydrophobicity and enhanced binding of both covalent and noncovalent constraints [248].

Efficient retinal delivery was achieved for apoliporotein-A1 when fused with penetratin and phospholipids containing high-density lipoprotein particles [249]. Significant therapeutic effect was observed in AMD murine model when pazopanib (an antiangiogenetic therapeutic) contained high-density lipoproteins microparticles along with penetratin [249–251].

5.7. Encapsulated Cell Technology

Encapsulated cell technology can become the alternative to intravitreal therapy, which uses the expression of protein molecules by providing continuous local production of proteins. Encapsulated cell technology uses permeable materials that allow the diffusion of nutrients, therapeutic factors, and waste products out of cells, thus protecting the cells from digestion by the host immune response. Prolonged release of vascular endothelial growth factor receptor protein (NT-503) and CNTF from implants encapsulating genetically altered human retinal pigment epithelial cells was observed without any retinal degeneration [252–254].

A study on long-term cell therapy on mouse eyes using genetically engineered microencapsulated ARPE-19 cells in alginate developed to produce complement receptor-2 fragment (CR2-fH) showed reduced corneal neovascularization and lesion size intravitreally and showed the presence of CR2-fH in the retinal pigment epithelial/choroid of treated mice with systemic expression of fusion proteins without producing any immune response [255,256].

5.8. Iontophoresis

Another noninvasive technique to transfer ionized molecules through biological membranes to the ocular tissues using a low electric current is iontophoresis, where the drugs can be transported across the membrane by migration or electro-osmotic processes. Dexamethasone phosphate [257], methylprednisolone [258], carboplatin [259], and methotrexate [260] showed successful delivery through the ocular iontophoretic technique via ocular tissues except therapeutic proteins. Using proper design of devices and probes, one can use iontophoretic technique via the transcorneal, corneoscleral, or transscleral route [261]. As the sclera has more surface area (17 cm^2) than the cornea (1.3 cm^2) and is more hydrated, presents fewer cells, and is more permeable to macromolecules having high molecular weight, the transscleral route is the preferred route for ocular delivery of macromolecules to the posterior segment. Moreover, the transscleral route is simple, nonintrusive, has a wide application, reduces the risk of toxicity, and is well tolerated by the patients [262].

The device used for the iontophoresis is flexible and placed under the eyelid to deliver ions through a small area of the eyeball, avoiding tissue damage [263]. Devices such as OcuPhore™ release the drug into the retina and choroid using an applicator, dispersive electrode, and a dose control for the transscleral iontophoresis; Visulex™ is used for the transscleral transport of ionized molecules such as dexamethasone and antisense oligodeoxynucleotides [264–266].

5.9. Ocular Microneedles

Ocular microneedles are popular delivery techniques exhibiting passive delivery of molecules via arrays of solid microneedles coated with drug formulations that dissolve a few minutes after insertion [267,268]. This technique is used as routine in clinic and is gaining popularity among formulators for having the potential to deliver ocular therapeutics, overcoming the transport barriers of epithelial tissues, eliminating clearance by conjunctival mechanisms, and minimizing retinal damage. For example, sunitinib malate containing microneedle pens showed suppression of corneal neovascularization [269].

5.10. Injectable Implants

With the aim of achieving sustained release in the vitreous and providing a long-term therapeutic effect from the polymeric network, intraocular implants are gaining popularity as drug delivery systems. Though it is an intrusive procedure, implants have shown several benefits such as bypassing the blood retinal barrier, avoiding burst release, reduction of the dose, and delivering therapeutics with a constant rate directly at the ocular site [230]. Nonbiodegradable and biodegradable implants are available in the market (see Table 3 and Figure 4) and can have a tunable delivery rate by changing the type and composition of the polymers or the delivery form, i.e., solid, semisolid, or a particulate-based system [270–272]. The mechanism of drug release from implants showed three phases, i.e., an early burst, a middle diffusive phase, and a final burst. Different polymers such as polylactic acid, polyglycolic acid, and polylactic-coglycolic acid are being used to prepare implants. Among the advantages of using implants are the no need to perform repeated injections intravitreally, increased half-life, reduced peak plasma level, and improved patient compliance. Nonetheless, the use of this type of device requires surgery or invasive implantation, which sometimes exerts certain ocular side effects. Incorporation of PEG400 and different block copolymers such as PLGA improves the burst release and provides prolonged release of therapeutic proteins [270,271]. Biodegradable implants offer several benefits, such as high payload, prolonged drug release, and minimal burst release, but a minor surgical procedure involves a skilled professional, leading to high treatment cost [273].

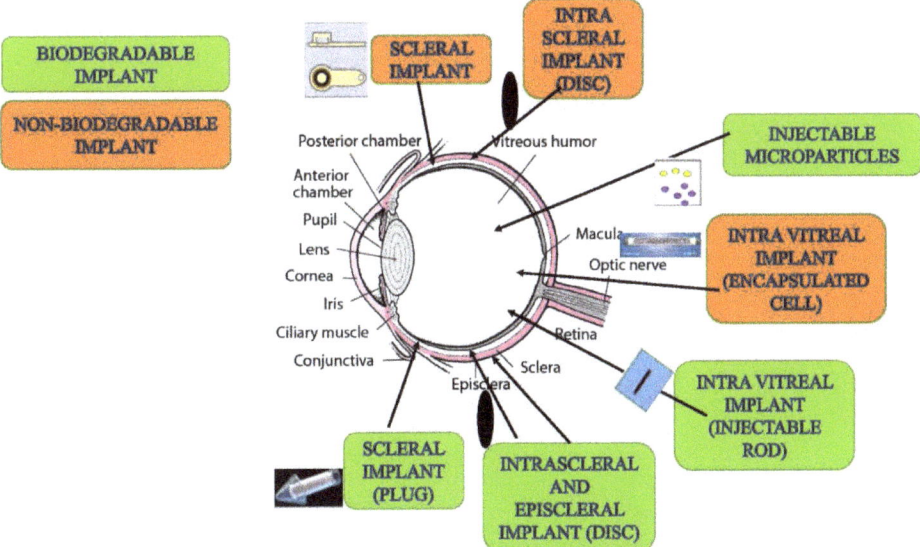

Figure 4. Biodegradable and nonbiodegradable implants for ocular delivery of therapeutic proteins.

FDA-approved biodegradable implants, namely, Ozurdex® based on PLGA and Iluvien® based on polyvinyl alcohol/fluocinolone acetonide in a polyamide tube, used for macular edema and noninfectious posterior uveitis showed sustained release of dexamethasone (0.7 mg) for up to 6 months in the vitreal cavity [274,275]. The short half-life (~3 h) of the corticosteroids leads to faster elimination from the vitreous, which can easily be administered by formulating into implants [276]. So far, no ocular implants have been approved for the delivery of ocular therapeutic proteins, but preclinical studies with human recombinant tissue plasminogen activator showed a release rate of 0.5µg/day in the vitreous for 14 days [277–281].

Nonbiodegradable implants provide more accurate, zero-order, and have longer release rates compared to biodegradable ones, but they require a surgical procedure for their removal, which involves associated risks.

An osmotic implant inserted into the subcutaneous region connected to the sclera using a brain infusion kit delivered IgG for up to 28 days [282]. Another nonbiodegradable implant containing a ranibizumab port delivery system from Genentech showed extended release in the vitreous [283].

Table 3. Examples of the most relevant results obtained with different formulation approaches used to improve the ocular delivery of therapeutic proteins.

Delivery System	Material	Molecule	Remarks	References
Microparticles	PLGA	Anti-VEGF aptamer EYE001	In vitro drug sustained release up to 20 days.	[178]
Microparticles	PLA nanoparticles in porous PLGA microparticles	Bevacizumab	In vivo sustained release after intravitreal injection in rats.	[214]
Microparticles	PLGA	Bevacizumab	In vitro drug sustained release for up to 91 days from the microparticles.	[284]
Microparticles	PLGA	Bevacizumab	In vivo sustained release after intravitreal injection to rabbit.	[285]
Microparticles	Silicon dioxide	Bevacizumab	In vitro sustained release for up to 165 days. From the porous silicon dioxide microparticles.	[286]
Microparticles/ Nanoparticles	PLGA-albumin	Bevacizumab	In vivo and ex vivo rabbit vitreous injection showed sustained release for up to 165 days from the developed PLGA-albumin microparticles (~197 nm).	[287]
Nanoparticles	HSA-PEG	Apatinib	Reduced leakage in vascular tissues with significant inhibition of hyperpermeability in streptozotocin-induced diabetic mice after intravitreal injection of apatinib-HAS-PEG nanoparticles.	[288]
Nanoparticles	Albuminated PLGA	Bevacizumab	Sustained release with antibody protection obtained with its stability intravitreally for about 8 weeks with vitreous concentration maintained above 500 ng/mL from the coumarin-6-loaded albuminated-PLGA-NPs.	[289]
Nanoparticles	CS-PLGA	Bevacizumab	Sustained and effective delivery of bevacizumab to posterior ocular tissues after subconjunctival administration and more reduction in VEGF level in retina than the topical or intravitreal administration.	[290]
Nanoparticles	CS-HA, Zinc sulphate	Bevacizumab	Sustained release for up to two months with reduced CNV from CS-loaded bevacizumab nanoparticles containing implants, when administered intravitreally.	[291]
Nanoparticles	PLGA	Connexin43mimetic peptide	Improved light sensitivity and suppression of inflammatory areas showing high concentration in ganglion cell layer and choroid within half an hour after intravitreal injection.	[292]
Nanoparticles	PLGA	Bevacizumab	Enhanced antiangiogenic effect and reduced toxicity of tissues after intravitreal injection in vivo	[293]

Table 3. Cont.

Delivery System	Material	Molecule	Remarks	References
Nanoparticles	ALBUMIN	Connexin43 mimetic peptide	Significant enhancement in protection against degradation and high retention in vitro with expression of CD44 cells in both retina and choroid.	[294]
Nanoparticles	CHITOSAN	Bevacizumab	VEGF expression inhibition after intravitreal injection.	[295]
Nanoparticles	PLA/PLA-PEO	C16Y Peptide	Sustained release and prolonged effect on suppression of CNV from NPs due to significant permeation to targeted tissues and reduced toxicity as compared to simple peptide solution after intravitreal injection.	[296]
Nanoparticles	12-7NH-12, DOPE, DPPC	Cy5-DNA	Concentration of drug found within 4 h postinjection intravitreally from nanoparticles located in NFL.	[297]
Nanoparticles	Chitosan	pDNA	Effective transfection in INL, IPL, and RGC layers after intravitreal injection.	[298]
Nanoparticles	PLGA	pDNA, shRNA	GFP expression effect is persistent with significant reduction in CNV, lesion thickness, and retinal damage for 4 weeks after intravitreal injection.	[299]
Nanoparticles	PLGA	pDNA	Significant reduction of vascular leakage CNV induced diabetic rats without tissue damage and effective K5 expression in the retinal layer for up to 4 weeks after intravitreal injection.	[300]
Nano-balls	bPEI	siRNA	Sustained release, longer retention with effective concentration in choroid and RPE target tissues for up to 2 weeks after intravitreal injection.	[301]
Nanoparticles	DOTAP, DOPE	pDNA	Transfection effect is increased significantly up to 6-fold in RPE as well as 2-fold in in vitro after intravitreal injection.	[302]
Lipid-nanoparticles	DOTAP, Cholesterol, PEG-DSPE	siRNA	VEGFR1 expression inhibited in ARPE-19 cell-lines showing no tissue damage and reduced CNV areas after intravitreal injection.	[303]
SLN	Precirol (ATO5), DOTAP, Tween 80 Dextran, HA	pDNA	High transfection efficiency in both PR and INL showing improvement in retinal structure after 2 weeks after intravitreal injection.	[304]
NLC	Monolaurin, Monostearin, Glyceryl tripalmitate, Palmitin Glyceryl stearate	Sorafenib	Demonstrated excellent physicochemical properties and good tolerance, sustained release, and enhanced ocular bioavailability in CNV after topical administration.	[305]
NLC	Glyceryl monostearate, lipoplysaccharides	Dasatinib	Observed sustained release, reduced ocular toxicity, and facilitated penetration into cornea via topical administration with effective inhibition of CNV.	[306]
Dendrimer	Lecithin	Anti-VEGF Plus Oligonucleotide 1	Topical delivery of dendrimers plus ODN-1 to the eyes of rats and inhibited laser-induced CNV for up to 6 months.	[307]

Table 3. Cont.

Delivery System	Material	Molecule	Remarks	References
Niosomes	DOTAP, squalene, Polysorbate 80	pDNA	Persistent protein expression after transfection intravitreally for at least 1 month after injection. Protection against enzymatic digestion, providing broad surface transfection in inner layer of retina with no cytotoxicity.	[224]
Liposomes	DOTMA, Cholesterol, DOPE	pDNA	Highest transfection effect with lower quantity of plasmid DNA in liposomes reached peak level within 3 days after intravitreal injection.	[228]
Liposomes	PC, Cholesterol, PEG-DSPE	Oligonucleotide	Sustained release in vitreous and retina–choroid from intravitreal injection of liposomal oligonucleotides showing protective effect against enzymatic degradation after intravitreal injection.	[229]
Liposomes	DPPC, EPC, Cholesterol	Bevacizumab	Significant improvement in mean residence time of bevacizumab after intravitreal injection.	[308]
Liposomes	EPC-Chol and DPC-Cholesterol	Bevacizumab	Showed sustained release of drug for up to 42 days after intravitreal injection.	[221]
Liposomes	PC-PS(Cholesterol)Toc	Bevacizumab-(annexin)	Liposomes showed 100 nm of size prepared with dehydration–rehydration technique and coated with annexin after intravitreal injection.	[220]
Liposomes	PC, Cholesterol	Vasoactive intestinal peptide	Reduced inflammation significantly with prolonged protection of peptide up to 14 days in vivo after intravitreal injection.	[225]
Biodegradable Implants	Molded hydrogel matrix	Bevacizumab	Implants prepared using PRINT technology from molded hydrogel showed sustained release of bevacizumab for 2 months after intravitreal administration.	[159]
Biodegradable implants	PCL	Ranibizumab	Film device containing nanopores on PCL provided sustained release of ranibizumab for 3 months after intravitreal injection.	[309]
Nonbiodegradable implants	Programmable micropump device	Ranibizumab	Micropump for posterior segment prepared using nonbiodegradable polymers showed long-term release of ranibizumab after intravitreal administration.	[310]
Implants	Port delivery system	Ranibizumab	Semipermeable refillable membrane providing long-term release of ranibizumab for 1 year after intravitreal administration.	[311]
Non-biodegradable implants	NT-503	VEGFR-Fc	Increased specific VEGFR binding observed with encapsulating cell showing continuous production of therapeutic proteins for two years after intravitreal administration.	[312]
Verisome IB20089	Biodegradable implant with liquid gel	Triamcinolone/ Ranibizumab	The formed spherules provided long term sustained release up to 1 year after intravitreal injection.	[313]
Microsphere in hydrogel	PNIPAAm	Ranibizumab and aflibercept	Sustained in vitro release for up to 196 days from thermosensitive hydrogel after intravitreal injection.	[180]
In situ hydrogel	HA(DEX)	Bevacizumab	Hydrogel formed by chemical crosslinking showed sustained release for up to 6 months in vivo administered intravitreal in rabbit model.	[146]

Table 3. Cont.

Delivery System	Material	Molecule	Remarks	References
Hydrogel	Alginate(Chitosan) hydrogel/PLGA microspheres	Bevacizumab/ Ranibizumab	Sustained release from intravitreally administered hydrogel observed for both bevacizumab and ranibizumab for up to 3 months.	[158]
Hydrogel	PLGA-mPEG	Bevacizumab	Sustained release for up to 1 month via intravitreal route in rabbits.	[159]
Hydrogel	PEOz(PCL)PEOz	Bevacizumab	Sustained release for up to 20 days in vitro.	[160]
Silk based hydrogels	Silk fibroin	Bevacizumab	Sustained release of bevacizumab from intravitreally administered hydrogel for 90 days in vitro as well as in vivo in Dutch-belted rabbits.	[161]
In situ gel	PCM(HEMA)	Bevacizumab	Provided in vivo retention for up to 2 months in SD rats via suprachoroidal route.	[162]
Hydrogel	PNIPAAm	Insulin	Sustained release of insulin for up to 30 days in vitro.	[163]
Hydrogel	PLGA–PEG	Ovalbumin (model protein)	Provided sufficient protein concentration for up to 14 days in ocular tissues via subconjunctival route.	[164]
Hydrogel	ESHU	Bevacizumab	Sustained release for up to 9 weeks via intravitreal route in rabbits.	[166]
Hydrogel	PEG-(ESHU)	Bevacizumab	Showed good in vitro and in vivo biocompatibility after intravitreal injection.	[167]
Hydrogel	PNIPAAm	Bevacizumab/ Ranibizumab	Provided good mechanical properties, biocompatibility from thermosensitive hydrogel after intravitreal injection.	[170]
Diels-alder hydrogels	PEG Macromonomers	Bevacizumab	Provided mechanical stability and long-term release for up to 6 weeks from the chemically crosslinked hydrogel after intravitreal injection.	[314]
Encapsulated cells	Polysulfone	CNTF	Continued clinical trials.	[315]
Retinal cells	HAS	Connexin43 mimetic peptide	Sustained release and prolonged retention with suppression of RGC and inflammation observed when intravitreally injected NPs encapsulating Cx43 MP were evaluated in a rat model of retinal ischemia-reperfusion injury.	[316]

Abbreviations: bPEI: Branched polyethylenimine; CNV: corneal neovascularization; CNTF: ciliary neurotrophic factor; DA: dexamethasone acetate; DDS: drug delivery systems; DEX: dexamethasone; DOPC: 1,2-Dioleoyl-sn-glycero-3-phosphocholine; DOPE: 1,2-Dioleoyl-sn-glycero-3-phospho-ethanol-amine; DOPG: 1,2-Dioleoyl-sn-glycero-3-phospho (10-rac-glycerol); DOTAP: 1,2-Dioleoyl-3-trimethyl-ammonium-propane; DOTMA: 1,2-Di-o-octadecanyl-3-tri-methyl-ammonium-propane; DPPC: 1,2-Dipalmitoyl-sn-glycero-3-phosphocholine; DR: diabetic retinopathy; DSPE (PEG): 1,2-Distearoyl-SN-Glycero-3-phosphoethanolamine-n(amino-polyethylene glycol); EAU: experimental autoimmune uveitis; EIU: endotoxin-induced uveitis; EPC: egg phosphatidylcholine; HA: hyaluronic acid; HAS: human serum albumin; HSPC: 1 (a)-Phosphatidyl-Choline-Hydrogenated soy; INL: inner nuclear layer; IPL: inner plexiform layer; mPEG (PCL): monomethoxy poly-ethylene glycol-poly-e-caprolactone; NDPR: nonproliferative diabetic retinopathy; NPs: nanoparticles; PCL: polycaprolactone; PC-PS-Toc: egg phosphatidylcholine-porcine brain phosphatidylserine-tocopherol; pDNA: plasmid deoxy-ribonucleic acid; PEG: polyethylene glycol; PEG-PHDC: poly(methoxy-poly(ethylene glycol)-cyanoacrylate-co-hexadecyl cyanoacrylate); PEO-PCL-PEO: poly(2-ethy-2-oxazoline)b-poly(caprolactone)-b-poly(2-ethyl-2-oxazoline); PLA: polylactic acid; PLA–PEO: poly lactic acid-polyethylene oxide; PLGA: poly-(lactide-coglycolide); PNIPAAm: poly (n-isopropylacrylamide); PSHU: poly (serinol hexamethylene urethane); RGC: retinal ganglion Cell; RPE: retinal pigment epithelium; RVO: retinal vein occlusion; SDS: Prague-Dawley; siRNA: small interfering ribonucleic acid; SLN: solid lipid nanoparticles; STZ: streptozotocin; VEGF: vascular endothelial growth factor; VIP: vasoactive intestinal peptide.

6. Conclusions

Recent developments in the medical biotechnology area promoted the use of therapeutic proteins to treat different ocular diseases and have changed the scenario in the research work carried out in last few decades. Optimal efficacy can be achieved with proper knowledge of ocular barriers, nature, and pharmacokinetics of therapeutic proteins along with reduction of the dosing frequency and use of novel or combination of technologies (e.g., nanocarriers included in hydrogel-based systems) or by adding penetration enhancers or enzyme inhibitors to the formulations. Future research must be conducted toward the development of more efficient, stable, noninvasive, and cost-effective formulations for ocular delivery of therapeutic proteins.

The development of effective delivery systems containing stable therapeutic proteins that can reach the eye topically, subconjunctivally, or periocularly remains challenging. There is a need to establish pharmacokinetic models that provide useful insights into the development of these ocular delivery systems, which can aid in preclinical to clinical translation and in predicting the dosing regimen.

Author Contributions: D.H.S. wrote the manuscript. A.C.S. and H.A. revised the manuscript. All authors have read and agreed to the published version of the manuscript.

Funding: This work was supported by the Applied Molecular Bio-sciences Unit-UCIBIO, which is financed by national funds from Fundação para a Ciência e a Tecnologia-FCT (UIDP/04378/2020 and UIDB/04378/2020) and CIBB (UIDB/04539/2020).

Institutional Review Board Statement: Not applicable.

Informed Consent Statement: Not applicable.

Data Availability Statement: Not applicable.

Acknowledgments: The authors are thankful to the Journal for inviting them to contribute the article.

Conflicts of Interest: The authors declared no conflict of Interests.

References

1. Sharma, D.S.; Wadhwa, S.; Gulati, M.; Ramanunny, A.K.; Awasthi, A.; Singh, S.K.; Khursheed, R.; Corrie, L.; Chitranshi, N.; Gupta, V.K.; et al. Recent advances in intraocular and novel drug delivery systems for the treatment of diabetic retinopathy. *Expert Opin. Drug Del.* **2021**, *18*, 553–576. [CrossRef]
2. Kim, H.M.; Woo, S.J. Ocular Drug Delivery to the Retina: Current Innovations and Future Perspectives. *Pharmaceutics* **2021**, *13*, 108. [CrossRef]
3. Bourne, R.R.A.; Flaxman, S.R.; Braithwaite, T.; Cicinelli, M.V.; Das, A.; Jonas, J.B.; Keeffe, J.; Kempen, J.H.; Leasher, J.; Limburg, H.; et al. Vision Loss Expert Group. Magnitude, temporal trends, and projections of the global prevalence of blindness and distance and near vision impairment: A systematic review and meta-analysis. *Lancet Glob. Health* **2017**, *5*, e888–e897. [CrossRef] [PubMed]
4. Claudio, F.; Francesco, B.; Michele, R.; Giovanni, A. Intravitreal Therapy for Diabetic Macular Edema: An Update. *J. Ophthalmol.* **2021**, *2021*, 6654168. [CrossRef]
5. Aiello, L.P. The potential role of PKC b in diabetic retinopathy and macular edema. *Survey Ophthalmol.* **2002**, *47* (Suppl. S2), 263–269. [CrossRef]
6. Alqahtani, F.Y.; Aleanizy, F.S.; El Tahir, E.; Alquadeib, B.T.; Alsarra, I.A.; Alanazi, J.S.; Abdelhady, H.G. Preparation, characterization, and antibacterial activity of diclofenac-loaded chitosan nanoparticles. *Saudi Pharm. J.* **2019**, *27*, 82–87. [CrossRef] [PubMed]
7. Hu, J.; Zhang, Y.; Li, X.; Han, W.; Zheng, J.; Yang, G.; Xu, A. Combination of Intrastromal and Intracameral Injections of Amphotericin B in the Treatment of Severe Fungal Keratitis. *J. Ophthalmol.* **2016**, *2016*, 3436415. [CrossRef]
8. Patel, P.B.; Shastri, D.H.; Shelat, P.K.; Shukla, A.K. Ophthalmic drug delivery system: Challenges and approaches. *Syst. Rev. Pharm.* **2010**, *1*, 113–120.
9. Liu, W.; Borrell, M.A.; Venerus, D.C.; Mieler, W.F.; Kang-Mieler, J.J. Characterization of Biodegradable Microsphere-Hydrogel Ocular Drug Delivery System for Controlled and Extended Release of Ranibizumab. *Transl. Vis. Sci. Technol.* **2019**, *8*, 12. [CrossRef]
10. Narayana, S.; Ahmed, M.G.; Gowda, B.H.J.; Shetty, P.K.; Nasrine, A.; Thriveni, M.; Noushida, N.; Sanjana, A. Recent advances in ocular drug delivery systems and targeting VEGF receptors for management of ocular angiogenesis: A comprehensive review. *Future J. Pharm. Sci.* **2021**, *7*, 186. [CrossRef]
11. Karasavvidou, E.M.; Tranos, P.; Panos, G.D. Brolucizumab for the Treatment of Degenerative Macular Conditions: A Review of Clinical Studies. *Drug Des. Devel. Ther.* **2022**, *16*, 2659–2680. [CrossRef] [PubMed]
12. Rosenfeld, P.J.; Brown, D.M.; Heier, J.S.; Boyer, D.S.; Kaiser, P.K.; Chung, C.Y.; Kim, R.Y.; Group, M.S. Ranibizumab for neovascular age-related macular degeneration. *N. Engl. J. Med.* **2006**, *355*, 1419–1431. [CrossRef] [PubMed]

13. Bakri, S.J.; Snyder, M.R.; Reid, J.M.; Pulido, J.S.; Ezzat, M.K.; Singh, R.J. Pharmacokinetics of intravitreal ranibizumab (Lucentis). *Ophthalmology* **2007**, *114*, 2179–2182. [CrossRef] [PubMed]
14. Krohne, T.U.; Liu, Z.; Holz, F.G.; Meyer, C.H. Intraocular pharmacokinetics of ranibizumab following a single intravitreal injection in humans. *Am. J. Ophthalmol.* **2012**, *154*, 682–686.e682. [CrossRef]
15. Gaudreault, J.; Fei, D.; Beyer, J.C.; Ryan, A.; Rangell, L.; Shiu, V.; Damico, L.A. Pharmacokinetics, and retinal distribution of ranibizumab, a humanized antibody fragment directed against VEGF-A, following intravitreal administration in rabbits. *Retina* **2007**, *27*, 1260–1266. [CrossRef]
16. Niwa, Y.; Kakinoki, M.; Sawada, T.; Wang, X.; Ohji, M. Ranibizumab and Aflibercept: Intraocular Pharmacokinetics and Their Effects on Aqueous VEGF Level in Vitrectomized and Nonvitrectomized Macaque Eyes. *Investig. Ophthalmol. Vis. Sci.* **2015**, *56*, 6501–6505. [CrossRef]
17. Park, S.J.; Choi, Y.; Na, Y.M.; Hong, H.K.; Park, J.Y.; Park, K.H.; Chung, J.Y.; Woo, S.J. Intraocular Pharmacokinetics of Intravitreal Aflibercept (Eylea) in a Rabbit Model. *Investig. Ophthalmol. Vis. Sci.* **2016**, *57*, 2612–2617. [CrossRef]
18. Bakri, S.J.; Snyder, M.R.; Reid, J.M.; Pulido, J.S.; Singh, R.J. Pharmacokinetics of intravitreal bevacizumab (Avastin). *Ophthalmology* **2007**, *114*, 855–859. [CrossRef]
19. Krohne, T.U.; Eter, N.; Holz, F.G.; Meyer, C.H. Intraocular pharmacokinetics of bevacizumab after a single intravitreal injection in humans. *Am. J. Ophthalmol.* **2008**, *146*, 508–512. [CrossRef]
20. Ahn, S.J.; Hong, H.K.; Na, Y.M.; Park, S.J.; Ahn, J.; Oh, J.; Chung, J.Y.; Park, K.H.; Woo, S.J. Use of Rabbit Eyes in Pharmacokinetic Studies of Intraocular Drugs. *J. Vis. Exp.* **2016**, *113*, e53878. [CrossRef]
21. Christoforidis, J.B.; Carlton, M.M.; Knopp, M.V.; Hinkle, G.H. PET/CT imaging of I-124-radiolabeled bevacizumab and ranibizumab after intravitreal injection in a rabbit model. *Investig. Ophthalmol. Vis. Sci.* **2011**, *5*, 5899–5903. [CrossRef]
22. Shelke, N.B.; Kadam, R.; Tyagi, P.; Rao, V.R.; Kompella, U.B. Intravitreal poly(L-lactide) microparticles sustain retinal and choroidal delivery of TG-0054, a hydrophilic drug intended for neovascular diseases. *Drug Deliv. Transl. Res.* **2011**, *1*, 76–90. [CrossRef]
23. Sinapis, C.I.; Routsias, J.G.; Sinapis, A.I.; Sinapis, D.I.; Agrogiannis, G.D.; Pantopoulou, A.; Theocharis, S.E.; Baltatzis, S.; Patsouris, E.; Perrea, D. Pharmacokinetics of intravitreal bevacizumab (Avastin(R)) in rabbits. *Clin. Ophthalmol.* **2011**, *5*, 697–704. [CrossRef]
24. Nomoto, H.; Shiraga, F.; Kuno, N.; Kimura, E.; Fujii, S.; Shinomiya, K.; Nugent, A.K.; Hirooka, K.; Baba, T. Pharmacokinetics of bevacizumab after topical, subconjunctival, and intravitreal administration in rabbits. *Investig. Ophthalmol. Vis. Sci.* **2009**, *50*, 4807–4813. [CrossRef] [PubMed]
25. Meyer, C.H.; Krohne, T.U.; Holz, F.G. Intraocular pharmacokinetics after a single intravitreal injection of 1.5 mg versus 3.0 mg of bevacizumab in humans. *Retina* **2011**, *31*, 1877–1884. [CrossRef]
26. Center for Drug Evaluation and Research Application Number 761125Orig1s000. Clinical Pharmacology Reviews. Available online: https://www.accessdata.fda.gov/drugsatfda_docs/nda/2019/761125Orig1s000ClinPharmR.pdf (accessed on 30 June 2022).
27. Ferro Desideri, L.; Traverso, C.E.; Nicolò, M. Abicipar pegol: An investigational anti-VEGF agent for the treatment of wet age-related macular degeneration. *Expert Opin. Investig. Drugs.* **2020**, *29*, 651–658. [CrossRef] [PubMed]
28. Nicolò, M.; Ferro Desideri, L.; Vagge, A.; Traverso, C.E. Faricimab: An investigational agent targeting the Tie-2/angiopoietin pathway and VEGF-A for the treatment of retinal diseases. *Expert Opin. Investig. Drugs.* **2021**, *30*, 193–200. [CrossRef]
29. Wykoff, C.C.; Abreu, F.; Adamis, A.P.; Basu, K.; Eichenbaum, D.A.; Haskova, Z.; Lin, H.; Loewenstein, A.; Mohan, S.; Pearce, I.A.; et al. Efficacy, durability, and safety of intravitreal faricimab with extended dosing up to every 16 weeks in patients with diabetic macular oedema (YOSEMITE and RHINE): Two randomised, double-masked, phase 3 trials. *Lancet* **2022**, *399*, 741–755. [CrossRef] [PubMed]
30. Zhou, P.; Zheng, S.; Wang, E.; Men, P.; Zhai, S. Conbercept for Treatment of Neovascular Age-Related Macular Degeneration and Visual Impairment due to Diabetic Macular Edema or Pathologic Myopia Choroidal Neovascularization: A Systematic Review and Meta-Analysis. *Front. Pharmacol.* **2021**, *12*, 696201. [CrossRef]
31. Zhou, B.; Wang, B. Pegaptanib for the treatment of age-related macular degeneration. *Exp. Eye Res.* **2006**, *83*, 615–619. [CrossRef]
32. Kourlas, H.; Schiller, D.S. Pegaptanib sodium for the treatment of neovascular age-related macular degeneration: A review. *Clin. Ther.* **2006**, *28*, 36–44. [CrossRef] [PubMed]
33. Mansour, S.E.; Browning, D.J.; Wong, K.; Flynn, H.W.; Bhavsar, A.R., Jr. The Evolving Treatment of Diabetic Retinopathy. *Clin. Ophthalmol.* **2020**, *14*, 653–678. [CrossRef] [PubMed]
34. Ng, E.W.; Adamis, A.P. Anti-VEGF aptamer (pegaptanib) therapy for ocular vascular diseases. *Ann. N. Y. Acad. Sci.* **2006**, *1082*, 151–171. [CrossRef]
35. Chen, W.; Yung, B.C.; Qian, Z.; Chen, X. Improving Long-Term Subcutaneous Drug Delivery by Regulating Material-Bioenvironment Interaction. *Adv. Drug Deliv. Rev.* **2018**, *127*, 20–34. [CrossRef]
36. Renukuntla, J.; Vadlapudi, A.D.; Patel, A.; Boddu, S.H.S.; Mitra, A.K. Approaches for Enhancing Oral Bioavailability of Peptides and Proteins. *Int. J. Pharm.* **2013**, *447*, 75–93. [CrossRef]
37. Faulds, D.; Goa, K.L.; Benfield, P. Cyclosporin. A review of its pharmacodynamic and pharmacokinetic properties, and therapeutic use in immunoregulatory disorders. *Drugs* **1993**, *45*, 953–1040. [CrossRef]
38. Brown, L.R. Commercial Challenges of Protein Drug Delivery. *Expert Opin. Drug Deliv.* **2005**, *2*, 29–42. [CrossRef]

39. Bhattacharya, M.; Sadeghi, A.; Sarkhel, S.; Hagström, M.; Bahrpeyma, S.; Toropainen, E.; Auriola, S.; Urtti, A. Release of functional dexamethasone by intracellular enzymes: A modular peptide-based strategy for ocular drug delivery. *J. Control. Release* **2020**, *327*, 584–594. [CrossRef]
40. Haddadzadegan, S.; Dorkoosh, F.; Bernkop-Schnürch, A. Oral delivery of therapeutic peptides and proteins: Technology landscape of lipid-based nanocarriers. *Adv. Drug Deliv. Rev.* **2022**, *182*, 114097. [CrossRef]
41. Lin, J. Pharmacokinetics of Biotech Drugs: Peptides, Proteins and Monoclonal Antibodies. *Curr. Drug Metab.* **2009**, *10*, 661–691. [CrossRef]
42. Ahmed, I.; Patton, T.F. Disposition of Timolol and Inulin in the Rabbit Eye Following Corneal versus Non-Corneal Absorption. *Int. J. Pharm.* **1987**, *38*, 9–21. [CrossRef]
43. Donovan, M.D.; Flynn, G.L.; Amidon, G.L. Absorption of Polyethylene Glycols 600 Through 2000: The Molecular Weight Dependence of Gastrointestinal and Nasal Absorption. *Pharm. Res. Off. J. Am. Assoc. Pharm. Sci.* **1990**, *7*, 863–868.
44. Shen, W.; Matsui, T. Intestinal Absorption of Small Peptides: A Review. *Int. J. Food Sci. Technol.* **2019**, *54*, 1942–1948. [CrossRef]
45. Xu, Q.; Boylan, N.J.; Suk, J.S.; Wang, Y.Y.; Nance, E.A.; Yang, J.C.; McDonnell, P.J.; Cone, R.A.; Duh, E.J.; Hanes, J. Nanoparticle Diffusion in, and Microrheology of, the Bovine Vitreous Ex Vivo. *J. Control. Release* **2013**, *167*, 76–84. [CrossRef] [PubMed]
46. Xu, J.; Heys, J.J.; Barocas, V.H.; Randolph, T.W. Permeability and Diffusion in Vitreous Humor: Implications for Drug Delivery. *Pharm. Res.* **2000**, *17*, 664–669. [CrossRef]
47. Balachandran, R.K.; Barocas, V.H. Contribution of Saccadic Motion to Intravitreal Drug Transport: Theoretical Analysis. *Pharm. Res.* **2011**, *28*, 1049–1064. [CrossRef]
48. Käsdorf, B.T.; Arends, F.; Lieleg, O. Diffusion Regulation in the Vitreous Humor. *Biophys. J.* **2015**, *109*, 2171–2181. [CrossRef]
49. Nakano, M.; Lockhart, C.M.; Kelly, E.J.; Rettie, A.E. Ocular Cytochrome P450s and Transporters: Roles in Disease and Endobiotic and Xenobiotic Disposition. *Drug Metab. Biophys. J. Rev.* **2014**, *46*, 247–260. [CrossRef]
50. Urtti, A. *Nanostructures Overcoming the Ocular Barrier: Drug Delivery Strategies*; Chapter 4.2.; Royal Society of Chemistry: London, UK, 2012; pp. 190–204.
51. DiCarlo, J.E.; Mahajan, V.B.; Tsang, S.H. Gene therapy and genome surgery in the retina. *J. Clin. Investig.* **2018**, *128*, 2177–2188. [CrossRef]
52. Sørensen, N.B. Subretinal Surgery: Functional and Histological Consequences of Entry into the Subretinal Space. *Acta Ophthalmol.* **2019**, *97*, 1–23. [CrossRef]
53. Subrizi, A.; del Amo, E.M.; Korzhikov-Vlakh, V.; Tennikova, T.; Ruponen, M.; Urtti, A. Design Principles of Ocular Drug Delivery Systems: Importance of Drug Payload, Release Rate, and Material Properties. *Drug Discov. Today.* **2019**, *24*, 1446–1457. [CrossRef]
54. Bachu, R.D.; Chowdhury, P.; Al-Saedi, Z.H.F.; Karla, P.K.; Boddu, S.H.S. Ocular Drug Delivery Barriers-Role of Nanocarriers in the Treatment of Anterior Segment Ocular Diseases. *Pharmaceutics* **2018**, *10*, 28. [CrossRef] [PubMed]
55. Muheem, A.; Shakeel, F.; Jahangir, M.A.; Anwar, M.; Mallick, N.; Jain, G.K.; Warsi, M.H.; Ahmad, F.J. A review on the strategies for oral delivery of proteins and peptides and their clinical perspectives. *Saudi Pharm. J.* **2016**, *24*, 413–428. [CrossRef] [PubMed]
56. Leclercq, B.; Mejlachowicz, D.; Behar-Cohen, F. Ocular Barriers and Their Influence on Gene Therapy Products Delivery. *Pharmaceutics* **2022**, *14*, 998. [CrossRef] [PubMed]
57. Tao, Y.; Li, X.X.; Jiang, Y.R.; Bai, X.B.; Wu, B.D.; Dong, J.Q. Diffusion of macromolecule through retina after experimental branch retinal vein occlusion and estimate of intraretinal barrier. *Curr. Drug Metab.* **2007**, *8*, 151–156. [CrossRef]
58. Jackson, T.L.; Antcliff, R.J.; Hillenkamp, J.; Marshall, J. Human retinal molecular weight exclusion limit and estimate of species variation. *Investig. Ophthalmol. Vis. Sci.* **2003**, *44*, 2141–2146. [CrossRef] [PubMed]
59. Blessing, C.I.; Charis, R.; Roel, F.M.; Mio, T.; Mei, C.; Wim, E.H. Hyaluronic Acid-PEG-Based Diels–Alder In Situ Forming Hydrogels for Sustained Intraocular Delivery of Bevacizumab. *Biomacromolecules* **2022**, *23*, 1525–7797.
60. Burgalassi, S.; Monti, D.; Nicosia, N.; Tampucci, S.; Terreni, E.; Vento, A.; Chetoni, P. Freeze-dried matrices for ocular administration of bevacizumab: A comparison between subconjunctival and intravitreal administration in rabbits. *Drug Deliv. Transl. Res.* **2018**, *8*, 461–472. [CrossRef]
61. Urtti, A. Challenges and obstacles of ocular pharmacokinetics and drug delivery. *Adv. Drug Deliv. Rev.* **2006**, *58*, 1131–1135. [CrossRef]
62. Levison, M.E.; Levison, J.H. Pharmacokinetics and pharmacodynamics of antibacterial agents. *Infect. Dis. Clini. N. Am.* **2009**, *23*, 791–815. [CrossRef]
63. Del Amo, E.M.; Urtti, A. Rabbit as an animal model for intravitreal pharmacokinetics: Clinical predictability and quality of the published data. *Exp. Eye. Res.* **2015**, *137*, 111–124. [CrossRef] [PubMed]
64. Sidman, R.L.; Li, J.; Lawrence, M.; Hu, W.; Musso, G.F.; Giordano, R.J.; Cardo-Vila, M.; Pasqualini, R.; Arap, W. The peptidomimetic Vasotide targets two retinal VEGF receptors and reduces pathological angiogenesis in murine and nonhuman primate models of retinal disease. *Sci. Transl. Med.* **2015**, *7*, 309. [CrossRef]
65. Pescina, S.; Ferrari, G.; Govoni, P.; Macaluso, C.; Padula, C.; Santi, P.; Nicoli, S. In-vitro permeation of bevacizumab through human sclera: Effect of iontophoresis application. *J. Pharm. Pharmacol.* **2010**, *62*, 1189–1194. [CrossRef] [PubMed]
66. Swami, R.; Shahiwala, A. Impact of physiochemical properties on pharmacokinetics of protein therapeutics. *Eur. J. Drug Metab. Pharmacokinetics.* **2013**, *38*, 231–239. [CrossRef] [PubMed]
67. Kuo, T.T.; Baker, K.; Yoshida, M.; Qiao, S.W.; Aveson, V.G.; Lencer, W.I.; Blumberg, R.S. Neonatal Fc receptor: From immunity to therapeutics. *J. Clin. Immunol.* **2010**, *30*, 777–789. [CrossRef] [PubMed]

68. Gaudana, R.; Ananthula, H.K.; Parenky, A.; Mitra, A.K. Ocular Drug Delivery. *AAPS J.* **2010**, *12*, 348–360. [CrossRef]
69. Edelhauser, H.F.; Rowe-Rendleman, C.L.; Robinson, M.R.; Dawson, D.G.; Chader, G.J.; Grossniklaus, H.E. Ophthalmic drug delivery systems for the treatment of retinal diseases: Basic research to clinical applications. *Investig. Ophthalmol. Vis. Sci.* **2010**, *51*, 5403–5420. [CrossRef] [PubMed]
70. Shen, J.; Durairaj, C.; Lin, T.; Liu, Y.; Burke, J. Ocular pharmacokinetics of intravitreally administered brimonidine and dexamethasone in animal models with and without blood-retinal barrier breakdown. *Investig. Ophthalmol. Vis. Sci.* **2014**, *55*, 1056–1066. [CrossRef]
71. Kim, Y.C.; Chiang, B.; Wu, X.; Prausnitz, M.R. Ocular delivery of macromolecules. *J. Con. Rel.* **2014**, *190*, 172–181. [CrossRef]
72. Joseph, R.R.; Venkatraman, S.S. Drug delivery to the eye: What benefits do nanocarriers offer? *Nanomedicine* **2017**, *12*, 683–702. [CrossRef]
73. Raghava, S.; Hammond, M.; Ub, K. Periocular routes for retinal drug delivery. *Expert Opin. Drug Deliv.* **2004**, *1*, 99–114. [CrossRef]
74. Puddu, A.; Sanguineti, R.; Montecucco, F.; Viviani, G.L. Retinal pigment epithelial cells express a functional receptor for glucagon-like peptide-1 (GLP-1). *Mediat. Inflamm.* **2013**, *2013*, 975032. [CrossRef] [PubMed]
75. Zelikin, A.N.; Ehrhardt, C.; Healy, A.M. Materials and methods for delivery of biological drugs. *Nat. Chem.* **2016**, *8*, 997–1007. [CrossRef] [PubMed]
76. Chang, J.H.; Garg, N.K.; Lunde, E.; Han, K.Y.; Jain, S.; Azar, D.T. Corneal neovascularization: An anti-VEGF therapy review. *Surv. Ophthalmol.* **2012**, *57*, 415–429. [CrossRef]
77. Vinores, S.A. Pegaptanib in the treatment of wet, age-related macular degeneration. *Int. J. Nanomed.* **2006**, *1*, 263–268.
78. Joseph, M.; Trinh, H.M.; Cholkar, K.; Pal, D.; Mitra, A.K. Recent perspectives on the delivery of biologics to back of the eye. *Expert Opin. Drug Deliv.* **2016**, *14*, 631–645. [CrossRef]
79. Xu, L.; Lu, T.; Tuomi, L.; Jumbe, N.; Lu, J.; Eppler, S.; Kuebler, P.; Damico-Beyer, L.A.; Joshi, A. Pharmacokinetics of ranibizumab in patients with neovascular age-related macular degeneration: A population approach. *Investig. Ophthalmol. Vis. Sci.* **2013**, *54*, 1616–1624. [CrossRef] [PubMed]
80. Vaishya, R.D.; Khurana, V.; Patel, S.; Mitra, A.K. Controlled ocular drug delivery with nanomicelles, Wiley interdisciplinary reviews. *Nanomed. Nanobiotechnol.* **2014**, *6*, 422–437. [CrossRef] [PubMed]
81. Moisseiev, E.; Waisbourd, M.; Ben-Artsi, E.; Levinger, E.; Barak, A.; Daniels, T.; Csaky, K.; Loewenstein, A.; Barequet, I.S. Pharmacokinetics of bevacizumab after topical and intravitreal administration in human eyes. *Graefe's Arch. Clin. Exp. Ophthalmol.* **2014**, *252*, 331–337.
82. Sharma, Y.R.; Venkatesh, P.; Gogia, V. Aflibercept—How does it compare with other Anti-VEGF Drugs? *Aust. J. Clin. Ophthalmol.* **2014**, *1*, 1–8.
83. Neri, P.; Lettieri, M.; Fortuna, C.; Zucchi, M.; Manoni, M.; Celani, S.A. Giovannini, Adalimumab (humira) in ophthalmology: A review of the literature. *Middle East Afr. J. Ophthalmol.* **2010**, *17*, 290–296. [CrossRef]
84. Rodrigues, E.B.; Farah, M.E.; Maia, M.; Penha, F.M.; Regatieri, C.; Melo, G.B.; Pinheiro, M.M.; Zanetti, C.R. Therapeutic monoclonal antibodies in ophthalmology. *Prog. Ret. Eye Res.* **2009**, *28*, 117–144. [CrossRef] [PubMed]
85. Khawli, L.A.; Goswami, S.; Hutchinson, R.; Kwong, Z.W.; Yang, J.; Wang, X.; Yao, Z.; Sreedhara, A.; Cano, T.; Tesar, D. Charge variants in IgG1: Isolation, characterization, In vitro binding properties and pharma-cokinetics in rats. *MAbs* **2010**, *2*, 613–624. [CrossRef]
86. Maurice, D.M.; Watson, P.G. The distribution and movement of serum albumin in the cornea. *Exp. Eye Res.* **1965**, *4*, 355–363. [CrossRef]
87. Kim, J.H.; Green, K.; Martinez, M.; Paton, D. Solute permeability of the corneal endothelium and Descemet's membrane. *Exp. Eye Res.* **1971**, *12*, 231–238. [CrossRef]
88. Olsen, T.W.; Edelhauser, H.F.; Lim, J.I.; Geroski, D.H. Human scleral permeability. Effects of age, cryotherapy, transscleral diode laser, and surgical thinning. *Investig. Ophthalmol. Vis. Sci.* **1995**, *36*, 1893–1903.
89. Mitragotri, S.; Burke, P.A.; Langer, R. Overcoming the challenges in administering biopharmaceuticals: Formulation and delivery strategies. *Nat. Rev. Drug Discov.* **2014**, *13*, 655–672. [CrossRef]
90. Duvvuri, S.; Majumdar, S.; Mitra, A.K. Drug delivery to the retina: Challenges and opportunities. *Expert Opin. Biol. Ther.* **2003**, *3*, 45–56. [CrossRef] [PubMed]
91. Manning, M.C.; Chou, D.K.; Murphy, B.M.; Payne, R.W.; Katayama, D.S. Stability of protein pharmaceuticals: An update. *Pharm. Res.* **2010**, *27*, 544–575. [CrossRef] [PubMed]
92. Li, S.K.; Liddell, M.R.; Wen, H. Effective electrophoretic mobilities and charges of anti-VEGF proteins determined by capillary zone electrophoresis. *J. Pharm. Biomed. Anal.* **2011**, *55*, 603–607. [CrossRef]
93. Kaja, S.; Hilgenberg, J.D.; Everett, E.; Olitsky, S.E.; Gossage, J.; Koulen, P. Effects of dilution and prolonged storage with preservative in a polyethylene container on Bevacizumab (Avastin) for topical delivery as a nasal spray in anti-hereditary hemorrhagic telangiectasia and related therapies. *Hum. Antibodies* **2011**, *20*, 95–101. [CrossRef] [PubMed]
94. Gregoritza, M.; Messmann, V.; Abstiens, K.; Brandl, F.P.; Goepferich, A.M. Controlled antibody release from degradable thermoresponsive hydrogels cross-linked by Diels-Alder chemistry. *Biomacromolecules* **2017**, *18*, 2410–2418. [CrossRef] [PubMed]
95. Jani, R.; Lang, J.; Rodeheaver, D.; Missel, P.; Roehrs, R.; Chowhan, M. *Design and Evaluation of Ophthalmic Pharmaceutical Products, Modern Pharmaceutics*, 4th ed.; CRC Press: Boca Raton, FL, USA, 2002.
96. Ali, Y.; Lehmussaari, K. Industrial perspective in ocular drug delivery. *Adv. Drug Deliv. Rev.* **2006**, *58*, 1258–1268. [CrossRef]

97. Subrizi, A.; Toropainen, E.; Ramsay, E.; Airaksinen, A.J.; Kaarniranta, K.; Urtti, A. Oxidative stress protection by exogenous delivery of rhHsp70 chaperone to the retinal pigment epithelium (RPE), a possible therapeutic strategy against RPE degeneration. *Pharm. Res.* **2015**, *32*, 211–221. [CrossRef]
98. Schymkowitz, J.; Rousseau, F. Protein aggregation: A rescue by chaperones. *Nat. Chem. Biol.* **2016**, *12*, 58–59. [CrossRef]
99. Angi, M.; Kalirai, H.; Coupland, S.E.; Damato, B.E.; Semeraro, F.; Romano, M.R. Proteomic Analyses of the Vitreous Humour. *Mediat. Inflamm.* **2012**, *2012*, 148039. [CrossRef]
100. Murthy, K.R.; Goel, R.; Subbannayya, Y.; Jacob, H.K.C.; Murthy, P.R.; Manda, S.S.; Patil, A.H.; Sharma, R.; Sahasrabuddhe, N.A.; Parashar, A.; et al. Proteomic Analysis of Human Vitreous Humor. *Clin. Proteom.* **2014**, *11*, 29. [CrossRef]
101. Babizhayev, M.A.; Burke, L.; Micans, P.; Richer, S.P. N-Acetylcarnosine Sustained Drug Delivery Eye Drops to Control the Signs of Ageless Vision: Glare Sensitivity, Cataract Amelioration and Quality of Vision Currently Available Treatment for the Challenging 50,000-Patient Population. *Clin. Interv. Aging* **2009**, *4*, 31–50. [CrossRef]
102. Peynshaert, K.; Devoldere, J.; Minnaert, A.K.; De Smedt, S.C.; Remaut, K. Morphology and Composition of the Inner Limiting Membrane: Species-Specific Variations and Relevance toward Drug Delivery Research. *Curr. Eye Res.* **2019**, *44*, 465–475. [CrossRef]
103. Boye, S.L.; Bennett, A.; Scalabrino, M.L.; McCullough, K.T.; Van Vliet, K.; Choudhury, S.; Ruan, Q.; Peterson, J.; Agbandje-McKenna, M.; Boye, S.E. Impact of Heparan Sulfate Binding on Transduction of Retina by Recombinant Adeno-Associated Virus Vectors. *J. Virol.* **2016**, *90*, 4215–4231. [CrossRef]
104. Bisht, R.; Rupenthal, I.D.; Sreebhavan, S.; Jaiswal, J.K. Development of a Novel Stability Indicating RP-HPLC Method for Quantification of Connexin43 Mimetic Peptide and Determination of Its Degradation Kinetics in Biological Fluids. *J. Pharm. Anal.* **2017**, *7*, 365–373. [CrossRef]
105. Stampfli, H.F.; Quon, C.Y. Polymorphic metabolism of flestolol and other ester containing compounds by a carboxylesterase in New Zealand white rabbit blood and cornea. *Res. Commun. Mol. Pathol. Pharmacol.* **1995**, *88*, 87–97. [PubMed]
106. Fosgerau, K.; Hoffmann, T. Peptide Therapeutics: Current Status and Future Directions. *Drug Discov. Today* **2015**, *20*, 122–128. [CrossRef] [PubMed]
107. Ambati, J.; Atkinson, J.P.; Gelfand, B.D. Immunology of age-related macular degeneration. *Nat. Rev. Immunol.* **2013**, *13*, 438–451. [CrossRef] [PubMed]
108. Radhakrishnan, K.; Sonali, N.; Moreno, M.; Nirmal, J.; Fernandez, A.A.; Venkatraman, S.; Agrawal, R. Protein delivery to the back of the eye: Barriers, carriers and stability of anti-VEGF proteins. *Drug Discov. Today.* **2017**, *22*, 416–423. [CrossRef]
109. Vaughan-Thomas, A.; Gilbert, S.J.; Duance, V.C. Elevated levels of proteolytic enzymes in the aging human vitreous. *Investig. Ophthalmol. Vis. Sci.* **2000**, *41*, 3299–3304.
110. Pescosolido, N.; Barbato, A.; Pascarella, A.; Giannotti, R.; Genzano, M.; Nebbioso, M. Role of Protease-Inhibitors in Ocular Diseases. *Molecules* **2014**, *19*, 20557–20569. [CrossRef]
111. Jwala, J.; Boddu, S.H.S.; Shah, S.; Sirimulla, S.; Pal, D.; Mitra, A.K. Ocular Sustained Release Nanoparticles Containing Stereoisomeric Dipeptide Prodrugs of Acyclovir. *J. Ocul. Pharmacol. Ther.* **2011**, *27*, 163–172. [CrossRef] [PubMed]
112. Brinckerhoff, L.H.; Kalashnikov, V.V.; Thompson, L.W.; Yamshchikov, G.V.; Pierce, R.A.; Galavotti, H.S.; Engelhard, V.H.; Slingluff, C.L. Terminal Modifications Inhibit Proteolytic Degradation of an Immunogenic MART-127-35 Peptide: Implications for Peptide Vaccines. *Int. J. Cancer* **1999**, *83*, 326–334. [CrossRef]
113. Werle, M.; Bernkop-Schnürch, A. Strategies to Improve Plasma Half Life Time of Peptide and Protein Drugs. *Amino Acids* **2006**, *30*, 351–367. [CrossRef]
114. Attar, M.; Shen, J.; Ling, K.H.J.; Tang-Liu, D. Ophthalmic Drug Delivery Considerations at the Cellular Level: Drug-Metabolising Enzymes and Transporters. *Expert Opin. Drug Deliv.* **2005**, *2*, 891–908. [CrossRef] [PubMed]
115. Schwartzman, M.L.; Masferrer, J.; Dunn, M.W.; Mcgiff, J.C.; Abraham, N.G. Cytochrome P450, Drug Metabolizing Enzymes and Arachidonic Acid Metabolism in Bovine Ocular Tissues. *Curr. Eye Res.* **1987**, *6*, 623–630. [CrossRef] [PubMed]
116. Hayasaka, S. Lysosomal Enzymes in Ocular Tissues and Diseases. *Surv. Ophthalmol.* **1983**, *27*, 245–258. [CrossRef] [PubMed]
117. Vandervoort, J.; Ludwig, A. Ocular Drug Delivery: Nanomedicine Applications. *Nanomedicine* **2007**, *2*, 11–21. [CrossRef] [PubMed]
118. Ferrara, N.; Adamis, A. Ten years of anti-vascular endothelial growth factor therapy. *Nat. Rev. Drug. Discov.* **2016**, *15*, 385–403. [CrossRef]
119. Traynor, K. Aflibercept approved for macular degeneration. *Am. J. Health Sys. Pharm.* **2012**, *69*, 6. [CrossRef]
120. Ng, E.W.; Shima, D.T.; Calias, P.; Cunningham, E.T.; Guyer, D.R.; Adamis, A.P. Pegaptanib, a targeted anti-VEGF aptamer for ocular vascular disease. *Nat. Rev. Drug Discov.* **2006**, *5*, 123–132. [CrossRef] [PubMed]
121. Theodossiadis, P.G.; Markomichelakis, N.N.; Sfikakis, P.P. Tumor necrosis factor antagonists: Preliminary evidence for an emerging approach in the treatment of ocular inflammation. *Retina* **2007**, *27*, 399–413. [CrossRef] [PubMed]
122. Haroomi, M.; Freilich, J.M.; Abelson, M.; Refojo, M. Efficacy of hyaluronidase in reducing increases in intraocular pressure related to the use of viscoelastic substances. *Arch. Ophthalmol.* **1998**, *116*, 1218–1221. [CrossRef]
123. Stern, R.; Jedrzejas, M.J. Hyaluronidases: Their genomics, structures, and mechanisms of action. *Chem. Rev.* **2006**, *106*, 818–839. [CrossRef]
124. Zhu, C.; Zhang, Y.; Pardridge, W.M. Widespread expression of an exogenous gene in the eye after intravenous administration. *Investig. Ophthalmol. Vis. Sci.* **2002**, *43*, 3075–3080.

125. Chandola, C.; Casteleijn, M.G.; Chandola, U.M.; Gopalan, L.N.; Urtti, A.; Neerathilingam, M. CD44 Aptamer Mediated Cargo Delivery to Lysosomes of Retinal Pigment Epithelial Cells to Prevent Age-Related Macular Degeneration. *Biochem. Biophys. Rep.* **2019**, *18*, 100642. [CrossRef]
126. Diaferia, C.; Morelli, G.; Accardo, A. Fmoc-Diphenylalanine as a Suitable Building Block for the Preparation of Hybrid Materials and Their Potential Applications. *J. Mater. Chem. B* **2019**, *7*, 5142–5155. [CrossRef] [PubMed]
127. Tadayoni, R.; Sararols, L.; Weissgerber, G.; Verma, R.; Clemens, A.; Holz, F.G. Brolucizumab: A Newly Developed Anti-VEGF Molecule for the Treatment of Neovascular Age-Related Macular Degeneration. *Ophthalmologica* **2021**, *244*, 93–101. [CrossRef] [PubMed]
128. Salazar, M.; Patil, P.N. An explanation for the long duration of mydriatic effect of atropine in eye. *Investig. Ophthalmol.* **1976**, *15*, 671–673.
129. Rimpelä, A.K.; Reinisalo, M.; Hellinen, L.; Grazhdankin, E.; Kidron, H.; Urtti, A.; del Amo, E.M. Implications of Melanin Binding in Ocular Drug Delivery. *Adv. Drug Deliv. Rev.* **2018**, *126*, 23–43. [CrossRef]
130. Bernstein, H.; Zvaifler, N.; Rubin, M.; Mansour, A.M. The Ocular Deposition of Chloroquine. *Investig. Ophthalmol.* **1963**, *2*, 384–392.
131. Robbie, S.J.; von Leithner, P.L.; Ju, M.; Lange, C.A.; King, A.G.; Adamson, P.; Lee, D.; Sychterz, C.; Coffey, P.; Ng, Y.S.; et al. Assessing a Novel Depot Delivery Strategy for Noninvasive Administration of VEGF/PDGF RTK Inhibitors for Ocular Neovascular Disease. *Investig. Ophthalmol. Vis. Sci.* **2013**, *54*, 1490–1500. [CrossRef] [PubMed]
132. Liao, D.S.; Grossi, F.V.; El Mehdi, D.; Gerber, M.R.; Brown, D.M.; Heier, J.S.; Wykoff, C.C.; Singerman, L.J.; Abraham, P.; Grassmann, F.; et al. Complement C3 Inhibitor Pegcetacoplan for Geographic Atrophy Secondary to Age-Related Macular Degeneration: A Randomized Phase 2 Trial. *Ophthalmology* **2020**, *127*, 186–195. [CrossRef]
133. Machinaga, N.; Ashley, G.W.; Reid, R.; Yamasaki, A.; Tanaka, K.; Nakamura, K.; Yabe, Y.; Yoshigae, Y.; Santi, D.V. A Controlled Release System for Long-Acting Intravitreal Delivery of Small Molecules. *Transl. Vis. Sci. Technol.* **2018**, *7*, 21. [CrossRef]
134. Mofidfar, M.; Abdi, B.; Ahadian, S.; Mostafavi, E.; Desai, T.A.; Abbasi, F.; Sun, Y.; Manche, E.E.; Flowers, C.W. Drug delivery to the anterior segment of the eye: A review of current and future treatment strategies. *Int. J. Pharm.* **2021**, *607*, 120924. [CrossRef] [PubMed]
135. Fishburn, C.S. The Pharmacology of PEGylation: Balancing PD with PK to Generate Novel Therapeutics. *J. Pharm. Sci.* **2008**, *97*, 4167–4183. [CrossRef] [PubMed]
136. Anand, B.; Nashed, Y.; Mitra, A. Novel dipeptide prodrugs of acyclovir for ocular herpes infections: Bioreversion, antiviral activity and transport across rabbit cornea. *Curr. Eye. Res.* **2003**, *26*, 151–163. [CrossRef]
137. Pudlarz, A.; Szemraj, J. Nanoparticles as Carriers of Proteins, Peptides and Other Therapeutic Molecules. *Open Life Sci.* **2018**, *13*, 285–298. [CrossRef]
138. Peyman, G.A.; Ganiban, G.J. Delivery systems for intraocular routes. *Adv. Drug Deliv. Rev.* **1995**, *16*, 107–123. [CrossRef]
139. Janoria, K.G.; Gunda, S.; Boddu, S.H.; Mitra, A.K. Novel approaches to retinal drug delivery. *Expert Opin. Drug Deliv.* **2007**, *4*, 371–388. [CrossRef]
140. Lambert, G.; Guilatt, R.L. Current ocular drug delivery challenges. *Drug Dev. Rep. Ind. Overv. Details* **2005**, *33*, 1–2.
141. Lang, J.C. Recent developments in ophthalmic drug delivery: Conventional ocular formulations. *Adv. Drug Deliv. Rev.* **1995**, *16*, 39–43. [CrossRef]
142. Kim, S.H.; GalbáN, C.J.; Lutz, R.J.; Dedrick, R.L.; Csaky, K.G.; Lizak, M.J.; Wang, N.S.; Tansey, G.; Robinson, M.R. Assessment of subconjunctival and intrascleral drug delivery to the posterior segment using dynamic contrast-enhanced magnetic resonance imaging. *Investig. Ophthalmol. Vis. Sci.* **2007**, *48*, 808–814. [CrossRef]
143. Rong, X.; Ji, Y.; Zhu, X.; Yang, J.; Qian, D.; Mo, X.; Lu, Y. Neuroprotective effect of insulin-loaded chitosan nanoparticles/PLGA-PEG-PLGA hydrogel on diabetic retinopathy in rats. *Int. J. Nanomed.* **2019**, *14*, 45–55. [CrossRef]
144. Vermonden, T.; Censi, R.; Hennink, W.E. Hydrogels for protein delivery. *Chem. Rev.* **2012**, *112*, 2853–2888. [CrossRef] [PubMed]
145. Kirchhof, S.; Goepferich, A.M.; Brandl, F.P. Hydrogels in ophthalmic applications. *Eur. J. Pharm. Biopharm.* **2015**, *95*, 227–238. [CrossRef] [PubMed]
146. Yu, Y.; Lau, L.C.; Lo, A.C.; Chau, Y. Injectable chemically crosslinked hydrogel for the controlled release of bevacizumab in vitreous: A 6-month in vivo study. *Transl. Vis. Sci. Technol.* **2015**, *4*, 5. [CrossRef]
147. Buwalda, S.J.; Bethry, A.; Hunger, S.; Kandoussi, S.; Coudane, J.; Nottelet, B. Ultrafast in situ forming poly(ethylene glycol)-poly(amido amine) hydrogels with tunable drug release properties via controllable degradation rates. *Eur. J. Pharm. Biopharm.* **2019**, *139*, 232–239. [CrossRef] [PubMed]
148. Buwalda, S.J.; Vermonden, T.; Hennink, W.E. Hydrogels for therapeutic delivery: Current developments and future directions. *Biomacromolecules* **2017**, *18*, 316–330. [CrossRef]
149. Bae, K.H.; Wang, L.S.; Kurisawa, M. Injectable biodegradable hydrogels: Progress and challenges. *J. Mater. Chem. B* **2013**, *1*, 5371. [CrossRef] [PubMed]
150. Franssen, O.; Vandervennet, L.; Roders, P.; Hennink, W.E. Degradable dextran hydrogels: Controlled release of a model protein from cylinders and microspheres. *J. Control. Release* **1999**, *60*, 211–221. [CrossRef]
151. Lin, C.C.; Metters, A.T. Hydrogels in controlled release formulations: Network design and mathematical modeling. *Adv. Drug Deliv. Rev.* **2006**, *58*, 1379–1408. [CrossRef]

152. Censi, R.; Vermonden, T.; Van, M.J. Photopolymerized thermosensitive hydrogels for tailorable diffusion-controlled protein delivery. *J. Control. Release.* **2009**, *140*, 230–236. [CrossRef]
153. Kirchhof, S.; Abrami, M.; Messmann, V. Diels-alder hydrogels for controlled antibody release: Correlation between mesh size and release rate. *Mol. Pharm.* **2015**, *12*, 3358–3368. [CrossRef]
154. Shastri, D.H.; Patel, L.D.; Parikh, R.K. Studies on *in situ* hydrogel: A smart way for safe and sustained ocular drug delivery. *J. Young Pharm.* **2010**, *2*, 116–120. [CrossRef]
155. Kanjickal, D.; Lopina, S.; Evancho-Chapman, M.M.; Schmidt, S.; Donovan, D. Effects of sterilization on poly(ethylene glycol) hydrogels. *J. Biomed. Mater. Res. A* **2008**, *87*, 608–617. [CrossRef] [PubMed]
156. Saher, O.; Ghorab, D.M.; Mursi, N.M. Preparation and in vitro/in vivo evaluation of antimicrobial ocular *in situ* gels containing a disappearing preservative for topical treatment of bacterial conjunctivitis. *Pharm. Dev. Technol.* **2016**, *21*, 600–610. [CrossRef] [PubMed]
157. Janet, T.; Stuart, W.; Kevin, H.; Gary, O.; Gabe, F.; Nicole, M.; Tomas, N.; Benjamin, M.; Benjamin, Y. In-vitro release of Bevacizumab from hydrogel-based drug delivery systems. *Investig. Ophthalmol. Vis. Sci.* **2015**, *56*, 222.
158. Blessing, C.I.; Arto, U.; Wim, E.H.; Tina, V. Intravitreal hydrogels for sustained release of therapeutic proteins. *J. Control. Release* **2020**, *326*, 419–441. [CrossRef]
159. Hu, C.C.; Chaw, J.R.; Chen, C.F.; Liu, H.W. Controlled release bevacizumab in thermoresponsive hydrogel found to inhibit angiogenesis. *Biomed. Mater. Eng.* **2014**, *24*, 1941–1950. [CrossRef]
160. Wang, C.H.; Hwang, Y.S.; Chiang, P.R.; Shen, C.R.; Hong, W.H.; Hsiue, G.H. Extended release of bevacizumab by thermosensitive biodegradable and biocompatible hydrogel. *Biomacromolecules* **2012**, *13*, 40–48. [CrossRef]
161. Lovett, M.L.; Wang, X.; Yucel, T.; York, L.; Keirstead, M.; Haggerty, L.; Kaplan, D.L. Silk hydrogels for sustained ocular delivery of anti-vascular endothelial growth factor (anti-VEGF) therapeutics. *Eur. J. Pharm. Biopharm.* **2015**, *95*, 271–278. [CrossRef]
162. Tyagi, P.; Barros, M.; Stansbury, J.W.; Kompella, U.B. Light activated, *in situ* forming gel for sustained suprachoroidal delivery of bevacizumab. *Mol. Pharm.* **2013**, *10*, 2858–2867. [CrossRef]
163. Misra, G.P.; Singh, R.S.J.; Aleman, T.S.; Jacobson, S.G.; Gardner, T.W.; Lowe, T.L. Subconjunctivally implantable hydrogels with degradable and thermoresponsive properties for sustained release of insulin to the retina. *Biomaterials* **2009**, *30*, 6541–6547. [CrossRef]
164. Rieke, E.R.; Amaral, J.; Becerra, S.P.; Lutz, R.J. Sustained subconjunctival protein delivery using a thermosetting gel delivery system. *J. Ocul. Pharmacol. Ther.* **2010**, *26*, 55–64. [CrossRef] [PubMed]
165. Alshaikh, A.R.; Christian, W.; Katie, B.R. Polymer based sustained drug delivery to the ocular posterior segment: Barriers and future opportunities for the treatment of neovascular pathologies. *Adv. Drug Deliv. Rev.* **2022**, *187*, 114–342. [CrossRef] [PubMed]
166. Rauck, B.M.; Friberg, T.R.; Medina Mendez, C.A.; Park, D.; Shah, V.; Bilonick, R.A.; Wang, Y. Biocompatible reverse thermal gel sustains the release of intravitreal bevacizumab in vivo. *Investig. Ophthalmol. Vis. Sci.* **2014**, *55*, 469–476. [CrossRef] [PubMed]
167. Park, D.; Wu, W.; Wang, Y. A functionalizable reverse thermal gel based on a polyurethane/PEG block copolymer. *Biomaterials* **2011**, *32*, 777–786. [CrossRef] [PubMed]
168. Cho, I.S.; Park, C.G.; Huh, B.K.; Cho, M.O.; Khatun, Z.; Li, Z.; Kang, S.W.; Choy, Y.B.; Huh, K.M. Thermosensitive hexanoyl glycol chitosan-based ocular delivery system for glaucoma therapy. *Acta Biomater.* **2016**, *39*, 124–132. [CrossRef]
169. Joseph, M.; Patel, S.P.; AGRAHARI, V.; Mitra, A.K. Pentablock Copolymer nano formulation for controlled Ocular Delivery of Protein Therapeutics. *Investig. Ophthalmol. Vis. Sci.* **2014**, *55*, 4629.
170. Alexander, A.; Ajazuddin, J.; Khan, J.; Saraf, S. Polyethylene glycol (PEG)-Poly(N-isopropylacrylamide) (PNIPAAm) based thermosensitive injectable hydrogels for biomedical applications. *Eur. J. Pharm. Biopharm.* **2014**, *88*, 575–585. [CrossRef]
171. López-Cano, J.J.; Sigen, A.; Andrés-Guerrero, V.; Tai, H.; Bravo-Osuna, I.; Molina-Martínez, I.T.; Wang, W.; Herrero-Vanrell, R. Thermo-Responsive PLGA-PEG-PLGA Hydrogels as Novel Injectable Platforms for Neuroprotective Combined Therapies in the Treatment of Retinal Degenerative Diseases. *Pharmaceutics* **2021**, *13*, 234. [CrossRef]
172. Cohen, S.; Yoshioka, T.; Lucarelli, M.; Hwang, L.H.; Langer, R. Controlled delivery systems for proteins based on poly(lactic/glycolic acid) microspheres. *Pharm. Res.* **1991**, *8*, 713–720. [CrossRef]
173. Ron, E.; Turek, T.; Mathiowitz, E.; Chasin, M.; Hageman, M.; Langer, R. Controlled release of polypeptides from polyanhydrides. *Proc. Natl. Acad. Sci. USA* **1993**, *90*, 4176–4180. [CrossRef]
174. Davis, M.E.; Brewster, M.E. Cyclodextrin-based pharmaceutics: Past, present and future. *Nat. Rev. Drug Discov.* **2004**, *3*, 1023–1035. [CrossRef]
175. Champion, J.A.; Mitragotri, S. Role of target geometry in phagocytosis. *Proc. Natl. Acad. Sci. USA* **2006**, *103*, 4930–4934. [CrossRef] [PubMed]
176. Burke, P.A.; Klumb, L.A.; Herberger, J.D.; Nguyen, X.C.; Harrell, R.A.; Zordich, M. Poly(lactide-co-glycolide) microsphere formulations of darbepoetin alfa: Spray drying is an alternative to encapsulation by spray-freeze drying. *Pharm. Res.* **2004**, *21*, 500–506. [CrossRef]
177. Vaishya, R.D.; Mandal, A.; Gokulgandhi, M.; Patel, S.; Mitra, A.K. Reversible hydrophobic ion-paring complex strategy to minimize acylation of octreotide during long-term delivery from PLGA microparticles. *Int. J. Pharm.* **2015**, *489*, 237–245. [CrossRef]
178. Carrasquillo, K.G.; Ricker, J.A.; Rigas, I.K.; Miller, J.W.; Gragoudas, E.S.; Adamis, A.P. Controlled delivery of the anti-VEGF aptamer EYE001 with poly(lactic-co-glycolic)acid microspheres. *Investig. Ophthalmol. Vis. Sci.* **2003**, *44*, 290–299. [CrossRef]

179. Cook, G.P.; Burgess, L.; Wing, J.; Dowie, T.; Calias, P.; Shima, D.T.; Campbell, K.; Allison, D.; Volker, S.; Schmidt, P. Preparation and Characterization of Pegaptanib Sustained Release Microsphere Formulations for Intraocular Application. *Investig. Ophthalmol. Vis. Sci.* **2006**, *47*, 5123.
180. Osswald, C.R.; Kang-Mieler, J.J. Controlled and Extended In vitro Release of Bioactive Anti-Vascular Endothelial Growth Factors from a Microsphere-Hydrogel Drug Delivery System. *Curr. Eye Res.* **2016**, *41*, 1216–1222. [CrossRef]
181. Vaishya, R.D.; Mandal, A.; Patel, S.; Mitra, A.K. Extended release microparticle-in-gel formulation of octreotide: Effect of polymer type on acylation of peptide during In vitro release. *Int. J. Pharm.* **2015**, *496*, 676–688. [CrossRef]
182. Mahlumba, P.; Choonara, Y.E.; Kumar, P.; du Toit, L.C.; Pillay, V. Stimuli-Responsive Polymeric Systems for Controlled Protein and Peptide Delivery: Future Implications for Ocular Delivery. *Molecules* **2016**, *21*, 2. [CrossRef]
183. Seah, I.; Zhao, X.; Lin, Q.; Liu, Z.; Su, S.Z.Z.; Yuetn, Y.S.; Hunziker, W.; Lingam, G.; Loh, X.J.; Su, X. Use of biomaterials for sustained delivery of anti-VEGF to treat retinal diseases. *Eye* **2020**, *34*, 1341–1356. [CrossRef]
184. Yang, F.; Pan, Y.F.; Wang, Z.Y.; Yang, Y.Q.; Zhao, Y.M.; Liang, S.Z.; Zhang, Y.M. Preparation and characteristics of interferon-alpha poly(lactic-co-glycolic acid) microspheres. *J. Microencap.* **2010**, *27*, 133–141. [CrossRef]
185. Pan, C.K.; Durairaj, C.; Kompella, U.B.; Agwu, O.; Oliver, S.C.; Quiroz-Mercado, H.; Mandava, N.; Olson, J.L. Comparison of long-acting bevacizumab formulations in the treatment of choroidal neovascularization in a rat model. *J. Ocul. Pharmacol. Ther.* **2011**, *27*, 219–224. [CrossRef]
186. Ramos, T.I.; Villacis-Aguirre, C.A.; Vispo, N.S.; Padilla, L.S.; Santana, S.P.; Parra, N.C.; Alonso, J.R.T. Forms and Methods for Interferon's Encapsulation. *Pharmaceutics* **2021**, *13*, 1533. [CrossRef] [PubMed]
187. Luaces-Rodríguez, A.; Mondelo, G.C.; Zarra-Ferro, I.; Barcia, M.; Aguiar, P.; Fernández-Ferreiro, A.; Otero-Espinar, F. Intravitreal anti-VEGF drug delivery systems for age-related macular degeneration. *Int. J. Pharm.* **2019**, *573*, 118767. [CrossRef] [PubMed]
188. Harish Prashanth, K.V.; Tharanathan, R.N. Depolymerized products of chitosan as potent inhibitors of tumor-induced angiogenesis. *Biochim. Et Biophys. Acta* **2005**, *1722*, 22–29. [CrossRef]
189. Khalili, H.; Lee, R.W.; Khaw, P.T.; Brocchini, S.; Dick, A.D.; Copland, D.A. An anti-TNF-alpha antibody mimetic to treat ocular inflammation. *Sci. Rep.* **2016**, *6*, 36905. [CrossRef] [PubMed]
190. Zamboulis, A.; Nanaki, S.; Michailidou, G.; Koumentakou, I.; Lazaridou, M.; Ainali, N.M.; Xanthopoulou, E.; Bikiaris, D.N. Chitosan and its Derivatives for Ocular Delivery Formulations: Recent Advances and Developments. *Polymers* **2020**, *12*, 1519. [CrossRef] [PubMed]
191. Zalevsky, J.; Chamberlain, A.K.; Horton, H.M.; Karki, S.; Leung, I.W.; Sproule, T.J.; Lazar, G.A.; Roopenian, D.C.; Desjarlais, J.R. Enhanced antibody half-life improves in vivo activity. *Nat. Biotech.* **2010**, *28*, 157–159. [CrossRef] [PubMed]
192. Sasahara, K.; McPhie, P.; Minton, A.P. Effect of dextran on protein stability and conformation attributed to macromolecular crowding. *J. Mol. Biol.* **2003**, *326*, 1227–1237. [CrossRef]
193. Sockolosky, J.T.; Szoka, F.C. The neonatal Fc receptor, FcRn, as a target for drug delivery and therapy. *Adv. Drug Deliv. Rev.* **2015**, *91*, 109–124. [CrossRef]
194. Bajracharya, R.; Song, J.G.; Back, S.Y.; Han, H.K. Recent Advancements in Non-Invasive Formulations for Protein Drug Delivery. *Comp. Struct. Biotech. J.* **2019**, *17*, 1290–1308. [CrossRef] [PubMed]
195. Webber, M.J.; Appel, E.A.; Vinciguerra, B.; Cortinas, A.B.; Thapa, L.S. Supramolecular PEGylation of biopharmaceuticals. *Proc. Natl. Acad. Sci. USA* **2016**, *113*, 14189–14194. [CrossRef] [PubMed]
196. Kim, H.; Robinson, S.B.; Csaky, K.G. Investigating the movement of intravitreal human serum albumin nanoparticles in the vitreous and retina. *Pharm. Res.* **2009**, *26*, 329–337. [CrossRef]
197. Hayashi, A.; Naseri, A.; Pennesi, M.E.; de Juan, E., Jr. Subretinal delivery of immunoglobulin G with gold nanoparticles in the rabbit eye. *Jap. J. Ophthalmol.* **2009**, *53*, 249–256. [CrossRef] [PubMed]
198. Zhang, K.; Zhang, L.; Weinreb, R.N. Ophthalmic drug discovery: Novel targets and mechanisms for retinal diseases and glaucoma. *Nat. Rev. Drug Discov.* **2012**, *11*, 541–559. [CrossRef]
199. Swed, A.; Cordonnier, T.; Fleury, F.; Boury, F. Protein Encapsulation into PLGA Nanoparticles by a Novel Phase Separation Method Using Non-Toxic Solvents. *J. Nanomed. Nanotechnol.* **2014**, *5*, 6. [CrossRef]
200. Zhang, L.; Li, Y.; Zhang, C.; Wang, Y.; Song, C. Pharmacokinetics, and tolerance study of intravitreal injection of dexamethasone-loaded nanoparticles in rabbits. *Int. J. Nanomed.* **2009**, *4*, 175–183. [CrossRef]
201. Carroll, R.; Bhatia, D.; Geldenhuys, W.; Bhatia, R.; Miladore, N.; Bishayee, A.; Sutariya, V. Brain-targeted delivery of tempol-loaded nanoparticles for neurological disorders. *J. Drug Target.* **2010**, *18*, 665–674. [CrossRef]
202. Makadia, H.K.; Siegel, S.J. Poly lactic-co-glycolic acid (plga) as biodegradable controlled drug delivery carrier. *Polymers.* **2011**, *3*, 1377–1397. [CrossRef]
203. De Negri Atanasio, G.; Ferrari, P.F.; Campardelli, R.; Perego, P.; Palombo, D. Poly (Lactic-co-Glycolic Acid) Nanoparticles and Nanoliposomes for Protein Delivery in Targeted Therapy: A Comparative In Vitro Study. *Polymers* **2020**, *12*, 2566. [CrossRef]
204. Feczko, T.; Toth, J.; Dosa, G.; Gyenis, J. Optimization of protein encapsulation in PLGA nanoparticles. *Chem. Eng. Process.* **2011**, *50*, 757–765. [CrossRef]
205. Li, H.; Tran, V.V.; Hu, Y.; Mark Saltzman, W.; Barnstable, C.J.; Tombran-Tink, J. A PEDF N- terminal peptide protects the retina from ischemic injury when delivered in PLGA nanospheres. *Exp. Eye Res.* **2006**, *83*, 824–833. [CrossRef] [PubMed]
206. Nayak, K.; Misra, M. A review on recent drug delivery systems for posterior segment of eye. *Biomed. Pharmacother.* **2018**, *107*, 1564–1582. [CrossRef] [PubMed]

207. Jin, J.; Zhou, K.K.; Park, K.; Hu, Y.; Xu, X.; Zheng, Z.; Tyagi, P.; Kompella, U.B.; Ma, J.X. Anti- inflammatory and antiangiogenic effects of nanoparticle-mediated delivery of a natural angiogenic inhibitor. *Investig. Ophthalmol. Vis. Sci.* **2011**, *52*, 6230–6237. [CrossRef] [PubMed]
208. O'Reilly, M.S.; Holmgren, L.; Shing, Y.; Chen, C.; Rosenthal, R.A.; Moses, M.; Lane, W.S.; Cao, Y.; Sage, E.H.; Folkman, J. Angiostatin: A novel angiogenesis inhibitor that mediates the suppression of metastases by a Lewis lung carcinoma. *Cell* **1994**, *79*, 315–328. [CrossRef] [PubMed]
209. Wang, Z.; Cheng, R.; Lee, K.; Tyagi, P.; Ding, L.; Kompella, U.B.; Chen, J.; Xu, X.; Ma, J.X. Nanoparticle-mediated expression of a Wnt pathway inhibitor ameliorates ocular neovascularization. *Arterioscler. Thromb. Vas. Bio.* **2015**, *35*, 855–864. [CrossRef] [PubMed]
210. Busik, J.V.; Grant, M.B. Wnting out ocular neovascularization: Using nanoparticle delivery of very-low density lipoprotein receptor extracellular domain as Wnt pathway inhibitor in the retina. *Arterioscler. Thromb. Vas. Bio.* **2015**, *35*, 1046–1047. [CrossRef]
211. Agrahari, V.; Hung, W.T.; Christenson, L.K.; Mitra, A.K. Composite Nano-formulation Therapeutics for Long-Term Ocular Delivery of Macromolecules. *Mol. Pharm.* **2016**, *13*, 2912–2922. [CrossRef]
212. Bisht, R.; Mandal, A.; Jaiswal, J.K.; Rupenthal, I.D. Nanocarrier mediated retinal drug delivery: Overcoming ocular barriers to treat posterior eye diseases. *WIREs Nanomed. Nanobiotechnol.* **2017**, *10*, e1473. [CrossRef]
213. Kelly, S.J.; Hirani, A.; Shahidadpury, V.; Solanki, A.; Halasz, K.; Varghese Gupta, S.; Madow, B.; Sutariya, V. Aflibercept Nanoformulation Inhibits VEGF Expression in Ocular In vitro Model: A Preliminary Report. *Biomedicines* **2018**, *6*, 92. [CrossRef]
214. Yandrapu, S.K.; Upadhyay, A.K.; Petrash, J.M.; Kompella, U.B. Nanoparticles in porous microparticles prepared by supercritical infusion and pressure quench technology for sustained delivery of bevacizumab. *Mol. Pharm.* **2013**, *10*, 4676–4686. [CrossRef] [PubMed]
215. Elsaid, N.; Jackson, T.L.; Elsaid, Z.; Alqathama, A.; Somavarapu, S. PLGA microparticles entrapping chitosan-based nanoparticles for the ocular delivery of ranibizumab. *Mol. Pharm.* **2016**, *13*, 2923–2940. [CrossRef]
216. Kim, H.; Choi, J.S.; Kim, K.S.; Yang, J.A.; Joo, C.K.; Hahn, S.K. Flt1 peptide-hyaluronate conjugate micelle-like nanoparticles encapsulating genistein for the treatment of ocular neovascularization. *Acta Biomater.* **2012**, *8*, 3932–3940. [CrossRef]
217. Mahaling, B.; Katti, D.S. Physicochemical properties of core-shell type nanoparticles govern their spatiotemporal biodistribution in the eye. *Nanomed. Nanotech. Bio. Med.* **2016**, *12*, 2149–2160. [CrossRef]
218. Chis, A.A.; Dobrea, C.; Morgovan, C.; Arseniu, A.M.; Rus, L.L.; Butuca, A.; Juncan, A.M.; Totan, M.; Vonica-Tincu, A.L.; Cormos, G.; et al. Applications and Limitations of Dendrimers in Biomedicine. *Molecules* **2020**, *25*, 3982. [CrossRef] [PubMed]
219. Wang, H.; Huang, Q.; Chang, H.; Xiao, J.; Cheng, Y. Stimuli-responsive dendrimers in drug delivery. *Biomater. Sci.* **2016**, *4*, 375–390. [CrossRef] [PubMed]
220. Davis, B.M.; Normando, E.M.; Guo, L.; Turner, A.; Nizari, S.; O'Shea, P.; Moss, S.E.; Somavarapu, S.; Cordeiro, M.F. Topical delivery of Avastin to the posterior segment of the eye in vivo using annexin A5-associated liposomes. *Small* **2014**, *10*, 1575–1584. [CrossRef]
221. Abrishami, M.; Zarei-Ghanavati, S.; Soroush, D.; Rouhbakhsh, M.; Jaafari, M.R.; Malaekeh-Nikouei, B. Preparation, characterization, and in vivo evaluation of nanoliposomes- encapsulated bevacizumab (avastin) for intravitreal administration. *Retina* **2009**, *29*, 699–703. [CrossRef]
222. Varela-Fernández, R.; García-Otero, X.; Díaz-Tomé, V.; Regueiro, U.; López-López, M.; González-Barcia, M.; Lema, M.I.; Otero-Espinar, F.J. Lactoferrin-loaded nanostructured lipid carriers (NLCs) as a new formulation for optimized ocular drug delivery. *Eur. J. Pharm. Biopharm.* **2022**, *172*, 144–156. [CrossRef]
223. Kazi, K.M.; Mandal, A.S.; Biswas, N.; Guha, A.; Chatterjee, S.; Behera, M.; Kuotsu, K. Niosome: A future of targeted drug delivery systems. *J. Adv. Pharm. Technol. Res.* **2010**, *1*, 374–380.
224. Puras, G.; Martínez-Navarrete, G.; Mashal, M.; Zárate, J.; Agirre, M.; Ojeda, E.; Grijalvo, S.; Eritja, R.; Diaz-Tahoces, A.; Avilés-Trigueros, M.; et al. Protamine/DNA/niosome ternary nonviral vectors for gene delivery to the retina: The role of protamine. *Mol. Pharm.* **2015**, *12*, 3658–3671. [CrossRef]
225. Camelo, S.; Lajavardi, L.; Bochot, A.; Goldenberg, B.; Naud, M.; Fattal, E.; Behar-Cohen, F.; De Kozak, Y. Ocular and systemic bio-distribution of rhodamine-conjugated liposomes loaded with VIP injected into the vitreous of Lewis rats. *Mol. Vis.* **2007**, *13*, 2263–2274.
226. Bochot, A.; Fattal, E. Liposomes for intravitreal drug delivery: A state of the art. *J. Control. Release* **2012**, *161*, 628–634. [CrossRef] [PubMed]
227. Mishra, G.P.; Bagui, M.; Tamboli, V.; Mitra, A.K. Recent applications of liposomes in ophthalmic drug delivery. *J. Drug. Deliv.* **2011**, *2011*, 863734. [CrossRef]
228. Kawakami, S.; Harada, A.; Sakanaka, K.; Nishida, K.; Nakamura, J.; Sakaeda, T.; Ichikawa, N.; Nakashima, M.; Sasaki, H. In vivo gene transfection via intravitreal injection of cationic liposome/plasmid DNA complexes in rabbits. *Int. J. Pharm.* **2004**, *278*, 255–262. [CrossRef]
229. Bochot, A.; Fattal, E.; Boutet, V.; Deverre, J.R.; Jeanny, J.C.; Chacun, H.; Couvreur, P. Intravitreal delivery of oligonucleotides by sterically stabilized liposomes. *Investig. Ophthalmol. Vis. Sci.* **2002**, *43*, 253–259.
230. Ben-Arzi, A.; Ehrlich, R.; Neumann, R. Retinal Diseases: The Next Frontier in Pharmacodelivery. *Pharmaceutics* **2022**, *14*, 904. [CrossRef] [PubMed]

231. Mandal, A.; Bisht, R.; Rupenthal, I.D.; Mitra, A.K. Polymeric micelles for ocular drug delivery: From structural frameworks to recent preclinical studies. *J. Control. Release.* **2017**, *48*, 96–116. [CrossRef]
232. Patel, S.P.; Vaishya, R.; Patel, A.; Agrahari, D.; Mitra, A.K. Optimization of novel pentablock copolymer based composite formulation for sustained delivery of peptide/protein in the treatment of ocular diseases. *J. Microencapsul.* **2016**, *33*, 103–113. [CrossRef]
233. Senturk, B.; Cubuk, M.O.; Ozmen, M.C.; Aydin, B.; Guler, M.O.; Tekinay, A.B. Inhibition of VEGF mediated corneal neovascularization by anti-angiogenic peptide nanofibers. *Biomaterials* **2016**, *107*, 124–132. [CrossRef] [PubMed]
234. Patel, S.P.; Vaishya, R.; Pal, D.; Mitra, A.K. Novel pentablock copolymer-based nanoparticulate systems for sustained protein delivery. *AAPS PharmSciTech.* **2015**, *16*, 327–343. [CrossRef]
235. Patel, S.P.; Vaishya, R.; Mishra, G.P.; Tamboli, V.; Pal, D.; Mitra, A.K. Tailor-made pentablock copolymer based formulation for sustained ocular delivery of protein therapeutics. *J. Drug Deliv.* **2014**, *2014*, 40174. [CrossRef]
236. Acharya, G.; Yuan, X.; Marcano, D.; Shin, C.; Hua, X. Nanowafer drug delivery to treat corneal neovascularization. *Investig. Ophthalmol. Vis. Sci.* **2015**, *56*, 5032.
237. Roman, V.M.; Peter, W.J.M.; Fraser, S.; Vitaliy, V.K. Penetration Enhancers in Ocular Drug Delivery. *Pharmaceutics.* **2019**, *11*, 321. [CrossRef]
238. Young, K.H.; Yum, Y.S.; Jang, G.; Ahn, D.R. Discovery of a non-cationic cell penetrating peptide derived from membrane-interacting human proteins and its potential as a protein delivery carrier. *Sci. Rep.* **2015**, *5*, 11719. [CrossRef] [PubMed]
239. De Cogan, F.; Hill, L.J.; Lynch, A.; Morgan-Warren, P.J.; Lechner, J.; Berwick, M.R.; Peacock, A.F.A.; Chen, M.; Scott, R.A.H.; Xu, H.; et al. Topical Delivery of Anti-VEGF Drugs to the Ocular Posterior Segment Using Cell-Penetrating Peptides. *Investig. Ophthalmol. Vis. Sci.* **2017**, *58*, 2578–2590. [CrossRef] [PubMed]
240. Wang, Y.; Lin, H.; Lin, S.; Qu, J.; Xiao, J.; Huang, Y.; Xiao, Y.; Fu, X.; Yang, Y.; Li, X. Cell-Penetrating Peptide TAT-Mediated Delivery of Acidic FGF to Retina and Protection against Ischemia-Reperfusion Injury in Rats. *J. Cell. Mol. Med.* **2010**, *14*, 1998–2005. [CrossRef]
241. Liu, C.; Tai, L.; Zhang, W.; Wei, G.; Pan, W.; Lu, W. Penetratin, a Potentially Powerful Absorption Enhancer for Noninvasive Intraocular Drug Delivery. *Mol. Pharm.* **2014**, *11*, 1218–1227. [CrossRef]
242. Mitchell, D.J.; Steinman, L.; Kim, D.T.; Fathman, C.G.; Rothbard, J.B. Polyarginine Enters Cells More Efficiently than Other Polycationic Homopolymers. *J. Pept. Res.* **2000**, *56*, 318–325. [CrossRef]
243. Vivès, E.; Brodin, P.; Lebleu, B. A Truncated HIV-1 Tat Protein Basic Domain Rapidly Translocates through the Plasma Membrane and Accumulates in the Cell Nucleus. *J. Biol. Chem.* **1997**, *272*, 16010–16017. [CrossRef]
244. Chu, Y.; Chen, N.; Yu, H.; Mu, H.; He, B.; Hua, H.; Wang, A.; Sun, K. Topical Ocular Delivery to Laser-Induced Choroidal Neovascularization by Dual Internalizing RGD and TAT Peptide-Modified Nanoparticles. *Int. J. Nanomed.* **2017**, *12*, 1353–1368. [CrossRef] [PubMed]
245. Li, Y.; Li, L.; Li, Z.; Sheng, J.; Zhang, X.; Feng, D.; Zhang, X.; Yin, F.; Wang, A.; Wang, F. Tat PTD-Endostatin-RGD: A Novel Protein with Anti-Angiogenesis Effect in Retina via Eye Drops. *Biochim. Biophys. Acta Gen. Subj.* **2016**, *1860*, 2137–2147. [CrossRef] [PubMed]
246. Bird, G.H.; Madani, N.; Perry, A.F.; Princiotto, A.M.; Supko, J.G.; He, X.; Gavathiotis, E.; Sodroski, J.G.; Walensky, L.D. Hydrocarbon double-stapling remedies the proteolytic instability of a lengthy peptide therapeutic. *Proc. Natl. Acad. Sci. USA* **2010**, *107*, 14093–14098. [CrossRef] [PubMed]
247. Chu, Q.; Moellering, R.E.; Hilinski, G.J.; Kim, Y.W.; Grossmann, T.N.; Yeh, G.L. Towards understanding cell penetration by stapled peptides. *Med. Chem. Comm.* **2015**, *6*, 111–119. [CrossRef]
248. Ho, J.; Uger, R.A.; Zwick, M.B.; Luscher, M.A.; Barber, B.H.; MacDonald, K.S. Conformational constraints imposed on a pan-neutralizing HIV-1 antibody epitope result in increased antigenicity but not neutralizing response. *Vaccine* **2005**, *23*, 1559–1573. [CrossRef] [PubMed]
249. Suda, K.; Murakami, T.; Gotoh, N.; Fukuda, R.; Hashida, Y.; Hashida, M.; Tsujikawa, A.; Yoshimura, N. High-Density Lipoprotein Mutant Eye Drops for the Treatment of Posterior Eye Diseases. *J. Control. Release* **2017**, *266*, 301–309. [CrossRef]
250. Tai, L.; Liu, C.; Jiang, K.; Chen, X.; Feng, L.; Pan, W.; Wei, G.; Lu, W. A Novel Penetratin-Modified Complex for Noninvasive Intraocular Delivery of Antisense Oligonucleotides. *Int. J. Pharm.* **2017**, *529*, 347–356. [CrossRef]
251. Jiang, K.; Gao, X.; Shen, Q.; Zhan, C.; Zhang, Y.; Xie, C.; Wei, G.; Lu, W. Discerning the Composition of Penetratin for Safe Penetration from Cornea to Retina. *Acta Biomater.* **2017**, *63*, 123–134. [CrossRef]
252. Emerich, D.F.; Thanos, C.G. NT-501: An ophthalmic implant of polymer-encapsulated ciliary neurotrophic factor-producing cells. *Curr. Opin. Mol. Ther.* **2008**, *10*, 506–515.
253. Kuno, N.; Fujii, S. Biodegradable intraocular therapies for retinal disorders: Progress to date. *Drugs Aging* **2010**, *27*, 117–134. [CrossRef]
254. Barar, J.; Aghanejad, A.; Fathi, M.; Omidi, Y. Advanced drug delivery and targeting technologies for the ocular diseases. *BioImpacts* **2016**, *6*, 49–67. [CrossRef] [PubMed]
255. Belhaj, M.; Annamalai, B.; Parsons, N.; Shuler, A.; Potts, J.; Rohrer, B. Encapsulated Cell Technology for the Delivery of Biologics to the Mouse Eye. *J. Vis. Exp.* **2020**. [CrossRef] [PubMed]
256. Annamalai, B.; Parsons, N.; Brandon, C.; Rohrer, B. The use of Matrigel combined with encapsulated cell technology to deliver a complement inhibitor in a mouse model of choroidal neovascularization. *Mol. Vis.* **2020**, *26*, 370–377. [PubMed]

257. Raiskup-Wolf, F.; Eljarrat-Binstock, E.; Rehak, M.; Domb, A.; Frucht-Pery, J. Transcorneal and transscleral iontophoresis of the dexamethasone phosphate into the rabbit eye. *Cesk. Slov. Oftalmol.* **2007**, *63*, 360–368.
258. Eljarrat-Binstock, E.; Orucov, F.; Frucht-Pery, J.; Pe'er, J.; Domb, A.J. Methylprednisolone delivery to the back of the eye using hydrogel iontophoresis. *J. Ocul. Pharmacol. Ther. Off. J. Assoc. Ocul. Pharmacol. Ther.* **2008**, *24*, 344–350. [CrossRef]
259. Eljarrat-Binstock, E.; Domb, A.J.; Orucov, F.; Dagan, A.; Frucht-Pery, J.; Pe'er, J. In vitro and in vivo evaluation of carboplatin delivery to the eye using hydrogel-iontophoresis. *Curr. Eye Res.* **2008**, *33*, 269–275. [CrossRef]
260. Eljarrat-Binstock, E.; Domb, A.J.; Frucht-Pery, J.; Pe'er, J. Methotrexate delivery to the eye using transscleral hydrogel iontophoresis. *Curr. Eye Res.* **2007**, *32*, 639–646. [CrossRef]
261. Molokhia, S.; Papangkorn, K.; Butler, C.; Higuchi, J.W.; Brar, B.; Ambati, B.; Li, S.K.; Higuchi, W.I. Transscleral Iontophoresis for Noninvasive Ocular Drug Delivery of Macromolecules. *J. Ocul. Pharmacol. Ther.* **2020**, *36*, 247–256. [CrossRef]
262. Zhang, Y.; Chen, Y.; Yu, X.; Qi, Y.; Chen, Y.; Hu, Z.; Li, Z. A flexible device for ocular iontophoretic drug delivery. *Biomicrofluidics* **2016**, *10*, 011911. [CrossRef]
263. Parkinson, T.M.; Ferguson, E.; Febbraro, S.; Bakhtyari, A.; King, M.; Mundasad, M. Tolerance of ocular iontophoresis in healthy volunteers. *J. Ocul. Pharmacol. Ther.* **2003**, *19*, 145–151. [CrossRef]
264. Vollmer, D.L.; Szlek, M.A.; Kolb, K.; Lloyd, L.B.; Parkinson, T.M. in vivo transscleral iontophoresis of amikacin to rabbit eyes. *J. Ocul. Pharmacol. Ther.* **2002**, *18*, 549–558. [CrossRef] [PubMed]
265. Eljarrat, B.E.; Raiskup, F.; Frucht, P.J.; Domb, A.J. Transcorneal and transscleral iontophoresis of dexamethasone phosphate using drug loaded hydrogel. *J. Control. Release* **2005**, *106*, 386–390. [CrossRef] [PubMed]
266. Stanley, T.C.; Liang, X.H.; Brenda, F.B.; Rosanne, M.C. Antisense technology: A review. *J. Bio. Chem.* **2021**, *296*. [CrossRef]
267. Gadziński, P.; Froelich, A.; Wojtyłko, M.; Białek, A.; Krysztofiak, J.; Osmałek, T.; Beilstein, J. Microneedle-based ocular drug delivery systems—Recent advances and challenges. *Beilstein J. Nanotechnol.* **2022**, *13*, 1167–1184. [CrossRef]
268. Thakur, R.R.; Fallows, S.J.; McMillan, H.L.; Donnelly, R.F.; Jones, D.S. Microneedle- mediated intrascleral delivery of in situ forming thermoresponsive implants for sustained ocular drug delivery. *J. Pharm. Pharmacol.* **2014**, *66*, 584–595. [CrossRef]
269. Song, H.B.; Lee, K.J.; Seo, I.H.; Lee, J.Y.; Lee, S.M. Impact insertion of transfer-molded microneedle for localized and minimally invasive ocular drug delivery. *J. Control. Release* **2015**, *209*, 272–279. [CrossRef]
270. García-Estrada, P.; García-Bon, M.A.; López-Naranjo, E.J.; Basaldúa-Pérez, D.N.; Santos, A.; Navarro-Partida, J. Polymeric Implants for the Treatment of Intraocular Eye Diseases: Trends in Biodegradable and Non-Biodegradable Materials. *Pharmaceutics* **2021**, *13*, 701. [CrossRef]
271. Procopio, A.; Lagreca, E.; Jamaledin, R.; La Manna, S.; Corrado, B.; Di Natale, C.; Onesto, V. Recent Fabrication Methods to Produce Polymer-Based Drug Delivery Matrices (Experimental and In Silico Approaches). *Pharmaceutics* **2022**, *14*, 872. [CrossRef]
272. Hippalgaonkar, K.; Adelli, G.R.; Hippalgaonkar, K.; Repka, M.A.; Majumdar, S. Indomethacin-loaded solid lipid nanoparticles for ocular delivery: Development, characterization, and In vitro evaluation. *J. Ocu. Pharmacol. Ther.* **2013**, *29*, 216–228. [CrossRef]
273. Yasukawa, T.; Ogura, Y.; Sakurai, E.; Tabata, Y.; Kimura, H. Intraocular sustained drug delivery using implantable polymeric devices. *Adv. Drug Deliv. Rev.* **2005**, *57*, 2033–2046. [CrossRef]
274. Malcles, A.; Dot, C.; Voirin, N.; Vie, A.L.; Agard, E.; Bellocq, D.; Denis, P.; Kodjikian, L. Safety of intravitreal Dexamethasone implant (OZURDEX): The SAFODEX study. Incidence and Risk Factors of Ocular Hypertension. *Retina* **2017**, *37*, 1352–1359. [CrossRef]
275. Christoforidis, J.B.; Chang, S.; Jiang, A.; Wang, J.; Cebulla, C.M. Intravitreal devices for the treatment of vitreous inflammation. *Mediat. Inflamm.* **2012**, *2012*, 126463. [CrossRef] [PubMed]
276. Torriglia, A.; Valamanesh, F.; Behar-Cohen Francine, F. On the Retinal Toxicity of Intraocular Glucocorticoids. *Biochem. Pharmacol.* **2010**, *80*, 1878–1886. [CrossRef]
277. Dugel, P.U.; Bandello, F.; Loewenstein, A. Dexamethasone Intravitreal Implant in the Treatment of Diabetic Macular Edema. *Clin. Ophthalmol.* **2015**, *9*, 1321–1335. [CrossRef] [PubMed]
278. Zhou, T.; Lewis, H.; Foster, R.E.; Schwendeman, S.P. Development of a multiple-drug delivery implant for intraocular management of proliferative vitreoretinopathy. *J. Control. Release* **1998**, *55*, 281–295. [CrossRef] [PubMed]
279. Bourges, J.L.; Bloquel, C.; Thomas, A.; Froussart, F.; Bochot, A.; Azan, F.; Gurny, R.; BenEzra, D.; Behar-Cohen, F. Intraocular implants for extended drug delivery: Therapeutic applications. *Adv. Drug Deliv. Rev.* **2006**, *58*, 1182–1202. [CrossRef] [PubMed]
280. Taban, M.; Lowder, C.Y.; Kaiser, P.K. Outcome of fluocinolone acetonide implant (Retisert) reimplantation for chronic noninfectious posterior uveitis. *Retina* **2008**, *28*, 1280–1288. [CrossRef]
281. Jaffe, G.J.; Martin, D.; Callanan, D.; Pearson, P.A.; Levy, B.; Comstock, T. Fluocinolone Acetonide Uveitis Study, Fluocinolone acetonide implant (Retisert) for noninfectious posterior uveitis: Thirty-four-week results of a multicenter randomized clinical study. *Ophthalmology* **2006**, *113*, 1020–1027. [CrossRef]
282. Ambati, J.; Gragoudas, E.S.; Miller, J.W.; You, T.T.; Miyamoto, K.; Delori, F.C.; Adamis, A.P. Transscleral delivery of bioactive protein to the choroid and retina. *Investig. Ophthalmol. Vis. Sci.* **2000**, *41*, 1186–1191.
283. Agarwal, P.; Rupenthal, I.D. Injectable implants for the sustained release of protein and peptide drugs. *Drug Disc. Today* **2013**, *18*, 337–349. [CrossRef]
284. Li, F.; Hurley, B.; Liu, Y.; Leonard, B.; Griffith, M. Controlled release of bevacizumab through nanospheres for extended treatment of age-related macular degeneration. *Open Ophthalmol. J.* **2012**, *6*, 54–58. [CrossRef] [PubMed]

285. Ye, Z.; Ji, Y.L.; Ma, X.; Wen, J.C.; Wei, W.; Huang, S.M. Pharmacokinetics, and distributions of bevacizumab by intravitreal injection of bevacizumab-PLGA microspheres in rabbits. *Int. J. Ophthalmol.* **2015**, *8*, 653–658. [PubMed]
286. Freeman, W.R.; Sailor, M.; Chen, M.; Cheng, L. Nanostructured Porous Silicon Dioxide Microparticles as an Intravitreal Injectable Drug Delivery System for Avastin (Bevacizumab) Lasting Six Months. *Investig. Ophthalmol. Vis. Sci.* **2012**, *53*, 456.
287. Varshochian, R.; Jeddi-Tehrani, M.; Mahmoudi, A.R.; Khoshayand, M.R.; Atyabi, F.; Sabzevari, A.; Esfahani, M.R.; Dinarvand, R. The protective effect of albumin on bevacizumab activity and stability in PLGA nanoparticles intended for retinal and choroidal neovascularization treatments. *Eur. J. Pharm. Sci.* **2013**, *50*, 341–352. [CrossRef]
288. Jeong, J.H.; Nguyen, H.K.; Lee, J.E.; Suh, W. Therapeutic effect of apatinib-loaded nanoparticles on diabetes-induced retinal vascular leakage. *Int. J. Nanomed.* **2016**, *11*, 3101–3109.
289. Varshochian, R.; Riazi-Esfahani, M.; Jeddi-Tehrani, M.; Mahmoudi, A.-R.; Aghazadeh, S.; Mahbod, M.; Movassat, M.; Atyabi, F.; Sabzevari, A.; Dinarvand, R. Albuminated PLGA nanoparticles containing bevacizumab intended for ocular neovascularization treatment. *J. Biomed. Mater. Res. A* **2015**, *103*, 3148–3156. [CrossRef]
290. Pandit, J.; Sultana, Y.; Aqil, M. Chitosan coated nanoparticles for efficient delivery of bevacizumab in the posterior ocular tissues via subconjunctival administration. *Carbohydr. Polym.* **2021**, *267*, 118217. [CrossRef]
291. Badiee, P.; Varshochian, R.; Rafiee-Tehrani, M.; Abedin Dorkoosh, F.; Khoshayand, M.R.; Dinarvand, R. Ocular implant containing Bevacizumab-loaded chitosan nanoparticles intended for choroidal neovascularization treatment. *J. Biomed. Mater. Res. A* **2018**, *106*, 2261–2271. [CrossRef]
292. Mat Nor, M.N.; Guo, C.X.; Rupenthal, I.D.; Chen, Y.-S.; Green, C.R.; Acosta, M.L. Sustained connexin43 mimetic peptide release from loaded nanoparticles reduces retinal and choroidal photodamage. *Investig. Ophthalmol. Vis. Sci.* **2018**, *59*, 36–82. [CrossRef]
293. Zhang, X.-P.; Sun, J.-G.; Yao, J.; Shan, K.; Liu, B.-H.; Yao, M.-D.; Ge, H.-M.; Jiang, Q.; Zhao, C.; Yan, B. Effect of nanoencapsulation using poly (lactide-co- glycolide) (PLGA) on anti-angiogenic activity of bevacizumab for ocular angiogenesis therapy. *Biomed. Pharmacother.* **2018**, *107*, 1056–1063. [CrossRef]
294. Huang, D.; Chen, Y.-S.; Rupenthal, I.D. Hyaluronic acid coated albumin nanoparticles for targeted peptide delivery to the retina. *Mol. Pharm.* **2017**, *14*, 533–545. [CrossRef] [PubMed]
295. Lu, Y.; Zhou, N.; Huang, X.; Cheng, J.-W.; Li, F.-Q.; Wei, R.-L.; Cai, J.-P. Effect of intravitreal injection of bevacizumab-chitosan nanoparticles on retina of diabetic rats. *Int. J. Ophthalmol.* **2014**, *7*, 1–7. [PubMed]
296. Kim, H.; Saky, K.G. Nanoparticle-integrin antagonist C16Y peptide treatment of choroidal neovascularization in rats. *J. Control. Release* **2010**, *142*, 286–293. [CrossRef] [PubMed]
297. Alqawlaq, S.; Sivak, J.; Huzil, J.T.; Ivanova, M.V.; Flanagan, J.G.; Beazely, M.A.; Foldvari, M. Preclinical development and ocular biodistribution of gemini-DNA nanoparticles after intravitreal and topical administration: Towards non-invasive glaucoma gene therapy. *Nanomed. Nanotechnol. Biol. Med.* **2014**, *10*, 1637–1647. [CrossRef] [PubMed]
298. Puras, G.; Zarate, J.; Aceves, M.; Murua, A.; Díaz, A.; Avilés-Triguero, M.; Fernández, E.; Pedraz, J. Low molecular weight oligochitosans for non-viral retinal gene therapy. *Eur. J. Pharm. Biopharm.* **2013**, *83*, 131–140. [CrossRef] [PubMed]
299. Zhang, C.; Wang, Y.-S.; Wu, H.; Zhang, Z.-X.; Cai, Y.; Hou, H.-Y.; Zhao, W.; Yang, X.-M.; Ma, J.-X. Inhibitory efficacy of hypoxia-inducible factor 1a short hairpin RNA plasmid DNA-loaded poly (D,L-lactide-co-glycolide) nanoparticles on choroidal neovascularization in a laser-induced rat model. *Gene Ther.* **2010**, *17*, 338–351. [CrossRef]
300. Park, K.; Chen, Y.; Hu, Y.; Mayo, A.S.; Kompella, U.B.; Longeras, R.; Ma, J.-X. Nanoparticle-mediated expression of an angiogenic inhibitor ameliorates ischemia-induced retinal neovascularization and diabetes-induced retinal vascular leakage. *Diabetes* **2009**, *58*, 1902–1913. [CrossRef]
301. Ryoo, N.-K.; Lee, J.; Lee, H.; Hong, H.K.; Kim, H.; Lee, J.B.; Woo, S.J.; Park, K.H.; Kim, H. Therapeutic effects of a novel siRNA-based anti-VEGF (siVEGF) nanoball for the treatment of choroidal neovascularization. *Nanoscale* **2017**, *9*, 15461–15469. [CrossRef]
302. Qin, Y.; Tian, Y.; Liu, Y.; Li, D.; Zhang, H.; Yang, Y.; Qi, J.; Wang, H.; Gan, L. Hyaluronic acid-modified cationic niosomes for ocular gene delivery: Improving transfection efficiency in retinal pigment epithelium. *J. Pharm. Pharmacol.* **2018**, *70*, 1139–1151. [CrossRef]
303. Liu, H.-A.; Liu, Y.-L.; Ma, Z.-Z.; Wang, J.-C.; Zhang, Q. A lipid nanoparticle system improves siRNA efficacy in RPE cells and a laser-induced murine CNV model. *Investig. Ophthalmol. Vis. Sci.* **2011**, *52*, 4789–4794. [CrossRef]
304. Apaolaza, P.S.; del Pozo-Rodriguez, A.; Solinís, M.A.; Rodríguez, J.M.; Friedrich, U.; Torrecilla, J.; Weber, B.H.; Rodríguez-Gascón, A. Structural recovery of the retina in a retinoschisin- deficient mouse after gene replacement therapy by solid lipid nanoparticles. *Biomaterials* **2016**, *90*, 40–49. [CrossRef] [PubMed]
305. Luo, Q.; Yang, J.; Xu, H.; Shi, J.; Liang, Z.; Zhang, R.; Lu, P.; Pu, G.; Zhao, N.; Zhang, J. Sorafenib-loaded nanostructured lipid carriers for topical ocular therapy of corneal neovascularization: Development, in vitro and in vivo study. *Drug Deliv.* **2022**, *29*, 837–855. [CrossRef] [PubMed]
306. Li, Q.; Yang, X.; Zhang, P. Dasatinib loaded nanostructured lipid carriers for effective treatment of corneal neovascularization. *Biomater Sci.* **2021**, *9*, 2571–2583. [CrossRef] [PubMed]
307. Marano, R.J.; Toth, I.; Wimmer, N.; Brankov, M.; Rakoczy, P.E. Dendrimer delivery of an anti-VEGF oligonucleotide into the eye: A long-term study into inhibition of laser induced CNV, distribution, uptake and toxicity. *Gene Ther.* **2005**, *12*, 1544–1550. [CrossRef]

308. Mu, H.; Wang, Y.; Chu, Y.; Jiang, Y.; Hua, H.; Chu, L.; Wang, K.; Wang, A.; Liu, W.; Li, Y.; et al. Multivesicular liposomes for sustained release of bevacizumab in treating laser-induced choroidal neovascularization. *Drug. Deliv.* **2018**, *25*, 1372–1383. [CrossRef]
309. Lance, K.D.; Bernards, D.A.; Ciaccio, N.A.; Good, S.D.; Mendes, T.S. In vivo and in vitro sustained release of ranibizumab from a nanoporous thin-film device. *Drug Deliv. Transl. Res.* **2016**, *6*, 771–780. [CrossRef]
310. Humayun, M.; Santos, A.; Altamirano, J.C.; Ribeiro, R.; Gonzalez, R.; de la Rosa, A.; Shih, J.; Pang, F.; Jiang, F.; Calvillo, P.; et al. Implantable Micropump for Drug Delivery in Patients with Diabetic Macular Edema. *Transl. Vis. Sci. Tech.* **2014**, *3*, 5. [CrossRef]
311. Wang, J.; Jiang, A.; Joshi, M.; Christoforidis, J. Drug delivery implants in the treatment of vitreous inflammation. *Mediat. Inflamm.* **2013**, *2013*, 780634. [CrossRef]
312. Smith, J.; Ward, D.; Michaelides, M.; Moore, A.T.; Simpson, S. New and emerging technologies for the treatment of inherited retinal diseases: A horizon scanning review. *Eye* **2015**, *29*, 131–1140. [CrossRef]
313. Lim, J.I.; Niec, M.; Wong, V. One year results of a phase 1 study of the safety and tolerability of combination therapy using sustained release intravitreal triamcinolone acetonide and ranibizumab for subfoveal neovascular AMD. *Brit. J. Ophthalmol.* **2015**, *99*, 618–623. [CrossRef]
314. Kirchhof, S.; Gregoritza, M.; Messmann, V.; Hammer, N.; Goepferich, A.M.; Brandl, F.P. Diels-Alder hydrogels with enhanced stability: First step toward controlled release of bevacizumab. *Eur. J. Pharm. Biopharm.* **2015**, *96*, 217–225. [CrossRef] [PubMed]
315. Zhang, K.; Hopkins, J.J.; Heier, J.S.; Birch, D.G.; Halperin, L.S.; Albini, T.A.; Brown, D.M.; Jaffe, G.J.; Tao, W.; Williams, G.A. Ciliary neurotrophic factor delivered by encapsulated cell intraocular implants for treatment of geographic atrophy in age-related macular degeneration. *Proc. Natl. Acad. Sci. USA* **2011**, *108*, 6241–6245. [CrossRef] [PubMed]
316. Huang, D.; Chen, Y.-S.; Green, C.R.; Rupenthal, I.D. Hyaluronic acid coated albumin nanoparticles for targeted peptide delivery in the treatment of retinal ischaemia. *Biomaterials* **2018**, *168*, 10–23. [CrossRef] [PubMed]

Disclaimer/Publisher's Note: The statements, opinions and data contained in all publications are solely those of the individual author(s) and contributor(s) and not of MDPI and/or the editor(s). MDPI and/or the editor(s) disclaim responsibility for any injury to people or property resulting from any ideas, methods, instructions or products referred to in the content.

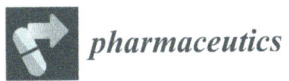

Review

Bioprinted Membranes for Corneal Tissue Engineering: A Review

Amin Orash Mahmoud Salehi [1], Saeed Heidari-Keshel [2], Seyed Ali Poursamar [3], Ali Zarrabi [4], Farshid Sefat [5,6], Narsimha Mamidi [1,*], Mahmoud Jabbarvand Behrouz [7] and Mohammad Rafienia [3,*]

1. Department of Chemistry and Nanotechnology, School of Engineering and Science, Tecnologico de Monterrey, Monterrey 64849, NL, Mexico
2. Department of Tissue Engineering and Applied Cell Sciences, School of Advanced Technologies in Medicine, Shahid Beheshti University of Medical Sciences, Tehran 1434875451, Iran
3. Biosensor Research Center, Isfahan University of Medical Sciences, Isfahan 8174673441, Iran
4. Department of Biomedical Engineering, Faculty of Engineering and Natural Sciences, Istinye University, Istanbul 34396, Turkey
5. Department of Biomedical and Electronics Engineering, School of Engineering, University of Bradford, Bradford BD7 1DP, UK
6. Interdisciplinary Research Centre in Polymer Science & Technology (Polymer IRC), University of Bradford, Bradford BD7 1DP, UK
7. Translational Ophthalmology Research Center, Farabi Eye Hospital, Tehran University of Medical Sciences, Tehran 1985717443, Iran
* Correspondence: nmamidi@tec.mx or narsimhachem06@gmail.com (N.M.); m_rafienia@med.mui.ac.ir (M.R.)

Abstract: Corneal transplantation is considered a convenient strategy for various types of corneal disease needs. Even though it has been applied as a suitable solution for most corneal disorders, patients still face several issues due to a lack of healthy donor corneas, and rejection is another unknown risk of corneal transplant tissue. Corneal tissue engineering (CTE) has gained significant consideration as an efficient approach to developing tissue-engineered scaffolds for corneal healing and regeneration. Several approaches are tested to develop a substrate with equal transmittance and mechanical properties to improve the regeneration of cornea tissue. In this regard, bioprinted scaffolds have recently received sufficient attention in simulating corneal structure, owing to their spectacular spatial control which produces a three-cell-loaded-dimensional corneal structure. In this review, the anatomy and function of different layers of corneal tissue are highlighted, and then the potential of the 3D bioprinting technique for promoting corneal regeneration is also discussed.

Keywords: corneal tissue engineering; epithelium; stroma; endothelium; 3D bioprinting

1. Introduction

The cornea, which is located in the anterior part of the eye, is a transparent layer and acts as the window of the eye [1–3]. The corneal structure contains three transparent layers, and two membranes [2]. The corneal structure transfers light into the eye's environment and protects the eye's structure from mechanical or chemical environmental injuries, UV light, and infection [4]. Corneal dysfunction causes corneal visual loss [5].

Corneal surgery and corneal transplantation are well-known therapies for corneal blindness [5]. According to the World Health Organization (WHO), about 10 million patients globally need healthy corneal donation [1]. Additionally, over 40,000 corneal transplantations are carried out in the United States annually [6]. However, corneal transplantation displayed several drawbacks including shortness of high-quality donor corneas, expensive surgery, and rejected tissue due to the immune system and weakness for long-term transplantation [7]. In addition, because aging diminishes the function of endothelial cells, the quality of the transplanted cornea is of utmost importance [8]. Furthermore, the tissue becomes ineligible for corneal transplantation by therapies that alter the corneal structure to improve vision, such as LASIK [9]. Scientists are utilizing stem cells and tissue-engineering techniques to generate bioengineered cornea, or even individual corneal layers, to address the shortage of eligible corneas for donation [10–12].

Tissue engineering utilizes cells, bioactive macromolecules, and scaffolds, or a blend of the mentioned factors [13–17]. Human corneal cell keratoplasty (HCCK) was recently chosen as an advanced corneal surgery technique. The HCCK technique includes transparent carriers to improve human corneal cell behavior [18–20]. These lamellar keratoplasties and tissue-engineered full-thickness are recognized as successful transplantations [5]. Although donor corneas are used in these approaches, they still possess some challenges such as allograft tissue availability and rejection [21]. Results have shown that the proliferative ability of cultured human corneal cells can be preserved; thus, cornea tissue engineering (CTE) is recognized as a suitable approach for reconstructing corneal damage [22]. A recent study revealed that human corneal cells (HCCs) have adequate efficacy for cell propagation, but they might show low biocompatibility, weak light transmittance, and poor mechanical properties [23–25]. There are several methods of producing tissue-engineered scaffolds that completely resemble corneal structures [9,26–29]. Among them, 3D bioprinting technology is one of the potential approaches for producing artificial target tissue scaffolds. For example, the advantage of choosing this method in scaffold construction is the induction of the natural process during embryogenetic tissue formation and imitation [30–32]. Overall, 3D printing is attractive due to its high spatial resolution, and the simultaneous processing of cells and materials [33]. The conventional 3D printer consists of a classic inkjet, nozzles, and printer heads with material loaded into the cartridges as bioinks [34–39]. Thus, this review paper will highlight the corneal anatomy and different corneal layers' functions, ocular disorders, and a summary of different approaches in scaffold constructions with a specific emphasis on 3D printed corneal tissue-engineered scaffolds.

2. Corneal Anatomy and Physiology

The cornea, known as the window of the eye, is optically transparent, including a special structure that is avascular anatomically. This dome-shaped and specialized tissue is located in the anterior part of the eye. Two major roles of the cornea are protecting the eye from harsh environments, and transmitting over 80% of light to inner portions (Figure 1A) [23]. As is evident in Figure 1B, the cornea is composed of three arranged and transparent layers, and two membranes: The cornea includes the outermost layer of epithelium, stroma, and the innermost layer of endothelium. Additionally, the epithelium and stroma are separated by Bowman's membrane. However, the stroma and endothelium are separated by Descemet's membrane (Figure 1B) [22]. Furthermore, the cornea acts as the last superficial barrier of the eye, providing safety from external potential dangers, and infections [40]. Moreover, to maintain and protect the integrity of the eye surface, corneal nerves play a vital role [23]. Consequently, corneal regeneration is obtained by nerve density, and corneal sensation factors after transplantation [4].

In addition, the aqueous humor is located at the eye's surface, and the function of the cornea depends on its malleability [41]. Moreover, it should be noted that the tear film is placed in the outermost portion of the eye, and acts as a reservoir for antibacterial and growth factors [9]. Additionally, one of the most critical roles of tear film in maintaining homeostasis, proliferation, and repair is covering the corneal surface. The anatomical importance of the cornea, which includes five transparent and arranged layers, corresponds to a wide-angle lens [13].

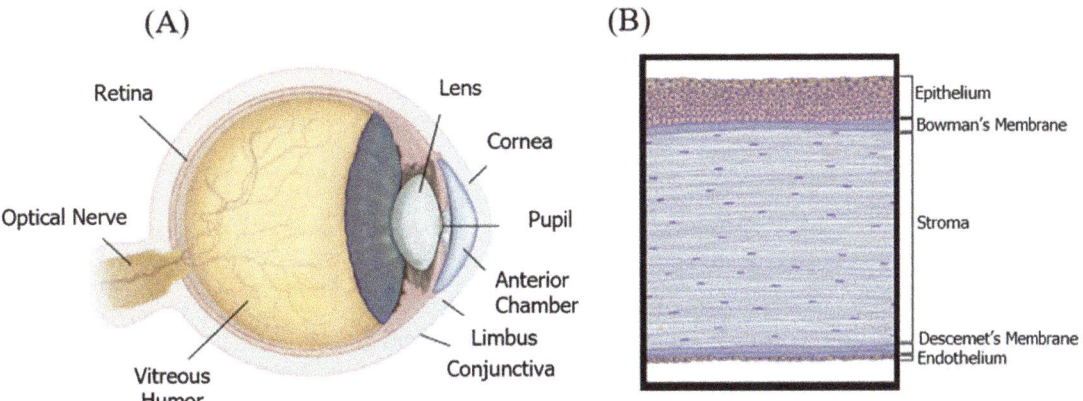

Figure 1. (**A**) The anatomy of the eye, cornea. (**B**) The cornea is an optically transparent multilayered structure consisting of three cell layers and two membranes. Adopted and modified from [1] (Chapter 67) with permission.

2.1. Corneal Epithelium

The epithelium is the outermost layer of the corneal tissue, and acts critically in the refraction of light into the eye [42–44]. The epithelium is a highly innervated tissue with nerve endings terminating at corneal epithelial layers [45]. The epithelium is a multilayered tissue and has five cell layers which occupy 10% of the corneal structure, and is about 50 µm thick [22]. The epithelium, a biological barrier, is responsible for the transfer of all soluble constituents and water out or into the stroma to maintain proper corneal light transparency, providing a smooth layer [23]. There are three cell types in the epithelial layer of the cornea. These cell types consist of 3–4 layers of flattened squamous cells, 1–3 layers of wing cells, and a single layer of columnar basal cells. It should be noted that these cells are held together by tight junctions [1]. These cell types are regenerated every 7–10 days continuously by the limbus stem cells (LSCs) [46].

There are some challenges in the regeneration of the epithelial layer by tissue engineering approaches, such as mimicking its arranged complexity, maintaining integrity as a sufficient barrier, and replacing epithelial cells continually [47–49]. In general, the epithelial layer, as the outermost layer, can keep the eye safe from mechanical damage, infection, and injuries [4]. In addition, it has a role in protecting the retina from UV damage [4].

2.2. Corneal Stroma

The stroma occupies 90% of the corneal tissue and 5% of corneal keratocyte cells (CKCs), and is an acellular layer but also a dense connective layer derived from neural crest cells [40]. The stroma comprises over 200 noncellular collagenous lamellae that are fully uniform, small, and aligned collagen fibers [7]. When injuries occur, flattened fibroblasts are activated. These lie quiescently, typically to produce collagen, then stabilize collagenous lamellae, and secrete the stromal components [2]. There are two important properties of a healthy stroma layer: optical transparency, and suitable mechanical strength [12–14]. Optical transparency is needed for biophysical properties, and suitable mechanical strength can be decreased when this organized structure is disturbed. Light transmittance can be reduced as a result of stromal damage and disruption. The stroma expresses two major challenges for the tissue engineer: equal mechanical stability, and high optical transparency [50].

2.3. Corneal Endothelium

Although the endothelium is the thinnest layer of the corneal tissue, it is important for maintaining function, and the ability to maintain corneal reproduction [1]. It is necessary to maintain dehydration by keeping optimal optical clarity [51]. Originally, the human endothelial cells (HECs) consist of about 5000 cells/mm^2, while the number of HECs shows loss with increasing age. In general, the major challenge for tissue-engineered transplantation is the HECs cell number of out 2500 cells/mm^2 [52]. The endothelium functions as a leaking pump of the corneal structure by leaking from the stroma layer in the presence of excessive stromal hydration (above 80%) [53]. The pumping-leak function process contains Na$^+$ and K$^+$-ATPase pumps that occupy the basolateral membrane. The main function of pumping-leak is to maintain stromal relative dehydration through transporting ions and water from the stroma to the tear film and aqueous humor [54–56]. The main characterization challenge is the efficiency measurement of the transplanted HECs [57]. There are some selective glucose transporters in this layer, permitting nutrition transformation from the aqueous humor to feed the epithelial and CKCs. Therefore, the main function of the endothelial layer is optical transparency with regulated hydrophilic proteoglycan and collagen interfibrillar spacing. In addition, endothelial distortion might lead to a loss in pump function [58].

3. Cells

3.1. Epithelium Cells

The corneal epithelial cells function as a physical barrier that resists the outer environment to maintain a healthy stroma layer. This effective corneal cell layer has a continuous turnover, with a lifespan of approximately 7 to 10 days (Figure 2). This turnover function is well described by the XYZ hypothesis [1]: X, the basal epithelial cells form the layer capable of proliferation properties; Y, migration centripetally of peripheral cells of new basal cells from the limbus to the cornea; and Z, loss of the epithelial cells from the surface. Generally, the epithelial cells shed constantly, and are substituted by a new cell sheet [59]. X + Y = Z describes the corneal epithelium's maintenance function: cell loss and replacement. These three stages describe the complete corneal wound healing process: Z represents the epithelial cell loss from the limbus, step Y describes the covering of the surface by the wound surface, and lastly, in the final step X, proliferation provides cells with the ability to replace the epithelial tissue. As a result, the intensity of the centripetal movement and enhancement of proliferation ability are reasons to promote corneal wound healing [60].

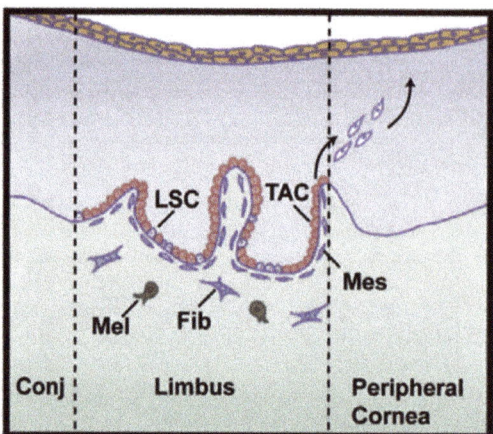

Figure 2. The major role of the limbus is to regenerate epithelium where the limbal stem cells (LSCs) reside. LSCs produce transient amplifying cells (TACs) that have a significant proliferation potential. Then, TACs migrate to epithelium which is responsible for producing epithelial cells and is replaced. Mes = mesenchymal cell, Mel = melanocyte, Fib = fibroblast, Conj = conjunctiva. Adopted and modified from [1] (Chapter 67) with permission.

3.2. Stroma Cells

The corneal stroma consists of both extracellular and cellular components [61]. Cellular components of the mature corneal stroma are CKCs. CKCs have a dendritic morphology and are responsible for the maintenance of the ECM of the stroma. CKCs generate keratocan and lumican, and they are the key factors in maintaining the shape and transparency of the stroma. These small leucine-rich protein family members (keratocan and lumican) are the most important keratan sulfate proteoglycans in the corneal stroma [62–64]. Keratocan is solely found as a proteoglycan in the cornea, while lumican may also exist in various tissues as a glycosylated protein [33]. Both keratocan and lumican interact with collagen fibrils, and regulate the structure of this tissue to fit within their limits for specific properties [4]. Based on previous evidence, keratocan plays a crucial role in preserving the corneal structure [9].

Wound healing processes change the dendritic morphology of CKCs to be fibroblastic in appearance [65]. Two important functions of the keratocyte—the expression of keratocan and keratan sulfate synthesis—are decreased during the fibroblast/myofibroblast transformation [9]. Both isolated keratocytes from the corneal stroma and cultured keratocytes exhibit fibroblastic/myofibroblast phenotypes, and, meanwhile, show decreased keratocan expression and keratan sulfate synthesis, similar to in vivo wound healing [66]. This demonstrates that keratocan can be regarded as an indication of the native keratocyte phenotype [2].

3.3. Endothelium Cells

The key function of the endothelial cells is to pump excess fluid from the stroma and epithelium into the superficial layer of the cornea to maintain optimum corneal nutrition, and hydration [67]. This is recognized as the "pump-leak hypothesis", preserving the cornea in a dehydrated state. It is worth mentioning that the hydration stage plays an important role in optical transparency (Figure 3) [60]. Endothelial cells are responsible for transporting proteins from inner layers using Na/K ATPase pumps. Thus, this gradient provides an osmotic pressure to maintain corneal stroma hydration, which is essential for endothelial cell growth [68].

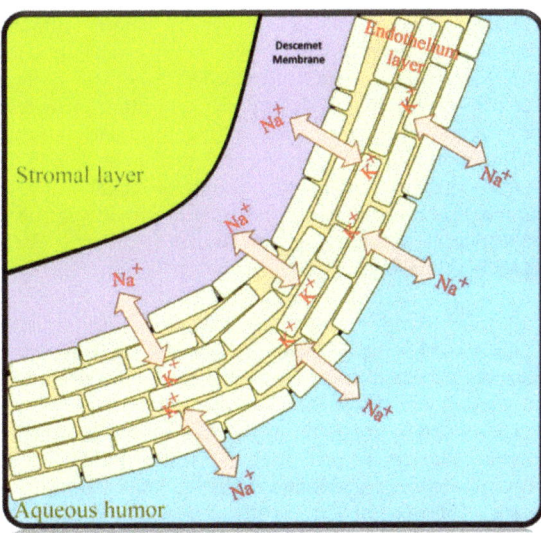

Figure 3. The corneal endothelial "pump-leak" hypothesis illustrated—basic principles [68].

4. Corneal Scarring

Understanding the processes of deficiency or disease in almost any aspect of the visual system necessitates an intensive investigation of the structural foundations of the cornea, hence necessitating a considerable emphasis on individualized medical and surgical regeneration therapy. Vision impairment and obstruction of light to the eye have revealed a lot of biological information about ophthalmic diseases, ranging from damaged superficial layers and limbal cells to corneal injuries [4].

4.1. Keratoconus

Overall, keratoconus involves a general weakness of the connective tissue of the cornea. It is a progressive, noninflammatory corneal dystrophy resulting in thinning and protrusion of the cornea, changing it from a dome shape to a conical shape with gradual bulging [69–71]. Initially, patients experience blurred vision with the same symptoms as irregular astigmatism and refractive defect [72–74]. Vision is obscured as keratoconus progresses. The extent of vision impairment is subject to the degree of progression.

As keratoconus progresses it can be more easily diagnosed, as patients experience impaired night vision, photophobia, severe headaches due to eye strain, and eye itching. Usually, the condition is bilateral, and begins in the early teenage years. Corneal scarring is seen in advanced keratoconus stages, and can contribute to further vision loss until it eventually progresses to the point that corneal transplantation is critical to repair vision [75–77]. Keratoconus is responsible for stromal scarring, axial thinning, the disintegration of the epithelial basement membrane, and breaks in the Bowman's membrane. According to the reported clinical case studies, the progression of keratoconus typically alters inevitable astigmatism from regular to irregular [4].

4.2. Dry Eye Disease

Dry eye has a wide range of eye surface diseases. According to a study reported in the 2007 international dry eye workshop, dry eye is a multidimensional disease, and its symptoms include tear instability, visual disturbance, eye discomfort, and potentially ocular surface damage [78]. According to data from previous studies, approximately 4.91 million Americans suffer from dry eye disease. Furthermore, there are tens of millions of less severe symptoms that can lead to dry eye failure if they are not followed up, which can trigger irritation—such as extended use of visual display terminals, or contact lens wear [79]. The pathophysiology involves either increased tear evaporation, decreased tear secretion, or both, resulting in hyperosmolarity of the tear film, and ocular surface inflammation. Corneal epithelial integrity can be seen in dry eye disease in its moderate to severe forms disrupted with punctate epithelial erosions; these erosions are detectable with fluorescein staining. The most common treatment for moderate to severe dry eyes is tearing supplementation, anti-inflammatory drops, eyelid hygiene, punctual plugs, and oral tetracycline [80].

4.3. Bacterial Keratitis

Bacterial keratitis is well-known as a devastating infection of the cornea, which can occur when the ocular defense is damaged. As a result, its spread causes inflammation, and gradual loss of vision. It is important to note that epithelial defects and decreased corneal sensitivity are prompting factors for severe ulcers, stromal necrosis, and bacterial growth. Failure in the protective mechanism and lack of ocular surface integrity causes the penetration of bacterial microbes into the cornea [81]. The most common causative organisms of bacterial keratitis include *Staphylococcus aureus, Streptococcus pneumonia*, and *Staphylococcus epidermidis* [82].

4.4. Light and Chemical Injuries

Clinically, exposure to UV light from a light source can damage the corneal epithelium, and cause fluorescein staining. Snow blindness, tanning bed use, direct lightening, and direct observation of the sun are some of the major causes of lesions on the corneal surface. Other important factors (such as chemical burns) can cause weakness in the cells of the corneal surface and affect the epithelial regeneration, even leading to potential blindness [83]. There are currently common treatments for superficial diseases that increase the ability of the corneal epithelium to recover. For extreme cases, cell-based restorative and repopulation treatments are necessary [21], which include techniques such as stem cell transplants, allografts, and limbal autografts to promote re-epithelialization [84].

4.5. Corneal Abrasion and Foreign Body

Corneal abrasions are more common in patients with symptoms in the epithelial layer, as they are more susceptible to injury. Abrasions typically occur with a range of symptoms, such as foreign body sensation, pain, tearing, sensitivity to light, and decreased vision, and it should be also noted that patients typically present with a history of trauma [85]. The presence of a foreign body within the corneal calls for immediate action to avoid permanent scarring, and serious loss of the epithelial cell surface. A deep wound with infected foreign material is likely to result in severe complications, initiating traumatic iritis, recurrent erosion syndrome, bacterial keratitis, and corneal ulcers [86].

5. Three-Dimensional Bioprinting

In general, the created scaffold structure is similar for all 3D printed models (Figure 4). First, the creation of a high-quality 3D model from the desired object is required. Then, the 3D structure should be printed in 2D layers of thickness, defined by the 3D image. The data will form the structure for layer-by-layer printing by transferring the command to the printer's desktop. The flexible manufacturing process allows it to be provided to the targeted tissue. In addition, graphical methods can be designed, including computer-aided design (CAD), and magnetic resonance imaging (MRI) of a structure similar to the data received from patients [33].

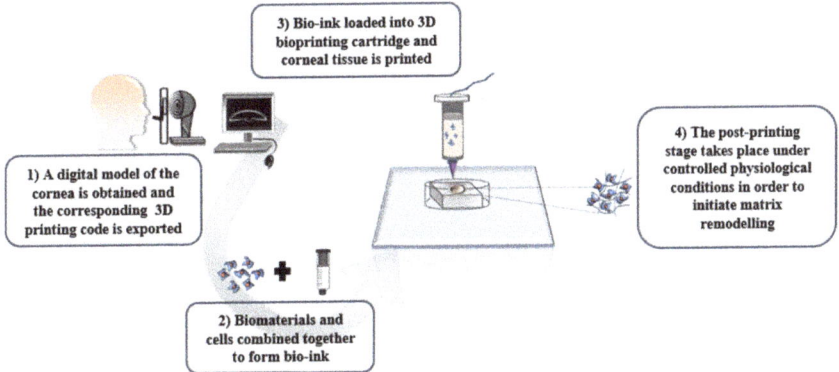

Figure 4. The path of making patient-specific devices via 3D printing [33] with permission.

Another consideration is bioprinting, which uses cellular encapsulated biological materials as bioinks [87]. Scaffolds printed with a cell are produced in situ. In this circumstance, the printing process must be carried out in disinfected conditions, and be compatible with the cell. The importance of maintaining structure and having mechanical properties in the printed structure are factors that limit the selection of cell-compatible materials [88]. It is also important to select the appropriate rheological parameter to reduce the shear pressure, which is required for the printing parameters [89]. Nevertheless, cell-loaded bioprinting reduces the resolution of the printed substrate. Secondly, the need to increase the cell density ratio relative to the surface area is of critical importance [90]. It should be noted that a healthy threshold of cell density in solid organs is considered to be about 10^9

to 10^{10} cells per cell culture well. Up until now, bioprinted hydrogel scaffolds only had a cell density ranging between 10^5 and 10^7 cells per cell culture well [91].

Bioprinting methods have successfully been applied by several researchers, and have demonstrated the reliable properties of bioprinting techniques to generate ex vivo constructs and membranes [92]. For example, scientists have obtained noticeable features by a microextrusion approach to produce a proper replacement for neural studies, generating 3D models of interacting human endothelial cells (HECs), and cancer studies by using a laser-based method, or even recreation of native ECM of cartilage by a droplet-based technique [93–95]. As a top-down approach, bioprinted scaffolds are known as a biofabrication technology for fabricating several types of ex vivo membranes and tissues artificially by consecutive deposition of cell-loaded layers [96–99]. Different approaches can be applied for fabricating bioprinted scaffolds such as laser-based, droplet-based, and extrusion-based techniques (Figure 5) [100]. These bioprinting techniques are compatible with several kinds of bioinks which can be crosslinked in different ways. However, optimizing bioink, according to the requirements of each of these bioprinting techniques, is associated with different challenges. An extrusion-based method is the most popular in comparison with other types of bioprinting approaches [101–103], since it is compatible with most injectable hydrogel platforms for biomedical engineering, and regeneration medicine applications [93,94,104]. In brief, this method contains pre-polymerized bioink which is extruded through a single nozzle under pressure. The pressurized air can be applied to the printer head to produce a 3D construct by extruding printing material layer by layer.

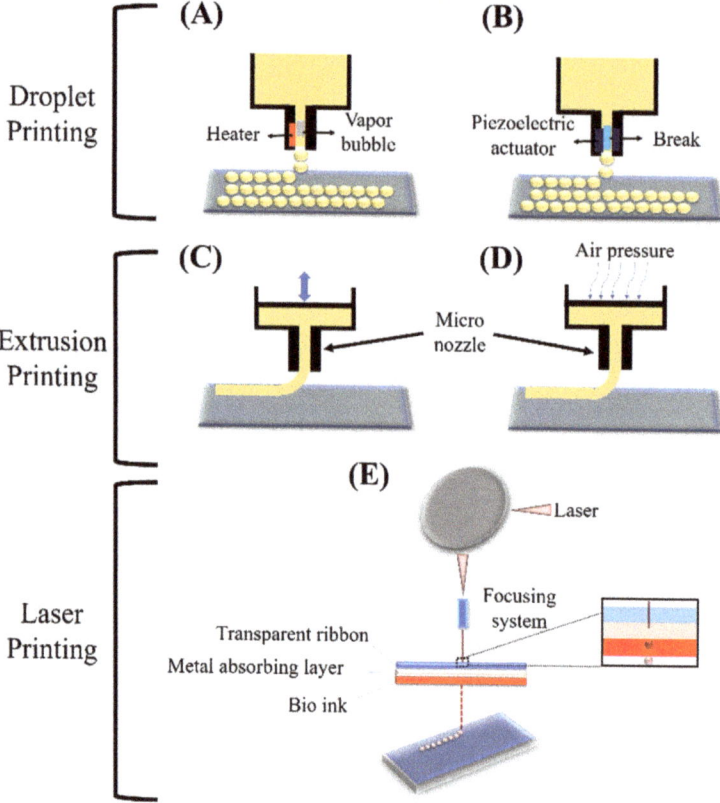

Figure 5. Schematic of the basic techniques of 3D printing: Droplet printing (thermal (**A**), piezoelectric (**B**)), Extrusion printing (piston (**C**), pneumatic (**D**)), and Laser printing (stereolithographic (**E**)) [100].

In addition to these three bioprinting methods, recent studies have demonstrated two more techniques that have illustrated interesting results. These techniques can be categorized into two major categories. Among these techniques, one involves using photocurable gels, and another is based on applying thermosensitive and natural (such as collagen) bioinks [105–108]. As a photocurable gel, both poly (ethylene glycol) diacrylate (PEGDA) and gelatin methacrylate (GelMA) can be crosslinked using lithium phenyl (2,4,6-trimethyl benzoyl) phosphinate (LAP) as a crosslinker under visible light. Bernal et al. [105] fabricated a GelMA-LAP bioink system to produce 3D printed osteogenic models by employing the volumetric method, setting 2D light with rotating and synchronously irradiated patterns. It should be noted that the volumetric bioprinting technique enables geometrically constructed production which aims to create centimeter-scale constructs at an unprecedented printing rate, opening new possibilities for upscaling the creation of the hydrogel-based structure. The result showed that the polymer was not cured evenly and only in some parts of the structure, preventing the gelation threshold as a result of increased absorption. Looking on the bright side, after fourteen days of continuous cell culturing, the tissue-engineered construct revealed enhanced alkaline phosphatase (ALP) expression, and mineral deposition. Another study by Grigoryan et al. [106] generated multi-vascular and intravascular structures via photopolymerizable gel with the addition of food dye for the stereolithography approach. Both studies illustrated that it is possible to fabricate a complex 3D construct via these methods, and demonstrate new possibilities for fabricating corneal tissue suitable for tissue transplant applications. The second category of bioprinting methods involves applying thermosensitive and natural bioinks [107,108]. Skylar-Scott et al. [107] generated a 3D printing scaffold with the sacrificial writing into functional tissue (SWIFT) approach. In the SWIFT technique, a high volume of cells are transferred into the engineered ECM during the bioprinting procedure. This technique contains a sacrificial gel that contains the cells. This gel is printed and after printing it is liquified by melting at room temperature; thus, the gel is removed creating a path for the medium to flow. The results have shown that after eight days of cell seeding cardiomyocyte cells showed a beating function, proving the successful functional application. Another study which was designed in the reverse order, in comparison to SWIFT, utilized freeform reversible embedding of suspended hydrogels (FRESH), supporting the 3D printed structure during the process which revealed positive results after 14 days of cell seeding [108]. Thus, the obtained results can be used for human corneal generation.

Corneal Bioprinting

In general, corneal bioprinting offers a wide range of possibilities to address current challenges and requirements of corneal tissue regeneration (i.e., controllable structure and properties, similar mechanical strength to withstand environmental as well as structural pressure, and fabricating a fully-organized corneal construct) [100]. As was addressed in Sections 2 and 3, the corneal structure consists of three transparent layers. The thickest layer of the cornea is the stromal layer (~500 μm), and the epithelium and endothelium are both delicate in structure (<50 μm) [109]. The stromal layer occupied over 90% of the corneal structure, and functionally is the most important tissue in CTE due to its transparency (as a result of aligned collagen lamellae and proteoglycan expressions) and mechanical performance (due to cross-linked collagen fibrils) [110]. In addition, the peripheral and central sections of the stromal layer show different mechanical properties, which play a crucial role in the orientation of collagen content, and corneal cell differentiation and alignment [111]. Therefore, to enhance the functionality of the stromal part, it is crucial to simulate the micro and macrostructure since the physical, mechanical, and chemical properties of the tissue-engineered structure directly and noticeably affect biological factors [9].

According to current studies, various bioprinting techniques for CTE have been considered (Table 1) [33,67,112–121]. Sorkio et al. [112] analyzed the feasibility of a laser-based bioprinting method to generate corneal tissue. In brief, the collagen type-I cell loaded enhanced LSCs cell attachment and proliferation. Although it is possible to print a tissue-like stromal layer, the tissue-engineered structure may not be appropriate in its structure and mechanical properties because of the very sensitive nature of CKCs. Additionally, the fabricated scaffold did not have proper transparency for corneal demands. Another study by Isaacson et al. [33] reported preparing bioink consisting of alginate-collagen type-I and CKCs. The prepared ink was injected into a 3D mold made by acrylonitrile butadiene styrene (ABS), and using the FRESH method. The final result was a structure similar to the 3D structure of corneal, with corneal tissue. Even though the produced construct showed suitable transparency, it could not support CKCs properly and the cells could not reach a dendritic shape.

Table 1. Summary of different experimental studies based on 3D printing techniques.

Corneal Layer	Bioprinting Method	Material	Cell Source	Results	Ref.
Stroma	Extrusion	ALG, COL bioink, FRESH support	CKCs	➢ Similar structure to native cornea architecture encapsulated stromal cells under COL-based bioink ➢ Stromal cells showed high cell viability	[33]
	Laser	Matrigel, COL bioink	LECs	➢ Printed membranes showed maintaining good cell viability and positive labeling for COL ➢ Suffered from lack of sufficient transparency	[112]
	Extrusion	COL, dC	CKCs	➢ The differentiation potential of hTMSCs just observed with the Dc-COL membrane ➢ Proper mechanical flexibility ➢ Improved transparency properties of COL-Dc in comparison with COL scaffold	[121]
	Droplet	COL, AG	CKCs	➢ Keeping native keratocyte phenotype as well as proper elongation ➢ Similar transparency in comparison with the stromal layer	[113]
	Extrusion	GelMa, reinforced with PEG, PCL Fibers	LSSCs	➢ Providing an ideal environment for the preservation of keratocyte phenotype	[120]
	Extrusion	GelMa	CKCs	➢ Keratocytes showed keeping of the phenotype ➢ Similar transparency with the native cornea ➢ Adequate mechanical stability	[118]
	Extrusion	dC	CKCs	➢ The optimal nozzle diameter for bioprinting cornea-like aligned collagen fibrils ➢ The optimal nozzle diameter to preserve the morphology and phenotype of keratocytes ➢ Excellent transparency ➢ Keeping the keratocyte phenotype	[122]
Endothelium	Extrusion	Gelatin, RGD bioink, amniotic membrane dC support	CECs	➢ Enhanced cell vitality and proliferation	[119]
Epithelium	Extrusion	GelMa bioink, GelMa dome-shaped mold	CEpCs	➢ Extremely transparent curved membrane through geometric fabricated features	[117]
	Extrusion	ALG, GelMa, COL	CEpCs	➢ Good printability and high transparency ➢ Enhanced cell viability and proliferation ➢ Controllable in vitro degradability ➢ Improved epithelial cells markers	[114]

The vitality and proliferation of CKCs are challenging, since this sensitive type of cell simply converts to scar-inducing stromal fibroblasts at non-desirable conditions. Recently, this challenge was overcome with the droplet-based printing technique, since it is more compatible with cells relating to laser-based or extrusion-based printing techniques. Campos et al. [113] printed collagen-type I-agarose bioink corneal construct with CKCs encapsulation to produce a dome-shaped structure in a layer-by-layer manner. The obtained results illustrated cell vitality and proliferation similar to the control sample, and showed positive expression for both lumican and keratocan markers.

From an anatomical standpoint, the stromal layer is difficult to regenerate with current techniques due to its highly complex microstructure, and it being made of randomly oriented collagen lamellae [120]. Additionally, the stromal mechanical strength and light transmittance performance are completely related to the stromal unique structure, which is fabricated from randomly oriented collagen fibrils [2]. Current research based on the fabrication of aligned PCL-PEG fibers with the incorporation of limbal stem cells (LSCs) and 15% GelMA gel to fabricate corneal tissue-engineered construct showed better mechanical strength with improved suture-ability, as well as improvement in expression of CKCs markers. Moreover, the scaffold illustrated high transparency and similar mechanical strength, in comparison with the native cornea [120]. Other studies have also been based on the advancement of bioprinting techniques for CTE by employing decellularized cornea gel or GelMA, showing improvement in CKCs differentiation, and better tensile strength. The printed scaffold improved filopodial elongations and phenotype maintenance similar to CKCs in vivo. The collected results motivated researchers to apply the bioprinting technique for the generation of CTE scaffolds due to their impact on architecture, transparency, mechanical strength, and cell/scaffold interactions [118,121].

After examining the aforementioned studies, it can be challenging to introduce the most promising technique to simulate corneal structure. For instance, enhanced mechanical features are possible with an extrusion-based approach, or improved elastic modulus can be achieved with a droplet-based technique; however, mechanical properties with a laser-based technique are not discussed yet. As reported in recent papers, the corneal stroma has about a 150–700 kPa elastic modulus [7]. Thus, the extrusion-based method would be the best candidate if mechanical properties have been chosen as the most important parameter. However, other properties such as microstructure and geometrical curvature are also prominent, which can be better satisfied using the droplet-based method. Furthermore, bioprinting considerably removes the possibility of human error, and it is superior to casting gels into molds in simulating native curvature of the corneal. Additionally, according to the microstructure, although it is not addressed by recent studies, future studies may be focused on the CKCs migration and orientation by employing smart fiber alignment [123].

6. Nanotechnology in CTE

Nanotechnology can be employed for the development of corneal scaffolds to enhance their physicochemical characteristics [9]. Nano scaffolds offer unique mechanical aspects that promote cell adhesion, proliferation, and differentiation, in addition to facilitating gas and nutrient exchange and waste removal [4]. For instance, dendrimers (~10 nm) are high-contrast polymers with a 3D ionic form, and many end groups [9]. The greatest benefits of dendritic systems are their high density of functional side chains, their capacity to manage network crosslinks, and their scalability across a broad range of sizes. It has been demonstrated that dendrimer-based hydrogels enhance the efficient healing of corneal fractures, without scarring or inflammation. Due to the ability to modulate the crosslinking process and alter the chemistry of crosslinking, it is feasible to influence the duration of resorption, and hence control the wound healing process over a longer period [124]. Thus, dendrimers are labile "smart" nanomaterials that can be employed for wound healing during long recovery periods, with a minimal likelihood of triggering an inflammatory reaction [124,125]. Combining nanotechnology and corneal tissue engineering with natural biomaterials could be a potential approach for reaching the current goal in this category [126]. For instance, to create biomaterials with the appropriate attributes, metal nanoparticles, graphene oxide, carbon nanotubes, and nanoliposomes can be combined. Enhancing the proliferation and functionality of additional stem cells is facilitated by their in situ transformation from sol to gel. Soft nanoparticles can interact with polymer chains and contribute to the hydrogel grid's subsequent crosslinking, hence enhancing its mechanical aspects [126–128]. In a study, Tayebi et al. [129] produced chitosan nanoparticles into chitosan/polycaprolactone membranes yielding a biodegradable, transparent scaffold for cultivating corneal endothelial cells. The chitosan nanoparticles/polycaprolactone, which have the lowest wettability, exhibited transparency comparable to human stromal tissue. The scaffold was non-cytotoxic, and enhanced the proliferation of CECs. The biophysical results revealed that CECs adhered to the scaffold, and formed a dense monolayer. Thus, the created scaffold appears to be appropriate for corneal endothelium regeneration. In another study, Chang et al. [130] developed a novel ophthalmic formulation based on moxifloxacin and dexamethasone-loaded nanostructured lipid carriers mixed with collagen/gelatin/alginate for the treatment of a corneal disorder, particularly bacterial keratitis. The nanoparticles had the following characteristics: average size: 132.1 ± 73.58 nm; zeta potential: 6.27 ± 4.95 mV; entrapment efficiency: $91.5 \pm 3.5\%$; and drug content: $18.1 \pm 1.7\%$. The findings indicated that the nanoparticles could release an effective working concentration in 60 min, and sustain the drug release for a minimum of 12 h. While the samples did not show any toxicities, the substrate enhanced the cell numbers of CEpCs. An animal study confirmed that it inhibits the growth of pathogen microorganisms, and promotes corneal wound healing. The results suggest that the nanoparticle formulation may be an effective anti-inflammatory agent for CTE. The application of nanoparticles, through using the bioprinting technique, permits tailored therapy for more precise and successful disease treatment [100]. Nanotechnology is predicted to be employed in the future to personalize regenerative medicine utilizing human stem cells, and to provide therapeutic tools to maintain a healthy environment for the growth and maturation of stem cells in the damaged area [131]. However, nanotechnology research in CTE is still in its infancy, and only limited in vivo investigations are reported. The behavior of corneal cells in tissue engineering constructions in corneal injury has been widely proven in vitro, but in vivo proof-of-concept investigations are lacking, leaving many concerns unanswered.

7. Conclusions and Future Progress

Recently, different studies on the advancement of CTE replacements are focused on analyzing various biomaterials, and fabrication methods. Although there are several studies on this subject, the prior studies displayed a lack of understanding of the corneal function and its structure; therefore, there is still significant room for progress in mimicking the native corneal properties, such as corneal physicochemical properties. Even though different studies have shown that biomaterials might have similar mechanical, optical, and physical properties to the natural cornea, it is challenging to arrange these biomaterials into the same well-organized structures as the natural cornea. Bioprinted tissue engineering scaffolds with proper orthogonal lamellae architecture can be a crucial step for the successful fabrication of CTE scaffolds. In this regard, the fabrication of a successful CTE scaffold will be mostly dependent on generating necessary features, such as releasing important functional biomolecules to improve corneal components, cells, and nerve regeneration. Furthermore, to produce a tissue-engineered scaffold adjusting mechanical and optical features is crucial as well. Research shows that bioprinted scaffolds equipped with nanotechnology components and nanoscale characteristics can improve the potential of CTE. The ultimate aim of CTE is to improve, preserve, and restore vision by developing nanotechnology-enabled regenerative therapies to heal damaged corneal tissues based on unique patient needs.

Funding: This research received no external funding.

Institutional Review Board Statement: Not applicable.

Informed Consent Statement: Not applicable.

Data Availability Statement: The data presented in this study are available on request from the corresponding author.

Conflicts of Interest: A.O.M.S., S.H.K., S.A.P., A.Z., F.S., N.M., M.J.B. and M.R. declare that they have no conflict of interest. This article does not contain any studies with human or animal subjects performed by any of the authors.

Abbreviations

Corneal keratocyte cells (CKCs), collagen (COL), limbal epithelial cells (LECs), alginate (ALG), agarose (AG), methacrylated gelatin (GelMa), limbal stromal stem cells (LSSCs), decellularized cornea (dC), corneal endothelial cells (CECs), corneal epithelial cells (CEpCs), human turbinate-derived mesenchymal stem cells (hTMSC).

References

1. Lanza, R.; Langer, R.; Vacanti, J.P.; Atala, A. *Principles of Tissue Engineering*; Academic Press: Cambridge, MA, USA, 2020.
2. Salehi, A.O.M.; Keshel, S.H.; Sefat, F.; Tayebi, L. Use of Polycaprolactone in Corneal Tissue Engineering: A Review. *Mater. Today Commun.* **2021**, *27*, 102402. [CrossRef]
3. Goodarzi, H.; Jadidi, K.; Pourmotabed, S.; Sharifi, E.; Aghamollaei, H. Preparation and in vitro characterization of cross-linked collagen–gelatin hydrogel using EDC/NHS for corneal tissue engineering applications. *Int. J. Biol. Macromol.* **2019**, *126*, 620–632. [CrossRef] [PubMed]
4. Yousaf, S.; Keshel, S.H.; Farzi, G.A.; Momeni-Moghadam, M.; Ahmadi, E.D.; Asencio, I.O.; Mozafari, M.; Sefat, F. Scaffolds for corneal tissue engineering. In *Handbook of Tissue Engineering Scaffolds*; Elsevier: Amsterdam, The Netherlands, 2021; Volume 2, pp. 649–672.
5. Chen, Z.; You, J.; Liu, X.; Cooper, S.; Hodge, C.; Sutton, G.; Crook, J.M.; Wallace, G.G. Biomaterials for corneal bioengineering. *Biomed. Mater.* **2018**, *13*, 032002. [CrossRef] [PubMed]
6. Chen, J.; Yan, C.; Zhu, M.; Yao, Q.; Shao, C.; Lu, W.; Wang, J.; Mo, X.; Gu, P.; Fu, Y. Electrospun nanofibrous SF/P (LLA-CL) membrane: A potential substratum for endothelial keratoplasty. *Int. J. Nanomed.* **2015**, *10*, 3337.
7. Wu, Z.; Kong, B.; Liu, R.; Sun, W.; Mi, S. Engineering of corneal tissue through an aligned PVA/collagen composite nanofibrous electrospun scaffold. *Nanomaterials* **2018**, *8*, 124. [CrossRef]
8. Akter, F. *Tissue Engineering Made Easy*; Academic Press: Cambridge, USA, 2016.
9. Ahearne, M.; Fernández-Pérez, J.; Masterton, S.; Madden, P.W.; Bhattacharjee, P. Designing Scaffolds for Corneal Regeneration. *Adv. Funct. Mater.* **2020**, *30*, 1908996. [CrossRef]
10. Koons, G.L.; Diba, M.; Mikos, A.G. Materials design for bone-tissue engineering. *Nat. Rev. Mater.* **2020**, *5*, 584–603. [CrossRef]
11. Guérin, L.-P.; Le-Bel, G.; Desjardins, P.; Couture, C.; Gillard, E.; Boisselier, É.; Bazin, R.; Germain, L.; Guérin, S.L. The Human Tissue-Engineered Cornea (hTEC): Recent Progress. *Int. J. Mol. Sci.* **2021**, *22*, 1291. [CrossRef]
12. Nosrati, H.; Abpeikar, Z.; Mahmoudian, Z.G.; Zafari, M.; Majidi, J.; Alizadeh, A.; Moradi, L.; Asadpour, S. Corneal epithelium tissue engineering: Recent advances in regeneration and replacement of the corneal surface. *Regen. Med.* **2020**, *15*, 2029–2044. [CrossRef]
13. Salehi, A.O.M.; Nourbakhsh, M.S.; Rafienia, M.; Baradaran-Rafii, A.; Keshel, S.H. Corneal stromal regeneration by hybrid oriented poly (ε-caprolactone)/lyophilized silk fibroin electrospun scaffold. *Int. J. Biol. Macromol.* **2020**, *161*, 377–388. [CrossRef]
14. Salehi, A.O.M.; Keshel, S.H.; Rafienia, M.; Nourbakhsh, M.S.; Baradaran-Rafii, A. Promoting keratocyte stem like cell proliferation and differentiation by aligned polycaprolactone-silk fibroin fibers containing Aloe vera. *Biomater. Adv.* **2022**, *137*, 212840. [CrossRef]
15. Janmohammadi, M.; Nazemi, Z.; Salehi, A.O.M.; Seyfoori, A.; John, J.V.; Nourbakhsh, M.S.; Akbari, M. Cellulose-based composite scaffolds for bone tissue engineering and localized drug delivery. *Bioact. Mater.* **2023**, *20*, 137–163. [CrossRef] [PubMed]
16. Movahedi, M.; Salehi, A.O.M.; Moezi, D.; Yarahmadian, R. In vitro and in vivo study of aspirin loaded, electrospun polycaprolactone–maltodextrin membrane for enhanced skin tissue regeneration. *Int. J. Polym. Mater. Polym. Biomater.* **2021**, *71*, 1334–1344. [CrossRef]
17. Movahedi, M.; Salehi, A.O.M.; Etemad, S. Casein release and characterization of electrospun nanofibres for cartilage tissue engineering. *Bull. Mater. Sci.* **2022**, *45*, 76. [CrossRef]
18. Biazar, E.; Baradaran-Rafii, A.; Heidari-Keshel, S.; Tavakolifard, S. Oriented nanofibrous silk as a natural scaffold for ocular epithelial regeneration. *J. Biomater. Sci. Polym. Ed.* **2015**, *26*, 1139–1151. [CrossRef] [PubMed]
19. Choi, J.H.; Jeng, B.H. Indications for keratoplasty in management of corneal ectasia. *Curr. Opin. Ophthalmol.* **2022**, *33*, 318–323. [CrossRef]
20. El Zarif, M.; Alió, J.L.; Alió del Barrio, J.L.; De Miguel, M.P.; Abdul Jawad, K.; Makdissy, N. Corneal stromal regeneration: A review of human clinical studies in keratoconus treatment. *Front. Med.* **2021**, *8*, 650724. [CrossRef]
21. Kumar, A.; Yun, H.; Funderburgh, M.L.; Du, Y. Regenerative therapy for the Cornea. *Prog. Retin. Eye Res.* **2021**, *87*, 101011. [CrossRef]
22. Ghezzi, C.E.; Rnjak-Kovacina, J.; Kaplan, D.L. Corneal tissue engineering: Recent advances and future perspectives. *Tissue Eng. Part B Rev.* **2015**, *21*, 278–287. [CrossRef]
23. Kong, B.; Mi, S. Electrospun scaffolds for corneal tissue engineering: A review. *Materials* **2016**, *9*, 614. [CrossRef]
24. Wicklein, V.J.; Singer, B.B.; Scheibel, T.; Salehi, S. Nanoengineered Biomaterials for Corneal Regeneration. In *Nanoengineered Biomaterials for Regenerative Medicine*; Elsevier: Amsterdam, The Netherlands, 2021; pp. 379–415.

25. Nosrati, H.; Alizadeh, Z.; Nosrati, A.; Ashrafi-Dehkordi, K.; Banitalebi-Dehkordi, M.; Sanami, S.; Khodaei, M. Stem cell-based therapeutic strategies for corneal epithelium regeneration. *Tissue Cell* **2021**, *68*, 101470. [CrossRef] [PubMed]
26. Bigham, A.; Salehi, A.O.M.; Rafienia, M.; Salamat, M.R.; Rahmati, S.; Raucci, M.G.; Ambrosio, L. Zn-substituted Mg2SiO4 nanoparticles-incorporated PCL-silk fibroin composite scaffold: A multifunctional platform towards bone tissue regeneration. *Mater. Sci. Eng. C* **2021**, *127*, 112242. [CrossRef] [PubMed]
27. Ulag, S.; Uysal, E.; Bedir, T.; Sengor, M.; Ekren, N.; Ustundag, C.B.; Midha, S.; Kalaskar, D.M.; Gunduz, O. Recent developments and characterization techniques in 3D printing of corneal stroma tissue. *Polym. Adv. Technol.* **2021**, *32*, 3287–3296. [CrossRef]
28. Mahdavi, S.S.; Abdekhodaie, M.J.; Mashayekhan, S.; Baradaran-Rafii, A.; Djalilian, A.R. Bioengineering approaches for corneal regenerative medicine. *Tissue Eng. Regen. Med.* **2020**, *17*, 567–593. [CrossRef] [PubMed]
29. Reddy, R.; Reddy, N. Biomimetic approaches for tissue engineering. *J. Biomater. Sci. Polym. Ed.* **2021**, *29*, 1667–1685. [CrossRef] [PubMed]
30. Sanie-Jahromi, F.; Eghtedari, M.; Mirzaei, E.; Jalalpour, M.H.; Asvar, Z.; Nejabat, M.; Javidi-Azad, F. Propagation of limbal stem cells on polycaprolactone and polycaprolactone/gelatin fibrous scaffolds and transplantation in animal model. *BioImpacts BI* **2020**, *10*, 45. [CrossRef] [PubMed]
31. Mahdavi, S.S.; Abdekhodaie, M.J.; Kumar, H.; Mashayekhan, S.; Baradaran-Rafii, A.; Kim, K. Stereolithography 3D bioprinting method for fabrication of human corneal stroma equivalent. *Ann. Biomed. Eng.* **2020**, *48*, 1955–1970. [CrossRef] [PubMed]
32. Miotto, M.; Gouveia, R.M.; Ionescu, A.M.; Figueiredo, F.; Hamley, I.W.; Connon, C.J. 4D corneal tissue engineering: Achieving time-dependent tissue self-Curvature through localized control of cell actuators. *Adv. Funct. Mater.* **2021**, *29*, 1807334. [CrossRef]
33. Isaacson, A.; Swioklo, S.; Connon, C.J. 3D bioprinting of a corneal stroma equivalent. *Exp. Eye Res.* **2021**, *173*, 188–193. [CrossRef]
34. Murphy, S.V.; Atala, A. 3D bioprinting of tissues and organs. *Nat. Biotechnol.* **2014**, *32*, 773–785. [CrossRef]
35. Kang, H.-W.; Lee, S.J.; Ko, I.K.; Kengla, C.; Yoo, J.J.; Atala, A. A 3D bioprinting system to produce human-scale tissue constructs with structural integrity. *Nat. Biotechnol.* **2016**, *34*, 312–319. [CrossRef] [PubMed]
36. Jeong, C.G.; Atala, A. 3D printing and biofabrication for load bearing tissue engineering. *Eng. Miner. Load Bear. Tissue* **2015**, *881*, 3–14.
37. Shafiee, A.; Atala, A. Printing technologies for medical applications. *Trends Mol. Med.* **2016**, *22*, 254–265. [CrossRef] [PubMed]
38. Colaco, M.; Igel, D.A.; Atala, A. The potential of 3D printing in urological research and patient care. *Nat. Rev. Urol.* **2021**, *15*, 213. [CrossRef] [PubMed]
39. Gillispie, G.J.; Han, A.; Uzun-Per, M.; Fisher, J.; Mikos, A.G.; Niazi, M.K.K.; Yoo, J.J.; Lee, S.J.; Atala, A. The Influence of Printing Parameters and Cell Density on Bioink Printing Outcomes. *Tissue Eng. Part A* **2020**, *26*, 1349–1358. [CrossRef]
40. Akter, F. Principles of Tissue Engineering. In *Tissue Engineering Made Easy*; Elsevier: Amsterdam, The Netherlands, 2016; pp. 3–16.
41. Sridhar, M.S. Anatomy of the cornea and ocular surface. *Ind. J. Ophthalmol.* **2021**, *66*, 190. [CrossRef]
42. Baradaran-Rafii, A.; Biazar, E.; Heidari-Keshel, S. Cellular response of limbal stem cells on polycaprolactone nanofibrous scaffolds for ocular epithelial regeneration. *Curr. Eye Res.* **2016**, *41*, 326–333. [CrossRef]
43. Palchesko, R.N.; Carrasquilla, S.D.; Feinberg, A.W. Natural biomaterials for corneal tissue engineering, repair, and regeneration. *Adv. Healthc. Mater.* **2021**, *7*, 1701434. [CrossRef]
44. Islam, M.M.; Sharifi, R.; Gonzalez-Andrades, M. Corneal Tissue Engineering. In *Corneal Regeneration*; Springer: Berlin/Heidelberg, Germany, 2019; pp. 23–37.
45. Stepp, M.A.; Tadvalkar, G.; Hakh, R.; Pal-Ghosh, S. Corneal epithelial cells function as surrogate Schwann cells for their sensory nerves. *Glia* **2017**, *65*, 851–863. [CrossRef]
46. Campbell, J.D.; Ahmad, S.; Agrawal, A.; Bienek, C.; Atkinson, A.; Mcgowan, N.W.; Kaye, S.; Mantry, S.; Ramaesh, K.; Glover, A. Allogeneic Ex Vivo Expanded Corneal Epithelial Stem Cell Transplantation: A Randomized Controlled Clinical Trial. *Stem Cells Transl. Med.* **2021**, *8*, 323–331. [CrossRef]
47. Arabpour, Z.; Baradaran-Rafii, A.; Bakhshaiesh, N.L.; Ai, J.; Ebrahimi-Barough, S.; Esmaeili Malekabadi, H.; Nazeri, N.; Vaez, A.; Salehi, M.; Sefat, F. Design and characterization of biodegradable multi layered electrospun nanofibers for corneal tissue engineering applications. *J. Biomed. Mater. Res. Part A* **2021**, *107*, 2340–2349. [CrossRef] [PubMed]
48. Hancox, Z.; Keshel, S.H.; Yousaf, S.; Saeinasab, M.; Shahbazi, M.-A.; Sefat, F. The progress in corneal translational medicine. *Biomater. Sci.* **2020**, *8*, 6469–6504. [CrossRef] [PubMed]
49. Kianersi, S.; Solouk, A.; Saber-Samandari, S.; Keshel, S.H.; Pasbakhsh, P. Alginate nanoparticles as ocular drug delivery carriers. *J. Drug Deliv. Sci. Technol.* **2021**, *66*, 102889. [CrossRef]
50. Fernández-Pérez, J.; Kador, K.E.; Lynch, A.P.; Ahearne, M. Characterization of extracellular matrix modified poly (ε-caprolactone) electrospun scaffolds with differing fiber orientations for corneal stroma regeneration. *Mater. Sci. Eng. C* **2020**, *108*, 110415. [CrossRef]
51. Kostenko, A.; Swioklo, S.; Connon, C.J. Alginate in corneal tissue engineering. *Biomed. Mater.* **2022**, *17*, 022004. [CrossRef]
52. Delaey, J.; De Vos, L.; Koppen, C.; Dubruel, P.; Van Vlierberghe, S.; Van den Bogerd, B. Tissue engineered scaffolds for corneal endothelial regeneration: A material's perspective. *Biomater. Sci.* **2022**, *10*, 2440–2461. [CrossRef]
53. Bosch, B.M.; Bosch-Rue, E.; Perpiñan-Blasco, M.; Perez, R.A. Design of functional biomaterials as substrates for corneal endothelium tissue engineering. *Regen. Biomater.* **2022**, *9*, rbac052. [CrossRef]
54. Takahashi, H. Corneal endothelium and phacoemulsification. *Cornea* **2016**, *35*, S3–S7. [CrossRef]

55. Eghrari, A.O.; Riazuddin, S.A.; Gottsch, J.D. Overview of the cornea: Structure, function, and development. In *Progress in Molecular Biology and Translational Science*; Elsevier: Amsterdam, The Netherlands, 2015; pp. 7–23.
56. El Zarif, M.; del Barrio, J.L.A.; Arnalich-Montiel, F.; De Miguel, M.P.; Makdissy, N.; Alió, J.L. Corneal stroma regeneration: A new approach for the treatment of cornea disease. *Asia-Pac. J. Ophthalmol.* **2020**, *9*, 571–579. [CrossRef]
57. Zhao, J.; Tian, M.; Li, Y.; Su, W.; Fan, T. Construction of tissue-engineered human corneal endothelium for corneal endothelial regeneration using a crosslinked amniotic membrane scaffold. *Acta Biomater.* **2022**, *147*, 185–197. [CrossRef]
58. Kim, D.K.; Sim, B.R.; Khang, G. Nature-derived aloe vera gel blended silk fibroin film scaffolds for cornea endothelial cell regeneration and transplantation. *ACS Appl. Mater. Interfaces* **2016**, *8*, 15160–15168. [CrossRef] [PubMed]
59. Sang, S.; Yan, Y.; Shen, Z.; Cao, Y.; Duan, Q.; He, M.; Zhang, Q. Photo-crosslinked hydrogels for tissue engineering of corneal epithelium. *Exp. Eye Res.* **2022**, *218*, 109027. [CrossRef] [PubMed]
60. Gandhi, S.; Jain, S. The Anatomy and Physiology of Cornea. In *Keratoprostheses and Artificial Corneas*; Springer: Berlin/Heidelberg, Germany, 2015; pp. 19–25.
61. Binte, M.; Yusoff, N.Z.; Riau, A.K.; Yam, G.H.; Binte Halim, N.S.H.; Mehta, J.S. Isolation and propagation of human corneal stromal keratocytes for tissue engineering and cell therapy. *Cells* **2022**, *11*, 178. [CrossRef]
62. Lagali, N. Corneal stromal regeneration: Current status and future therapeutic potential. *Curr. Eye Res.* **2020**, *45*, 278–290. [CrossRef]
63. Matthyssen, S.; Van den Bogerd, B.; Dhubhghaill, S.N.; Koppen, C.; Zakaria, N. Corneal regeneration: A review of stromal replacements. *Acta Biomater.* **2021**, *69*, 31–41. [CrossRef]
64. Del Barrio, J.L.A.; Arnalich-Montiel, F.; De Miguel, M.P.; El Zarif, M.; Alió, J.L. Corneal stroma regeneration: Preclinical studies. *Exp. Eye Res.* **2021**, *202*, 108314. [CrossRef]
65. Wang, Y.; Xu, L.; Zhao, J.; Liang, J.; Zhang, Z.; Li, Q.; Zhang, J.; Wan, P.; Wu, Z. Reconstructing auto tissue engineering lamellar cornea with aspartic acid modified acellular porcine corneal stroma and preconditioned limbal stem cell for corneal regeneration. *Biomaterials* **2022**, *289*, 121745. [CrossRef] [PubMed]
66. Formisano, N.; van der Putten, C.; Grant, R.; Sahin, G.; Truckenmüller, R.K.; Bouten, C.V.; Kurniawan, N.A.; Giselbrecht, S. Mechanical Properties of Bioengineered Corneal Stroma. *Adv. Healthc. Mater.* **2021**, *10*, 2100972. [CrossRef] [PubMed]
67. Khalili, M.; Asadi, M.; Kahroba, H.; Soleyman, M.R.; Andre, H.; Alizadeh, E. Corneal endothelium tissue engineering: An evolution of signaling molecules, cells, and scaffolds toward 3D bioprinting and cell sheets. *J. Cell. Physiol.* **2021**, *236*, 3275–3303. [CrossRef] [PubMed]
68. Klyce, S.D. 12. Endothelial pump and barrier function. *Exp. Eye Res.* **2020**, *198*, 108068. [CrossRef] [PubMed]
69. Atalay, E.; Özalp, O.; Yıldırım, N. Advances in the diagnosis and treatment of keratoconus. *Ther. Adv. Ophthalmol.* **2021**, *13*, 25158414211012796. [CrossRef] [PubMed]
70. Tafti, M.F.; Aghamollaei, H.; Moghaddam, M.M.; Jadidi, K.; Alio, J.L.; Faghihi, S. Emerging tissue engineering strategies for the corneal regeneration. *J. Tissue Eng. Regen. Med.* **2022**, *16*, 683–706. [CrossRef] [PubMed]
71. Niazi, S.; Niknejad, H.; Niazi, F.; Doroodgar, F.; Sanginabadi, A. Tissue-engineered recombinant human collagen-based corneal substitutes in end-stage keratoconus. *Investig. Ophthalmol. Vis. Sci.* **2021**, *60*, 5105.
72. Sharif, R.; Priyadarsini, S.; Rowsey, T.G.; Ma, J.-X.; Karamichos, D. Corneal tissue engineering: An in vitro model of the stromal-nerve interactions of the human cornea. *JoVE J. Vis. Exp.* **2021**, *131*, e56308. [CrossRef] [PubMed]
73. Bhattacharjee, P.; Ahearne, M. Significance of crosslinking approaches in the development of next generation hydrogels for corneal tissue engineering. *Pharmaceutics* **2021**, *13*, 319. [CrossRef]
74. Qin, J.; Yin, N. Tobramycin Collagen Fast Dissolving Ocular Films for Corneal Tissue Engineering of Keratoconus. *J. Biomater. Tissue Eng.* **2021**, *9*, 804–809. [CrossRef]
75. Alió del Barrio, J.L.; Alió, J.L. Cellular therapy of the corneal stroma: A new type of corneal surgery for keratoconus and corneal dystrophies. *Eye Vis.* **2021**, *5*, 1–10. [CrossRef]
76. Jadidi, K.; Mosavi, S.A.; Nejat, F.; Aghamolaei, H.; Pirhadi, S. Innovative intra-corneal ring-supported graft surgery for treatment of keratoconus and cornea regeneration: Surgical technique and case report. *Ind. J. Ophthalmol.* **2022**, *70*, 3412–3415.
77. Teo, A.W.J.; Mansoor, H.; Sim, N.; Lin, M.T.-Y.; Liu, Y.-C. In Vivo Confocal Microscopy Evaluation in Patients with Keratoconus. *J. Clin. Med.* **2022**, *11*, 393. [CrossRef]
78. Veernala, I.; Jaffet, J.; Fried, J.; Mertsch, S.; Schrader, S.; Basu, S.; Vemuganti, G.; Singh, V. Lacrimal gland regeneration: The unmet challenges and promise for dry eye therapy. *Ocul. Surf.* **2022**, *25*, 129–141. [CrossRef]
79. Gong, Q.; Zhang, S.; Jiang, L.; Lin, M.; Xu, Z.; Yu, Y.; Wang, Q.; Lu, F.; Hu, L. The effect of nerve growth factor on corneal nerve regeneration and dry eye after LASIK. *Exp. Eye Res.* **2021**, *203*, 108428. [CrossRef] [PubMed]
80. Lu, Q.; Al-Sheikh, O.; Elisseeff, J.H.; Grant, M.P. Biomaterials and tissue engineering strategies for conjunctival reconstruction and dry eye treatment. *Middle East Afr. J. Ophthalmol.* **2015**, *22*, 428. [PubMed]
81. Hill, L.J.; Moakes, R.J.; Vareechon, C.; Butt, G.; Ng, A.; Brock, K.; Chouhan, G.; Vincent, R.C.; Abbondante, S.; Williams, R.L. Sustained release of decorin to the surface of the eye enables scarless corneal regeneration. *NPJ Regen. Med.* **2021**, *3*, 1–12. [CrossRef] [PubMed]
82. Tabbara, K.F.; El-Asrar, A.M.A.; Khairallah, M. *Ocular Infections*; Springer: Berlin/Heidelberg, Germany, 2014.
83. Xenoulis, P.G.; Steiner, J.M. Lipid metabolism and hyperlipidemia in dogs. *Vet. J.* **2010**, *183*, 12–21. [CrossRef] [PubMed]

84. Huang, T.; Wang, Y.; Zhang, H.; Gao, N.; Hu, A. Limbal allografting from living-related donors to treat partial limbal deficiency secondary to ocular chemical burns. *Arch. Ophthalmol.* **2011**, *129*, 1267–1273. [CrossRef] [PubMed]
85. Wipperman, J.; Dorsch, J.N. Evaluation and management of corneal abrasions. *Am. Fam. Physician* **2013**, *87*, 114–120. [PubMed]
86. Shahid, S.M.; Harrison, N. Corneal abrasion: Assessment and management. *InnovAiT* **2013**, *6*, 551–554. [CrossRef]
87. Wang, Y.; Wang, J.; Ji, Z.; Yan, W.; Zhao, H.; Huang, W.; Liu, H. Application of Bioprinting in Ophthalmology. *Int. J. Bioprinting* **2022**, *8*, 552. [CrossRef]
88. Song, Y.; Hua, S.; Sayyar, S.; Chen, Z.; Chung, J.; Liu, X.; Yue, Z.; Angus, C.; Filippi, B.; Beirne, S. Corneal bioprinting using a high concentration pure collagen I transparent bioink. *Bioprinting* **2022**, *28*, e00235. [CrossRef]
89. Stafiej, P.; Küng, F.; Thieme, D.; Czugala, M.; Kruse, F.E.; Schubert, D.W.; Fuchsluger, T.A. Adhesion and metabolic activity of human corneal cells on PCL based nanofiber matrices. *Mater. Sci. Eng. C* **2017**, *71*, 764–770. [CrossRef]
90. Zhang, M.; Yang, F.; Han, D.; Zhang, S.Y.; Dong, Y.; Li, X.; Ling, L.; Deng, Z.; Cao, X.; Tian, J. 3D Bioprinting of Corneal Decellularized Extracellular Matrix (CECM): GelMA Composite Hydrogel for Corneal Stroma Engineering. 2022. Available online: https://ssrn.com/abstract=4246348 (accessed on 20 October 2022).
91. Kim, J.I.; Kim, J.Y.; Park, C.H. Fabrication of transparent hemispherical 3D nanofibrous scaffolds with radially aligned patterns via a novel electrospinning method. *Sci. Rep.* **2021**, *8*, 3424. [CrossRef] [PubMed]
92. Chameettachal, S.; Pati, F. *Preparation and Characterization of Decellularized Corneal Matrix Hydrogel for Different Clinical Indications and 3D Bioprinting Applications*; RAIITH: Kirkcaldy, UK, 2022.
93. Lindsay, C.D.; Roth, J.G.; LeSavage, B.L.; Heilshorn, S.C. Bioprinting of stem cell expansion lattices. *Acta Biomater.* **2021**, *95*, 225–235. [CrossRef] [PubMed]
94. Phamduy, T.B.; Sweat, R.S.; Azimi, M.S.; Burow, M.E.; Murfee, W.L.; Chrisey, D.B. Printing cancer cells into intact microvascular networks: A model for investigating cancer cell dynamics during angiogenesis. *Integr. Biol.* **2015**, *7*, 1068–1078. [CrossRef] [PubMed]
95. Betsch, M.; Cristian, C.; Lin, Y.Y.; Blaeser, A.; Schöneberg, J.; Vogt, M.; Buhl, E.M.; Fischer, H.; Duarte Campos, D.F. Incorporating 4D into bioprinting: Real-time magnetically directed collagen fiber alignment for generating complex multilayered tissues. *Adv. Healthc. Mater.* **2021**, *7*, 1800894. [CrossRef] [PubMed]
96. Leberfinger, A.N.; Dinda, S.; Wu, Y.; Koduru, S.V.; Ozbolat, V.; Ravnic, D.J.; Ozbolat, I.T. Bioprinting functional tissues. *Acta Biomater.* **2021**, *95*, 32–49. [CrossRef] [PubMed]
97. Atala, A. *Introduction: 3D Printing for Biomaterials*; ACS Publications: Washington, DC, USA, 2020.
98. Murphy, S.V.; De Coppi, P.; Atala, A. Opportunities and challenges of translational 3D bioprinting. *Nat. Biomed. Eng.* **2020**, *4*, 370–380. [CrossRef] [PubMed]
99. Smith, B.T.; Bittner, S.M.; Watson, E.; Smoak, M.M.; Diaz-Gomez, L.; Molina, E.R.; Kim, Y.S.; Hudgins, C.D.; Melchiorri, A.J.; Scott, D.W. Multimaterial dual gradient three-dimensional printing for osteogenic differentiation and spatial segregation. *Tissue Eng. Part A* **2020**, *26*, 239–252. [CrossRef]
100. Zhang, B.; Xue, Q.; Li, J.; Ma, L.; Yao, Y.; Ye, H.; Cui, Z.; Yang, H. 3D bioprinting for artificial cornea: Challenges and perspectives. *Med. Eng. Phys.* **2021**, *71*, 68–78. [CrossRef]
101. Dubbin, K.; Tabet, A.; Heilshorn, S.C. Quantitative criteria to benchmark new and existing bio-inks for cell compatibility. *Biofabrication* **2017**, *9*, 044102. [CrossRef]
102. Cidonio, G.; Glinka, M.; Dawson, J.; Oreffo, R. The cell in the ink: Improving biofabrication by printing stem cells for skeletal regenerative medicine. *Biomaterials* **2021**, *209*, 10–24. [CrossRef]
103. Liu, W.; Heinrich, M.A.; Zhou, Y.; Akpek, A.; Hu, N.; Liu, X.; Guan, X.; Zhong, Z.; Jin, X.; Khademhosseini, A. Extrusion bioprinting of shear-thinning gelatin methacryloyl bioinks. *Adv. Healthc. Mater.* **2017**, *6*, 1601451. [CrossRef] [PubMed]
104. Foster, A.A.; Marquardt, L.M.; Heilshorn, S.C. The diverse roles of hydrogel mechanics in injectable stem cell transplantation. *Curr. Opin. Chem. Eng.* **2017**, *15*, 15–23. [CrossRef] [PubMed]
105. Bernal, P.N.; Delrot, P.; Loterie, D.; Li, Y.; Malda, J.; Moser, C.; Levato, R. Volumetric bioprinting of complex living-tissue constructs within seconds. *Adv. Mater.* **2021**, *31*, 1904209. [CrossRef] [PubMed]
106. Grigoryan, B.; Paulsen, S.J.; Corbett, D.C.; Sazer, D.W.; Fortin, C.L.; Zaita, A.J.; Greenfield, P.T.; Calafat, N.J.; Gounley, J.P.; Ta, A.H. Multivascular networks and functional intravascular topologies within biocompatible hydrogels. *Science* **2021**, *364*, 458–464. [CrossRef] [PubMed]
107. Skylar-Scott, M.A.; Uzel, S.G.; Nam, L.L.; Ahrens, J.H.; Truby, R.L.; Damaraju, S.; Lewis, J.A. Biomanufacturing of organ-specific tissues with high cellular density and embedded vascular channels. *Sci. Adv.* **2021**, *5*, eaaw2459. [CrossRef] [PubMed]
108. Lee, A.; Hudson, A.; Shiwarski, D.; Tashman, J.; Hinton, T.; Yerneni, S.; Bliley, J.; Campbell, P.; Feinberg, A. 3D bioprinting of collagen to rebuild components of the human heart. *Science* **2021**, *365*, 482–487. [CrossRef] [PubMed]
109. Meek, K.M.; Knupp, C. Corneal structure and transparency. *Prog. Retin. Eye Res.* **2015**, *49*, 1–16. [CrossRef]
110. Mohan, R.R.; Kempuraj, D.; D'Souza, S.; Ghosh, A. Corneal stromal repair and regeneration. *Prog. Retin. Eye Res.* **2022**, *91*, 101090. [CrossRef]
111. Gouveia, R.M.; Lepert, G.; Gupta, S.; Mohan, R.R.; Paterson, C.; Connon, C.J. Assessment of corneal substrate biomechanics and its effect on epithelial stem cell maintenance and differentiation. *Nat. Commun.* **2021**, *10*, 1496. [CrossRef]
112. Sorkio, A.; Koch, L.; Koivusalo, L.; Deiwick, A.; Miettinen, S.; Chichkov, B.; Skottman, H. Human stem cell based corneal tissue mimicking structures using laser-assisted 3D bioprinting and functional bioinks. *Biomaterials* **2021**, *171*, 57–71. [CrossRef]

113. Duarte Campos, D.F.; Rohde, M.; Ross, M.; Anvari, P.; Blaeser, A.; Vogt, M.; Panfil, C.; Yam, G.H.F.; Mehta, J.S.; Fischer, H. Corneal bioprinting utilizing collagen-based bioinks and primary human keratocytes. *J. Biomed. Mater. Res. Part A* **2021**, *107*, 1945–1953. [CrossRef] [PubMed]
114. Wu, Z.; Su, X.; Xu, Y.; Kong, B.; Sun, W.; Mi, S. Bioprinting three-dimensional cell-laden tissue constructs with controllable degradation. *Sci. Rep.* **2016**, *6*, 24474. [CrossRef] [PubMed]
115. Kutlehria, S.; Dinh, T.C.; Bagde, A.; Patel, N.; Gebeyehu, A.; Singh, M. High-throughput 3D bioprinting of corneal stromal equivalents. *J. Biomed. Mater. Res. Part B Appl. Biomater.* **2020**, *108*, 2981–2994. [CrossRef] [PubMed]
116. Osidak, E.O.; Kozhukhov, V.I.; Osidak, M.S.; Domogatsky, S.P. Collagen as Bioink for Bioprinting: A Comprehensive Review. *Int. J. Bioprinting* **2020**, *6*, 270.
117. Zhang, B.; Xue, Q.; Hu, H.-Y.; Yu, M.-F.; Gao, L.; Luo, Y.-C.; Li, Y.; Li, J.-T.; Ma, L.; Yao, Y.-F. Integrated 3D bioprinting-based geometry-control strategy for fabricating corneal substitutes. *J. Zhejiang Univ. Sci. B* **2021**, *20*, 945–959. [CrossRef]
118. Bektas, C.K.; Hasirci, V. Cell loaded 3D bioprinted GelMA hydrogels for corneal stroma engineering. *Biomater. Sci.* **2020**, *8*, 438–449. [CrossRef]
119. Kim, K.W.; Lee, S.J.; Park, S.H.; Kim, J.C. Ex vivo functionality of 3D bioprinted corneal endothelium engineered with ribonuclease 5-overexpressing human corneal endothelial cells. *Adv. Healthc. Mater.* **2021**, *7*, 1800398. [CrossRef]
120. Kong, B.; Chen, Y.; Liu, R.; Liu, X.; Liu, C.; Shao, Z.; Xiong, L.; Liu, X.; Sun, W.; Mi, S. Fiber reinforced GelMA hydrogel to induce the regeneration of corneal stroma. *Nat. Commun.* **2020**, *11*, 1435. [CrossRef]
121. Kim, H.; Park, M.-N.; Kim, J.; Jang, J.; Kim, H.-K.; Cho, D.-W. Characterization of cornea-specific bioink: High transparency, improved in vivo safety. *J. Tissue Eng.* **2021**, *10*, 2041731418823382. [CrossRef]
122. Kim, H.; Jang, J.; Park, J.; Lee, K.-P.; Lee, S.; Lee, D.-M.; Kim, K.H.; Kim, H.K.; Cho, D.-W. Shear-induced alignment of collagen fibrils using 3D cell printing for corneal stroma tissue engineering. *Biofabrication* **2021**, *11*, 035017. [CrossRef]
123. Gouveia, R.M.; Koudouna, E.; Jester, J.; Figueiredo, F.; Connon, C.J. Template curvature influences cell alignment to create improved human corneal tissue equivalents. *Adv. Biosyst.* **2017**, *1*, 1700135. [CrossRef] [PubMed]
124. Trujillo-de Santiago, G.; Sharifi, R.; Yue, K.; Sani, E.S.; Kashaf, S.S.; Alvarez, M.M.; Leijten, J.; Khademhosseini, A.; Dana, R.; Annabi, N. Ocular adhesives: Design, chemistry, crosslinking mechanisms, and applications. *Biomaterials* **2021**, *197*, 345–367. [CrossRef] [PubMed]
125. Koppa Raghu, P.; Bansal, K.K.; Thakor, P.; Bhavana, V.; Madan, J.; Rosenholm, J.M.; Mehra, N.K. Evolution of nanotechnology in delivering drugs to eyes, skin, and wounds via topical route. *Pharmaceuticals* **2020**, *13*, 167. [CrossRef] [PubMed]
126. Patra, H.K.; Azharuddin, M.; Islam, M.M.; Papapavlou, G.; Deb, S.; Osterrieth, J.; Zhu, G.H.; Romu, T.; Dhara, A.K.; Jafari, M.J.; et al. Rational Nanotoolbox with Theranostic Potential for Medicated Pro-Regenerative Corneal Implants. *Adv. Funct. Mater.* **2021**, *29*, 1903760. [CrossRef]
127. Krishna, L.; Dhamodaran, K.; Jayadev, C.; Chatterjee, K.; Shetty, R.; Khora, S.S.; Das, D. Nanostructured scaffold as a determinant of stem cell fate. *Stem Cell Res. Ther.* **2016**, *7*, 188. [CrossRef]
128. Motealleh, A.; Kehr, N.S. Nanocomposite hydrogels and their applications in tissue engineering. *Adv. Healthc. Mater.* **2017**, *6*, 1600938. [CrossRef] [PubMed]
129. Tayebi, T.; Baradaran-Rafii, A.; Hajifathali, A.; Rahimpour, A.; Zali, H.; Shaabani, A.; Niknejad, H. Biofabrication of chitosan/chitosan nanoparticles/polycaprolactone transparent membrane for corneal endothelial tissue engineering. *Sci. Rep.* **2021**, *11*, 7060. [CrossRef]
130. Chang, M.-C.; Kuo, Y.-J.; Hung, K.-H.; Peng, C.-L.; Chen, K.-Y.; Yeh, L.-K. Liposomal dexamethasone–moxifloxacin nanoparticle combinations with collagen/gelatin/alginate hydrogel for corneal infection treatment and wound healing. *Biomed. Mater.* **2020**, *15*, 055022. [CrossRef]
131. Anitua, E.; Muruzabal, F.J.; De La Fuente, M.; Merayo, J.; Durán, J.; Orive, G. Plasma rich in growth factors for the treatment of ocular surface diseases. *Curr. Eye Res.* **2016**, *41*, 875–882. [CrossRef]

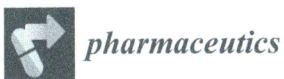

Review

Fluorescent Nanosystems for Drug Tracking and Theranostics: Recent Applications in the Ocular Field

Elide Zingale [1,†], Alessia Romeo [1,†], Salvatore Rizzo [1], Cinzia Cimino [1], Angela Bonaccorso [1,2], Claudia Carbone [1,2], Teresa Musumeci [1,2] and Rosario Pignatello [1,2,*]

1. Department of Pharmaceutical and Health Sciences, University of Catania, 95124 Catania, Italy; elide.zingale@gmail.com (E.Z.); alessia.romeo@phd.unict.it (A.R.); salvo_rizzo@outlook.it (S.R.); cinzia.cimino@phd.unict.it (C.C.); angela.bonaccorso@unict.it (A.B.); ccarbone@unict.it (C.C.); teresa.musumeci@unict.it (T.M.)
2. NANO-i—Research Center for Ocular Nanotechnology, University of Catania, 95124 Catania, Italy
* Correspondence: rosario.pignatello@unict.it
† These authors contributed equally to this work.

Abstract: The greatest challenge associated with topical drug delivery for the treatment of diseases affecting the posterior segment of the eye is to overcome the poor bioavailability of the carried molecules. Nanomedicine offers the possibility to overcome obstacles related to physiological mechanisms and ocular barriers by exploiting different ocular routes. Functionalization of nanosystems by fluorescent probes could be a useful strategy to understand the pathway taken by nanocarriers into the ocular globe and to improve the desired targeting accuracy. The application of fluorescence to decorate nanocarrier surfaces or the encapsulation of fluorophore molecules makes the nanosystems a light probe useful in the landscape of diagnostics and theranostics. In this review, a state of the art on ocular routes of administration is reported, with a focus on pathways undertaken after topical application. Numerous studies are reported in the first section, confirming that the use of fluorescent within nanoparticles is already spread for tracking and biodistribution studies. The first section presents fluorescent molecules used for tracking nanosystems' cellular internalization and permeation of ocular tissues; discussions on the classification of nanosystems according to their nature (lipid-based, polymer-based, metallic-based and protein-based) follows. The following sections are dedicated to diagnostic and theranostic uses, respectively, which represent an innovation in the ocular field obtained by combining dual goals in a single administration system. For its great potential, this application of fluorescent nanoparticles would experience a great development in the near future. Finally, a brief overview is dedicated to the use of fluorescent markers in clinical trials and the market in the ocular field.

Keywords: nanotechnology; fluorescence; ocular delivery; probes; diagnostics; PKs

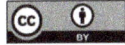

1. Introduction

In recent years, vision-related problems have acquired a greater relevance due to the ageing of the world's population, which leads to an increase in visual problems, such as cataracts, glaucoma, age-related macular degeneration and diabetic retinopathy, occurring more frequently among over-60s [1,2]. Many visual diseases are associated with neurodegenerative disorders [3,4]. Young people over the age of 18 also suffer from visual problems, which increase especially with the growing use of electronic devices [5]. The rising number of people with vision impairment leads to a greater interest in dedicated care and treatments. This situation increases the costs in the global economy destined for the care of these disorders [6]. In addition, ocular therapy is a serious challenge because of the difficulty in targeting a drug to the appropriate ocular tissues.

In this landscape, technological research is actively involved, with the aim of developing innovative systems for targeted drug delivery [7]. The eye is a very complex structure, both anatomically and physiologically, and the treatment of pathologies affecting this organ is therefore not simple [8–10]. This is related to the various aspects that limit the transportation of drugs to the target site: anatomical barriers, physiological processes, mechanisms and metabolic aspects [11,12]. Reaching the target becomes more complicated if therapy is addressed to the posterior segment of the eye [13–16]. For this purpose, the major administration route remains intravitreal injection, which is invasive and produces undesirable effects such as pain and discomfort, inducing patient noncompliance [17,18]. The preferred route of administration would undoubtedly be the topical one, but conventionally it is used to treat diseases of the anterior eye. In fact, it is estimated that only a very small percentage of the drug instilled in the eye surface reaches the anterior chamber (around 5%) and even less in the posterior segment [19–21].

Nanotechnology represents a field of recent interest to overcome these issues. One potential strategy for improving drug delivery to the different eye tissues uses nanocarriers with specific size and surface properties, designed to ensure successful achievement of the drug to the target tissue, as well as the potential for a controlled release of the loaded drug, reducing the frequency of treatment and improving the retention time on the corneal surface [22–24]. Currently, the most widely studied nanosystems are used in the treatment of anterior eye diseases such as cataracts [25], glaucoma [26], dry eye syndrome [27], keratitis [28], conjunctivitis [29] and uveitis [30], but also posterior eye diseases such as retinitis [31], macular degeneration [32], endophthalmitis [33] and ocular tumors [34]. Suitable drug nanocarriers possess a mean size in the nanometric range (around 200 nm) and are classified according to their structural composition and the materials used, which must be biodegradable and biocompatible [35,36]. Many reviews focus on the development of nanosystems designed for ocular delivery, but none on the ophthalmic use of fluorescent nanocarriers. It is not certain that after their administration, the drug effectively reaches the target site; therefore, during its design, tracking studies are necessary to demonstrate its distribution and positioning.

One possible strategy is to follow the nanosystem movements using a fluorescent probe. Fluorescence is a simple and non-invasive way to track the drug through the eye tissues, and it is also widely used in diagnostics to visualize diseased tissues, lesions and pathological markers. The development of personalized medicine and the need for early intervention in the diagnosis and treatment of specific diseases have promoted the birth and development of a new discipline: theranostics [37]. It can be defined as the combination of diagnostics with a specific therapeutic treatment. In vitro diagnostics and prognostics, in vivo molecular imaging, molecular therapeutics, image-guided therapy, biosensors, nanobiosensors and bioelectronics, system biology and translational medicine and point-of-care are some recent application examples.

This review deals with the use of fluorescent probes in the last 5 years applied to nanomedicine in the ophthalmic field. The aim is to illustrate state-of-the-art fluorescent nanosystems divided according to their application: fluorescent nanosystems for biodistribution studies to clarify the best performing nanoparticle design and delivery strategies able to address specific ocular diseases, for diagnostics and finally, for the emerging field of theranostics. PubMed database was used to perform an advanced search. The time frame included the range from January 2017 to February 2022. The keywords used were "fluorescence", "nanoparticles", "ocular" and "delivery", "theranostics", "diagnostics". Articles were limited to "Free full text" and "Full text" articles in the English language published in journals with an impactor factor not less than 4. The same process was repeated on ScienceDirect database. Reference lists of articles were also reviewed for additional citations.

General Aspect of the Human Eye

The eyeball consists of three chambers: anterior, posterior (containing the aqueous humor) and the vitreous chamber (containing the vitreous body). The wall is composed of three tunics [8,38]. The first, called external, is composed anteriorly of the cornea and for the remaining part of the sclera. The middle tunic (uvea) is richly vascularized and pigmented and includes the iris, the ciliary body and the choroid. Finally, the internal or nervous tunic is represented by the retina [39]. The sclera is anteriorly lined by the conjunctiva. Its function is to maintain the shape of the bulb and to provide attachment to the tendons of the striated muscles of the eye [40]. The cornea is a transparent lamina without vessels (necessary conditions for the passage of light). A cross-section of the corneal tissues is shown in Figure 1. Under the cornea, there is the iris, a sphincter of pigmented smooth muscle that regulates pupillary caliber. Trophism in this district is provided by the aqueous humor [41]. The ciliary body is an ocular anatomical structure responsible for both the production of aqueous humor and the control of accommodation. The ciliary body is located immediately posterior to the iris and anterior to the choroid. Posterior to the iris and in front of the vitreous body is where the crystalline is situated, which transmits and focuses light onto the retina. It consists of a single layer of epithelial cells that, during fetal development, migrate laterally toward the equator of the lens where it inverts, elongates, synthesizes large amounts of specific proteins and finally, degrades organelles so as to increase transparency [20]. From a physiological perspective, there are two reflexes involved in vision: lens accommodation (regulates convexity) and pupillary reflex (regulates pupil caliber). The accommodation allows the focal point to fall always at the level of the retina, allowing both short- and long-distance vision. Furthermore, the pupillary reflex regulates the intensity of incoming light. Finally, the transduction of light impulses at the retinal level into visual images is mediated by photoreceptors which generate nerve stimuli that reach the contralateral posterior cortex through the optic nerve [42–44]. The delivery of a drug into the eye tissues is related to two different routes of administration, which are divided into invasive and non-invasive routes. A list of these routes is shown in Table 1.

Table 1. Conventional route of ocular delivery: benefits and limits.

Administration Route	Benefits	Limits	Ocular Anterior/Posterior Target	References
Oral	• Non-invasive. • Increased compliance.	• Difficult achievement of the anterior and posterior tracts of the eye. • Possible degradation by digestive fluids. • Possible low absorption and bioavailability. • Hepatic first-pass metabolism. • Presence of anatomical barriers (blood-aqueous barrier and the blood-retinal barrier).	Potentially both	[45–48]
Systemic (Intravenous and intramuscular)	• Avoided first-pass metabolism.	• Difficult achievement of the anterior or posterior segment of the eye. • Lower compliance. • Presence of anatomical barriers (blood-aqueous barrier and the blood-retinal barrier). • Sterility of the final form	Potentially both	[48,49]
Parenteral (intravitreal, subretinal, suprachoroidal, subconjunctival, intracameral, intrascleral, and intrastromal)	• Deposit of the therapeutic agent in the eye, in some cases directly at the site of action. • Increased local concentration of the drug. • Reduced required dose and avoided off-target actions. • Bypassing of ocular epithelium and other barriers, resulting in increased bioavailability.	• Administration performed by specialized personnel. • Invasive technique. • Short-term complications, including retinal damage, endophthalmitis, haemorrhage, intraocular inflammation, and increased Intraocular Pressure (IOP). • Sterility of the final form	Posterior	[50–55]

Table 1. Cont.

Administration Route	Benefits	Limits	Ocular Anterior/Posterior Target	References
Topical	• Over 90% of the ophthalmic product on the market.	• Rapid precorneal elimination of the drug due to eyelid reflex, tear drainage, dilution by tears, and systemic absorption from the conjunctival sac. • Misapplication of the product to the ocular surface. • Presence of corneal epithelial barrier. • Narrow barriers at the front and back of the eye (limit and regulate fluid and solute uptake). • Complex kinetic processes of absorption, distribution and elimination, influenced by physiology, the physicochemical properties of the drug (lipophilicity, charge, size and shape of the molecule) and the formulation (pH, buffer, tonicity, viscosity, possible presence of preservatives and stabilizers). • Allowed permeation of small lipophilic molecules through the cornea and of larger or hydrophilic compounds through the conjunctiva and the sclera. • Achievement of the anterior segment for only 1% of the administered dose segment, and an even smaller percentage to the posterior segment. • Sterility of the final form	Both	[56–64]

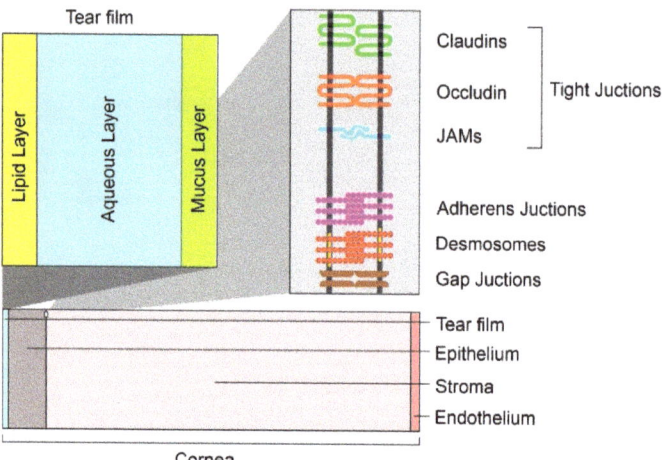

Figure 1. Cross-section of corneal tissues: barriers to drug penetration after topical instillation.

The corneal epithelium and endothelium (lipophilic in nature) consist of cells connected by tight junctions that limit the passage of large molecules (Figure 1). The hydrophilic stroma consists of tightly packed collagen. The epithelium, however, provides the greatest resistance to diffusion. The paracellular pathway through the intercellular pores is allowed for small ionic and hydrophilic molecules of size <350 Da, whereas the transcellular pathway allows the passage of larger lipophilic molecules. The variations in lipophilicity of the corneal layers allowed the realization of a parabolic relationship

2.1. The Coumarins Family

Coumarins have a conjugated double ring system. In the industry, coumarins find application as cosmetic ingredients, perfumers, food additives and in synthetic pharmaceuticals. In nature, coumarins are found in a wide variety of plants: tonka bean (*Dipteryx odorata*), sweet wood (*Galium odoratum*), vanilla grass (*Anthoxanthum odoratum*) and sweet grass (*Hierochloe odorata*) [73]. Among the different synthetic derivatives, Coumarin-6 (C6) exhibits acid-base properties. In the study of Duong et al., a membrane with C6 demonstrated to exhibit colorimetric and ratiometric fluorescence properties with a dynamic pH range between 4.5 and 7.5 (the study uses blue nile in parallel) [74].

2.2. Fluorescein Family

Fluorescein is a xanthene dye with yellowish-green fluorescence. It was firstly synthesized in 1871 by von Bayer via Friedel's acylation/cyclodegradation reaction using resorcinol and phthalic anhydride [75]. It has a rigid tricyclic-coplanar structure with two aryl groups fused to a pyran ring. It has two distinct structures, an open fluorescent ring in the carboxylic acid form and a closed non-fluorescent ring in the spirocyclic lactone form. The open-closed equilibrium in the structure of fluorescein makes it sensitive to the pH of the medium [76]. Among the amine derivatives of fluorescein, those with one or two NH_2 groups in the phthalic residue are of particular interest. The corresponding (di)anions do not show intense fluorescence unless the amine groups are involved in new covalent bonds. In alcohols, the quantum yield, φ, is quite low. In dimethylsulfoxide (DMSO), acetone and other hydrogen bond donor solvents, φ values approach dianionic values [77]. Its sodium salt form finds wide use in angiography [78,79] and glioma studies [80]. Fluorescein 5(6)-isothiocyanate has been used for fluorescence labeling of bacteria, exosomes, proteins (immunofluorescence) and H Protein for gel chromatography. The 5-(iodoacetamido)-fluorescein is used for the synthesis of fluorescently labeled organelles, proteins, peptides and enzymes. Finally, the 5(6)-carboxyfluorescein, a fluorescent polyanionic probe, was used to measure changes in intracellular pH and to highlight processes such as dendrimer aggregation and absorption [81].

2.3. Rhodamine Family

These compounds were discovered in 1887. In the 4–10 pH range, their fluorescence spectra are unaffected by changes. The typical chemical structure of rhodamines involves three benzene rings, whose spirocyclic/open-ring conversion results in their off/on fluorescence [82]. In nonpolar solvents, they exist as spironolactone forms with very low φ due to disruption of p-conjugation of the xanthene core. In polar solutions, the lactone form undergoes charge separation to form a zwitterion [68]. In open-loop forms, rhodamine dyes exist as ammonium cations that can be driven into mitochondria via MMP (Matrix MetalloProteinase). A famous example is rhodamine 123, which forms the basis of the Mito-Tracker dye [83]. Lastly, the rhodamine 6G is a rhodamine analog useful in Pgp (P-glycoprotein) efflux assays, and it has been used to characterize the kinetics of MRP1 (multidrug resistance protein 1)- mediated efflux. An in vivo study of rhodamine B-labeled polymeric nanoparticles was conducted by Bonaccorso et al. to evaluate the distribution in brain areas after intranasal administration of the formulation [84].

2.4. Cyanine Family

Cyanine dyes are among the most widely used families of fluorophores. Cyanine 5 (Cy5) has five carbon atoms in the bridge. It becomes reversibly photocommutable between a bright and dark state in the presence of a primary thiol [85]. Cy5 excited by visible light undergoes thiolation with a thiol anion and transforms into a non-fluorescent thiolated Cy5. The thiolated Cy5 returns to the light-emitting dethiolated form simply by UV irradiation [86]. The photophysical properties of organic dyes with rotatable bonds are strongly governed by their internal rotation in the excited state since rotation can greatly affect molecular conformation and bond conjugation [87]. In the biological field, it

Table 2. Cont.

Probe	Chemical Structure	Molar Mass (g mol^{-1})	Solubility in Water	Excitation (nm)	Fluorescence (nm)
5-aminofluorescein		347.32	Soluble	450–490	500–550
Fluorescein-5-isothiocyanate		389.38	Insoluble	495	519
5-(iodoacetamido)fluorescein		515.25	Insoluble	492	518
5(6)-carboxyfluorescein		376.32	Low	495	520
Nile Red		318.37	Insoluble	543–633	550–700
Rhodamine B		479.01	Soluble	488–530	600–633
Rhodamine B isothiocyanate		536.08	Insoluble	553	563–650
Rhodamine 123		380.82	Low	488	515–575
Rhodamine 6G		479.01	Soluble	480	530
Toluidine Blue O		305.83	Soluble	595	626

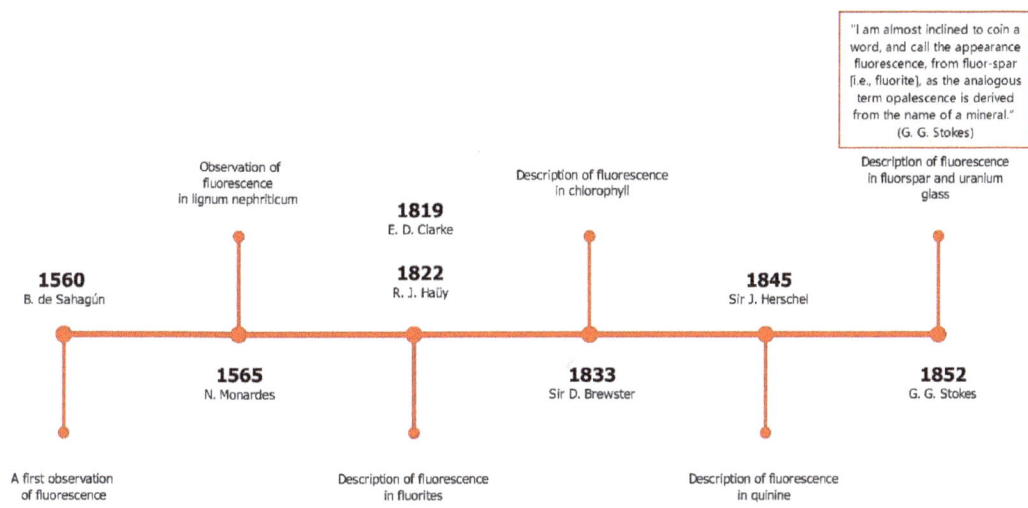

Figure 2. Timeline of the fluorescence discovery.

The following section delineates the family of fluorescent probes reported in reviewed studies, while Table 2 gathers the probes that are used in the experimental papers cited in this review.

Table 2. Physico-chemical properties of the main fluorescent probes used in ocular bioimaging.

Probe	Chemical Structure	Molar Mass (g mol^{-1})	Solubility in Water	Excitation (nm)	Fluorescence (nm)
Coumarin-6		350.43	Insoluble	488–666	502–649
Curcumin		368.38	Insoluble	300–470	571
Cyanine 5-phosphoramidite		944.21	Insoluble	649	666
1,1'-dioctadecyl-3,3,3',3'-tetramethylindocarbocyanine perchlorate		933.87	Low	550	565–588
Fluorescein		332.31	Insoluble	465–490	494
Fluorescein sodium salt		376.27	Soluble	460	512

between corneal permeability and diffusion coefficient. pH is another important factor in corneal permeability [38]. Many studies that have examined permeability across conjunctiva, tenon and sclera have shown that the conjunctiva is more permeable to hydrophilic molecules than the cornea. The greater surface area (in humans, about 17 times bigger than the cornea) and the presence of larger pore sizes promote increased permeability compared to the cornea. However, mucus and the presence of lymphatics and vasculature increases systemic leakage [24,38]. In ocular topical administration, reaching the posterior portion is size-dependent [65]. Nanocarriers with a diameter of 20–200 nm are suitable for retinal-targeted delivery. Small nanoparticles (20 nm) are able to cross the sclera and are rapidly eliminated due to periocular circulation. The larger ones (200 nm) do not cross the sclera or the sclera-choroid-retinal pigment epithelium (RPE) and remain in the periocular site releasing their contents even for long periods. Even in the case of intravitreal administration, the kinetics are size-dependent. Nanocarriers with a diameter of 2 µm remain in the vitreous cavity or migrate into the trabeculae. Those with a diameter of less than 200 nm reach the retina [66]. In order to discuss the application of nanosystems in the ocular field, an emergent role is represented by fluorescent nanosystems. The tailor ability of design, architecture and photophysical properties has attracted the attention of many research groups, resulting in numerous reports related to novel nanosensors to analyze a great variety of biological analytes.

2. Fluorescent Probes in Ocular Applications

Before focusing on the published experimental studies, in this section, a brief discussion on fluorescence and on the molecules applied in the ocular field is given.

Absorption of a photon from a fluorescent chemical species causes a transition to an excited state of the same multiplicity (spin) as the fundamental state (S0). In solution, Sn states (with n > 1) rapidly relax to S1 through nonradiative processes. Ultimately, relaxation from S1 to S0 causes the emission of a photon with an energy lower than the absorbed photon. The fluorescence quantum yield (φ), one of the most important parameters, provides the efficiency of the fluorescence process; it is defined as the ratio between the number of photons emitted to those absorbed.

$$\varphi = \frac{Number\ of\ photons\ emitted}{Number\ of\ photons\ absorbed}$$

In Figure 2, we reproduce a brief history of the discovery of the fluorescence phenomenon. This discovery enabled the development of fluorescent probes that achieve single-molecule sensitivity. The figure shows that the first observation of a fluorescence phenomenon was described in 1560 by Bernardino de Sahagun; the same experiment was repeated by Nicolas Monardes in 1565. The fluorescence of the infusion known as lignum nephriticum was observed. This phenomenon was caused by the fluorescence of the oxidation product of one of the flavonoids present in those woods: matlaline. In the middle of the nineteenth century, George Gabriel Stokes coined the term fluorescence, derived from fluorite. The knowledge of atomic structure needed to understand and describe the nature of the phenomenon was not acquired until the beginning of the 20th century. By providing detailed information, this technique has enormous advantages over classical microscopy techniques [67]. In fact, literature is plentiful of studies dealing with the design of new fluorescent probes such as (bio)sensors to detect (even with the naked eye) enzymes, metals, biomaterials and others. Since 1945, the ability of analytes to promote the opening of rhodamine spirolactams has been exploited to design probes that detect metal ions and biological targets [68,69]. The pH sensitivity of fluorescein can be used to detect changes in a specific environment. By controlling the balance of ring-opening and ring-closing, following the interaction with specific targets, it can be used to detect metal ions from industrial and commercial specimens [70]. Curcumin is also widely used as a fluorescent probe for different applications, from producing drug carriers to the realization of specific sensors for ions and biomolecules [71,72].

finds use in comparative genomic hybridization, transcriptomics in proteomics, and RNA localization [88]. Moreover, DiI is a cyanine-derived dialkyl carbon sensitive to the polarity of the environment. It is weakly fluorescent in water but highly fluorescent in nonpolar solvents. It is commonly used as a lipophilic marker for fluorescence microscopy in the biological field. DiI molecules penetrate in cell membranes with the 2 long alkyl chains (12 carbons) immersed in the bilayer and the rings parallel to the bilayer surface. The dye emits characteristic bright red fluorescence when its alkyl chains are incorporated into membranes making it particularly useful for tracking in the biological membrane [89]. In the study by Musumeci et al. the 1-1′-dioctadecyl-3,3,3′,3′-tetramethylindotricarbocyanine iodide dye was used to label polymeric nanoparticles and study their cerebral delivery after intranasal administration [90].

2.5. Nile Red

Nile red is a hydrophobic dye of recent interest in the identification of microplastics [91]. It is widely used in biophysical studies focusing on proteins, lipids and live-cell analysis. Depending on the environment, Nile Red shows different absorption and fluorescence spectra. In particular, in organic solvents or nonpolar environments, it shows strong fluorescence that changes depending on the environment, presenting shifts toward blue emission in nonpolar environments [92].

2.6. Curcumin

Curcumin is the main natural polyphenol found in the rhizome of *Curcuma longa* (turmeric) and in others *Curcuma* spp. Its countless benefits in the treatment of inflammatory states, metabolic syndrome, pain and inflammatory-degenerative conditions of the eyes are related to its antioxidant and anti-inflammatory effects [93]. Theoretical studies have predicted that its wide absorption band (410 and 430 nm) is due to the π-π* transition, while the maximum absorption between 389 and 419 nm is related to the keto and enol form, respectively [67].

2.7. Toluidine Blue O

Toluidine blue (TB) is a thiazine-based metachromatic dye. It has a high affinity for acidic tissue components. This characteristic allows colorimetric identification of DNA- and RNA-rich tissues [94]. In the ocular field, Navahi et al. performed a study on the use of TB in the diagnosis of ocular surface squamous neoplasm (OSSN) [95]. In the Su et al. study, in vivo antibacterial efficacy of TB-mediated photodynamic therapy on bacterial keratitis by *Staphylococcus aureus* in a rabbit was demonstrated. This provides a new option for the clinical treatment of bacterial keratitis [96].

3. Fluorescent Nanosystems in Ocular Application

The following section is focused on recently investigated fluorescent nanomaterials and nanosystems for ocular applications. The reviewed works have been divided according to the use of such fluorescent nanosystems. Most studies concern the use of probes to assess nanosystems distribution within the ocular tissues. Among the most investigated fluorescent nanosystems, there are lipid-based nanocarriers—such as nanostructured lipid carriers (NLCs) and solid lipid nanoparticles (SLNs), polymeric nanoparticles and nanocapsules, hybrid nanoparticles, cubosomes, emulsomes, nanoemulsions, niosomes, liposomes, films, nanomicelles and hydrogels. Fluorescence is introduced through the methods commonly used to prepare nanosystems [97,98]. The fluorescent nanosystems are essentially divided into (i) probe-loaded, in which the dye or probe is encapsulated into the system mostly during the formulation processes, and (ii) labeled/grafted, in which the probe is covalently bound to the surface of the nanosystem (often linked to some matrix component, such as polymers or lipids), always forming an adduct (Figure 3).

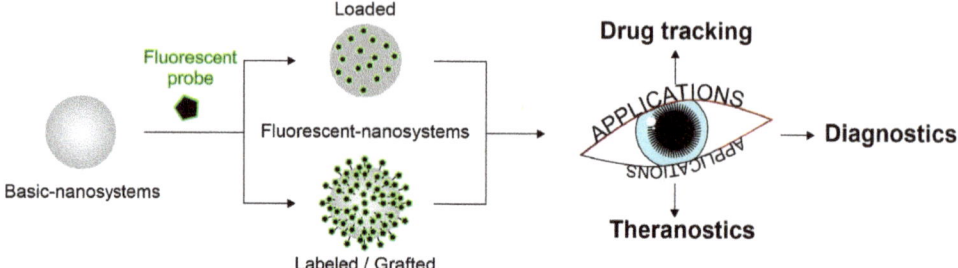

Figure 3. Schematic structure of fluorescent nanosystems for ocular applications.

3.1. Biodistribution

As above cited, the tissues that compose the eye are many and with different properties. The difficulty for a nanosystem to reach the target tissue is high; thus, the profile of drug delivery is not always predictable. When the target is located in deeper ocular tissues, it is even more difficult to predict the ideal pathways followed by the carriers in vivo and through the ocular barriers. Tracking the drug after topical administration is important for several factors. Firstly, it allows for assessment of the effective achievement of the target site in order to accomplish the desired therapeutic action. Another factor to consider is the non-productive distribution of the drug in non-desired tissues, which could lead to the possible occurrence of side effects in addition to reducing the effective drug concentration. Furthermore, studying the pathways followed by the nanosystems is necessary to avoid issues related to barriers, tight junctions and physiological phenomena (tear flow and blinking), which could impair the routes. Size, surface charge and morphology of the nanocarriers have a great influence on their biodistribution, clearance and cellular uptake [99–102]. Before performing biodistribution studies, it is important to characterize the system and to proceed with in vitro and in vivo assays. For instance, mean size measurement, zeta potential, mucoadhesion studies and morphological analyses are, of course, also required to make the system as conformable as possible to a correct drug release. Tracking of nanosystems can be carried out in two ways, invasive and non-invasive; bioimaging using fluorescent molecules is a non-invasive method [103,104]. Among the most important characteristics that the nanosystem should have are small size, necessary to enter cells for allowing bioimaging, high sensitivity for effective detection, fast response, compatibility, absence of toxicity, good dispersibility in the biological environment and highly selective detection in the tissues. In Figure 4, a summary is gathered of the fluorescent probes used in the studied nanosystems discussed in Sections 3.1–3.3.

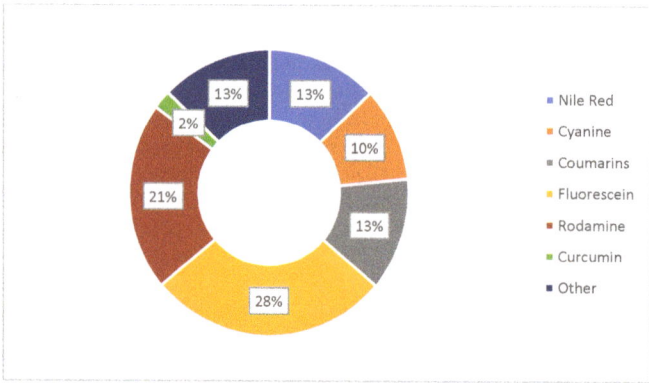

Figure 4. Graphical analysis of the fluorescent probes discussed in this review.

3.1.1. Fluorescent Lipid-Based Nanosystems

Lipid systems are of great interest for drug delivery in ocular tissues; their biocompatible and biodegradable composition makes them technologically safe, while their lipidic nature and structural characteristics allow them to pass through the corneal layers and achieve an efficient drug dosage even in the deepest tissues of the eye. The distribution of these systems occurs mainly in lipophilic layers, with minimal involvement of the stroma, since it has hydrophilic nature, and the lipid systems are difficult to distribute there. This was confirmed in the work of Namprem et al., in which confocal scanning microfluorometer (CSMF) analysis confirmed poor penetration of NLC labeled with Nile Red in hydrophilic compartments such as the stroma compared to corneal layers [105]. Due to eye barriers and obstacles to ocular administration, understanding the path taken by the designed nanosystem is necessary, especially if it is targeted to the back of the eye. The main route through which lipid systems reach the deeper tissues is the transcorneal one. There is growing evidence that successful drug delivery by functionalized nanocarriers depends largely on their efficient intra/paracellular transport, a process that is not fully understood yet. Therefore, the development of new imaging and diagnostic techniques is very important, particularly in a complex biological system such as the eye. Due to its lipophilic nature, one of the most used dyes for the preparation of fluorescent-lipid nanosystems is Nile Red (NR) Cubosomes labeled with Nile Red were prepared in the work of El Gendy et al. to assess the role of nine different lipids as penetration enhancers. The type of lipid used in the preparation plays an important role in tissue distribution. Among the prepared lipid systems, fluorescence analysis showed that the combination of oleic acid, Captex® 8000 and Capmul® MCM improved the penetration of the systems into the mucosa by increasing diffusivity due to both surfactant properties and the ability to disrupt the organization of the lipid bilayer [106]. Once again, Nile Red was used in the work of Kapadia et al. in order to visualize drug-loaded emulsomes. For the physico-chemical characterization and subsequent analyses, the nanosystems were loaded with triamcinolone acetonide, while for the studies of precorneal retention and ocular distribution, the fluorescent dye was loaded instead of the drug. The study revealed that after topical administration, the pathways taken to reach the back of the eye were basically three: corneal (via the iris and aqueous humor), conjunctival and systemic. The drug may diffuse through the sclera by lateral diffusion, followed by penetration of Bruch's membrane and retinal pigment epithelium (RPE). To a lesser extent, the drug may be absorbed into the systemic circulation either through the conjunctival vessels and the nasolacrimal duct, and gain systemic access to the retinal vessel [107]. Another lipophilic DiI dye (1,1-dioctadecyl-3,3,3 tetramethyl indocarbocyanine perchlorate) was used to label lipid nanocapsules (LNCs) fluorescently. An important finding was made in the study by Eldesouky et al., where, despite the lipophilic nature of the dye, better penetration was achieved by encapsulation in lipid systems compared to simple dispersion. Fluorescence analysis showed that, without the use of lipid nanocarriers, the dye is unable to cross the hydrophobic corneal layer [108]. Mucoadhesion plays a key role in the enhancement of bioavailability. Efforts are made to design systems that have the ability to improve retention on the ocular surface. In this respect, the use of chitosan to improve the delivery of drugs into the eye tissues for its properties as a mucoadhesive agent, controlled drug release and permeation enhancer is interesting [24]. It is used in conjugation with a drug, such as in the study of Dubashynskaya et al., to improve the intravitreal delivery of dexamethasone [109]. In the major cases, it was used as a coating of nanocarriers to promote intraocular penetration, as reported by which designed modified NLCs with three different types of chitosan: chitosan acetyl-L-cysteine (CS-NAC), chitosan oligosaccharides (COS) and carboxymethyl chitosan (CMCS). The distribution profile was evaluated by loading the hydrophobic dye C6 into the NLCs. It was revealed through CLSM analysis that only NLCs modified with COS and CS-NAC were able to pass the cornea through the opening of tight junctions between epithelial cells [110]. Rhodamine-labeled NLCs were used to assess the corneal retention of such lipid nanocarriers, modified with a complex containing boronic acid, which is able to bind with high affinity the sialic acids of mucin. The NLCs were loaded with dexamethasone and designed for the treatment of dry eye syndrome. Fluorescence marking revealed the increased retention time due to the mucoadhesive property of the nanosystem, which also proved to be a potential not irritant treatment for dry eye syndrome [111]. Another key factor that improves retention time on the ocular surface is the positive charge of nanosystems interacting with the negative charges of mucin. The addition of octa-arginine (R8) to the nanoemulsions prepared by Liu et al. imparted a positive charge to the system with the aim of increasing eye retention. Once again, C6 was used to label lipid emulsions of disulfiram. In particular, the permeation of these systems under the influence of particle size and the presence of R8 was investigated and revealed that the addition of R8 and a size of ~50 nm improved the ocular delivery performance of nanosystems. In addition, the study showed that C6 passed through the corneal epithelium mainly by paracellular pathways, but there was also a fluorescent signal in the cytoplasm, indicating a transport also by transcellular pathways [112]. The internalization of lipid nanoparticles occurs mainly through an endocytosis mechanism. This is in fact the route taken by the mRNA-based solid lipid nanoparticles prepared by Gómez-Aguado et al. The SLN were developed in order to produce IL-10 to treat corneal inflammation and was loaded with Nile Red to assess cellular uptake in corneal epithelial cells (HCE-2 cells). This platform could also be used as a theranostic model as GFP (green fluorescent protein) is produced inside the cells, so the intensity of the fluorescence is indicative of the amount of protein produced. Since GFP, once produced, remains at the intracellular level, instillation on the ocular surface of mice of the samples permitted the identification of the corneal layers where transfection occurred. All the prepared mRNA-based SLN formulations showed higher fluorescence intensity than naked mRNA, demonstrating the enhancement of their targeting ability [113]. Fluorescein is one of the most widely used fluorescent dyes for drug tracking and visualization of ocular damage following treatment. In Section 4, some clinical trials using fluorescein as a fluorescent in the study will be proposed. Fluorescein was used by Jounaki et al. for tracking vancomycin loaded NLCs. The aim of the work is the idea that NLCs for topical use could be a valid substitute of intravitreal injection in the treatment of bacterial endophthalmitis caused especially by *Staphylococcus*. Both drug-loaded and fluorescein-loaded NLCs (0.2 mg/mL) were prepared by cold homogenization technique and were used to evaluate precorneal retention with an inverted fluorescent microscope. The increased fluorescence found in the corneal epithelium demonstrated that dye-loaded, stearylamine-coated NLCs were retained more in the ocular surface. Indeed, the cationic lipid stearylamine is trapped in the mucin layer and retained due to the interaction between the fillers, facilitating the penetration and delivery of the drug to the intraocular tissues [101]. In the work of Kakkar et al., fluorescein was also used in concentrations almost like the previous work (0.25 mg/mL) to track hybrid nanoparticles. Solid lipid nanoparticles were prepared and then coated with PEG in order to encapsulate the antimycotic fluconazole. Analysis to assess the penetration into the ocular internal layers revealed that fluorescence was observed in the vitreous humor, retina, sclera and choroid after instillation of a single drop of Fluconazole-SLNs into the rat eye. In addition, the ex vivo study showed that the system exhibited a 164.64% higher flux through the porcine cornea when compared to the commercial drops ZoconVR [114]. In addition to coating the nanosystems, fluorescein was used to label them binding it covalently to the material of the nanosystem. In the work of Puglia et al. [66] an adduct is prepared between fluorescein and stearic acid named ODAF (N-(30,60-dihydroxy-3-oxospiro[isobenzofuran-1(3H),90-[9H]xanthen]-5-yl)-octadecanamide). In this case, the dye was grafted (and not loaded) and the conjugation of the lipid with the dye leads to a fluorescent probe. Solvent-diffusion technique was used to prepare SLNs of about 120 nm. The in vivo distribution from 1 h to 16 h was evaluated in rabbits and the results showed that, after ocular instillation, ODAF SLNs were mostly located in the cornea (up to 2 h), whereas over a longer time (from the second hour to the eighth hour) the fluorescent signal gradually extended toward the back of the eye, confirming the ability of controlled delivery by the lipid nanosystems [66].

Considering that the influence of blinking and tearing on ocular drug absorption was rarely evaluated in studies, Pretor et al. evaluated absorption of two lipid-based formulations, a liposome and a SLN, in presence of these two physiological conditions. The SLNs were also labeled with a fluorescent phospholipid, thus constituting another example of a grafted nanosystem. From the study, using C6 as the fluorescent compound, it is evaluated that liposomes are shown to provide a greater absorption, despite the influence of blinking (shear stress of 0.1 Pa.) and tear flow. This interesting study was carried out by coupling the use of microfluidics with channels and cultured HCE-T cells as well as the use of a fluorescent dye to simulate the physiological mechanisms; it could be useful to add this kind of assay to the basic characterization of the nanosystem addressed to ocular targets [115]. In the rhodamine family, Rhodamine B is widely available and low-cost. The following two studies promote the use of this molecule for tracking nanosystems. The first is focused on the preparation of lipid systems (niosomes vesicles) and Eudragit nanoparticles for the treatment of eye fungal infections. Encapsulation of fluconazole within these systems resulted in being a good way to increase the bioavailability of the drug compared to free drugs. The systems obtained were innovative in terms of formulation as there is a triple step: the drug was first complexed using β-cyclodextrin, then encapsulated into niosomes, and the niosomes were finally incorporated into an in-situ gelling system made by Poloxamer, HPMC and chitosan. Niosomes were labeled with Rhodamine B and then were compared to labeled polymeric nanoparticles. The fluorescent signal of CLSM analysis increased in intensity when the NPs were incorporated into the hydrogel, whereas the signal of the pure dye was limited to the superficial epithelial layers, suggesting effective permeation of the nanosystems into the inner tissues [116]. Rhodamine B was also used to study the transport of curcumin as a model drug in multilamellar liposomes. These were coated with sodium alginate grafted acrylic acid conjugated with riboflavin. These multi-dye vesicles (rhodamine and curcumin), prepared using the lipid film hydration technique, have proven to be excellent carriers for drug delivery to the retina. The study evaluated both the encapsulation efficiency of the two dyes and their in vitro release. The release test in pH 7.4 medium demonstrated time-depended release, which was faster for rhodamine than for curcumin. An extended-release profile was obtained using fluorescence, red for rhodamine and green for curcumin, showing greater entrance into the cell at 12 h than at 3 h, and greater endocytosis for smaller, more spherical particles [117].

3.1.2. Polymer-Based Nanocarriers

Topical delivery of polymeric nanosystems is useful to improve corneal penetration and prolong the therapeutic response of several drugs. Nanocarriers need to be evaluated to find clinical application; specifically, their distribution in biological environment should be examined in order to understand the most appropriate strategy to address specific ocular pathologies. Plausible routes of topically instilled drug delivery for the treatment of ocular diseases involving the posterior segment include several pathways, including corneal, non-corneal and uveal routes. Successful nanocarrier development, therefore, involves fluorescent labeling useful for investigating mechanisms and biodistribution profiles of the designed systems. Polymeric nanostructures to be used as imaging diagnostic agents include various kinds of systems, such as nanoparticles, niosomes, film and nanomicelles and in-situ gel. The review of Swetledge et al. offers a detailed discussion on the biodistribution of polymer nanoparticles in major ocular tissues [118]. To improve retention time on the ocular surface, release profile and mucoadhesion performance, nanocarriers are often coated with polymers. Poly-lactide (PLA), polyglycolide (PGA), poly-lactide-co-glycolide (PLGA) and chitosan, Eudragit®, but also different copolymers such as PLGA-PEG, poly-(3-hydroxybutyrate-co-3-hydroxyvalerate) (PHBV) constituted by hydroxybutyrate (HB) and hydroxyvalerate (HV) and chitosan modified copolymer are some of these. Among them, many polysaccharides are used as a useful coating for nanocarriers. Some of these, including chitosan, alginate sodium, hyaluronate sodium and cellulose derivatives, are approved for ophthalmic use by the FDA and are already present in the composition of ophthalmic products on the market [119]. Depending on the type of polymer, the most suitable fluorescent probe should be chosen. A study conducted by Zhukova et al. focused on understanding the interactions between probes, polymeric nanoparticles and the biological environment. Four dyes with different degrees of hydrophobicity were encapsulated (C6, rhodamine 123, DiI) or covalently bound to the polymer (amine Cyanin 5.5, Cy5.5) in order to label PLGA nanoparticles. To increase the accuracy of the interpretation of in vivo biodistribution data, dual-labeled nanoparticles were administered, using C6 as the encapsulated label and Cy5.5 as the grafted label. Neuroimaging results showed that the signal of the nanoparticles bounded with Cy5.5 was detected in retinal vessels, whereas the signal of the encapsulated C6 was found outside of blood vessels and in tissue background. The extra vasal distribution of C6 could falsify the data interpretation, leading to erroneous assumptions that the nanoparticles could efficiently cross the blood-retinal barrier. Assessing the affinity of the dye to the polymer and the lipophilic structures could be useful in scaling up these issues. Although C6 has not proved to be an ideal label, it aided in explaining the phenomenon whereby drugs are delivered to tissues through encapsulation in nanocarriers without involving any nanoparticle penetration [120]. Similar results were obtained by Zhang et al. tracking in vivo the distribution of PLGA-NPs in the retinal blood circulation after intravenous injection. NPs were labeled with lipophilic perchlorate carbocyanins (DiI) or hydrophilic rhodamine 123 (Rho123). DiI fluorescent signal was detected for a long time (>90 min) in retinal vessels, in contrast with Rho123 whose fluorescence was short (>15 min), due to diffusion from particles and elimination from the blood circulation. To avoid artefacts, dual-labeled nanoparticles were also injected intravenously in rats. Colocalization of fluorescent markers was performed by conjugating the polymer with Cy5.5 and loading the systems with probes (DiI/Rho 123). Cy5.5 signal was detected for both cargoes in retinal vessels for more than 90 min; however, colocalization was observed only for lipophilic DiI dye, which was more closely related to the hydrophobic polymer matrix. These findings further confirm that the affinity of the dye for the polymer and cell membranes played a key role in biodistribution kinetics [121]. The hydrophilic properties of rhodamine B make it a suitable fluorescent candidate for polymers of a hydrophilic nature such as chitosan, whose mucoadhesive qualities have been exploited by X et al. for the design of topical films for the treatment of glaucoma. Corneal permeation studies demonstrated the mucoadhesive efficacy of polymeric films in transporting rhodamine B molecules through the cornea with a high permeation rate [122]. A water-insoluble derivative of the rhodamine family is rhodamine B isothiocyanate, which has affinity for hydrophobic polymers. This dye was used as a label for nanoparticles consisting of hydrophobic PHBV polymer to obtain information regarding the depth and rate of penetration after topical administration. Confocal analysis showed improved penetration deepness of encapsulated marker compared to the free one, used as a control [123]. Recently, hydrophobic C6 was doubly used as a model drug and a fluorescent marker to track surface-modified PLGA-NPs with chitosan, glycol chitosan and polysorbate 80 in retinal tissues. Tracking of NPs after topical instillation was performed by fluorescence microscopy, revealing intense staining throughout the whole eyeball, anterior segment including cornea and conjunctiva, lens, iris/ciliary body and retina, with a peak at 30 min after administration and the disappearance of the signal after 60 min. Ocular tissue autofluorescence was distinct around the outer segments of the photoreceptor. Based on the average size of the NPs (<200 nm), the specific pathway of the NPs to the retina did not exclude any of the plausible routes of delivery to the posterior segment (corneal, noncorneal or uveal pathways) [124]. C6 was also used to label polymeric nanomicelles designed for the topical treatment of fungal keratitis. The nanomicelles consisted of a chitosan oligosaccharide-vitamin E copolymer conjugated to phenylboronic acid (PBA-CS-VE) to enhance corneal retention. C6 delivery through a monolayer of HCE-T cells and 3D cell spheroids demonstrated strong corneal penetration ability. Several characteristics of the polymer were able to influence nanomicelle uptake, but the key role in the process of cellular endocytosis was attributed to the high-affinity interaction between the PBA portion and sialic acid on the surface of the cell membrane [125].

Another study using C6 as a fluorescent probe was reported by Sai et al., aiming to evaluate the corneal transportation of an in-situ gelling system based on mixed micelles. This formulation designed for curcumin was composed of micelles, consisting of 1,2-distearoyl-sn-glycero-3-phosphoethanolamine-N-[methoxy(polyethyleneglycol)-2000] (PEG-DSPE) and poly(oxyethylene) esters of 12-hydroxystearic acid (Solutol HS 15), incorporated in a gellan gum gel. Incubation of human corneal epithelial cells (HCEC) with the fluorescently labeled systems showed time-dependent and improved absorption for the encapsulated dye, compared to free C6. Transcorneal penetration was investigated in vivo by CLSM and results suggested that curcumin was able to penetrate more effectively when incorporated into the gelled systems, probably due to the increased retention time conferred by the gellan gum, which was five-fold higher than the mixed micelles alone [126]. A pilot study with C6 was performed to evaluate the feasibility of the approach in assessing the biodistribution of PLGA-PEG nanoparticles suspended in hydrogels. The preliminary study showed an important limitation due to the high green autofluorescence of the examined ocular tissues. To deal with the drawbacks highlighted by the pilot study, PLGA nanoparticles in the full study were labeled with Cy-5, a far-red fluorophore that did not overlap with the natural autofluorescence of the ocular tissues. Results from the full study showed that topical application allowed the nanoparticles to be distributed into the outer ocular tissues (cornea, episcleral tissue and sclera) and the choroid was the only internal tissue to show a slight increased fluorescence, probably attributed to the permeation of [118]. Another dye recently used as a model drug to label mucoadhesive films with a hydrophilic nature based on chitosan and poly(2-ethyl-2-oxazoline) is fluorescein sodium. To avoid precipitation of complexes between the negatively charged dye and the positively charged chitosan backbones, concentrations less than 0.1 mg/mL were used. Films tested by ex vivo (bovine cornea) and in vivo (chinchilla rabbits) studies showed excellent corneal adhesion (up to 50 min) [127]. From this review of recently published papers, it emerged that, to ascertain the applicability of nanosystems to biodistribution studies, it was necessary to (i) take in account the degree of affinity and interference between probe, polymeric carriers and cell membranes, and (ii) accurately interpret the data by selecting an effective labeling method upstream. The most reliable way to track the pathways of the systems remains the conjugation of the fluorescent dye to the polymeric core. Therefore, colocalization by double labeling may be the most appropriate technique to minimize errors in the interpretation of fluorescence signals. Currently, there is no unique approach to fluorescent polymer nanosystems that can be used for all types of labeling systems and probes.

3.1.3. Metallic-Based and Inorganic-Based Nanosystems

Inorganic nanodevices became of great interest in ocular delivery due to their unique properties such as low cost, easy preparation methods, small size, tuneable porosity, high surface-volume and robust stability. Fluorescent labeling has been applied to these delivery systems to assess their ability to cross ocular barriers and provide therapeutic efficacy [128]. Corneal barrier functions were investigated by Mun et al. using two types of silica nanoparticles (thiolate and PEGylated) fluorescently labeled with 5-(iodoacetamido)-fluorescein (5-IAF). Permeation studies were performed in vitro on intact or β-cyclodextrin pretreated bovine corneas. To provide experimental parameters close to in vivo conditions and to avoid artifacts such as the potential risk of corneal swelling when using Franz diffusion cells, the "whole-eye" method was used. 5-IAF-loaded thiolate silica nanoparticles, PEG-grafted silica nanoparticles (5-IAF-PEG), sodium fluorescein and fluorescein isothiocyanate dextran solutions were tested. It resulted that fluorescein salt (376 Da) did not uniformly penetrate the cornea; however, the dye was detected in the stroma. Larger molecules such as FITC-dextran (400 Da) and 5-IAF-PEG formed a layer on the corneal surface with no permeation of the epithelial membrane. β-cyclodextrin pre-treatment disrupted the integrity of the cornea by providing homogeneous permeation of the low-molecular-weight dye, although it did not improve the penetration of larger molecules. Concerning NPs, no permeation was reported regardless of surface modification, particle size and pre-treatment with β-cyclodextrin, thus suggesting that the tight junctions of the corneal epithelium acted as the main barrier to permeation. The absence of penetration and confinement on the corneal surface was observed for thiolated NPs because of the formation of disulfide bonds between the NPs thiol groups and the cysteine domains of the mucus glycoprotein layer. The interaction between mucin and -SH thiol groups remained a limiting permeation factor even after the removal of the epithelial layer. NPs PEGylation was able to mask thiol groups, allowing passage into the stroma [129]. Baran-Rachwalska et al. designed a novel platform consisting of hybrid silicon-lipid nanoparticles, aiming to deliver siRNA to the cornea by topical administration. A fluorescent oligonucleotide duplex, siRNA transfection indicator (siGLO), was employed as a tracking probe to assess in vitro cellular uptake on a human corneal epithelial cell line (HCE-S) and in vivo corneal penetration on wild-type mice. Red fluorescence of the oligonucleotide marker allowed detection of nanoparticles in all layers of the cornea 3 h after instillation, in contrast to the control siGLO. The tracking of biodegradable nanosystems in corneal tissues was confirmed by the reduction of protein expression in the corneal epithelium, making them ideal candidates for therapeutic oligonucleotide delivery [130]. Biodegradable mesoporous silica nanoparticles (MSNs) loaded with carboplatin were designed by Qu et al. for the treatment of retinoblastoma. Carboplatin, being an anticancer drug, causes severe side effects; therefore, it is necessary to focus the action strictly on the target site. For this purpose, MSNs were surface modified by conjugation with an ideal target, epithelial cell adhesion molecule (EpCAM), in order to increase specificity as well as therapeutic efficacy. To assess the targeting efficacy of the designed systems, the authors evaluated the cellular uptake of untargeted and targeted MSNs in retinoblastoma Y79 tumor cells. Rhodamine B and Lysotracker Green were used as fluorescent probes to track cellular and subcellular uptake of the vectors. Increased cellular uptake for targeted MSNs was attributed to EpCAM-specific receptor-mediated cellular internalization. Lysosomal localization of MSNs confirmed that the nanosystems followed the endocytosis pathway for drug delivery [131]. A hexa-histidine with metal ions nanosystem was designed to deliver Avastin in the treatment of corneal neovascularization (CNV). Pre-corneal retention time and ability to cross ocular barriers were studied on a rat CNV model induced by alkaline burns by FITC labeling the systems. Avastin encapsulated in the vectors showed a longer precorneal adhesion time compared to the free drug. These innovative systems have emerged as a promising platform for ocular topical delivery of protein drugs [132]. An interesting zirconium-porphyrin metal-organic framework (NPMOF) has been designed for drug tracking and delivery. The bright fluorescence self-emitted by the metal-organic framework qualifies the carriers to be applied for imaging. NPMOF was used as a skeleton for the delivery of methylprednisolone, a very efficacious corticosteroid in the treatment of retinal degenerative diseases. Adult zebrafish with photoreceptor degeneration induced by high-intensity light exposure were used to test in vivo distribution and therapeutic efficacy. Red fluorescence signals were detected in choroid, retina, photoreceptors and retinal pigment epithelium for up to 7 days. Recovery of visual function by rapid regeneration of photoreceptors and proliferation of Müller's glia and retinal regeneration were reached after a single intravitreal injection. NPMOF vectors represent a novel delivery system for the treatment of diseases affecting the posterior eye segment [133].

3.1.4. Protein-Based Nanosystems

Protein-based nanosystems have attracted considerable interest in recent years and are designed for drug delivery, diagnostics and bioimaging. These highly bio-compatible systems, which have been extensively studied in the biomedical field, owe their properties to the protein they are composed of. Among the proteins used in their preparation, there are antibodies, enzymes, animal and plant proteins, collagen, plasma proteins, gelatin and proteins derived from virus capsids [134]. Fluorescent proteins are usually used to monitor protein-protein interactions, protein localization and gene expression. However, without any carrier, the fluorescent efficiency of a single protein is relatively low. The use of fluorescent protein-labeled nanomaterials improves loading due to increased surface area and allows the development of fluorescent nanosystems useful in bioimaging and biosensing. In the study carried out by Yang et al., nanoparticles were prepared from regenerated silk fibroin. This protein, which is the most abundant in silk, is considered to have high biocompatibility and degradability properties. In the biomedical field, it has been used for drug delivery in small nanosystems, biological drug delivery, gene therapy, wound healing and bone regeneration. The formulation is targeted for intravitreal injection with the aim of increasing the bioavailability of the drug in the retina. Fluorescein isothiocyanate labeled bovine serum albumin (FITC-BSA) has been encapsulated as a model drug. In vitro cytotoxicity studies were conducted on ARPE-19 cells, showing that these nanosystems were very compatible. In addition, in vivo comparison of the biodistribution in posterior ocular tissues in rabbits revealed increased retention in the retina due to encapsulation in the nanosystem rather than with a solution of model drug [135,136]. Albumin is widely used in the preparation of ocular nanosystems [137]. In a recent study, bovine serum albumin nanoparticles loaded with apatinib were prepared for the treatment of diabetic retinopathy. In contrast to the previous study, in this disease, invasive administration has to be avoided, so topical administration is the ultimate goal. The nanoparticles were coated with hyaluronic acid (HA) to increase mucoadhesion. The biodistribution study in retinal tissue was carried out by preparing fluorescent nanosystems with 1,1'-dioctadecyl-3,3,3',3'-tetramethylindodicarbocyanine, 4-chlorobenzenesulfonate salt (DiD) solution in ethanol (0.5 mg/mL), which was added during the formulation phase. Through the comparative in vivo biodistribution study, it was shown that HA-coated nanoparticles demonstrate higher fluorescence in retinal tissue compared to uncoated nanoparticles, thus representing a viable alternative to intravitreal injection, maintaining comparable perfusion and bioavailability [138]. Another study involved the preparation of nanoparticles using pseudo-proteins for the potential treatment of ophthalmic diseases. Ten types of nanoparticles obtained by precipitation of pseudo-proteins were prepared, then they were loaded, and some of them were also pegylated; finally, they were labeled with a fluorescent probe, fluorescein diacetate (FDA) or rhodamine 6G (Rh6G), to assess ocular penetration. Corneal fluorescence was obtained as expected, while surprising results were the reaching of tissues such as the sclera and retina. Thus, they proved to be a promising delivery system for topical use in chronic eye diseases [139].

3.2. Diagnostics

Labeling nanoparticles with fluorescent probes was demonstrated to be a useful approach to improve the effectiveness of some diagnostic tests aimed to detect ocular pathologies. In fact, some eye diseases require a prompt diagnosis in order to contain possible damages related to the ongoing pathways involved. Age-related macular degeneration (AMD) is the main cause of vision loss for over-65-year-olds [37]; this pathology has often been analyzed to improve diagnostic techniques since it has several predisposing factors, and early detection is crucial to avoid degeneration toward blindness [140]. AMD has an unclear etiology, although oxidative stress is considered one of the main risk factors [141]; as a matter of fact, clinical studies demonstrated the importance of supplementation with antioxidants in order to slow down the progression of AMD [142,143]. Physiological antioxidant patterns involve metallothioneins (MT), low molecular mass proteins characterized by the presence of cysteine sulfur ligands, which are able to scavenge free radicals, thus protecting cells and tissues. The retina is particularly subject to oxidative stress due to visible and UV light exposure; moreover, age progression involves a reduction of MT expression, predisposing to AMD [144]. For this reason, bioimaging these proteins in ocular tissues could be an important tool useful to highlight the tendency to develop AMD. For this purpose, fluorescent gold nanoclusters involving Cu and Zn and bioconjugated with specific primary antibodies were developed by Cruz-Alonso and coworkers [145]. Laser ablation (LA)-inductively coupled plasma (ICP)-mass spectrometry (MS) technique was used to identify $^{63}Cu^+$ and $^{64}Zn^+$ in the retina of post-mortem donors since MT bind both Cu and Zn [146]. This method showed results comparable with conventional immunohistochemistry for MT proteins, with amplification of signals related to the presence of nanoclusters, which allowed the obtainment of higher resolution bioimages. An in vivo model of human "wet" AMD is laser-induced choroidal neovascularization (mouse LCNV) mouse, in which the inflammatory biomarker vascular cell adhesion molecule-1 (VCAM-1) is highly expressed. Gold nanoparticles functionalized with anti-sense DNA complementary to VCAM-1 mRNA were developed by Uddin et al., who aimed to detect this molecule, thus assessing the occurrence of oxidative stress [147]. The fluorescence in-situ hybridization (FISH) technique was used to perform photothermal-optical coherence tomography (PT-OCT) involving a fluorescent probe (Alexafluor-647) bonded to 3' end of anti-sense DNA in order to highlight its interaction with the target mRNA. The conjugation of anti-sense DNA to gold nanoparticles proved to protect from the degradation performed by DNase while enhancing the uptake, probably through endocytosis, as suggested by transmission electron microscopic (TEM) images of retinal cells; moreover, it was verified that no inference in the fluorescence was produced due to low pH, which is characteristic of inflamed tissues. Compared to the control group, in vivo systemic injection in mice confirmed the enhancement in the fluorescent signal for anti-sense DNA coupled with nanoparticles, which mostly depended on VCAM-1 mRNA hybridization, thus demonstrating the potentiality of the developed platform as a tool to obtain direct images of endogenous mRNA in a tissue. In some cases, this pathology requires transplantation of photoreceptor precursors (PRPs) in the subretinal space, which was successfully performed, guaranteeing a certain vision restoration [148]. For a certain period, monitoring of the efficiency of the transplantations needs to be performed. As confirmed by Chemla and coworkers [149], gold nanoparticles could be transplanted together with photoreceptor precursors cells labeled with a fluorescent probe (Alexa 594) in order to ameliorate the efficiency of computed tomography (CT) and optical coherence tomography (OCT) in assessing the success of the transplant. The nanoparticles were firstly characterized in order to assess their safety, thus demonstrating no toxicity toward the transplanted cells and no occurrence of inflammation in the retina and vitreous. Furthermore, this platform demonstrated to enhance X-ray signal detected by CT and related to cell survival without interference from the particles secreted from the cells [150]; moreover, they were also able to increase optical signal for OCT by up to 1.4-fold and track cells migration toward layers deeper than the injection site. These results confirm the efficiency of such a platform in the monitoring of transplantation but also suggest a potential use for ameliorating existent molecular imaging in cell therapy and diagnostic. Another important diagnostic test is fundus fluorescein angiography (FFA), which allows highlighting vascular leakages in retinal and choroidal pathologies [151]. This clinical tool is useful to diagnose several ocular diseases: age-related macular degeneration, which is characterized by hemorrhaging and exudation in the retina [140]; diabetic retinopathy, which involves retinal damages related to microvascular modification which are clinically not revealable in the early stages [152]; diabetic macular edema, whose pathophysiology implicates modifications of choroidal and retinal vasculature due to BRB impairment [153]. Furthermore, the aforementioned diseases are characterized by alterations of ocular vessels, and share the consequent compromission of visual activity, if not quickly detected and treated. Fluorescein sodium (FS) is injected intravenously to perform this analysis, diffusing in the blood vessels, thus allowing us to observe them through a confocal scanning laser ophthalmoscopy system. Despite it being considered relatively safe, nausea and vomiting frequently occur, while severe effects such as anaphylaxis are rare. The main drawbacks are the diffusion of FS into normal tissues and cellular absorption, with long retention, which were overcome using nanoparticles. Cai et al. coworkers developed a high molecular weight polyethyleneimine (PEI) nanoparticles which demonstrated to successfully couple fluorescein [151]; moreover, in vitro studies showed good cytocompatibility, no significant difference in apoptosis rates considering various concentration tested, no genotoxicity, and no morphological changes or significant difference in endothelial tube formation. Cellular uptake assays, carried on with different concentrations of free FS and FS-NP, confirmed similar rapid uptake by cells, with a concentration-dependent and time-dependent fluorescence of main retinal vessels and microvessels. Furthermore, free FS was longer retained in cells when compared to FS-NP, as highlighted by in vivo fluorescence studies, suggesting a potential decrease in FS toxicity. These results confirm the potentiality of this platform as a diagnostic tool to detect retinal vessels; moreover, PEI enhances fluorescein metabolism, thus reducing its toxicity. Other polymeric nanoparticles developed as a potential diagnostic tool are composed of copolymerized glycerol mono methacrylate (GMMA), glycidyl methacrylate (GME) and ethylene glycol dimethacrylate (EGDMA), which were functionalized with Vancomycin, Polymyxin B or Amphotericin B, in order to detect the presence of Gram-positive bacteria, Gram-negative bacteria and fungi through a specific bond with the respective antibiotic or antimycotic [154]. The occurrence of such bonds was differently highlighted using fluorescent Vancomycin, and probes such as fluorescein isothiocyanate (FITC) and Calcofluor White. Tests conducted on various microbiological strains showed a proportional increase in the fluorescence signal with the increase in the number of organisms involved; moreover, the presence of functionalized polymers favored the microorganism bonding. Besides the biocompatibility of this platform, another advantage of this platform is the possibility to be shaped as a contact lens requiring only a 30-min exposure to efficiently detect the occurrence of infection, thus demonstrating to be a promising approach for an easy diagnosis of corneal infections.

3.3. Nanotheranostics

The recent development of systems that integrate the treatment of diseases with their diagnostics is referred to as theranostics. When the system is in a nanoscale range, it is called nanotheranostics. Figure 5 shows prototypes of nanosystems suitable for theranostic purposes.

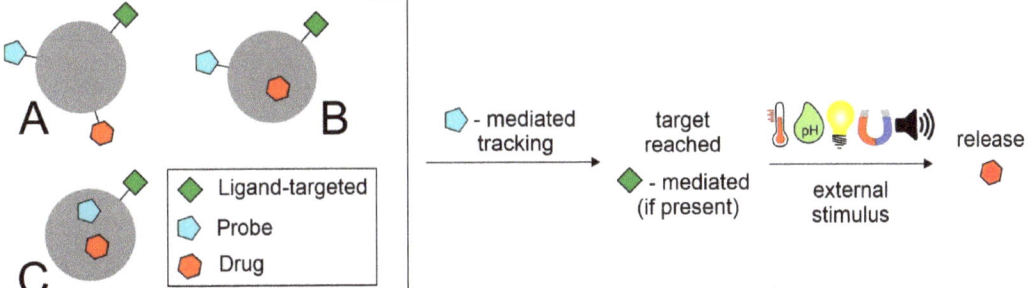

Figure 5. Prototypes of theranostic nanosystems and their mechanism of action. In figure: (**A**) labeling of both probe and drug; (**B**) loading of drug and labeling of probe; (**C**) co-loading of drug and probe.

The development of these applications has given researchers a new way of diagnosing and treating diseases such as cancer, diabetic retinopathy and age-related macular degeneration [37,155]. Among the major chronic eye diseases, diabetic retinopathy is the most prevalent. Angiogenesis in the posterior eye segment is the main cause of retinal impairment. Clinical management consists of pathological diagnosis and intravitreal injections of vascular endothelial growth factor (VEGF) inhibitors to suppress neovascularization. The development of innovative nanotheranostic systems is emerging to overcome these critical problems with less invasive methods to diagnose and treat ocular angiogenesis synergistically. Silicon nanoparticles conjugated to the peptide Cyclo-(Arg-Gly-Asp-d-Tyr-Cys) (c-(RGDyC)) (SiNP-RGD) were designed by Tang et al. with the dual action of imaging and treating ocular neovascularization. The effective anti-angiogenic capability of these biocompatible theranostic nanoprobes was based on the combination of a specific detection by labeling endothelial cells and angiogenic blood vessels and a selective inhibition of neovascularization [156]. Metal NPs are receiving a lot of attention as carriers for the delivery of biomolecules, among which silver NPs (AgNPs) have found numerous applications. Stati et al. designed curcumin stabilized AgNPs using a green and cost-effective method to exploit the promising characteristics of this polyphenol in the in vivo treatment of human pterygo. Curcumin is a molecule suitable for theranostic application, as widely reported in the work of Shabbir et al. [157]. Pterygo is a progressive eye disease that could culminate in an irreversible impairment of visual function. Available treatments require invasive surgical procedures, such as excision, which often leads to a worsening of the clinical picture. Spectroscopic techniques revealed a strong plasmonic resonance between the silver nuclei and the curcumin molecule, demonstrating the presence of the polyphenol on the surface of AgNPs. The biological efficacy of the formulation was tested in vitro on human keratinocytes derived from pterygium explants, showing decreased cell viability in treated samples compared to controls. Although no studies have been conducted to track the fate of NPs, the fluorescent emission of the samples could be exploited for bioimaging applications [158]. Fluorescent silicon nanoparticles modified with Vancomycin were designed by Zhang et al. for the simultaneous non-invasive diagnosis and treatment of keratitis induced by Gram-positive bacteria. These nanotheranostic agents have demonstrated, in combination with strong antimicrobial activity against *Staphylococcus aureus*, a rapid (<10 min) imaging capability both in vitro and in vivo. The rapidity with which bacterial keratitis was diagnosed at an early stage suggests that these devices may be useful in preventing the progress of the disease, which could impair visual function if not treated [159]. Oliveira et al. designed hybrid theranostic systems consisting of a lipid matrix of 1,2-dipalmitoyl-sn-glycero-3-phosphatidylcholine (DPPC), coated with Pluronic® F127, covalently bound with the fluorescent probe 5(6)-carboxyfluorescein and loaded with the photosensitizing agent verteporfin. Preliminary studies on a glioblastoma cell line (T98G) were conducted to evaluate the potential application as theranostic nanodevices. The fluorescence of the systems revealed on the cancer cell membrane and the 98% reduction in cell viability of T98G cells encouraged further investigation of such multifunctional platforms for the treatment and diagnosis of ophthalmic diseases [160]. Photothermal therapy has been making inroads into the eye sector for a couple of years now. Heat therapy refers to the use of heat as a therapeutic tool to treat diseases such as tumors. In the recent work of Li et al., an approach to treat choroidal melanoma using nanocomposites was designed. Nanosystems were synthesized based on hydrogel, which is itself based on rare-earth nanoparticles. These platforms emit fluorescence in an NIR-II region. Characterized by their tiny size of less than 5 nm, they are targeted for the treatment and simultaneous bioimaging of choroidal melanoma. They have been incorporated into biodegradable hydrogels based on PNIPAM dual response, which could release the drug in a controlled manner by responding to heat and glutathione in the tumor microenvironment. The nanocomposites were then further decorated with indocyanine green (ICS) and folic acid (FA) to enhance therapeutically and to target specificity and the possibility of achieving photothermal therapy [161]. A lot of studies showed the potential of therapeutic contact lenses in the management of eye disease [162]. Infectious endophthalmitis is a growing concern that causes irreversible damage to intraocular tissue and the optic nerve. The work of Huang et al. focuses on the design of contact lenses consisting of hybrid hydrogels based on quaternized chitosan composite (HTCC), silver nanoparticles and graphene oxide (GO). Fungal keratitis infection often leads to the formation of a biofilm, which is particularly difficult to be penetrated by antifungal agents, especially through eye drops. In addition, the bioavailability of a drug such as Voriconazole is very limited. The function of these nanoparticles is not only to deliver Voriconazole in the treatment of fungal keratitis, but also to act as an antimicrobial agent due to its properties. In fact, the materials used, such as quaternized chitosan, have inherent antimicrobial capabilities. The dual functionality makes this system a useful theranostic approach for the treatment of eye infections [163]. The study by Jin et al. reports a therapeutic nanoplatform based on UiO-66-NH$_2$ to combine photodynamic therapy (PDT) and targeting lipopolysaccharides (LPS) through polypeptide modification (YVLWKRKFCFI-NH$_2$). The fluorescent used was Toluidine blue (TB), which acted as a photosensitiser (PS) and was loaded into UiO-66-NH$_2$ nanoparticles (NPs). The dye acts both as a tracer and as a therapeutic agent through photodynamics. The release of the fluorescent is pH-dependent. The study proved beneficial against *Pseudomonas aeruginosa* and *Staphylococcus epidermidis*, and the in vivo model showed positive results in the treatment of endophthalmitis [164].

4. Fluorescent Status for Ocular Therapies in Clinical Trials and Market

Scientific progress in the field of ocular nanomedicine is constantly advancing, many nanoformulations for the treatment of ophthalmic diseases have been clinically investigated, and some have already been introduced to the market. A list of nanomedicines for eye diseases in clinical trials and approved by the Food and Drug Administration (FDA) is discussed in the review provided by Khiev et al. [165].

Novel nanosystems on the market included NorFLO, a dietary supplement based on a patented curcuma-phospholipid formula (iphytoone®). Phospholipids enhanced the targeted distribution of curcumin in the eye, and the efficacy of the formulation has been demonstrated in over 40 studies in processes triggered or sustained by chronic inflammation, found to be the cause of many eye diseases. Prolidofta is another supplement marketed as an ocular spray to counteract inflammatory processes affecting the palpebral component and restore any functional and structural changes. This spray consists of small vesicles (50–500 nm) made up of a double layer of phospholipids surrounding an aqueous core for the delivery of vitamins A and E. OMK1-LF is an ophthalmic liposomal solution based on citicolin, an endogenous molecule that restores the damage caused by glaucoma in the cell membranes and hyaluronic acid, which acts to hydrate, protect and lubricate the tear film. TriMix is an eye drop with cross-linked Hyaluronic Acid, Trehalose and Stearylamine Liposome indicated to counteract dryness and eye irritation.

Regarding imaging in surgery, near-infrared fluorescence (NIRF) with the dye indocyanine green has been widely used. Indocyanine green (ICG) is a clinically approved NIRF dye in ophthalmology for imaging retinal blood vessels; an overview of surgical applications using indocyanine green fluorescence imaging has been proposed by Alander et al. [166]. Based on clinicaltrials.gov, a website database of clinical trials conducted around the world (as accessed on 1 April 2022), since 2010 fluorescence imaging has been used in clinical trials to assess the integrity or damage of ocular surfaces after administration of novel nanosystems. Green dye fluorescein was used in 13 clinical trials for the evaluation of nanosystems with different ocular indications, from dry eye to autoimmune Sjögren's syndrome. The role of the dye and details of the studies are given in Table 3.

Table 3. Use of Fluorescein dye in clinical trials of drug delivery systems for eye diseases.

Role of Molecule in the Study	Name and Type of Formulation Tested	Name of the Study	Pathologies	Status	Identified Number of the Study
Evaluate corneal and conjunctival damage	LAMELLEYE Liposomal suspension	Lamelleye vs. Comparator for the Treatment of Dry Eye Disease	Dry Eye Syndromes	Completed	NCT03052140
Evaluate tear break up time and corneal damage	AQUORAL LIPO (liposomal solution) in contact lens	Efficacy of "Aquoral Lipo" Artificial Tears in Contact Lens Wearers With Discomfort	Contact Lens Complication	New study (March, 2022) not yet recruiting	NCT05290727
Evaluate corneal and conjunctival damage	LAMELLEYE Liposomal suspension	LAMELLEYE for the Treatment of Dry Eye Symptoms in pSS Patients	Primary Sjögren Syndrome	Unknown	NCT03140111
Evaluate corneal damage	LIPOSIC AND TEARS NATURALE FORTE (liposomal suspension)	Comparison of the Effects of Two Tear Substitutes in Patients with Dry Eye Syndrome	Dry eye	Completed	NCT03211351
Evaluate ocular surface damage	TEARS AGAIN (liposomal spray)	Dry Eye Treatment with Artificial Tears	Dry eye	Completed	NCT02420834

Table 3. Cont.

Role of Molecule in the Study	Name and Type of Formulation Tested	Name of the Study	Pathologies	Status	Identified Number of the Study
Evaluate the absence of anterior chamber cells	OCS-01 (Dexamethasone Cyclodextrin Nanoparticle Ophthalmic Suspension 1.5%)	OCS-01 in Treating Inflammation and Pain in Post-cataract Patients (SKYGGN)	Inflammation and pain following cataract surgery	Completed	NCT04130802
Evaluate corneal damage	Intravenous Administration of Secukinumab (AIN457) or Canakinumab (ACZ885) solution	The Effects of a Single Intravenous Administration of Secukinumab (AIN457) or Canakinumab (ACZ885) in Dry Eye Patients	Dry eye	Completed	NCT01250171
Evaluate corneal and conjunctival damages	Tanfanercept (HL036) Topical Ophthalmic Solution	A Study to Assess the Efficacy and Safety of Tanfanercept (HL036) Ophthalmic Solution in Participants With Dry Eye (VELOS-3)	Dry eye	Recruiting. Phase III	NCT05109702
Evaluate conjunctival damage	HL036 0.10 percent (%) ophthalmic solution as topical ophthalmic drops	A Study to Assess Efficacy of HL036 in Subjects With Dry Eyes (VELOS-1)	Dry eye	Completed. Phase II	NCT03334539
Evaluate changes in inferior cornea	NCX 4251 (fluticasone propionate nanocrystal)	Study Evaluating the Safety and Efficacy of NCX 4251 Ophthalmic Suspension for the Treatment of Blepharitis	Blepharitis	Completed	NCT04675242
Evaluate tear film break-up time	SYSTANE® Complete Nanoemulsion ocular lubricant (Propylene glycol-based eye drops)	Study of Efficacy and Tolerability of SYSTANE Complete in Patients with Dry Eye Disease	Dry eye	Completed	NCT03492541
Evaluate corneal damage	TJO-087 Cyclosporine ophthalmic Nanoemulsion (0.08%)	Evaluating the Efficacy and Safety of TJO-087 in Moderate to Severe Dry Eye Disease Patients	Dry eye	Recruiting	NCT05245604
Evaluate corneal damage	OCU300 Brimonidine Tartrate Nanoemulsion	Study of Brimonidine Tartrate Nanoemulsion Eye Drops in Patients With Ocular Graft-vs-Host Disease	Ocular Graft Versus Host Disease	Completed	NCT03591874

Fluorescence for the development and clinical investigation of innovative ocular nanosystems seems to be a promising strategy to increase the number of formulations able to reach market commercialization. In Table 4, few products with fluorescein approved by the FDA are reported.

Table 4. FDA-approved products with fluorescein.

Name	Active Ingredients	Company	Description	NDA
Altafluor Benox	Benoxinate Hydrochloride; Fluorescein Sodium (0.4%; 0.25%)	Altaire Pharms Inc. (Aquibogue, NY, USA)	Solution/Drops; Ophthalmic	208582
Fluorescein Sodium And Benoxinate Hydrochloride	Benoxinate Hydrochloride; Fluorescein Sodium (0.4%; 0.3%)	Bausch & Lomb (Dublin, Ireland)	Solution/Drops; Ophthalmic	211039

5. Challenges and Future Perspectives

The growing number of people who have blindness and visual impairment indicates a continuous increase in the need for care and treatment. Given this evidence, urgent action is required to address this largely preventable global problem and provide adequate eye care services. There are still many gaps in the literature regarding optimal design and traffic pathways within the eye. In particular, further research is needed to unravel the transport mechanisms across certain barriers in the eye. Moreover, rapid clearance remains a challenge for nanosystems as they need to release their payload before being eliminated from the eye. Many studies focus on assessing the distribution in various tissues once the formulation has been instilled into the eye [106–132,134,137–139]. Unfortunately, few studies focus on assessing how mechanisms including blinking, tear drainage and ocular metabolism may interact with nanosystems [66,115]. Among other things, a very important aspect is the evaluation of the toxicity and the actual applicability of these systems. In fact, many of them are quite complex, and the applicability, especially in the theranostic field, is not entirely easy. The evaluation has to be as precise as possible because many eye studies use rodent models; this is highly questionable, especially in the quantification of distribution and kinetic properties of nanoparticles in the eye, as there are many significant differences between the rodent and human eye. Therefore, the most impactful future studies on this topic will come from larger animal models with eyes that are physiologically and anatomically more similar to ours.

The increasing use of fluorescent probes in the realization of biosensors for colorimetric and radiometric identification of specific targets is a great step forward since the fluorescence represents a non-invasive diagnostic method. This has important benefits in early diagnosis through self-medication screening based on membranes or other platforms containing the appropriate fluorescent probe. These tools are also applicable in epidemics through the realization of specific self-tests based on ELISA or other strategies able to identify the etiological agent selectively. A large and growing field is the use of these probes as part of theranostic photo switch structures, able to change their structure after light stimulus, releasing the therapeutic agent and activating or switching off the fluorescence of the probe. Thus, fluorescence allows accurate and quantitative identification (under certain conditions even by the naked eye as also through in vitro tests) of the drug release process. Therefore, the use of fluorescent probes is finding increasing use in experimental and advanced ocular chemotherapy using photo-activated systems.

6. Conclusions

The eye has a complex anatomical structure, representing the main difficulty for drugs to achieve this target. Nanomedicine has made it possible to overcome several difficulties related to the administration of this almost isolated compartment. The study of the pathways followed by the nanosystems makes it possible to assess the effective achievement of the target site and to consider any non-productive distribution in undesirable tissues with the possible onset of side effects. The biodistribution study also allows the correlation between the chemico-physical parameters of the nanosystems (e.g., ZP, size, morphology, mucoadhesive properties, etc.) and the paths followed by them. This investigation is also aimed at evaluating and developing strategies to bypass physiological barriers of the eye, including tight junctions, tearing and blinking, that could compromise targeting effectiveness. The development of bioimaging mediated by fluorescent probes has improved the efficiency of some diagnostic tests for eye diseases. It is known that early (or rather preventive) diagnosis is a necessity to limit the damage, especially in the long term, caused by specific diseases. The involvement of fluorescent nanoparticles as diagnostics demonstrated to be suitable for detecting the occurrence of pathological pathways, ameliorating techniques already employed in ocular diagnostic, thus providing better results through equipment of common use (OCT, CT, FFA, etc.). This is where the important contribution of fluorescent probes to nanotheranostic approaches becomes relevant since, in these systems, diagnostic and therapy coexist. Tracking the nanoparticles makes it possible to highlight the effective achievement of the target, thus following the release of the therapeutic agent through an external stimulus (e.g., ultrasounds, magnetic fields, light, etc.). In conclusion, as highlighted in this review, the potential applications of fluorescence in the ocular field have been demonstrated as a useful strategy for translating nanoformulations into marketable drug candidates. In addition, to the best of our knowledge, there are no reviews focused on this topic, so this work aims to raise awareness and summarize the use of fluorescents in the ocular field.

Author Contributions: Conceptualization, R.P.; data curation, C.C. (Cinzia Cimino), S.R., A.R. and E.Z.; writing—original draft preparation, C.C. (Cinzia Cimino), A.R. and E.Z.; writing—review and editing, A.B., C.C. (Claudia Carbone), T.M. and R.P.; visualization C.C. (Cinzia Cimino) and E.Z.; funding, T.M.; supervision, R.P.; project administration, R.P. All authors have read and agreed to the published version of the manuscript.

Funding: The work was partially financed under the 3N-ORACLE project (University of Catania, PIACERI—Linea 2 funding program 2020–2022).

Institutional Review Board Statement: Not applicable.

Informed Consent Statement: Not applicable.

Data Availability Statement: Not applicable.

Acknowledgments: C.C. (Cinzia Cimino) was supported by the PhD program in Biotechnology, XXXVI cycle, University of Catania; A.R. was supported by the International PhD program in Neurosciences, XXXV cycle, University of Catania and E.Z. was supported by the International PhD program in Neurosciences, XXXVII cycle, University of Catania. A.B. is a researcher at the University of Catania within the EU-funded PON REACT project (Azione IV.4—"Dottorati e contratti di ricerca su tematiche dell'innovazione", nuovo Asse IV del PON Ricerca e Innovazione 2014–2020 "Istruzione e ricerca per il recupero—REACT—EU"; Progetto "Approcci terapeutici innovativi per il targeting cerebrale di farmaci e materiale genico", CUP E65F21002640005).

Conflicts of Interest: The authors declare no conflict of interest.

References

1. Flaxman, S.R.; Bourne, R.R.A.; Resnikoff, S.; Ackland, P.; Braithwaite, T.; Cicinelli, M.V.; Das, A.; Jonas, J.B.; Keeffe, J.; Kempen, J.; et al. Global causes of blindness and distance vision impairment 1990–2020: A systematic review and meta-analysis. *Lancet Glob. Health* **2017**, *5*, e1221–e1234. [CrossRef]
2. Marques, A.P.; Ramke, J.; Cairns, J.; Butt, T.; Zhang, J.H.; Muirhead, D.; Jones, I.; Tong, B.A.M.A.; Swenor, B.K.; Faal, H.; et al. Global economic productivity losses from vision impairment and blindness. *EClinicalMedicine* **2021**, *35*, 100852. [CrossRef]
3. Nagarajan, N.; Assi, L.; Varadaraj, V.; Motaghi, M.; Sun, Y.; Couser, E.; Ehrlich, J.R.; Whitson, H.; Swenor, B.K. Vision impairment and cognitive decline among older adults: A systematic review. *BMJ Open* **2022**, *12*, e047929. [CrossRef] [PubMed]
4. Lorenzo-Veiga, B.; Alvarez-Lorenzo, C.; Loftsson, T.; Sigurdsson, H.H. Age-related ocular conditions: Current treatments and role of cyclodextrin-based nanotherapies. *Int. J. Pharm.* **2021**, *603*, 120707. [CrossRef] [PubMed]
5. Pacheco, E.; Lips, M.; Yoong, P. Transition 2.0: Digital technologies, higher education, and vision impairment. *Internet High. Educ.* **2018**, *37*, 1–10. [CrossRef]
6. Bourne, R.R.A.; Steinmetz, J.D.; Saylan, M.; Mersha, A.M.; Weldemariam, A.H.; Wondmeneh, T.G.; Sreeramareddy, C.T.; Pinheiro, M.; Yaseri, M.; Yu, C.; et al. Causes of blindness and vision impairment in 2020 and trends over 30 years, and prevalence of avoidable blindness in relation to VISION 2020: The Right to Sight: An analysis for the Global Burden of Disease Study. *Lancet Glob. Health* **2021**, *9*, e144–e160. [CrossRef]
7. Lyu, Q.; Peng, L.; Hong, X.; Fan, T.; Li, J.; Cui, Y.; Zhang, H.; Zhao, J. Smart nano-micro platforms for ophthalmological applications: The state-of-the-art and future perspectives. *Biomaterials* **2021**, *270*, 120682. [CrossRef] [PubMed]
8. Kels, B.D.; Grzybowski, A.; Grant-Kels, J.M. Human ocular anatomy. *Clin. Dermatol.* **2015**, *33*, 140–146. [CrossRef]
9. Jonas, J.B.; Ohno-Matsui, K.; Panda-Jonas, S. Myopia: Anatomic changes and consequences for its etiology. *Asia-Pac. J. Ophthalmol.* **2019**, *8*, 355–359. [CrossRef] [PubMed]
10. Lindfield, D.; Das-Bhaumik, R. Emergency department management of penetrating eye injuries. *Int. Emerg. Nurs.* **2009**, *17*, 155–160. [CrossRef] [PubMed]
11. Maulvi, F.A.; Shetty, K.H.; Desai, D.T.; Shah, D.O.; Willcox, M.D.P. Recent advances in ophthalmic preparations: Ocular barriers, dosage forms and routes of administration. *Int. J. Pharm.* **2021**, *608*, 121105. [CrossRef] [PubMed]
12. Suri, R.; Beg, S.; Kohli, K. Target strategies for drug delivery bypassing ocular barriers. *J. Drug Deliv. Sci. Technol.* **2020**, *55*, 101389. [CrossRef]
13. Varela-Fernández, R.; Díaz-Tomé, V.; Luaces-Rodríguez, A.; Conde-Penedo, A.; García-Otero, X.; Luzardo-álvarez, A.; Fernández-Ferreiro, A.; Otero-Espinar, F.J. Drug delivery to the posterior segment of the eye: Biopharmaceutic and pharmacokinetic considerations. *Pharmaceutics* **2020**, *12*, 269. [CrossRef]
14. Madni, A.; Rahem, M.A.; Tahir, N.; Sarfraz, M.; Jabar, A.; Rehman, M.; Kashif, P.M.; Badshah, S.F.; Khan, K.U.; Santos, H.A. Non-invasive strategies for targeting the posterior segment of eye. *Int. J. Pharm.* **2017**, *530*, 326–345. [CrossRef] [PubMed]
15. Bansal, P.; Garg, S.; Sharma, Y.; Venkatesh, P. Posterior Segment Drug Delivery Devices: Current and Novel Therapies in Development. *J. Ocul. Pharmacol. Ther.* **2016**, *32*, 135–144. [CrossRef] [PubMed]
16. Kamaleddin, M.A. Nano-ophthalmology: Applications and considerations. *Nanomed. Nanotechnol. Biol. Med.* **2017**, *13*, 1459–1472. [CrossRef]

17. Yorston, D. Intravitreal injection technique. *Community Eye Health J.* **2014**, *27*, 47. [CrossRef]
18. Seah, I.; Zhao, X.; Lin, Q.; Liu, Z.; Su, S.Z.Z.; Yuen, Y.S.; Hunziker, W.; Lingam, G.; Loh, X.J.; Su, X. Use of biomaterials for sustained delivery of anti-VEGF to treat retinal diseases. *Eye* **2020**, *34*, 1341–1356. [CrossRef] [PubMed]
19. Jumelle, C.; Gholizadeh, S.; Annabi, N.; Dana, R. Advances and limitations of drug delivery systems formulated as eye drops. *J. Control. Release* **2020**, *321*, 1–22. [CrossRef] [PubMed]
20. Shiels, A.; Hejtmancik, J.F. Biology of Inherited Cataracts and Opportunities for Treatment. *Annu. Rev. Vis. Sci.* **2019**, *5*, 123–149. [CrossRef]
21. Al-Ghananeem, A.M.; Crooks, P.A. Phase I and phase II ocular metabolic activities and the role of metabolism in ophthalmic prodrug and codrug design and delivery. *Molecules* **2007**, *12*, 373–388. [CrossRef]
22. Tang, Z.; Fan, X.; Chen, Y.; Gu, P. Ocular Nanomedicine. *Adv. Sci.* **2022**, *2003699*, 1–36. [CrossRef] [PubMed]
23. Leonardi, A.; Bucolo, C.; Drago, F.; Salomone, S.; Pignatello, R. Cationic solid lipid nanoparticles enhance ocular hypotensive effect of melatonin in rabbit. *Int. J. Pharm.* **2015**, *478*, 180–186. [CrossRef] [PubMed]
24. Burhan, A.M.; Klahan, B.; Cummins, W.; Andrés-Guerrero, V.; Byrne, M.E.; O'reilly, N.J.; Chauhan, A.; Fitzhenry, L.; Hughes, H. Posterior segment ophthalmic drug delivery: Role of muco-adhesion with a special focus on chitosan. *Pharmaceutics* **2021**, *13*, 1685. [CrossRef] [PubMed]
25. Gautam, D.; Pedler, M.G.; Nair, D.P.; Petrash, J.M. Nanogel-facilitated in-situ delivery of a cataract inhibitor. *Biomolecules* **2021**, *11*, 1150. [CrossRef]
26. Gagandeep, G.T.; Malik, B.; Rath, G.; Goyal, A.K. Development and characterization of nano-fiber patch for the treatment of glaucoma. *Eur. J. Pharm. Sci.* **2014**, *53*, 10–16. [CrossRef] [PubMed]
27. Ghosh, A.K.; Thapa, R.; Hariani, H.N.; Volyanyuk, M.; Ogle, S.D.; Orloff, K.A.; Ankireddy, S.; Lai, K.; Žiniauskaitė, A.; Stubbs, E.B.; et al. Poly(Lactic-co-glycolic acid) nanoparticles encapsulating the prenylated flavonoid, xanthohumol, protect corneal epithelial cells from dry eye disease-associated oxidative stress. *Pharmaceutics* **2021**, *13*, 1362. [CrossRef] [PubMed]
28. Shi, L.; Li, Z.; Liang, Z.; Zhang, J.; Liu, R.; Chu, D.; Han, L.; Zhu, L.; Shen, J.; Li, J. A dual-functional chitosan derivative platform for fungal keratitis. *Carbohydr. Polym.* **2022**, *275*, 118762. [CrossRef]
29. Liu, Y.C.; Lin, M.T.Y.; Ng, A.H.C.; Wong, T.T.; Mehta, J.S. Nanotechnology for the treatment of allergic conjunctival diseases. *Pharmaceuticals* **2020**, *13*, 351. [CrossRef]
30. Nirbhavane, P.; Sharma, G.; Singh, B.; Begum, G.; Jones, M.C.; Rauz, S.; Vincent, R.; Denniston, A.K.; Hill, L.J.; Katare, O.P. Triamcinolone acetonide loaded-cationic nano-lipoidal formulation for uveitis: Evidences of improved biopharmaceutical performance and anti-inflammatory activity. *Colloids Surfaces B Biointerfaces* **2020**, *190*, 110902. [CrossRef]
31. Du, S.; Wang, H.; Jiang, F.; Wang, Y. Diabetic Retinopathy Analysis—Effects of Nanoparticle-Based Triamcinolone. *J. Nanosci. Nanotechnol.* **2020**, *20*, 6111–6115. [CrossRef] [PubMed]
32. Suri, R.; Neupane, Y.R.; Mehra, N.; Nematullah, M.; Khan, F.; Alam, O.; Iqubal, A.; Jain, G.K.; Kohli, K. Sirolimus loaded chitosan functionalized poly (lactic-co-glycolic acid) (PLGA) nanoparticles for potential treatment of age-related macular degeneration. *Int. J. Biol. Macromol.* **2021**, *191*, 548–559. [CrossRef] [PubMed]
33. Youssef, A.; Dudhipala, N.; Majumdar, S. Ciprofloxacin Loaded Nanostructured Lipid Carriers Incorporated into In-Situ Gels to Improve Management of Bacterial Endophthalmitis. *Pharmaceutics* **2020**, *12*, 572. [CrossRef] [PubMed]
34. Tabatabaei, S.N.; Derbali, R.M.; Yang, C.; Superstein, R.; Hamel, P.; Chain, J.L.; Hardy, P. Co-delivery of miR-181a and melphalan by lipid nanoparticles for treatment of seeded retinoblastoma. *J. Control. Release* **2019**, *298*, 177–185. [CrossRef] [PubMed]
35. Allyn, M.M.; Luo, R.H.; Hellwarth, E.B.; Swindle-Reilly, K.E. Considerations for Polymers Used in Ocular Drug Delivery. *Front. Med.* **2022**, *8*, 1–25. [CrossRef]
36. Toropainen, E.; Fraser-Miller, S.J.; Novakovic, D.; Del Amo, E.M.; Vellonen, K.S.; Ruponen, M.; Viitala, T.; Korhonen, O.; Auriola, S.; Hellinen, L.; et al. Biopharmaceutics of topical ophthalmic suspensions: Importance of viscosity and particle size in ocular absorption of indomethacin. *Pharmaceutics* **2021**, *13*, 452. [CrossRef]
37. Divya, K.; Yashwant, V.P.; Kevin, B.S. Theranostic Applications of Nanomaterials for Ophthalmic Applications. *Int. J. Sci. Adv.* **2021**, *2*, 354–364. [CrossRef]
38. Awwad, S.; Mohamed Ahmed, A.H.A.; Sharma, G.; Heng, J.S.; Khaw, P.T.; Brocchini, S.; Lockwood, A. Principles of pharmacology in the eye. *Br. J. Pharmacol.* **2017**, *174*, 4205–4223. [CrossRef]
39. Dosmar, E.; Walsh, J.; Doyel, M.; Bussett, K.; Oladipupo, A.; Amer, S.; Goebel, K. Targeting Ocular Drug Delivery: An Examination of Local Anatomy and Current Approaches. *Bioengineering* **2022**, *9*, 41. [CrossRef]
40. Atta, G.; Tempfer, H.; Kaser-Eichberger, A.; Traweger, A.; Heindl, L.M.; Schroedl, F. Is the human sclera a tendon-like tissue? A structural and functional comparison. *Ann. Anat.* **2022**, *240*, 151858. [CrossRef]
41. Lopes, B.T.; Bao, F.; Wang, J.; Liu, X.; Wang, L.; Abass, A.; Eliasy, A.; Elsheikh, A. Review of in-vivo characterisation of corneal biomechanics. *Med. Nov. Technol. Devices* **2021**, *11*, 100073. [CrossRef]
42. Zénon, A. Eye pupil signals information gain. *Proc. R. Soc. B Biol. Sci.* **2019**, *286*, 20191593. [CrossRef] [PubMed]
43. Domkin, D.; Forsman, M.; Richter, H.O. Effect of ciliary-muscle contraction force on trapezius muscle activity during computer mouse work. *Eur. J. Appl. Physiol.* **2019**, *119*, 389–397. [CrossRef] [PubMed]
44. Chow, L.S.; Paley, M.N.J. Recent advances on optic nerve magnetic resonance imaging and post-processing. *Magn. Reson. Imaging* **2021**, *79*, 76–84. [CrossRef]

45. Kaur, I.P.; Smitha, R.; Aggarwal, D.; Kapil, M. Acetazolamide: Future perspective in topical glaucoma therapeutics. *Int. J. Pharm.* **2002**, *248*, 1–14. [CrossRef]
46. Nielsen, L.H.; Keller, S.S.; Boisen, A. Microfabricated devices for oral drug delivery. *Lab Chip* **2018**, *18*, 2348–2358. [CrossRef]
47. Underhill, G.H.; Khetani, S.R. Advances in engineered human liver platforms for drug metabolism studies. *Drug Metab. Dispos.* **2018**, *46*, 1626–1637. [CrossRef]
48. Pitkänen, L.; Ranta, V.P.; Moilanen, H.; Urtti, A. Permeability of retinal pigment epithelium: Effects of permeant molecular weight and lipophilicity. *Investig. Ophthalmol. Vis. Sci.* **2005**, *46*, 641–646. [CrossRef]
49. Reinholz, J.; Landfester, K.; Mailänder, V. The challenges of oral drug delivery via nanocarriers. *Drug Deliv.* **2018**, *25*, 1694–1705. [CrossRef]
50. Kim, Y.C.; Chiang, B.; Wu, X.; Prausnitz, M.R. Ocular delivery of macromolecules. *J. Control. Release* **2014**, *190*, 172–181. [CrossRef]
51. Urtti, A. Challenges and obstacles of ocular pharmacokinetics and drug delivery. *Adv. Drug Deliv. Rev.* **2006**, *58*, 1131–1135. [CrossRef] [PubMed]
52. Falavarjani, K.G.; Nguyen, Q.D. Adverse events and complications associated with intravitreal injection of anti-VEGF agents: A review of literature. *Eye* **2013**, *27*, 787–794. [CrossRef] [PubMed]
53. Ibrahim, S.S. The Role of Surface Active Agents in Ophthalmic Drug Delivery: A Comprehensive Review. *J. Pharm. Sci.* **2019**, *108*, 1923–1933. [CrossRef]
54. Liebmann, J.M.; Barton, K.; Weinreb, R.N.; Eichenbaum, D.A.; Gupta, P.K.; McCabe, C.M.; Wolfe, J.D.; Ahmed, I.; Sheybani, A.; Craven, E.R. Evolving Guidelines for Intracameral Injection. *J. Glaucoma* **2020**, *29*, 1–7. [CrossRef] [PubMed]
55. Takahashi, K.; Morizane, Y.; Hisatomi, T.; Tachibana, T.; Kimura, S.; Hosokawa, M.M.; Shiode, Y.; Hirano, M.; Doi, S.; Toshima, S.; et al. The influence of subretinal injection pressure on the microstructure of the monkey retina. *PLoS ONE* **2018**, *13*, e0209996. [CrossRef] [PubMed]
56. Sebbag, L.; Moody, L.M.; Mochel, J.P. Albumin levels in tear film modulate the bioavailability of medically-relevant topical drugs. *Front. Pharmacol.* **2020**, *10*, 1–9. [CrossRef] [PubMed]
57. Järvinen, K.; Järvinen, T.; Urtti, A. Ocular absorption following topical delivery. *Adv. Drug Deliv. Rev.* **1995**, *16*, 3–19. [CrossRef]
58. Patere, S.; Newman, B.; Wang, Y.; Choi, S.; Vora, S.; Ma, A.W.K.; Jay, M.; Lu, X. Influence of Manufacturing Process Variables on the Properties of Ophthalmic Ointments of Tobramycin. *Pharm. Res.* **2018**, *35*, 1–6. [CrossRef]
59. Lazcano-Gomez, G.; Castillejos, A.; Kahook, M.; Jimenez-Roman, J.; Gonzalez-Salinas, R. Videographic assessment of glaucoma drop instillation. *J. Curr. Glaucoma Pract.* **2015**, *9*, 47–50. [CrossRef]
60. Taneja, M.; Chappidi, K.; Harsha Ch, S.N.S.; Richhariya, A.; Mohamed, A.; Rathi, V.M. Innovative bulls eye drop applicator for self-instillation of eye drops. *Contact Lens Anterior Eye* **2020**, *43*, 256–260. [CrossRef]
61. Davies, I.; Williams, A.M.; Muir, K.W. Aids for eye drop administration. *Surv. Ophthalmol.* **2017**, *62*, 332–345. [CrossRef]
62. Hornof, M.; Toropainen, E.; Urtti, A. Cell culture models of the ocular barriers. *Eur. J. Pharm. Biopharm.* **2005**, *60*, 207–225. [CrossRef] [PubMed]
63. Juretić, M.; Cetina-Čižmek, B.; Filipović-Grčić, J.; Hafner, A.; Lovrić, J.; Pepić, I. Biopharmaceutical evaluation of surface active ophthalmic excipients using in vitro and ex vivo corneal models. *Eur. J. Pharm. Sci.* **2018**, *120*, 133–141. [CrossRef] [PubMed]
64. Li, Q.; Weng, J.; Wong, S.N.; Thomas Lee, W.Y.; Chow, S.F. Nanoparticulate Drug Delivery to the Retina. *Mol. Pharm.* **2021**, *18*, 506–521. [CrossRef] [PubMed]
65. Karki, R.; Meena, M.; Prakash, T.; Rajeswari, T.; Goli, D.; Kumar, S. Reduction in drop size of ophthalmic topical drop preparations and the impact of treatment. *J. Adv. Pharm. Technol. Res.* **2011**, *2*, 192. [CrossRef]
66. Puglia, C.; Santonocito, D.; Romeo, G.; Intagliata, S.; Romano, G.L.; Strettoi, E.; Novelli, E.; Ostacolo, C.; Campiglia, P.; Sommella, E.M.; et al. Lipid nanoparticles traverse non-corneal path to reach the posterior eye segment: In vivo evidence. *Molecules* **2021**, *26*, 4673. [CrossRef]
67. Bechnak, L.; El Kurdi, R.; Patra, D. Fluorescence Sensing of Nucleic Acid by Curcumin Encapsulated Poly(Ethylene Oxide)-Block-Poly(Propylene Oxide)-Block-Poly(Ethylene Oxide) Based Nanocapsules. *J. Fluoresc.* **2020**, *30*, 547–556. [CrossRef] [PubMed]
68. Beija, M.; Afonso, C.A.M.; Martinho, J.M.G. Synthesis and applications of rhodamine derivatives as fluorescent probes. *Chem. Soc. Rev.* **2009**, *38*, 2410–2433. [CrossRef] [PubMed]
69. Han, Z.X.; Zhang, X.B.; Li, Z.; Gong, Y.J.; Wu, X.Y.; Jin, Z.; He, C.M.; Jian, L.X.; Zhang, J.; Shen, G.L.; et al. Efficient fluorescence resonance energy transfer-based ratiometric fluorescent cellular imaging probe for Zn^{2+} using a rhodamine spirolactam as a trigger. *Anal. Chem.* **2010**, *82*, 3108–3113. [CrossRef] [PubMed]
70. Keerthana, S.; Sam, B.; George, L.; Sudhakar, Y.N.; Varghese, A. Fluorescein Based Fluorescence Sensors for the Selective Sensing of Various Analytes. *J. Fluoresc.* **2021**, *31*, 1251–1276. [CrossRef]
71. El Khoury, E.; Patra, D. Length of hydrocarbon chain influences location of curcumin in liposomes: Curcumin as a molecular probe to study ethanol induced interdigitation of liposomes. *J. Photochem. Photobiol. B Biol.* **2016**, *158*, 49–54. [CrossRef] [PubMed]
72. Khorasani, M.Y.; Langari, H.; Sany, S.B.T.; Rezayi, M.; Sahebkar, A. The role of curcumin and its derivatives in sensory applications. *Mater. Sci. Eng. C* **2019**, *103*, 109792. [CrossRef] [PubMed]
73. Carneiro, A.; Matos, M.J.; Uriarte, E.; Santana, L. Trending topics on coumarin and its derivatives in 2020. *Molecules* **2021**, *26*, 501. [CrossRef] [PubMed]
74. Duong, H.D.; Shin, Y.; Rhee, J. Il Development of novel optical pH sensors based on coumarin 6 and nile blue A encapsulated in resin particles and specific support materials. *Mater. Sci. Eng. C* **2020**, *107*, 110323. [CrossRef] [PubMed]

75. Grimm, J.B.; Lavis, L.D. Synthesis of rhodamines from fluoresceins using pd-catalyzed c-n cross-coupling. *Org. Lett.* **2011**, *13*, 6354–6357. [CrossRef] [PubMed]
76. Rajasekar, M. Recent development in fluorescein derivatives. *J. Mol. Struct.* **2021**, *1224*, 129085. [CrossRef]
77. McHedlov-Petrossyan, N.O.; Cheipesh, T.A.; Roshal, A.D.; Shekhovtsov, S.V.; Moskaeva, E.G.; Omelchenko, I.V. Aminofluoresceins Versus Fluorescein: Peculiarity of Fluorescence. *J. Phys. Chem. A* **2019**, *123*, 8860–8870. [CrossRef]
78. Zhao, X.; Belykh, E.; Cavallo, C.; Valli, D.; Gandhi, S.; Preul, M.C.; Vajkoczy, P.; Lawton, M.T.; Nakaji, P. Application of Fluorescein Fluorescence in Vascular Neurosurgery. *Front. Surg.* **2019**, *6*, 52. [CrossRef]
79. Küçükyürük, B.; Korkmaz, T.Ş.; Nemayire, K.; Özlen, F.; Kafadar, A.M.; Akar, Z.; Kaynar, M.Y.; Sanus, G.Z. Intraoperative Fluorescein Sodium Videoangiography in Intracranial Aneurysm Surgery. *World Neurosurg.* **2021**, *147*, e444–e452. [CrossRef]
80. Bömers, J.P.; Danielsen, M.E.; Schulz, M.K.; Halle, B.; Kristensen, B.W.; Sørensen, M.D.; Poulsen, F.R.; Pedersen, C.B. Sodium fluorescein shows high surgeon-reported usability in glioblastoma surgery. *Surgeon* **2020**, *18*, 344–348. [CrossRef]
81. Voronin, D.V.; Kozlova, A.A.; Verkhovskii, R.A.; Ermakov, A.V.; Makarkin, M.A.; Inozemtseva, O.A.; Bratashov, D.N. Detection of rare objects by flow cytometry: Imaging, cell sorting, and deep learning approaches. *Int. J. Mol. Sci.* **2020**, *21*, 2323. [CrossRef] [PubMed]
82. Wang, L.; Du, W.; Hu, Z.; Uvdal, K.; Li, L.; Huang, W. Hybrid Rhodamine Fluorophores in the Visible/NIR Region for Biological Imaging. *Angew. Chem.-Int. Ed.* **2019**, *58*, 14026–14043. [CrossRef] [PubMed]
83. Marnett, L.J. Synthesis of 5- and 6-Carboxy-X-rhodamines. *Org. Lett.* **2008**, *10*, 4799–4801.
84. Bonaccorso, A.; Musumeci, T.; Serapide, M.F.; Pellitteri, R.; Uchegbu, I.F.; Puglisi, G. Nose to brain delivery in rats: Effect of surface charge of rhodamine B labeled nanocarriers on brain subregion localization. *Colloids Surf. B Biointerfaces* **2017**, *154*, 297–306. [CrossRef] [PubMed]
85. Dempsey, G.T.; Bates, M.; Kowtoniuk, W.E.; Liu, D.R.; Tsien, R.Y.; Zhuang, X. Photoswitching mechanism of cyanine dyes. *J. Am. Chem. Soc.* **2009**, *131*, 18192–18193. [CrossRef]
86. Lim, E.; Kwon, J.; Park, J.; Heo, J.; Kim, S.K. Selective thiolation and photoswitching mechanism of Cy5 studied by time-dependent density functional theory. *Phys. Chem. Chem. Phys.* **2020**, *22*, 14125–14129. [CrossRef]
87. Bae, S.; Lim, E.; Hwang, D.; Huh, H.; Kim, S.K. Torsion-dependent fluorescence switching of amyloid-binding dye NIAD-4. *Chem. Phys. Lett.* **2015**, *633*, 109–113. [CrossRef]
88. Blower, M.D.; Feric, E.; Weis, K.; Heald, R. Genome-wide analysis demonstrates conserved localization of messenger RNAs to mitotic microtubules. *J. Cell Biol.* **2007**, *179*, 1365–1373. [CrossRef]
89. Martos, A.; Berger, M.; Kranz, W.; Spanopoulou, A.; Menzen, T.; Friess, W.; Wuchner, K.; Hawe, A. Novel High-Throughput Assay for Polysorbate Quantification in Biopharmaceutical Products by Using the Fluorescent Dye DiI. *J. Pharm. Sci.* **2020**, *109*, 646–655. [CrossRef] [PubMed]
90. Musumeci, T.; Serapide, M.F.; Pellitteri, R.; Dalpiaz, A.; Ferraro, L.; Dal Magro, R.; Bonaccorso, A.; Carbone, C.; Veiga, F.; Sancini, G.; et al. Oxcarbazepine free or loaded PLGA nanoparticles as effective intranasal approach to control epileptic seizures in rodents. *Eur. J. Pharm. Biopharm.* **2018**, *133*, 309–320. [CrossRef]
91. Capolungo, C.; Genovese, D.; Montalti, M.; Rampazzo, E.; Zaccheroni, N.; Prodi, L. Photoluminescence-Based Techniques for the Detection of Micro- and Nanoplastics. *Chem.-A Eur. J.* **2021**, *27*, 17529–17541. [CrossRef]
92. Sancataldo, G.; Avellone, G.; Vetri, V. Nile Red lifetime reveals microplastic identity. *Environ. Sci. Process. Impacts* **2020**, *22*, 2266–2275. [CrossRef]
93. Hewlings, S.J.; Kalman, D.S. Curcumin: A review of its effects on human health. *Foods* **2017**, *6*, 92. [CrossRef] [PubMed]
94. Sridharan, G.; Shankar, A.A. Toluidine blue: A review of its chemistry and clinical utility. *J. Oral Maxillofac. Pathol.* **2012**, *16*, 251–255. [CrossRef] [PubMed]
95. Aliakbar Navahi, R.; Hosseini, S.B.; Kanavi, M.R.; Rakhshani, N.; Aghaei, H.; Kheiri, B. Comparison of toluidine blue 1% staining patterns in cytopathologically confirmed ocular surface squamous neoplasias and in non-neoplastic lesions. *Ocul. Surf.* **2019**, *17*, 578–583. [CrossRef]
96. Su, G.; Wei, Z.; Wang, L.; Shen, J.; Baudouin, C.; Labbé, A.; Liang, Q. Evaluation of toluidine blue-mediated photodynamic therapy for experimental bacterial keratitis in rabbits. *Transl. Vis. Sci. Technol.* **2020**, *9*, 1–10. [CrossRef] [PubMed]
97. Craparo, E.F.; Musumeci, T.; Bonaccorso, A.; Pellitteri, R.; Romeo, A.; Naletova, I.; Cucci, L.M.; Cavallaro, G.; Satriano, C. Mpeg-plga nanoparticles labeled with loaded or conjugated rhodamine-b for potential nose-to-brain delivery. *Pharmaceutics* **2021**, *13*, 1508. [CrossRef]
98. Turcsányi, Á.; Ungor, D.; Csapó, E. Fluorescent labeling of hyaluronic acid-chitosan nanocarriers by protein-stabilized gold nanoclusters. *Crystals* **2020**, *10*, 1113. [CrossRef]
99. Romero, G.B.; Keck, C.M.; Müller, R.H.; Bou-Chacra, N.A. Development of cationic nanocrystals for ocular delivery. *Eur. J. Pharm. Biopharm.* **2016**, *107*, 215–222. [CrossRef]
100. Pignatello, R.; Corsaro, R.; Santonocito, D. Chapter A Method for Efficient Loading of Ciprofloxacin Hydrochloride in Cationic Solid Lipid Nanoparticles. *Nanomaterials* **2018**, *8*, 304. [CrossRef]
101. Jounaki, K.; Makhmalzadeh, B.S.; Feghhi, M.; Heidarian, A. Topical ocular delivery of vancomycin loaded cationic lipid nanocarriers as a promising and non-invasive alternative approach to intravitreal injection for enhanced bacterial endophthalmitis management. *Eur. J. Pharm. Sci.* **2021**, *167*, 105991. [CrossRef] [PubMed]

102. Vaishya, R.D.; Khurana, V.; Patel, S.; Mitra, A.K. Controlled ocular drug delivery with nanomicelles. *Wiley Interdiscip. Rev. Nanomed. Nanobiotechnology* **2014**, *6*, 422–437. [CrossRef] [PubMed]
103. Zhang, W.H.; Hu, X.X.; Zhang, X.B. Dye-doped fluorescent silica nanoparticles for live cell and in vivo bioimaging. *Nanomaterials* **2016**, *6*, 81. [CrossRef]
104. Siddique, S.; Chow, J.C.L. Application of nanomaterials in biomedical imaging and cancer therapy. *Nanomaterials* **2020**, *10*, 1700. [CrossRef] [PubMed]
105. Niamprem, P.; Srinivas, S.P.; Tiyaboonchai, W. Penetration of Nile red-loaded nanostructured lipid carriers (NLCs) across the porcine cornea. *Colloids Surf. B Biointerfaces* **2019**, *176*, 371–378. [CrossRef] [PubMed]
106. El-Gendy, M.A.; Mansour, M.; El-Assal, M.I.A.; Ishak, R.A.H.; Mortada, N.D. Delineating penetration enhancer-enriched liquid crystalline nanostructures as novel platforms for improved ophthalmic delivery. *Int. J. Pharm.* **2020**, *582*, 119313. [CrossRef]
107. Kapadia, R.; Parikh, K.; Jain, M.; Sawant, K. Topical instillation of triamcinolone acetonide-loaded emulsomes for posterior ocular delivery: Statistical optimization and in vitro-in vivo studies. *Drug Deliv. Transl. Res.* **2021**, *11*, 984–999. [CrossRef] [PubMed]
108. Eldesouky, L.M.; El-Moslemany, R.M.; Ramadan, A.A.; Morsi, M.H.; Khalafallah, N.M. Cyclosporine lipid nanocapsules as thermoresponsive gel for dry eye management: Promising corneal mucoadhesion, biodistribution and preclinical efficacy in rabbits. *Pharmaceutics* **2021**, *13*, 360. [CrossRef] [PubMed]
109. Dubashynskaya, N.V.; Bokatyi, A.N.; Golovkin, A.S.; Kudryavtsev, I.V.; Serebryakova, M.K.; Trulioff, A.S.; Dubrovskii, Y.A.; Skorik, Y.A. Synthesis and characterization of novel succinyl chitosan-dexamethasone conjugates for potential intravitreal dexamethasone delivery. *Int. J. Mol. Sci.* **2021**, *22*, 10960. [CrossRef] [PubMed]
110. Li, J.; Tan, G.; Cheng, B.; Liu, D.; Pan, W. Transport mechanism of chitosan-N-acetylcysteine, chitosan oligosaccharides or carboxymethyl chitosan decorated coumarin-6 loaded nanostructured lipid carriers across the rabbit ocular. *Eur. J. Pharm. Biopharm.* **2017**, *120*, 89–97. [CrossRef] [PubMed]
111. Tan, G.; Li, J.; Song, Y.; Yu, Y.; Liu, D.; Pan, W. Phenylboronic acid-tethered chondroitin sulfate-based mucoadhesive nanostructured lipid carriers for the treatment of dry eye syndrome. *Acta Biomater.* **2019**, *99*, 350–362. [CrossRef] [PubMed]
112. Liu, C.; Lan, Q.; He, W.; Nie, C.; Zhang, C.; Xu, T.; Jiang, T.; Wang, S. Octa-arginine modified lipid emulsions as a potential ocular delivery system for disulfiram: A study of the corneal permeation, transcorneal mechanism and anti-cataract effect. *Colloids Surf. B Biointerfaces* **2017**, *160*, 305–314. [CrossRef] [PubMed]
113. Gómez-Aguado, I.; Rodríguez-Castejón, J.; Beraza-Millor, M.; Vicente-Pascual, M.; Rodríguez-Gascón, A.; Garelli, S.; Battaglia, L.; Del Pozo-Rodríguez, A.; Solinís, M.Á. Mrna-based nanomedicinal products to address corneal inflammation by interleukin-10 supplementation. *Pharmaceutics* **2021**, *13*, 1472. [CrossRef] [PubMed]
114. Kakkar, S.; Singh, M.; Mohan Karuppayil, S.; Raut, J.S.; Giansanti, F.; Papucci, L.; Schiavone, N.; Nag, T.C.; Gao, N.; Yu, F.S.X.; et al. Lipo-PEG nano-ocular formulation successfully encapsulates hydrophilic fluconazole and traverses corneal and non-corneal path to reach posterior eye segment. *J. Drug Target.* **2021**, *29*, 631–650. [CrossRef]
115. Pretor, S.; Bartels, J.; Lorenz, T.; Dahl, K.; Finke, J.H.; Peterat, G.; Krull, R.; Dietzel, A.; Bu, S.; Behrends, S.; et al. Cellular Uptake of Coumarin-6 under Microfluidic Conditions into HCE-T Cells from Nanoscale Formulations. *Mol. Pharm.* **2015**, *12*, 34–45. [CrossRef] [PubMed]
116. Elmotasem, H.; Awad, G.E.A. A stepwise optimization strategy to formulate in situ gelling formulations comprising fluconazole-hydroxypropyl-beta-cyclodextrin complex loaded niosomal vesicles and Eudragit nanoparticles for enhanced antifungal activity and prolonged ocular delivery. *Asian J. Pharm. Sci.* **2020**, *15*, 617–636. [CrossRef] [PubMed]
117. Anishiya chella daisy, E.R.; Rajendran, N.K.; Jeyaraj, M.; Ramu, A.; Rajan, M. Retinal photoreceptors targeting SA-g-AA coated multilamellar liposomes carrier system for cytotoxicity and cellular uptake evaluation. *J. Liposome Res.* **2021**, *31*, 203–216. [CrossRef]
118. Swetledge, S.; Carter, R.; Stout, R.; Astete, C.E.; Jung, J.P.; Sabliov, C.M. Stability and ocular biodistribution of topically administered PLGA nanoparticles. *Sci. Rep.* **2021**, *11*, 1–11. [CrossRef]
119. Dubashynskaya, N.; Poshina, D.; Raik, S.; Urtti, A.; Skorik, Y.A. Polysaccharides in ocular drug delivery. *Pharmaceutics* **2020**, *12*, 22. [CrossRef]
120. Zhukova, V.; Osipova, N.; Semyonkin, A.; Malinovskaya, J.; Melnikov, P.; Valikhov, M.; Porozov, Y.; Solovev, Y.; Kuliaev, P.; Zhang, E.; et al. Fluorescently labeled plga nanoparticles for visualization in vitro and in vivo: The importance of dye properties. *Pharmaceutics* **2021**, *13*, 1145. [CrossRef]
121. Zhang, E.; Zhukova, V.; Semyonkin, A.; Osipova, N.; Malinovskaya, Y.; Maksimenko, O.; Chernikov, V.; Sokolov, M.; Grigartzik, L.; Sabel, B.A.; et al. Release kinetics of fluorescent dyes from PLGA nanoparticles in retinal blood vessels: In vivo monitoring and ex vivo localization. *Eur. J. Pharm. Biopharm.* **2020**, *150*, 131–142. [CrossRef] [PubMed]
122. Li, B.; Wang, J.; Gui, Q.; Yang, H. Drug-loaded chitosan film prepared via facile solution casting and air-drying of plain water-based chitosan solution for ocular drug delivery. *Bioact. Mater.* **2020**, *5*, 577–583. [CrossRef] [PubMed]
123. Álvarez-Álvarez, L.; Barral, L.; Bouza, R.; Farrag, Y.; Otero-Espinar, F.; Feijóo-Bandín, S.; Lago, F. Hydrocortisone loaded poly-(3-hydroxybutyrate-co-3-hydroxyvalerate) nanoparticles for topical ophthalmic administration: Preparation, characterization and evaluation of ophthalmic toxicity. *Int. J. Pharm.* **2019**, *568*, 118519. [CrossRef] [PubMed]
124. Tahara, K.; Karasawa, K.; Onodera, R.; Takeuchi, H. Feasibility of drug delivery to the eye's posterior segment by topical instillation of PLGA nanoparticles. *Asian J. Pharm. Sci.* **2017**, *12*, 394–399. [CrossRef] [PubMed]

125. Sun, X.; Sheng, Y.; Li, K.; Sai, S.; Feng, J.; Li, Y.; Zhang, J.; Han, J.; Tian, B. Mucoadhesive phenylboronic acid conjugated chitosan oligosaccharide-vitamin E copolymer for topical ocular delivery of voriconazole: Synthesis, in vitro/vivo evaluation, and mechanism. *Acta Biomater.* **2022**, *138*, 193–207. [CrossRef]
126. Sai, N.; Dong, X.; Huang, P.; You, L.; Yang, C.; Liu, Y.; Wang, W.; Wu, H.; Yu, Y.; Du, Y.; et al. A novel gel-forming solution based on PEG-DSPE/Solutol HS 15 mixed micelles and gellan gum for ophthalmic delivery of curcumin. *Molecules* **2020**, *25*, 81. [CrossRef]
127. Abilova, G.K.; Kaldybekov, D.B.; Ozhmukhametova, E.K.; Saimova, A.Z.; Kazybayeva, D.S.; Irmukhametova, G.S.; Khutoryanskiy, V.V. Chitosan/poly(2-ethyl-2-oxazoline) films for ocular drug delivery: Formulation, miscibility, in vitro and in vivo studies. *Eur. Polym. J.* **2019**, *116*, 311–320. [CrossRef]
128. Chi, H.; Gu, Y.; Xu, T.; Cao, F. Multifunctional organic–inorganic hybrid nanoparticles and nanosheets based on chitosan derivative and layered double hydroxide: Cellular uptake mechanism and application for topical ocular drug delivery. *Int. J. Nanomedicine* **2017**, *12*, 1607–1620. [CrossRef]
129. Mun, E.A.; Morrison, P.W.J.; Williams, A.C.; Khutoryanskiy, V.V. On the barrier properties of the cornea: A microscopy study of the penetration of fluorescently labeled nanoparticles, polymers, and sodium fluorescein. *Mol. Pharm.* **2014**, *11*, 3556–3564. [CrossRef]
130. Baran-Rachwalska, P.; Torabi-Pour, N.; Sutera, F.M.; Ahmed, M.; Thomas, K.; Nesbit, M.A.; Welsh, M.; Moore, C.B.T.; Saffie-Siebert, S.R. Topical siRNA delivery to the cornea and anterior eye by hybrid silicon-lipid nanoparticles. *J. Control. Release* **2020**, *326*, 192–202. [CrossRef]
131. Qu, W.; Meng, B.; Yu, Y.; Wang, S. EpCAM antibody-conjugated mesoporous silica nanoparticles to enhance the anticancer efficacy of carboplatin in retinoblastoma. *Mater. Sci. Eng. C* **2017**, *76*, 646–651. [CrossRef] [PubMed]
132. Xu, H.; Tang, B.; Huang, W.; Luo, S.; Zhang, T.; Yuan, J.; Zheng, Q.; Zan, X. Deliver protein across bio-barriers via hexa-histidine metal assemblies for therapy: A case in corneal neovascularization model. *Mater. Today Bio* **2021**, *12*, 100143. [CrossRef] [PubMed]
133. Wang, Y.; Liu, W.; Yuan, B.; Yin, X.; Li, Y.; Li, Z.; Cui, J.; Yuan, X.; Li, Y. The application of methylprednisolone nanoscale zirconium-porphyrin metal-organic framework (MPS-NPMOF) in the treatment of photoreceptor degeneration. *Int. J. Nanomedicine* **2019**, *14*, 9763–9776. [CrossRef] [PubMed]
134. Ding, S.; Zhang, N.; Lyu, Z.; Zhu, W.; Chang, Y.C.; Hu, X.; Du, D.; Lin, Y. Protein-based nanomaterials and nanosystems for biomedical applications: A review. *Mater. Today* **2021**, *43*, 166–184. [CrossRef]
135. Nguyen, T.P.; Nguyen, Q.V.; Nguyen, V.H.; Le, T.H.; Huynh, V.Q.N.; Vo, D.V.N.; Trinh, Q.T.; Kim, S.Y.; Van Le, Q. Silk fibroin-based biomaterials for biomedical applications: A review. *Polymers* **2019**, *11*, 1933. [CrossRef]
136. Yang, P.; Dong, Y.; Huang, D.; Zhu, C.; Liu, H.; Pan, X.; Wu, C. Silk fibroin nanoparticles for enhanced bio-macromolecule delivery to the retina. *Pharm. Dev. Technol.* **2019**, *24*, 575–583. [CrossRef]
137. Tiwari, R.; Sethiya, N.K.; Gulbake, A.S.; Mehra, N.K.; Murty, U.S.N.; Gulbake, A. A review on albumin as a biomaterial for ocular drug delivery. *Int. J. Biol. Macromol.* **2021**, *191*, 591–599. [CrossRef]
138. Radwan, S.E.S.; El-Kamel, A.; Zaki, E.I.; Burgalassi, S.; Zucchetti, E.; El-Moslemany, R.M. Hyaluronic-coated albumin nanoparticles for the non-invasive delivery of apatinib in diabetic retinopathy. *Int. J. Nanomed.* **2021**, *16*, 4481–4494. [CrossRef]
139. Zhang, W.; Kantaria, T.; Zhang, Y.; Kantaria, T.; Kobauri, S.; Tugushi, D.; Brücher, V.; Katsarava, R.; Eter, N.; Heiduschka, P. Biodegradable Nanoparticles Based on Pseudo-Proteins Show Promise as Carriers for Ophthalmic Drug Delivery. *J. Ocul. Pharmacol. Ther.* **2020**, *36*, 421–432. [CrossRef]
140. Thomas, C.J.; Mirza, R.G.; Gill, M.K. Age-Related Macular Degeneration. *Med. Clin. North Am.* **2021**, *105*, 473–491. [CrossRef]
141. Hanus, J.; Anderson, C.; Wang, S. RPE necroptosis in response to oxidative stress and in AMD. *Ageing Res. Rev.* **2015**, *24*, 286–298. [CrossRef] [PubMed]
142. Hammond, B.R.; Johnson, M.A. The age-related eye disease study (AREDS). *Nutr. Rev.* **2002**, *60*, 283–288. [CrossRef] [PubMed]
143. Gregori, N.Z.; Goldhardt, R. Nutritional Supplements for Age-Related Macular Degeneration. *Curr. Ophthalmol. Rep.* **2015**, *3*, 34–39. [CrossRef] [PubMed]
144. Álvarez-Barrios, A.; Álvarez, L.; García, M.; Artime, E.; Pereiro, R.; González-Iglesias, H. Antioxidant defenses in the human eye: A focus on metallothioneins. *Antioxidants* **2021**, *10*, 89. [CrossRef] [PubMed]
145. Cruz-Alonso, M.; Fernandez, B.; Álvarez, L.; González-Iglesias, H.; Traub, H.; Jakubowski, N.; Pereiro, R. Bioimaging of metallothioneins in ocular tissue sections by laser ablation-ICP-MS using bioconjugated gold nanoclusters as specific tags. *Microchim. Acta* **2018**, *185*, 1–9. [CrossRef]
146. Osredkar, J. Copper and Zinc, Biological Role and Significance of Copper/Zinc Imbalance. *J. Clin. Toxicol.* **2011**, *3*, 1–18. [CrossRef]
147. Uddin, M.I.; Kilburn, T.C.; Yang, R.; McCollum, G.W.; Wright, D.W.; Penn, J.S. Targeted imaging of VCAM-1 mRNA in a mouse model of laser-induced choroidal neovascularization using antisense hairpin-DNA-functionalized gold-nanoparticles. *Mol. Pharm.* **2018**, *15*, 5514–5520. [CrossRef]
148. Pearson, R.A.; Barber, A.C.; Rizzi, M. Restoration of vision after transplantation of photoreceptors. *Nature* **2012**, *485*, 99–103. [CrossRef]
149. Chemla, Y.; Betzer, O.; Markus, A.; Farah, N.; Motiei, M.; Popovtzer, R.; Mandel, Y. Gold nanoparticles for multimodal high-resolution imaging of transplanted cells for retinal replacement therapy. *Nanomedicine* **2019**, *14*, 1857–1871. [CrossRef]

150. Meir, R.; Shamalov, K.; Betzer, O.; Motiei, M.; Horovitz-Fried, M.; Yehuda, R.; Popovtzer, A.; Popovtzer, R.; Cohen, C.J. Nanomedicine for Cancer Immunotherapy: Tracking Cancer-Specific T-Cells in Vivo with Gold Nanoparticles and CT Imaging. *ACS Nano* **2015**, *9*, 6363–6372. [CrossRef] [PubMed]
151. Cai, W.; Chen, M.; Fan, J.; Jin, H.; Yu, D.; Qiang, S.; Peng, C.; Yu, J. Fluorescein sodium loaded by polyethyleneimine for fundus fluorescein angiography improves adhesion. *Nanomedicine* **2019**, *14*, 2595–2611. [CrossRef] [PubMed]
152. Safi, H.; Safi, S.; Hafezi-Moghadam, A.; Ahmadieh, H. Early detection of diabetic retinopathy. *Surv. Ophthalmol.* **2018**, *63*, 601–608. [CrossRef]
153. Wang, X.; Li, S.; Li, W.; Hua, Y.; Wu, Q. Choroidal Variations in Diabetic Macular Edema: Fluorescein Angiography and Optical Coherence Tomography. *Curr. Eye Res.* **2018**, *43*, 102–108. [CrossRef] [PubMed]
154. Shivshetty, N.; Swift, T.; Pinnock, A.; Pownall, D.; Neil, S.M.; Douglas, I.; Garg, P.; Rimmer, S. Evaluation of ligand modified poly (N-Isopropyl acrylamide) hydrogel for etiological diagnosis of corneal infection. *Exp. Eye Res.* **2022**, *214*, 108881. [CrossRef] [PubMed]
155. Ladju, R.B.; Ulhaq, Z.S.; Soraya, G.V. Nanotheranostics: A powerful next-generation solution to tackle hepatocellular carcinoma. *World J. Gastroenterol.* **2022**, *28*, 176–187. [CrossRef] [PubMed]
156. Tang, M.; Ji, X.; Xu, H.; Zhang, L.; Jiang, A.; Song, B.; Su, Y.; He, Y. Photostable and Biocompatible Fluorescent Silicon Nanoparticles-Based Theranostic Probes for Simultaneous Imaging and Treatment of Ocular Neovascularization. *Anal. Chem.* **2018**, *90*, 8188–8195. [CrossRef] [PubMed]
157. Shabbir, U.; Rubab, M.; Tyagi, A.; Oh, D.H. Curcumin and its derivatives as theranostic agents in alzheimer's disease: The implication of nanotechnology. *Int. J. Mol. Sci.* **2021**, *22*, 196. [CrossRef] [PubMed]
158. Stati, G.; Rossi, F.; Trakoolwilaiwan, T.; Tung, L.D.; Mourdikoudis, S.; Thanh, N.T.K.; Di Pietro, R. Development and Characterization of Curcumin-Silver Nanoparticles as a Promising Formulation to Test on Human Pterygium-Derived Keratinocytes. *Molecules* **2022**, *27*, 282. [CrossRef] [PubMed]
159. Zhang, L.; Ji, X.; Su, Y.; Zhai, X.; Xu, H.; Song, B.; Jiang, A.; Guo, D.; He, Y. Fluorescent silicon nanoparticles-based nanotheranostic agents for rapid diagnosis and treatment of bacteria-induced keratitis. *Nano Res.* **2021**, *14*, 52–58. [CrossRef]
160. de Oliveira, D.C.S.; de Freitas, C.F.; Calori, I.R.; Goncalves, R.S.; Cardinali, C.A.E.F.; Malacarne, L.C.; Ravanelli, M.I.; de Oliveira, H.P.M.; Tedesco, A.C.; Caetano, W.; et al. Theranostic verteporfin-loaded lipid-polymer liposome for photodynamic applications. *J. Photochem. Photobiol. B Biol.* **2020**, *212*, 112039. [CrossRef]
161. Li, L.; Zeng, Z.; Chen, Z.; Gao, R.; Pan, L.; Deng, J.; Ye, X.; Zhang, J.; Zhang, S.; Mei, C.; et al. Microenvironment-triggered degradable hydrogel for imaging diagnosis and combined treatment of intraocular choroidal melanoma. *ACS Nano* **2020**, *14*, 15403–15416. [CrossRef] [PubMed]
162. Maulvi, F.A.; Desai, D.T.; Shetty, K.H.; Shah, D.O.; Willcox, M.D.P. Advances and challenges in the nanoparticles-laden contact lenses for ocular drug delivery. *Int. J. Pharm.* **2021**, *608*, 121090. [CrossRef] [PubMed]
163. Huang, J.F.; Zhong, J.; Chen, G.P.; Lin, Z.T.; Deng, Y.; Liu, Y.L.; Cao, P.Y.; Wang, B.; Wei, Y.; Wu, T.; et al. A Hydrogel-Based Hybrid Theranostic Contact Lens for Fungal Keratitis. *ACS Nano* **2016**, *10*, 6464–6473. [CrossRef] [PubMed]
164. Jin, Y.; Wang, Y.; Yang, J.; Zhang, H.; Yang, Y.W.; Chen, W.; Jiang, W.; Qu, J.; Guo, Y.; Wang, B. An Integrated Theranostic Nanomaterial for Targeted Photodynamic Therapy of Infectious Endophthalmitis. *Cell Reports Phys. Sci.* **2020**, *1*, 100173. [CrossRef]
165. Khiev, D.; Mohamed, Z.A.; Vichare, R.; Paulson, R.; Bhatia, S.; Mohapatra, S.; Lobo, G.P.; Valapala, M.; Kerur, N.; Passaglia, C.L.; et al. Emerging nano-formulations and nanomedicines applications for ocular drug delivery. *Nanomaterials* **2021**, *11*, 173. [CrossRef]
166. Alander, J.T.; Kaartinen, I.; Laakso, A.; Tommi, P.; Spillmann, T.; Tuchin, V.V.; Venermo, M.; Petri, V. A Review of Indocyanine Green Fluorescent Imaging in Surgery. *Int. J. Biomed. Imaging* **2012**, *2012*, 7. [CrossRef] [PubMed]

MDPI
St. Alban-Anlage 66
4052 Basel
Switzerland
Tel. +41 61 683 77 34
Fax +41 61 302 89 18
www.mdpi.com

Pharmaceutics Editorial Office
E-mail: pharmaceutics@mdpi.com
www.mdpi.com/journal/pharmaceutics

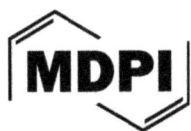

www.ingramcontent.com/pod-product-compliance
Lightning Source LLC
LaVergne TN
LVHW070500100526
838202LV00014B/1761